Recent Concepts in Gastrointestinal (GI) Surgery

Mohammad Ibrarullah
Editor

Recent Concepts in Gastrointestinal (GI) Surgery

Springer

Editor
Mohammad Ibrarullah
Department of Surgical Gastroenterology
Apollo Hospitals
Bhubaneswar, Odisha, India

ISBN 978-981-92-1117-3 ISBN 978-981-92-1118-0 (eBook)
https://doi.org/10.1007/978-981-92-1118-0

This Springer imprint is published by the registered company Springer Nature Singapore Pte Ltd.
The registered company address is: 152 Beach Road, #21-01/04 Gateway East, Singapore 189721, Singapore

Foreword

In my capacity as his mentor during his training at the Sanjay Gandhi Postgraduate Institute of Medical Sciences (SGPGIMS), Lucknow, and as the co-author of his first publications—a case report on agenesis of the gallbladder, published in the *Japanese Journal of Surgery* in 1991, and an original article on Mirizzi syndrome, published in the *Australia & New Zealand Journal of Surgery* in 1993—I have the honor and pleasure of writing this Foreword for *Recent Concepts in Gastrointestinal (GI) Surgery*, edited by Dr. Mohammad Ibrarullah.

It is not without reason that it is said that the "morning shows the day." We all knew that Ibrar, as we all fondly called him, was going to become a prolific writer—he is a virtual "publications churning out machine." He was one of the few residents (MCh students) who exploited the huge clinical database of the Department to the maximum and produced a large number of highly cited publications, most as the first author. After obtaining his MCh in Surgical Gastroenterology from the SGPGIMS, Dr. Ibrarullah served in academic positions at the SCB Medical College, Cuttack; SV Institute of Medical Science (SVIMS), Tirupati; and the Sri Ramchandra Medical College (SRMC), Chennai, before he settled in his current position as a Professor and Senior Consultant, Department of Surgical Gastroenterology at the Apollo Hospitals, Bhubaneswar. But the move from the academic institutions to a corporate hospital did not subdue his academic "itch," and he has continued to write and publish.

Being one of the few surgeons who also dabble in endoscopy (including therapeutic interventions), it was no wonder that he produced an *Atlas of Diagnostic Endoscopy*, published by CRC and running in its third edition. His passion for advocating and training for an injury-free cholecystectomy resulted in a richly illustrated atlas on Safe Laparoscopic Cholecystectomy—a virtual treatise on the subject containing numerous tips and tricks to keep the procedure safe—a must-read for every surgeon.

Dr. Ibrarullah has now published his third book, *Recent Concepts in Gastrointestinal (GI) Surgery*. Although it does not claim to be a textbook, the book covers nearly all aspects of GI and HPB surgery. Dedicated chapters on the surgical anatomy of the liver, biliary system, and pancreas are especially welcome in a surgical text. Clinical dilemmas, such as pancreatic head masses, receive special attention. Uncommon topics, e.g., small bowel diverticulum, short bowel syndrome, small bowel transplant, cholangiohepatitis, pancreas and islet transplant, splenectomy for hematological disorders, and splenic preservation, which would likely occupy only a page or a paragraph in other books, are covered in separate chapters. Unconventional but important topics, such as indocyanine green, tumor markers, and statistics, also find a place in the book. The special section on tropical diseases, including enteric fever, hydatid, and ascaris, will be especially useful to students in India and other developing and underdeveloped countries. Although titled *Recent Concepts in Gastrointestinal (GI) Surgery*, the chapters also cover nonsurgical management in adequate detail.

The contributing authors, who range from young residents to senior consultants, are from several prestigious institutions and hospitals of India, indicating the respect Dr. Ibrarullah commands among his peers in GI & HPB Surgery and include some leading authorities on the topics they have written about.

Dr. Mohammad Ibrarullah's *Recent Concepts in Gastrointestinal (GI) Surgery* is a must-read for all general surgical postgraduates and can serve as a quick revision for the fellows in GI and HPB surgery; it should find a place on the shelves in all institutional and departmental libraries.

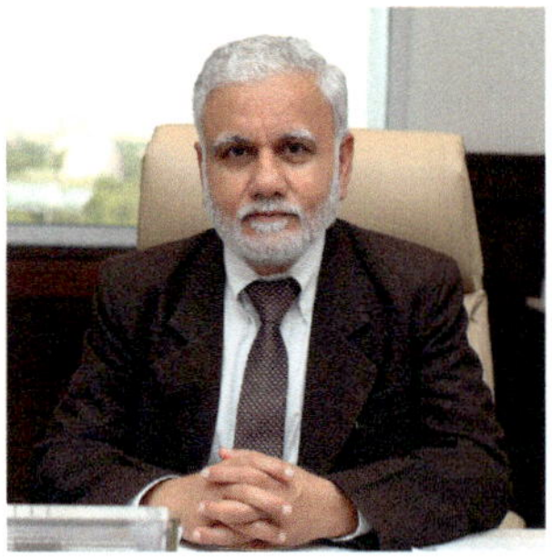

V. K. Kapoor, MS, FACS, FRCS

Former Professor and Head of the Department of Surgical Gastroenterology
Sanjay Gandhi Postgraduate Institute of
Medical Sciences (SGPGIMS)
Lucknow, India

Professor of Surgical Gastroenterology, Pro Vice Chancellor
Mahatma Gandhi University of Medical
Sciences & Technology (MGUMST)
Jaipur, India

Preface

The practice of surgery has seen a paradigm shift in recent times. Though the diseases do not change, the understanding of them and their management does. Molecular biology and advanced imaging have ushered in an era of better understanding of the disease process and precision in diagnosis. With the advent of minimally invasive surgery, robotic surgery, and telesurgery, the popular adage, "big surgeons give big incisions," is now considered obsolete. A constant upgradation of knowledge and skills is, therefore, expected of every trainee and practicing surgeon. *Recent Concepts in Gastrointestinal (GI) Surgery* is an effort in that direction. The book covers all possible developments in gastrointestinal surgery. The chapters are organized systematically (organ-wise). The presentation is concise and up to date, enabling the readers to take a holistic view of the subject. It covers all surgical aspects of the disease and its updated management. The presentation is concise and crisp, enriched with high-resolution digital images and sketches, and concludes with key points/take-home messages at the end of each chapter. The book is expected to prepare students for both clinical and academic challenges (to crack qualifying exams).

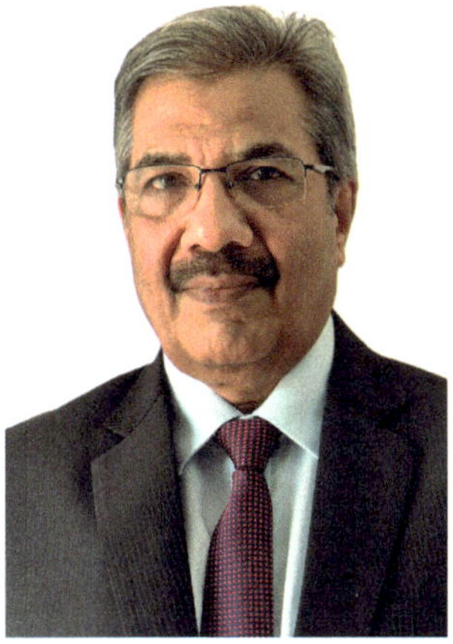

Bhubaneswar, Odisha, India — Mohammad Ibrarullah

Contents

Contributors

Younis Ahmad Sher-i-Kashmir Institute of Medical Sciences, Srinagar, Jammu and Kashmir, India

Sadaf Ali Sher-i-Kashmir Institute of Medical Sciences, Srinagar, Jammu and Kashmir, India

N. Ananthakrishnan Jawaharlal Institute of Post-Graduate Medical Education and Research (JIPMER), Puducherry, India

Vikeerna Bharti All India Institute of Medical Sciences, Bhubaneswar, India

Kaushik Bhattacharya Mata Gujri Memorial Medical College and LSK Hospital, Kishanganj, Bihar, India

Sanjay Debakshi Calcutta Medical Research Institute, Kolkata, West Bengal, India

Govindraj Dessai KEM Hospital, Mumbai, India

Vidyachandra Gandhi Ruby Hall Clinic, Pune, India

Nalini Kanta Ghosh Fortis Hospital, Noida, India

Amit Gupta All India Institute of Medical Sciences, Rishikesh, India

Subash Gupta Max Super Speciality Hospital, Saket, New Delhi, India

Sunita Gupta All India Institute of Medical Sciences, Bhubaneswar, Odisha, India

Vishal Gupta Department of Surgical Gastroenterology, All India Institute of Medical Sciences, Bhopal, India

Yashika Gupta G B Pant Institute of Postgraduate Medical Education and Research (GIPMER), New Delhi, India

Nissar Hussain Hamdani Government Medical College, Srinagar, Jammu and Kashmir, India

Mohammad Ibrarullah Department of Surgical Gastroenterology, Apollo Hospitals, Bhubaneswar, Odisha, India

Shridhar G. Iyer National University of Singapore, Mount Elizabeth Medical Centre, ALPS Clinic, Mount Elizabeth, Singapore

Gaurav Jain Arora St Lukes Medical Center, Milwaukee, WI, India

Nikhil Jillawar D Y Patil Medical College, Hospital and Research Centre, Pune, India

R. Kalayarasan Jawaharlal Institute of Post-Graduate Medical Education and Research (JIPMER), Puducherry, India

Anchin Kalia Mahatma Gandhi University of Medical Sciences and Technology (MGUMST), Jaipur, Rajasthan, India

Chetan V. Kantharia Seth GS Medical College & KEM Hospital, Mumbai, India

Sharad C. Kantharia Seth GS Medical College & KEM Hospital, Mumbai, India

Vikram Kate Jawaharlal Institute of Post-Graduate Medical Education and Research (JIPMER), Puducherry, India

Ragini Kilambi Institute of Liver and Biliary Sciences, New Delhi, India

Pothugunta Sai Krishna Jawaharlal Institute of Post-Graduate Medical Education and Research (JIPMER), Puducherry, India

Ajit Kumar All India Institute of Medical Sciences, Rishikesh, India

Prashant Kumar Sakra World Hospital, Bangalore, India

Sai Kumar Asian Institute of Gastroenterology, Hyderabad, India

Aditya R. Kunte Tata Memorial Hospital, Mumbai, India

Sean Siwei Li Lee Kong Chain School of Medicine, Nanyang Technological University, Singapore, Singapore

Shao Qian Lian Lee Kong Chain School of Medicine, Nanyang Technological University, Singapore, Singapore

Matthias Yi Quan Liau Lee Kong Chian School of Medicine, Nanyang Technological University, Singapore, Singapore

Kausar Makki Fortis Hospital, Noida, India

Naren Mandalapu Institute of Liver and Biliary Sciences, New Delhi, India

Deep Mashru Tata Memorial Hospital, Mumbai, India

Ajeet P. Maurya Department of General Surgery, All India Institute of Medical Sciences, Bhopal, India

Akash Mishra Mahatma Gandhi University of Medical Sciences and Technology (MGUMST), Jaipur, Rajasthan, India

Banabihari Mishra Srirama Chandra Bhanja Medical College and Hospital, Cuttack, India

Laxminarayan Mohanty Srirama Chandra Bhanja Medical College and Hospital, Cuttack, India

Swati Mohanty Department of Surgical Gastroenterology, Apollo Hospitals, Bhubaneswar, India

Ashutosh Mohapatra Sai Institute of Gastroenterology and Liver Sciences, Bhubaneswar, India

Sonmoon Mohapatra Sai Institute of Gastroenterology and Liver Sciences, Bhubaneswar, India

Murugappan Nachiappan Valluvanad Hospital, Ottapalam, Palakkad, India

H. H. Nag G B Pant Institute of Postgraduate Medical Education and Research (GIPMER), New Delhi, India

Samiran Nundy Sir Ganga Ram Hospital, New Delhi, India

Siba Narayan Padhi All India Institute of Medical Sciences, Bhubaneswar, Odisha, India

Hirak Pahari Sir Ganga Ram Hospital, New Delhi, India

Partha Pal Asian Institute of Gastroenterology, Hyderabad, India

Saneya Pandrowala Tata Memorial Hospital, Mumbai, India

Rajesh Panwar Department of GI Surgery & Liver Transplantation, All India Institute of Medical Sciences, New Delhi, India

Krunal Patel Mahatma Gandhi University of Medical Sciences and Technology (MGUMST), Jaipur, Rajasthan, India

Ranjan Patel All India Institute of Medical Sciences, Bhubaneswar, Odisha, India

Bramhadatta Pattnaik All India Institute of Medical Sciences, Bhubaneswar, Odisha, India

Monika Pohekar Tata Memorial Hospital, Mumbai, India

Biju Pottakkat Jawaharlal Institute of Post-Graduate Medical Education and Research (JIPMER), Puducherry, India

Ramkrishna Prabhu KEM Hospital, Mumbai, India

Sharvari G. Pujari Seth GS Medical College & KEM Hospital, Mumbai, India

Ankur Punia Mahatma Gandhi University of Medical Sciences and Technology (MGUMST), Jaipur, India

Govind K. Purushothaman Paalana Institute of Medical Sciences, Palakkad, Kerala, India

Sumyra Qadri Sher-i-Kashmir Institute of Medical Sciences, Srinagar, Jammu and Kashmir, India

Manmohan Rajpoot Mahatma Gandhi University of Medical Sciences and Technology (MGUMST), Jaipur, India

Phani Krishna Ravula Pace Hospitals, Hyderabad, India

Soumen Roy Apollo Hospitals, Bhubaneswar, India

Peush Sahni Centre for Liver and Biliary Sciences, Max Super Speciality Hospital, Saket, New Delhi, India

Manash Ranjan Sahoo All India Institute of Medical Sciences, Bhubaneswar, India

Rupashree Sahoo Srirama Chandra Bhanja Medical College and Hospital, Cuttack, India

Vivek Sanjekar All India Institute of Medical Sciences, Rishikesh, India

Senthil Muthuraman Institute of Abdominal Organ & Multivisceral Transplant CareVue Health/ MGM Healthcare, Chennai, Tamilnadu, India

Suresh Sepuri Pace Hospitals, Hyderabad, India

Tashmeen Kaur Sethi All India Institute of Medical Sciences, Jodhpur, India

S. Sankar Sri Ramachandra Medical College, Chennai, Tamil Nadu, India

Ajay Sharma Mahatma Gandhi University of Medical Sciences and Technology (MGUMST), Jaipur, India

Neha Sharma Max Institute of Cancer Care, Vaishali, Ghaziabad, Uttar Pradesh, India

Paresh Sharma Mahatma Gandhi University of Medical Sciences and Technology (MGUMST), Jaipur, India

Vishal G. Shelat Department of General Surgery, Surgical Science Training Centre, Tan Tock Seng Hospital, Singapore, Singapore

Rajesh S. Shinde Tata Memorial Hospital, Mumbai, India

Shailesh V. Shrikhande Tata Memorial Hospital, Mumbai, India

Sadiq S. Sikora Sakra World Hospital, Bangalore, India

Sanjamjot Singh All India Institute of Medical Sciences, Jodhpur, India

S Sreejith Max Super Speciality Hospital, Saket, New Delhi, India

Ritu Thakur All India Institute of Medical Sciences, Rishikesh, India

Mahesh Thombare D Y Patil Medical College, Hospital and Research Centre, Pune, India

Shikhar Tripathi Sir Ganga Ram Hospital, New Delhi, India

Anil Vaidya Institute of Abdominal Organ & Multivisceral Transplant CareVue Health/ MGM Healthcare, Chennai, Tamilnadu, India

Peeyush Varshney All India Institute of Medical Sciences, Jodhpur, India

Venkatesh Balaraman Sundararajan Institute of Abdominal Organ & Multivisceral Transplant CareVue Health/ MGM Healthcare, Chennai, Tamilnadu, India

Vivek Vij Fortis Hospital, Noida, India

Hamza Wani Government Medical College, Jammu, India

Erin Yan Qing Wee Lee Kong Chian School of Medicine, Nanyang Technological University, Singapore, Singapore

Amitabh Yadav Sir Ganga Ram Hospital, New Delhi, India

Keng Xin Yi Lee Kong Chain School of Medicine, Nanyang Technological University, Singapore, Singapore

Part I

Esophagus, Stomach, and Duodenum

Gastroesophageal Reflux Disease and Hiatus Hernia

1

Swati Mohanty and Mohammad Ibrarullah

Abstract

Gastroesophageal reflux disease (GERD) is characterized by a symptom complex resulting from the reflux of gastric contents into the esophagus and beyond through the lower esophageal sphincter (LES). An interplay between protective mechanisms and aggravating factors is implicated in the genesis of GERD. Hiatus hernia is a common cause for GERD. Medical management comprising lifestyle management and proton-pump inhibitor often controls the symptoms in the majority. Failure of medical management and complications of long-standing GERD are main indications of surgery. Laparoscopic Nissen's fundoplication is currently the surgical treatment of choice.

Keywords

GERD · Hiatus hernia

Gastroesophageal reflux disease (GERD) is characterized by a symptom complex resulting from the reflux of gastric contents into the esophagus and beyond through the lower esophageal sphincter (LES). Nearly one-third of the population in Europe and America, and about 10% in Asia, are affected by GERD. Often considered a mostly benign lifestyle disease, atypical presentations such as noncardiac chest pain or pulmonary symptoms can be problematic and cause confusion in diagnosis and treatment. A rising incidence of adenocarcinoma of the distal esophagus has also been linked to GERD and Barrett's esophagus.

1.1 Pathophysiology

An interplay between protective mechanisms and aggravating factors is implicated in the genesis of GERD. The gastroesophageal junction (GEJ) is 2.5–4.5 cm long and is located between the lower end of the esophagus and the cardia of the stomach. The LES is a functional sphincter that prevents gastric acidic contents from regurgitating into the esophagus. Its action is maintained by gastric cardia fibers that loop around the esophagus, the angle of His, the abdominal esophagus, the diaphragmatic crura, and the phreno-esophageal membrane (PEM). GERD occurs when any of these factors become disturbed. Increased gastric acidity is observed in about 30% of patients with GERD. Helicobacter pylori is associated with decreased acidity, thus protecting against GERD. Saliva has a protective effect on the esophageal mucosa. Esophageal peristalsis facilitates the clearance of refluxate. Therefore, reduced salivation or peristalsis, as seen in connective tissue disorders, may precipitate GERD. Increased intra-abdominal pressure caused by pregnancy, obesity, pyloric obstruction, or gastrectomy can also lead to GERD.

Hiatal hernia (HH) results from weakening or widening of the crural hiatus and PEM. A defect in the PEM causes the gastroesophageal junction (GEJ) to herniate into the mediastinum. HH is classified into four types based on the defect in the PEM and the herniating organ(s) (Fig. 1.1 and Table 1.2).

S. Mohanty · M. Ibrarullah (✉)
Department of Surgical Gastroenterology, Apollo Hospitals, Bhubaneswar, Odisha, India

M. Ibrarullah (ed.), *Recent Concepts in Gastrointestinal (GI) Surgery*, https://doi.org/10.1007/978-981-92-1118-0_1

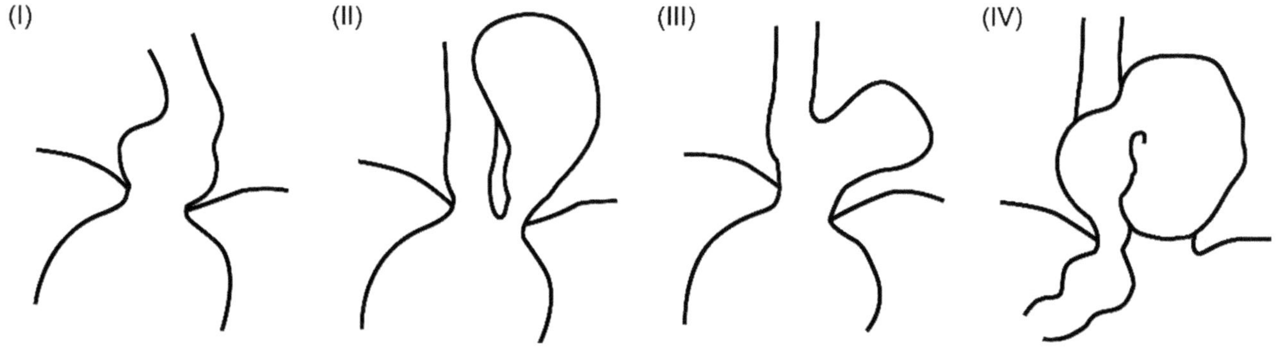

Fig. 1.1 Types of hiatus hernia (see Table 1.2 for details)

Table 1.1 GERD: Protecting and aggravating factors

Protecting factors	Aggravating factors
LES mechanism comprising: *Gastric cardia oblique fibers around the esophagus* *Angle of His* *Intra-abdominal length of the esophagus* *Pinchcock action of the diaphragmatic crura* *Phreno-esophageal membrane*	Compromised LES mechanism
Esophageal peristalsis	Hiatus hernia
Saliva	Increased abdominal/gastric pressure
Helicobacter pylori infection	Increased gastric acidity
	Compromised esophageal peristalsis

Table 1.2 Types of hiatus hernia

Hiatus hernia	Types	Pathology
Sliding hernia	I	Circumferential defect in PEM, GEJ migrates above the diaphragm
Paraesophageal hernia	II	Partially weak PEM, GEJ below the diaphragm, part of the stomach herniates
	III	Migration of GEJ and fundus above the diaphragm
	IV	Migration of GEJ, stomach, and/or part of the bowel into the mediastinum

PEM phreno-esophageal membrane, *GEJ* gastroesophageal junction

1.2 Progression of GERD

Natural history:

- Categorical disorder: Classified as either Nonerosive Reflux Disease (NERD) or Erosive Reflux Disease (ERD).
- Spectrum disorder: With NERD at one spectrum and Barrett's esophagus and adenocarcinoma at another end, the disease progresses over time.

There is clinical evidence to support the spectrum disorder concept, which is further classified as follows:

1. NERD
2. Mild ERD: Defined as healing of esophagitis using proton pump inhibitor (PPI) therapy
3. Severe ERD: Characterized by nonhealing esophagitis despite PPI therapy
4. Barrett's esophagus

1.3 Clinical Features

GERD is considered clinically relevant when mild symptoms occur at least twice a week, or moderate to severe symptoms occur at least once a week, or if there are complications from reflux of gastric contents into the esophagus or beyond, such as the oral cavity or lungs (Table 1.3).

Table 1.3 Symptoms of GERD

Typical esophageal symptoms	*Prevalence (%)*
Heartburn	80
Regurgitation	54
Water brash	
Atypical esophageal symptoms	
Dysphagia for solids	23
Epigastric pain	29
Bloating	15
Belching	15
Extraesophageal symptoms	
Cough	27
Hoarseness	21
Aspiration	14
Wheezing	07
Throat pain and globus	04

1.4 Diagnosis

Diagnosis of GERD is based on clinical presentation supported by investigations.

1.4.1 Esophagogastroduodenoscopy

Esophagogastroduodenoscopy (EGD) is performed to identify evidence of reflux-related mucosal changes (Table 1.4). While detecting these changes supports the diagnosis, their absence does not exclude the possibility of GERD (Figs. 1.2 and 1.3).

Table 1.4 Los Angeles endoscopic grading of esophagitis

Grade A: One or more mucosal break(s) no longer than 5 mm that do not extend between the top of two mucosal folds
Grade B: One or more mucosal break(s) >5 mm long not extending between the tops of two mucosal folds.
Grade C: One or more mucosal breaks between the top of two or more mucosal folds involving <75% of the circumference.
Grade D: One or more mucosal break(s) involving at least 75% of the esophageal circumference

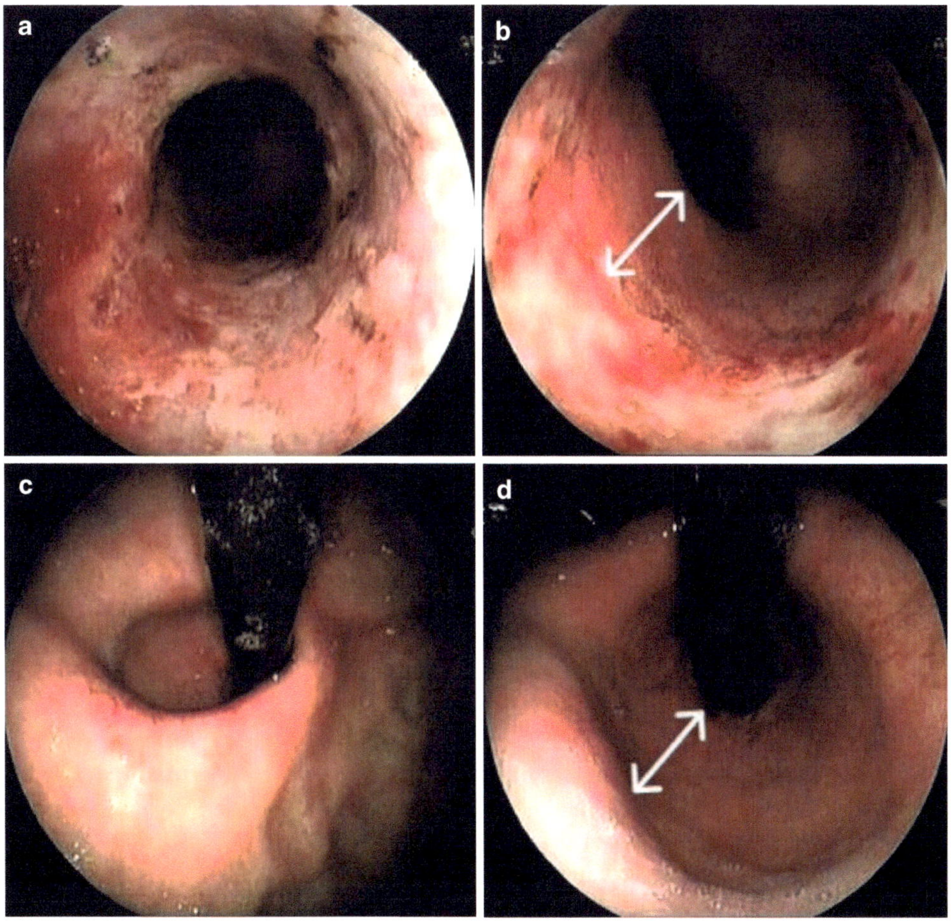

Fig. 1.2 (**a**) Sliding hiatus hernia with erosive esophagitis. (**b–d**) Endoscopic diagnosis of hiatus hernia: The distance between the squamo-columnar junction and the diaphragmatic indentation (arrow) is greater than 2 cm (normal <0.5 cm). On retroflexion, the diaphragmatic indentation does not snugly fit around the endoscope. The 'bell'-like appearance represents the hiatal sac. Gastric mucosa appears drawn into the hiatal sac

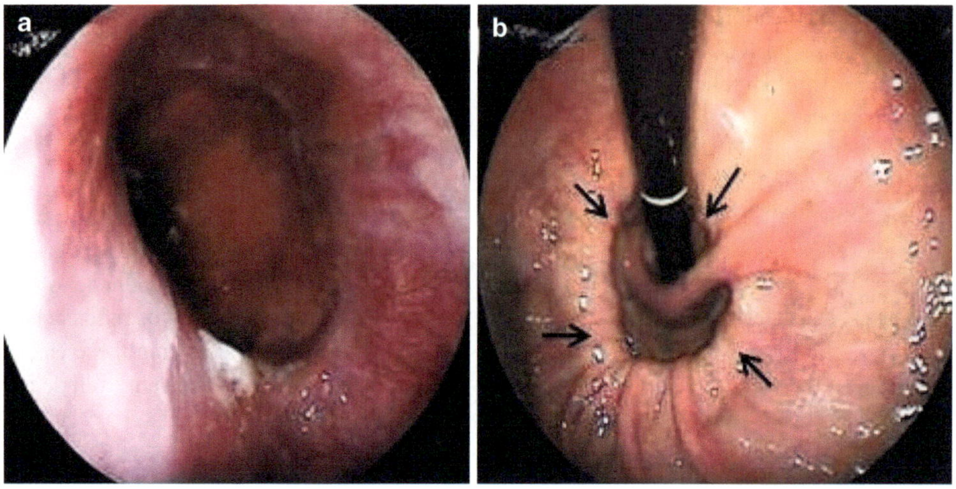

Fig. 1.3 Paraesophageal hernia. (**a**) Hiatus hernia diagnosed on forward view. (**b**) On retroflexion, note the diaphragmatic indentation (arrows) and the herniating gastric pouch alongside the GEJ

1.4.2 High-Resolution Manometry and Ambulatory pH and Impedance Monitoring

Ambulatory pH monitoring is crucial for a definitive diagnosis of GERD, especially in patients with atypical symptoms or when endoscopy results are inconclusive. Prior High-Resolution Manometry (HRM) is recommended to (i) identify different esophageal segments and pressure zones for correct placement of the pH probe, (ii) rule out motility disorders that may mimic GERD symptoms, and (iii) assess esophageal motility, which affects the choice of anti-reflux procedures. Two devices are available for esophageal pH monitoring: the catheter-based device and the capsule-based device, recording data for 24 and 96 hours, respectively. The pH probe is positioned above the LES, identified by HRM. Patients are asked to record their symptoms throughout the study to allow correlation with pH data. A scoring system (see below), based on six parameters, is used to evaluate the severity of GERD (Table 1.5).

pH-impedance monitoring can differentiate between weakly acidic and acidic reflux, evaluate baseline mucosal impedance, and identify the upper extent of refluxate. Conversely, ambulatory (capsule) pH monitoring enables up to 96 hours of pH data collection, helping to account for daily reflux variability, and may assist in guiding PPI discontinuation if reflux levels are normal.

1.4.3 Barium Esophagogram

A barium contrast study is rarely used as a primary treatment for GERD. However, it can be a helpful investigation to provide morphological and functional details of the stomach and esophagus. While this study cannot confirm or rule out GERD, it offers additional information about conditions such as esophageal diverticula, tumors, peptic strictures, dysmotility, achalasia, and gastroparesis.

Table 1.5 Johnson–DeMeester scoring system to assess the severity of GERD based on ambulatory pH monitoring

Total number of reflux episodes
Number of episodes lasting >5 minutes
Longest reflux episode duration
Percentage of time esophageal pH is <4
Percentage of time pH < 4 in the upright position
Percentage of time pH < 4 in the supine position

1.5 Management

The majority of patients have mild symptoms that are effectively managed with lifestyle modification and acid suppression therapy.

1.5.1 Lifestyle Modification

- Weight loss
- Cessation of alcohol and tobacco
- Earlier evening meal to prevent nighttime acid exposure
- Elevation of the head end of the bed (6–10 inches) and sleeping in the left lateral position
- Avoid chocolate, peppermint, fat, onions, garlic, alcohol, caffeine, and nicotine

1.5.2 Optimization of Antisecretory Therapy

- Optimal timing of PPI administration is 30–60 minutes before meals.
- PPI taken as the first meal of the day.

- Confirm medication adherence and timing.
- In refractory GERD, the dosage should be twice daily for optimal symptom relief, healing esophagitis, and decreasing acid burden.
- Higher potency PPIs: Esomeprazole, Dexlansoprazole, and Rabeprazole are more potent than Omeprazole and Lansoprazole.
- Vonoprazan, the potassium-competitive antagonist (P-CAB), is a potent new molecule that is likely to replace PPIs as the preferred drug for acid suppression.
- Reflux inhibitors and mucosal protective agents: Baclofen reduces transient LES relaxations (TLESRs). Antacid preparations combined with alginate (Gaviscon Advance), along with a hyaluronic acid-chondroitin sulfate-based bioadhesive formulation (Esox), have shown benefits when used as an addition to PPI therapy compared to placebo with or without PPI. Gastric prokinetics such as Itopride, Domperidone, Metoclopramide, Levosulpiride, and others also increase LES pressure and are commonly prescribed alongside PPI therapy.

1.6 Operative Management of GERD

Laparoscopic fundoplication and its variants have become the 'gold standard' in surgical treatment of GERD. The traditional open transabdominal approach (Nissen) is suitable only for a select few, while the transthoracic approach has largely become outdated and is now regarded as historical. In confirmed cases of GERD, surgery has demonstrated long-term effectiveness comparable to PPI therapy in several randomized trials. This benefit also extends to patients with refractory GERD who do not respond to optimized PPI therapy. In a 17-year follow-up, surgery showed sustained benefits, with at least 60% of patients able to stop taking antisecretory medication.

1.6.1 Laparoscopic Fundoplication

1.6.1.1 Indications

- Patients with esophageal or extraesophageal GERD symptoms who respond to but are not fully relieved by PPI
- Patient experiencing heartburn who responds to PPI but has ongoing regurgitation
- Patients with well-documented reflux events prior to symptoms such as chest pain, cough, and wheeze
- GERD complications such as stricture, Barrett's esophagus, or recurrent laryngitis while taking PPI twice a day, as well as recurrent aspiration or pneumonia
- Symptomatic paraesophageal hernia
- Young age (to avoid long-term undesirable side effects of PPI)
- Intolerance to PPI treatment (Fig. 1.4 and Table 1.6)

1.6.1.2 Contraindications

- Surgically unfit and unable to tolerate general anaesthesia
- Previous upper abdominal surgery*
- Morbid obesity
- Severe esophagitis +/− stricture*
- Short oesophagus*
- Large paraesophageal hernia*

**Open surgery is desirable.*

1.6.2 Indications of Partial Fundoplication

- Impaired esophageal clearance due to a motility disorder
- Severe aerophagia associated with belching, especially during daytime reflux
- Insufficient gastric fundus to perform a tension-free total fundoplication

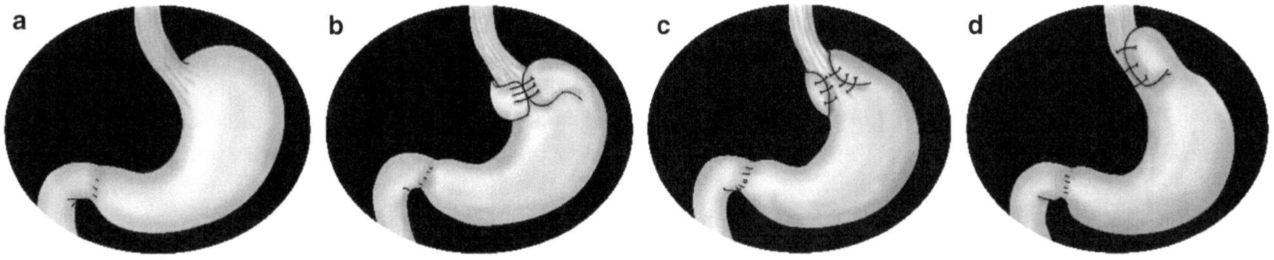

Fig. 1.4 Types of fundoplication: (**a**) Normal anatomy, (**b**) complete fundoplication, (**c**) partial fundoplication, (**d**) anterior fundoplication

Table 1.6 Types of fundoplication

Procedure	Type	Degree of wrap	Position
Nissen's	Complete	360°	Circumferential
Dor	Partial	180–200°	Anterior
Thal	Partial	90°	Anterior
Toupet	Partial	270°	Posterior
Watson	Partial	120°	Anterolateral

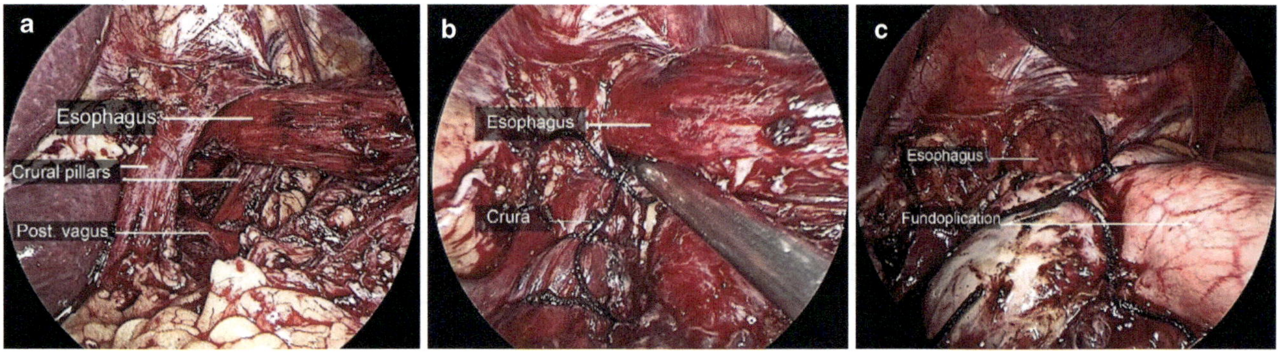

Fig. 1.5 Laparoscopic Nissen fundoplication. (**a**) Mobilization of abdominal esophagus and hiatal dissection. (**b**) Hiatal closure with interrupted silk suture. Note the small gap between the esophagus and the reconstituted hiatus. (**c**) Complete fundal wrap around the esophagus

- Psychological abnormality in tolerating the side effects of fundoplication
- Concomitant Heller myotomy for achalasia

1.6.3 Key Points for an Optimal Fundoplication

- Identify the GE junction: the collar of Helvetius or the loop of Willis, where the circular muscle fibers of the esophagus meet the oblique fibers of the stomach, and the gastroesophageal fat pad are the two key points for identification.
- Circumferential dissection near crura and esophagus.
- Avoid injury to the esophagus and vagus nerve.
- Dissection of the gastrohepatic ligament (pars flaccida) is performed above the hepatic branch of the vagus nerve, which may contain an aberrant left hepatic artery.
- Achieve 2–3 cm of intra-abdominal esophagus without applying traction.
- Division of short gastric vessels and posterior attachments to the pancreas when necessary.
- Closure of hiatal defect with interrupted sutures.
- Create a short (2 cm), floppy (tension-free) fundoplication around the esophagus.
- Fundoplication involves using the fundus as the wrap (not any other part of the stomach) around the esophagus (not around the proximal body of the stomach).

Table 1.7 Postoperative complications

Mortality	<1%
Perioperative morbidity	8–17%
Conversion to open fundoplication	2.5%
Early complications	
Bowel injury	0–4%
Bleeding and splenic injury	<1%
Pneumothorax	0–1.5%
Severe postoperative nausea and vomiting	2–5%
Late complications	
Gas-bloat syndrome	Up to 85%
Dysphagia	
Early	10–50%
Late	03–24%
Diarrhoea	18–33%
Recurrent heartburn	10–62%

- Fundoplication should remain in the abdomen without tension, and the crura should prevent the stomach or fundoplication from moving into the chest (Fig. 1.5 and Table 1.7).

Gas-Bloat Syndrome The proposed mechanisms of gas-bloat syndrome are (i) the inability of the surgically altered GEJ to relax in response to gastric distention or food intake, (ii) aerophagia, and (iii) iatrogenic injury to vagus nerve fibers resulting in altered gastric emptying and abnormal belching reflux. Most patients recover with conservative treatment. Measures that may help in more severe cases include (i) avoiding gas-producing foods and carbonated beverages, (ii) eating slowly to prevent aerophagia, (iii) avoiding smoking, (iv) using gastric prokinetic drugs, (v) taking antiflatulent agents such as simethicone and charcoal, and (vi) biofeedback techniques to retrain patients to decrease swallowing frequency. Severe and persistent symptoms may require revision surgery, such as conversion to partial fundoplication or gastric drainage procedures for confirmed cases of gastroparesis.

Dysphagia Most cases of dysphagia are temporary and result from postoperative inflammation and swelling; they tend to improve over time. Persistent dysphagia lasting more than 3–6 months should be evaluated. Possible causes include a too tight wrap or crural closure, an unrecognized motility disorder, a peptic stricture, a paraesophageal hernia, a slipped fundoplication into the chest, or distally onto the stomach. Initial treatment involves esophageal dilatation; if this is unsuccessful, revision surgery may be necessary.

Failed Fundoplication About 90% of patients recover well after laparoscopic fundoplication. The surgery usually fails within 2 years, presenting symptoms such as gas-bloat, dysphagia, or recurrent heartburn. Failure often results from missed underlying issues or incorrect surgical technique during the initial procedure. Technical failure is categorized as follows:

Type 1A: Herniation of both the wrap and GEJ into the chest.
Type 1B: Hernia recurs, but the wrap stays below the diaphragm.
Type II: Presence of paraesophageal hernia.
Type III: Malposition of the wrap on or below the gastric cardia.

Revision surgery requires a thorough workup, including endoscopy, barium esophagogram, esophageal manometry, and motility studies. Specialists should perform reoperation, and the procedure must be tailored to the specific pathology.

1.7 Nonsurgical Antireflux Procedures

The magnetic sphincter augmentation device (MSAD), also known as LINX, is a magnetic ring made of interconnected titanium beads that is surgically placed around the GEJ. The device improves the LES function and reduces reflux. MSAD is considered a less invasive alternative to fundoplication. Patients often experience significant symptom improvement after implantation, with PPI use decreasing from 100% to 15% and regurgitation symptoms from 57% to 1%. Less common complications include mild dysphagia, gas-bloat, inability to belch or vomit, and device erosion or migration.

Endoscopic Procedures Several endoscopic techniques have been described as alternatives to surgery for treating GERD. Some of the more recent techniques include:

- Transoral incisionless fundoplication (TIF): Using an endoscopic device (EsophyX), the LES is reinforced through plication, forming a 3 cm valve with a 270° circumferential wrap from inside.
- Endoscopic fundoplication with the Medigus Ultrasonic Endostapling System (MUSE): The stapler is inserted transorally into the stomach, and after retroflexion, the anchoring stapler is positioned between the fundus and the esophagus at the left lateral side, with stapling performed between 60° and 180° around the GEJ circumference.
- Endoscopic plication with the GERDx device: Full-thickness plication of the GEJ using endoscopic suturing to strengthen the LES.
- Antireflux mucosectomy (ARMS) causes scarring around the GEJ by performing crescentic or circumferential mucosal resection. The circumferential scar strengthens the LES.
- Antireflux Band Mucosectomy (ARBM) and Antireflux Mucosal Ablation (ARMA) using argon plasma coagulation.
- A pooled success rate of 73.8% has been reported over short-term follow-up with antireflux mucosal interventions. Post-procedure dysphagia requiring dilation was reported by 10%, while perforation occurred in 2.2%.
- Endoscopic bulking techniques to augment the LES are performed using various products such as Enteryx (biopolymer augmentation), PMMA (polymethylmethacrylate), and hydrogel prostheses.

All these endoscopic procedures have been proposed over time as less invasive alternatives to surgery. However, none has yet proven to be consistently accepted or effective. These procedures are technically demanding and constantly evolving and require specialized devices and expertise that may not be readily available. Therefore, there is no substantial experience or long-term data on any endoscopic procedure to justify its equivalence or superiority over established surgical methods.

Key Points

- The lower esophageal sphincter mechanism includes the gastric cardia oblique fibers, the angle of His, the intra-abdominal esophagus, the pinchcock action of the diaphragmatic crura, and the phreno-esophageal membrane.
- GERD occurs when any of these areas becomes impaired.
- Heartburn is the most typical presenting symptom.
- Extraesophageal symptoms such as recurrent cough, hoarseness, and noncardiac chest pain can create confusion in diagnosis.
- Endoscopy can diagnose esophageal mucosal changes due to GERD, but the absence of it does not rule out reflux.
- Ambulatory pH monitoring is the most accurate test to diagnose GERD.
- The majority of patients respond to medical management that includes PPI and lifestyle modification.
- Antireflux surgery is indicated in patients who present with PPI failure or complications of GERD.
- Laparoscopic fundoplication is considered the 'gold standard' for antireflux surgery.
- Fundal wrap can be either complete or partial; the partial option is recommended for patients with concomitant motility disorder.
- Gas-bloat and dysphagia are common self-limiting complications after surgery.
- Persistent symptoms beyond 3–6 months may require revision surgery.
- A detailed workup, including endoscopy, barium esophagogram, esophageal manometry, and motility studies, must be performed before proceeding with revision surgery.

Selected Reading

1. Richter JE. Gastroesophageal reflux disease treatment: side effects and complications of fundoplication. Clin Gastroenterol Hepatol. 2013;11:465–71.
2. Moore M, Afaneh C, Benhuri D, et al. Gastroesophageal reflux disease: a review of surgical decision making. World J Gastrointest Surg. 2016;8(1):77–83. https://doi.org/10.4240/wjgs.v8.i1.77.
3. Lopes SO, Gonçalves AR, Guilherme Macedo G, Santos-Antunes J. Endoscopic treatment of gastroesophageal reflux: a narrative review. Porto Biomed J. 2023;8(4):e226. https://doi.org/10.1097/j.pbj.0000000000000226.
4. Davis TA, Gyawali CP. Refractory gastroesophageal reflux disease: diagnosis and management. J Neurogastroenterol Motil. 2024;30:1728. https://doi.org/10.5056/jnm23145.

Motility Disorders of the Esophagus and Achalasia Cardia

2

Swati Mohanty, Sai Kumar, and Partha Pal

Abstract

Achalasia cardia is the most common esophageal motility disorder affecting adults of all age groups, with no gender predilection. Primarily involving the lower esophageal sphincter (LES), it is characterized by increased LES pressure that fails to relax, along with a secondary loss of peristalsis in the esophageal body. Esophageal manometry is essential for diagnosis and to guide management. Laparoscopic Heller's cardiomyotomy and peroral endoscopic myotomy (POEM) are currently the most accepted forms of treatment.

Keywords

Achalasia cardia · Heller's operation · POEM

Achalasia cardia, with an incidence of 0.6–1% per 100,000 people, is the most common esophageal motility disorder (EMD) affecting adults of all age groups, with no gender predilection. Primarily involving the lower esophageal sphincter (LES), it is characterized by increased LES pressure that fails to relax, along with a secondary loss of peristalsis in the esophageal body. These features vary in severity and form the basis for classifying achalasia cardia (Tables 2.1 and 2.2).

Table 2.1 Etiological classification of esophageal motility disorder

Primary	Secondary
Achalasia	Scleroderma
Diffuse esophageal spasm	Dermatomyositis
Nutcracker esophagus	Polymyositis
Hypertensive LES	Lupus erythematosus
Ineffective esophageal motility	Chagas disease
	Myasthenia gravis

LES lower esophageal sphincter

Table 2.2 Chicago classification of esophageal motility disorder based on high-resolution manometry

Disorders of EGJ outflow	Disorders of peristalsis
Achalasia I	Absent contractility
Achalasia II	Diffuse esophageal spasm
Achalasia III	Hypercontractile esophagus
EGJ outflow obstruction	Ineffective esophageal spasm

EGJ esophagogastric junction

2.1 Pathogenesis

Achalasia is believed to result from degeneration of the myenteric plexus and vagus nerve fibers in the LES. The loss of inhibitory neurons containing vasoactive intestinal peptide (VIP) and nitric oxide synthase in the esophageal myenteric plexus, and in severe cases, the involvement of cholinergic neurons, has been linked to infection, genetic inheritance, autoimmune disease, or neuronal degeneration.

2.2 Clinical Features

The common symptoms of achalasia include dysphagia, regurgitation, chest pain, and weight loss. Contrary to traditional teachings, dysphagia can happen with both solids and liquids, not just liquids. It may come and go, worsen with the consumption of hot or cold liquids, or be triggered by emotional stress. Regurgitation is usually spontaneous and can be

S. Mohanty (✉)
Department of Surgical Gastroenterology, Apollo Hospitals, Bhubaneswar, India

S. Kumar · P. Pal
Asian Institute of Gastroenterology, Hyderabad, India

M. Ibrarullah (ed.), *Recent Concepts in Gastrointestinal (GI) Surgery*, https://doi.org/10.1007/978-981-92-1118-0_2

Table 2.3 Clinical presentation of achalasia cardia

Symptoms	Incidence (%)
Dysphagia (solid and liquid)	90
Regurgitation	76–91
Nocturnal cough	30
Chronic aspiration	8
Chest pain	25–64
Burning sensation	18–52
Weight loss	35–91

Table 2.4 Eckardt score indicating achalasia severity: a score higher than 3 suggests the need for intervention, while a score below 3 indicates successful therapy after treatment

Symptoms/signs	Score 0	1	2	3
Recent weight loss (kg)	None	<5	5–10	>10
Dysphagia	None	Occasional	Daily	With each meal
Chest pain	None	Occasional	Daily	Several times a day
Regurgitation	None	Occasional	Daily	With each meal

observed as soiling of the pillow during sleep. Weight loss may occur due to limited food intake or, in rare cases, be a sign of an underlying cancer (Tables 2.3 and 2.4).

2.3 Diagnosis

Diagnosis of achalasia cardia is based on clinical symptoms supported by imaging and manometry (Table 2.5).

Functional Luminal Imaging Probe (FLIP) EndoFLIP is an innovative device that assesses the esophagogastric junction (EGJ) using a balloon catheter. The catheter has 8 or 16 impedance sensors attached to a balloon that is gradually filled with saline. The balloon distends the distal esophagus and EGJ, enabling the sensors to measure the cross-sectional area, compliance, and distensibility. The recorded rhythmic secondary peristaltic patterns aid in classifying esophageal motility, similar to manometry. EndoFLIP helps confirm the presence and subtypes of achalasia, as well as identify obstructions that HRM may have missed. Additionally, intraoperative EndoFLIP allows for tailoring the myotomy and assessing its effectiveness after therapy. A distensibility index (DI) at the GEJ > 2.8 mm^2/mm Hg, a diameter >13 mm, and repeated anterograde contractions in response to distention are considered normal. A DI < 2 mm^2/mm Hg indicates achalasia, while values between 2 and 3 are indeterminate (Figs. 2.1, 2.2, and 2.3).

Table 2.5 Diagnostic tests for achalasia cardia

Tests	Findings
UGI endoscopy	Dilated esophagus with retained saliva and food residue Presence of stasis changes in the mucosa and occasional candidiasis The LES shows transient resistance and relaxes with gentle pressure Malignancy superimposed or causing secondary achalasia when present
Barium esophagogram and timed barium esophagogram (TBE)	Dilated esophagus with retained food and contrast Lack of peristaltic stripping waves Narrowed GEJ causing a 'bird beak' appearance The Type III variant may present a corkscrew appearance Multiple images at specific intervals (e.g., 1, 2, and 5 minutes) are taken to observe the passage of barium through the esophagus and confirm delayed or absent emptying Absence of gastric air bubble
High-resolution manometry (HRM)	A mean integrated relaxation pressure greater than normal and absent peristalsis Incomplete LES relaxation Type I: Absent peristalsis may take the form of 100% failed peristalsis[a] Type II: Pan-esophageal pressurization with >20% of swallows with no normal peristalsis[b] Type III: >20% of swallows are associated with premature contraction with no normal peristalsis[c]
Contrast-enhanced CT scan	Primarily used to distinguish primary from secondary achalasia, which can be caused by a soft tissue mass at the GE junction. Additionally, it may detect mediastinal lymphadenopathy, lung, liver, or bone metastasis when present

[a]Moderate response to surgery
[b]Best response to surgery
[c]Poor response to surgery

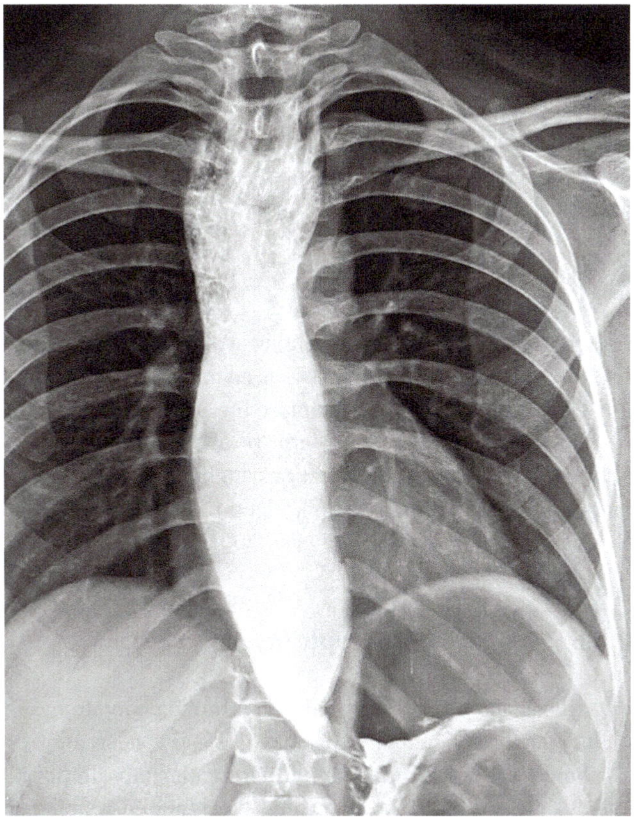

Fig. 2.1 Barium esophagogram showing a dilated esophagus with a distal 'bird beak' appearance, indicative of achalasia cardia

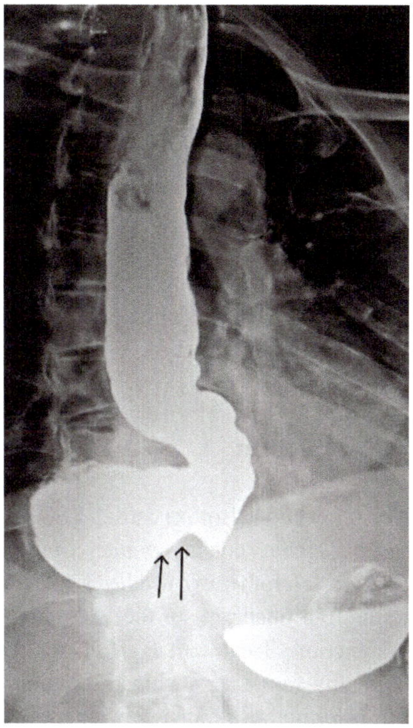

Fig. 2.2 Achalasia cardia with a large epiphrenic diverticulum (arrow)

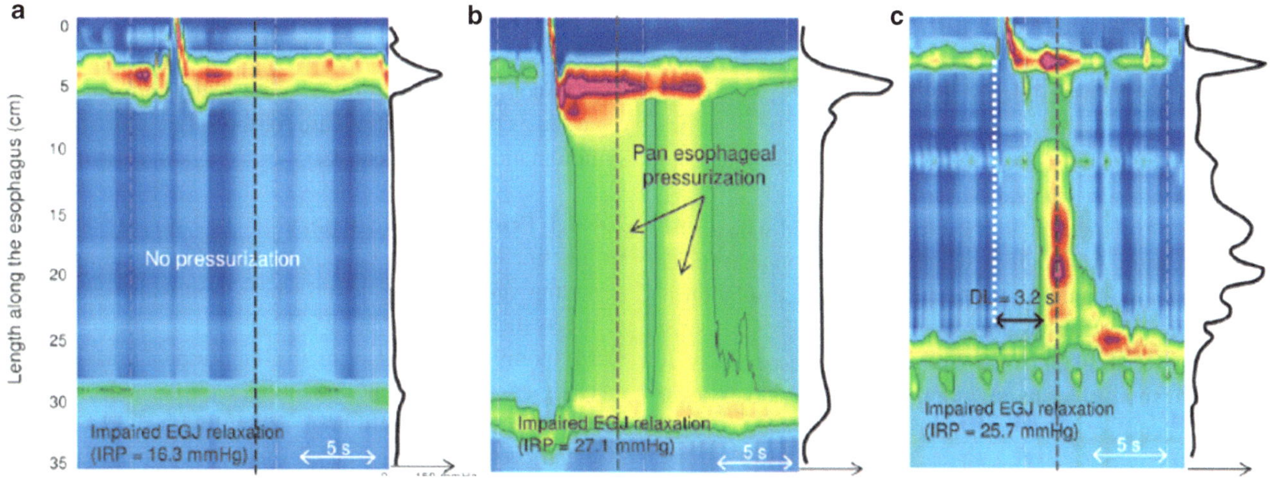

Fig. 2.3 Classification of achalasia cardia based on manometric findings. (**a**) Type I: Absent peristalsis, which may consist of 100% failed peristalsis. (**b**) Type II: Panesophageal pressurization with over 20% of swallows showing no normal peristalsis. (**c**) Type III: More than 20% of swallows are associated with premature contractions and no normal peristalsis

2.4 Treatment

2.4.1 Medical Management

Various smooth muscle relaxants have been used with limited success in treating achalasia cardia. The response is often unpredictable, short-term, and accompanied by side effects such as hypotension, dizziness, headache, and pedal edema. Therefore, while awaiting definitive therapy, these medications are usually given as a temporary measure or for preoperative preparation (Table 2.6).

2.4.2 Botox Injection

Botulinum toxin injection (Botox) causes LES relaxation by blocking the neurogenic, not myogenic, component of the sphincter. Using a sclerotherapy needle, a total of 100 U is injected into the four quadrants of the LES above the squamocolumnar junction. Treatment is often temporary, with symptoms typically returning within 6–12 months. It provides short-term symptom relief, with relapse occurring in 50% of patients within 1 year. The scar that forms in the submucosal layer makes subsequent myotomy more difficult, with an estimated 30% risk of perforation. Therefore, this method is only recommended for high-risk patients who are poor surgical candidates, as a bridge to surgery, or to treat residual spastic contractions above the myotomy site or LES. Successful Botox therapy also suggests favorable long-term relief after adequate dilatation or myotomy.

2.4.3 Pneumatic Dilatation

Pneumatic dilatation is performed using a balloon catheter with graded sizes (Rigiflex dilator, 30, 35, and 40 mm). The balloon is positioned across the LES and inflated with air for 15–60 seconds. A straightened balloon waist, visible under fluoroscopy, indicates complete dilation. Graded dilation is performed and evaluated after 4–6 weeks. Success rates for single and serial dilations are 28% and 44%, respectively. A positive response is more common in individuals over 45 years old, females, those with post-dilation LES pressure below 10 mm Hg, and patients with type 2 achalasia. Perforation has been reported in 0–16% of cases, often requiring surgical repair. Therefore, poor cardiopulmonary status or other comorbidities that prevent surgery (in case of perforation) may be contraindications to pneumatic dilatation.

Table 2.6 Pharmacological agents and their mechanisms of action

Drug	Mechanism of action
Calcium channel blocker: Nifedipine	Inhibits the L-type calcium channel and relaxes the LES
Nitrates: Carvasin	Increases nitric oxide in and relaxes the LES
Anticholinergics: Cetobromide, ammonium bromide	Relaxes the LES
PDE4 inhibitors: Sildenafil	Prevents nitric oxide degradation and prolongs LES relaxation

2.4.4 Esophageal Stents

A temporary self-expanding metallic stent, either partially or fully covered (20–30 mm), serves as an indwelling LES dilator. The stent is usually kept in place for about 1–4 weeks. In limited experience, the short-term results of stenting seem promising. Reported complications include stent displacement, regurgitation, perforation, bleeding, and stent-related tissue proliferation, which may lead to new stenosis.

2.4.5 Peroral Endoscopic Myotomy (POEM)

POEM, an endoscopic equivalent of surgical myotomy, is mainly performed in four steps: mucosal incision, creation of a submucosal tunnel, division of the circular muscle fibers, and closure of the mucosal incision. The reported benefits of the procedure include a short procedure time, less blood loss, a brief hospital stay, improved short-term Eckardt scores, and reduced postoperative pain (Fig. 2.4; Tables 2.7 and 2.8).

2.4.6 Surgery: Heller Cardiomyotomy

Laparoscopic Heller cardiomyotomy with fundoplication is regarded as the standard of care for the surgical treatment of symptomatic achalasia cardia.

2.4.6.1 Principles of Surgery

- Identification of the EJG by the gastric fat pad and palisading veins at the junction where the tubular esophagus meets the stomach.
- Myotomy involves splitting the longitudinal muscle fibers using controlled, blunt dissection. Circular muscle fibers are lifted with an endo-hook and cut with short bursts of electric current, being careful to avoid contact with the mucosa.
- The myotomy is extended proximally for about 5–6 cm on the esophagus and 2–3 cm distally onto the stomach.
- Myotomy is tested with air insufflation for leaks and repaired if any are detected.
- Partial fundoplication (Dor or Toupet) is performed. The gastric flap should be short (<2 cm) and anchored with both margins of the myotomy through stitches that pass through the crura (Fig. 2.5).

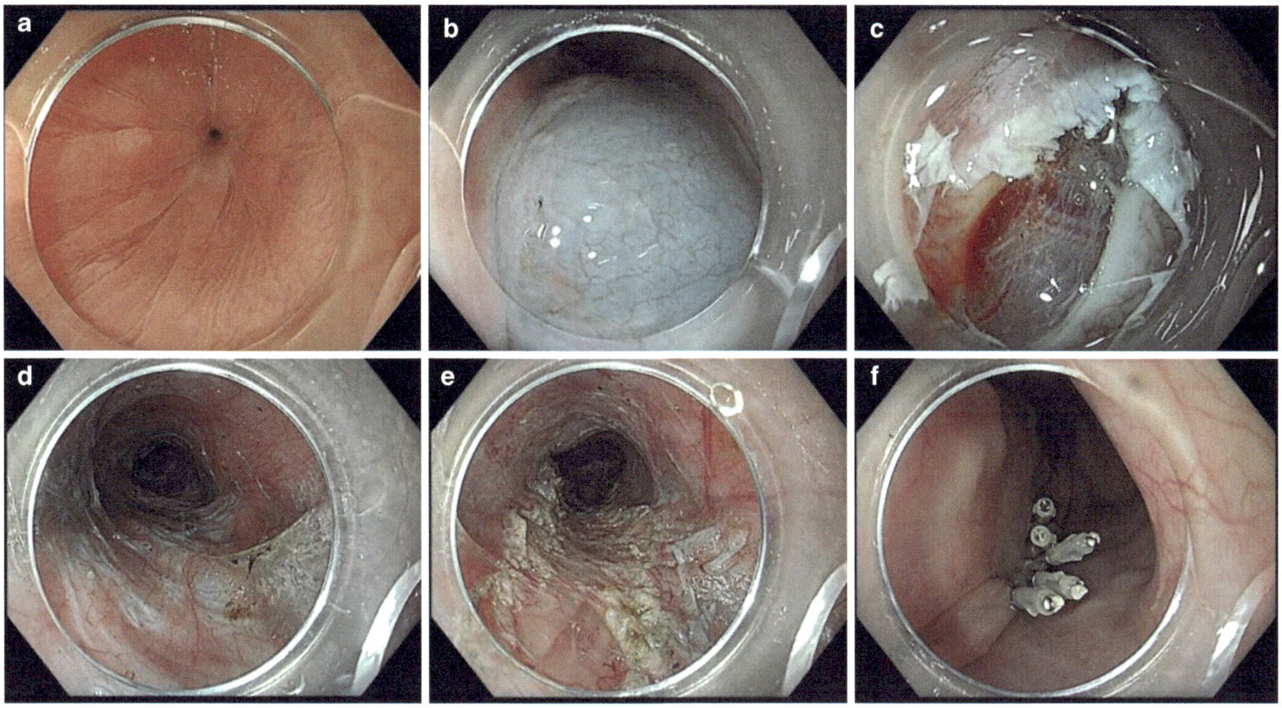

Fig. 2.4 POEM—posterior approach. (**a**) UGI endoscopy shows a tight LES and a dilated esophageal lumen. (**b**) Normal saline mixed with indigo carmine is injected at the 5 o'clock position, 8 cm above the EJG. (**c**) A 1 cm mucosal incision is made. (**d**) A submucosal tunnel is created. (**e**) A 5 cm myotomy is performed at the esophagus and 2 cm at the cardia. (**f**) The mucosal entry site is closed with endoclips. (Image courtesy: Sonmoon Mohapatra, Asutosh Mohapatra)

Table 2.7 Indications and contraindications of POEM

Indications	Contraindication
Type III achalasia requiring a long myotomy	Sigmoid esophagus
Nutcracker esophagus	Large epiphrenic diverticulum
Hypertensive LES	
Failed surgical myotomy	

Table 2.8 Complications of POEM

Intraoperative	Incidence (%)	Postoperative	Incidence (%)
Bleeding	1.4	Gastroesophageal reflux[b]	≈15
Mucosal injury[a]	4.8	Esophagitis	28
Perforation	0.2	Abnormal pH study	55
Subcutaneous emphysema	7.5	Postoperative pain	79
Pneumothorax	1.2	Postoperative leak	
Pneumomediastinum	1.1		
Pneumoperitoneum	6.8		
Pleural effusion	1.2		
Conversion to surgery	0.1		

[a]Predisposing factors include submucosal fibrosis, previous myotomy, mucosal edema, and a long submucosal tunnel >13 cm

[b]A modified technique called sling fiber-preserving POEM reduces postoperative reflux-induced esophagitis from 44.1% to 18.5%

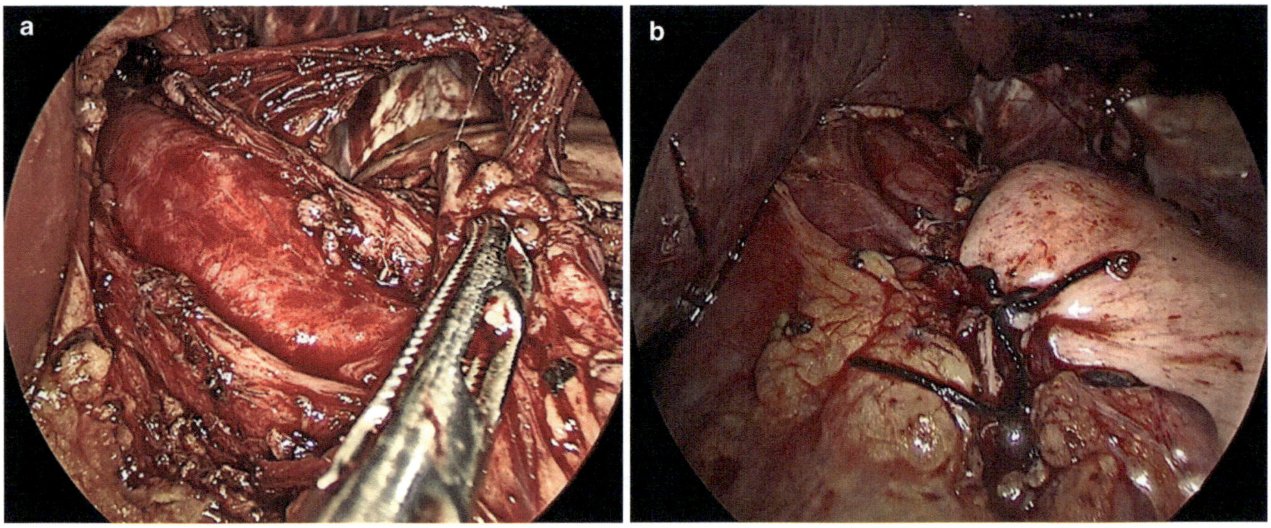

Fig. 2.5 (**a**) Laparoscopic Heller's cardiomyotomy; (**b**) Dor fundoplication after myotomy

2.4.6.2 Complications

- Perforation: Mucosal injury caused by dissection or cautery burn may occur during surgery or shortly after. The incidence ranges from 3% to 6% in primary procedures and can reach up to 30% in redo Heller's myotomy. If identified during surgery, it should be repaired with fine (3-0 or 4-0) sutures and reinforced with an anterior gastric flap (Dor fundoplication). If detected afterward, the repair should be supported with an omental flap.
- Persistent dysphagia: Dysphagia may continue or worsen after myotomy. This might be caused by incomplete myotomy, unnoticed malignancy, or a tight fundal wrap and should initially be managed conservatively. Persistent dysphagia can be treated with dilation or revision of the myotomy. Esophagectomy may be considered for a failed myotomy in the sigmoid esophagus or in cases with concurrent malignancy. The Table 2.9 below outlines the causes of dysphagia based on the timeframe and the recommended treatments.
- Gastroesophageal reflux and reflux-induced stricture: Extending the myotomy too far onto the stomach can cause gastroesophageal reflux and esophagitis. In open surgery, it is recommended to extend it by no more than 1 cm onto the stomach to reduce reflux and prevent a fundal wrap. In laparoscopic surgery, the recommended myotomy extension is at least 2–3 cm, which requires an anti-reflux procedure. Fundoplication decreases the incidence of reflux from 30% to 9%.
- Recently, a complication seen in both Heller's myotomy and POEM is 'blown out myotomy (BOM),' which is defined radiologically as a wide-mouthed outpouching or pseudo-diverticulum that causes more than a 50% increase in esophageal diameter. It is more common in Heller myotomy compared to POEM and also occurs in patients with persistently high intragastric resting pressure (IRP).

Table 2.9 Dysphagia after myotomy: causes and treatment

Dysphagia	Differential diagnosis	Suggested treatment
Persistent	Incomplete myotomy Tight fundoplication Failed myotomy	Dilatation/POEM/ revision myotomy Dilatation /revision surgery Esophagectomy
Early recurrence	Transdiaphragmatic herniation Food impaction	Revision surgery Endoscopic removal
Late recurrence	Transdiaphragmatic herniation Food impaction Gastroesophageal reflux Esophageal stricture End-stage achalasia Malignancy	Revision surgery Endoscopic removal Revision surgery Dilatation/revision surgery Esophagectomy Esophagectomy

2.4.6.3 Postop Care and Follow-Up for POEM and Heller Myotomy

- Water-soluble contrast esophagogram on POD 1. If there is no leak or obstruction, the patient will start a clear liquid diet, then switch to a pureed diet, and finally progress to a regular diet within 1 week.
- Routine follow-up in 4 weeks with UGI endoscopy.
- A timed barium swallow and pHmetry planned around 6 months.
- Screening endoscopies every 5 years due to the increased risk of cancer.

Table 2.10 Pneumatic dilation vs Lap Heller myotomy vs POEM

	Pneumatic dilatation	Lap Heller myotomy	POEM
Treatment efficacy	44–84% Best result in type II Poor results in young males <40 years and type I/III variants	57.0–89.3% Best results in the type II variant	75–97% Better than other modalities for type III with long myotomy
Post-procedure GERD	2–3%	2–33% Significantly reduced by fundoplication	20–54%
Procedure-related complications	Esophageal perforation (3–5%) Hematoma Diverticula formation	Perforation Recurrent dysphagia Inadvertent vagotomy and its consequences Splenic injury	Insufflation-related adverse events Bleeding (early and delayed) Mucosal perforation
Limitations	Redilatation required in approx. 1/3	Suboptimal results in sigmoid esophagus and type III achalasia	High rates of GERD Requires expertise in third-space endoscopy

2.4.6.4 POEM Versus Laparoscopic Heller's Myotomy

Both procedures provide relief from dysphagia in approximately 90–95% of patients with achalasia cardia. POEM is associated with higher reflux rates compared to Heller's myotomy with fundoplication. Most cases are classified as grade 1 esophagitis, which is clinically silent but can be identified during endoscopy. Severe esophagitis (grades C and D) occurs with equal frequency (around 5%) in both procedures. Twenty-four-hour ambulatory pH monitoring shows that elevated acid exposure time is observed in 30% of patients following either procedure. However, the increased incidence of reflux is mostly asymptomatic and may not be clinically significant (Table 2.10).

Key Points

- Dysphagia, chest pain, painless regurgitation, and weight loss are the primary symptoms of achalasia cardia.
- Diagnosis is suspected with UGI endoscopy and confirmed by a timed barium swallow and high-resolution manometry (HRM).
- Increased LES pressure, failure to relax, and disordered peristalsis are characteristic features of achalasia.
- HRM classifies achalasia into three types and differentiates it from other esophageal motility disorders.
- Medical management is generally ineffective, but Botox injection may offer short-term relief.
- Pneumatic dilatation, POEM, and laparoscopic Heller's myotomy provide long-term relief in 90–95% of cases.
- Causes of persistent or recurrent dysphagia after POEM or Heller's myotomy include incomplete myotomy, tight fundal wrap, stricture, and superimposed malignancy.
- Gastroesophageal reflux following a therapeutic procedure is usually asymptomatic.
- Esophagectomy may be necessary for failed myotomy, sigmoid esophagus, end-stage achalasia, and superimposed malignancy.

Selected Reading

1. Kahrilas PJ, Bredenoord AJ, Fox M, et al. The Chicago classification of esophageal motility disorders, v3.0. Neurogastroenterol Motil. 2015;27:160–74.
2. Patel DA, Yadlapati R, Vaezi MF. Esophageal motility disorders: current approach to diagnostics and therapeutics. Gastroenterology. 2022;162(6):1617–34.
3. Vasireddy AR, Leggett CL, Kamboj AK. Esophageal motility disorders: a concise review on classification, diagnosis, and management. Mayo Clin Proc. 2025;100(2):332–9.
4. Li MY, Wang QH, Chen RP, Su XF, Wang DY. Pathogenesis, clinical manifestations, diagnosis, and treatment progress of achalasia of cardia. World J Clin Cases. 2023;11(8):1741–52.
5. Mari A, Khoury T, Sweis R. Achalasia: beyond the basics. Front Gastroenterol. 2025;16:59–71.

Corrosive Injury of the UGI Tract

3

R. Kalayarasan, Vikram Kate, and N. Ananthakrishnan

Abstract

Corrosive ingestion in children is mainly accidental. In adults, it may be accidental or intentional, frequently linked to suicidal attempts. Acute corrosive injury is managed conservatively unless it presents with esophageal or gastric necrosis and perforation. Esophageal stricture, a long-term consequence of corrosive injury, is initially managed with endoscopic dilatation. Failure or an undilatable stricture is an indication for reconstructive surgery. Colon is the most suitable organ for esophagogastric replacement.

Keywords

Corrosive injury · esophageal stricture

Corrosive injuries of the esophagus, though less common in developed countries, remain a leading cause of benign esophageal strictures in many parts of the developing world, including India. The severe and often devastating effects of corrosive ingestion on the upper gastrointestinal tract pose significant diagnostic and treatment challenges. Managing these patients often requires substantial healthcare resources, as the treatment process is lengthy and frequently complicated by recurring issues or new symptoms over time. Every clinical decision, from initial response to corrosive exposure to long-term management, greatly influences the outcome and quality of life for these patients.

3.1 Pathophysiology

Corrosive substances are generally divided into acids and alkalis, with the term "lye" often used to refer to strong alkali agents. Common alkali substances involved in corrosive poisoning include sodium hydroxide-based cleaners, drain openers, bleaches, toilet bowl cleaners, dishwashing liquids, and detergents. Conversely, widely used acidic agents that cause corrosive injuries include toilet bowl cleaners containing sulfuric or hydrochloric acid, rust removers with hydrochloric, oxalic, or hydrofluoric acid, swimming pool cleaners with hydrofluoric acid, vinegar containing acetic acid, and formic acid used in the rubber tanning industry.

Corrosive injuries affect both children and adults, with distinct patterns of cause. In children, corrosive ingestion is mainly accidental, often due to their natural curiosity and tendency to explore household items. In adults, corrosive ingestion can be accidental or intentional, frequently linked to suicidal attempts. Suicidal ingestions tend to cause more severe injuries, especially in the proximal gastrointestinal tract, such as the pharynx or proximal esophagus, often because of hesitant consumption of the corrosive fluid. Conversely, accidental ingestions usually involve larger volumes, resulting in more serious gastric injuries. The severity and extent of injury after corrosive ingestion depend on the type, concentration, and amount of the substance ingested. Alkali agents, which are frequently colorless, tasteless, and less odorous, are often consumed in larger quantities. These agents cause liquefaction necrosis, leading to deep tissue damage and potential transmural injuries. For example, sodium hydroxide can cause full-thickness necrosis of the esophagus within seconds of exposure. Additionally, injuries caused by alkali are more likely to involve tissues surrounding the esophagus and nearby organs, such as the respiratory tract.

Acids typically cause coagulation necrosis, creating a protective coagulum that limits deeper tissue damage. However, concentrated acids in large amounts can lead to severe transmural injuries and even perforation. Acid ingestion usually results in more gastric than esophageal injuries, often affecting the gastric antrum or body, depending on whether the person is fasting at the time. The saying that "acid licks the esophagus and bites the stomach" has been questioned, as significant esophageal injuries can also occur with acid inges-

R. Kalayarasan · V. Kate (✉) · N. Ananthakrishnan
Jawaharlal Institute of Post-Graduate Medical Education and Research (JIPMER), Puducherry, India

M. Ibrarullah (ed.), *Recent Concepts in Gastrointestinal (GI) Surgery*, https://doi.org/10.1007/978-981-92-1118-0_3

tion. Small bowel injuries are rare because reflex pyloric spasm prevents corrosives from passing beyond the stomach. However, in cases of severe ingestion or previous gastric surgeries bypassing the pylorus, corrosives can cause notable small bowel injuries. The outcomes of corrosive injuries depend directly on the severity of the initial damage. Milder injuries limited to the mucosa usually heal without complications, whereas moderate injuries may lead to esophageal strictures. Severe injuries can cause acute perforation or dense, unexpandable strictures in the chronic phase.

3.2 Acute Corrosive Injury

3.2.1 Clinical Features

The clinical presentation varies depending on the severity of the injury. In its mildest form, the patient may be asymptomatic or exhibit minor symptoms such as mild throat discomfort and slight erythema of the oral mucosa. In cases of moderate to severe injury, symptoms become more prominent. Odynophagia and dysphagia often indicate significant esophageal involvement, while hoarseness or stridor suggests injury to the upper airway. Symptoms like epigastric pain and hematemesis are signs of gastric involvement. It is important to recognize that symptom overlap is common, and clinical signs alone are not always reliable for pinpointing the exact site of injury. Severe cases may present with respiratory distress, tachycardia, and excessive salivation, indicating more extensive damage. Abdominal tenderness or signs of peritonitis are concerning signs of gastric necrosis. Perforation of the esophagus or stomach generally occurs within the first 2 weeks after ingestion, with the highest risk between days 3 and 12. A sudden change in clinical status, such as worsening abdominal pain suggesting gastric perforation or new chest pain indicating esophageal perforation, requires prompt radiological assessment to guide further management.

3.2.2 Investigations

The role of investigations in acute corrosive injury primarily involves assessing the extent of damage. Upper gastrointestinal endoscopy remains a crucial tool for evaluating caustic ingestion and guiding treatment decisions. However, there is ongoing debate regarding the optimal timing for performing endoscopy. Some experts recommend early endoscopy within 24 hours of ingestion, as it allows for prompt injury assessment, facilitating early discharge of patients without significant injury and enabling timely intervention for those with severe damage. Conversely, a more common approach is to delay endoscopy until 48–72 hours after ingestion, to avoid underestimating the injury's depth due to swelling and to reduce procedural risks. Studies show that endoscopy can be safely performed up to 96 hours post-ingestion without increasing complications. Notably, endoscopy is contraindicated between days 5 and 15 after ingestion because of the higher risk of iatrogenic perforation during this period. Modern, flexible, slender endoscopes used by experienced operators have decreased the risk of perforation, allowing a thorough evaluation of the esophagus and stomach. This contrasts with earlier practices, where the procedure has been halted at the first sign of injury. The Zargar classification is commonly used to grade endoscopic findings (Figs. 3.1 and 3.2; Table 3.1).

Patients with Grade 1 or 2a injuries typically recover without complications, while Grade 2b injuries and survivors of Grade 3 injuries often develop strictures that require endoscopic or surgical treatment. A major limitation of endoscopy in assessing acute corrosive injuries is its inability to accurately determine the depth of necrosis, which can lead to unnecessary surgery or inappropriate conservative management, potentially impacting patient outcomes. Additionally, endoscopic grading is subjective and susceptible to interobserver variability. To address these limitations, contrast-enhanced computed tomography (CECT) has become a valuable tool for more precisely grading corrosive injuries (Table 3.2).

CT Grade 1 indicates mild injuries observed in endoscopic Grade 1–2a, while CT Grade 2 corresponds to more severe endoscopic Grade 2b–3b injuries. CT Grade 3 always matches very severe endoscopic Grade 3b injuries. This grading system supports endoscopic findings and offers important insights into the extent of transmural injury, aiding accurate decision-making and improving patient management.

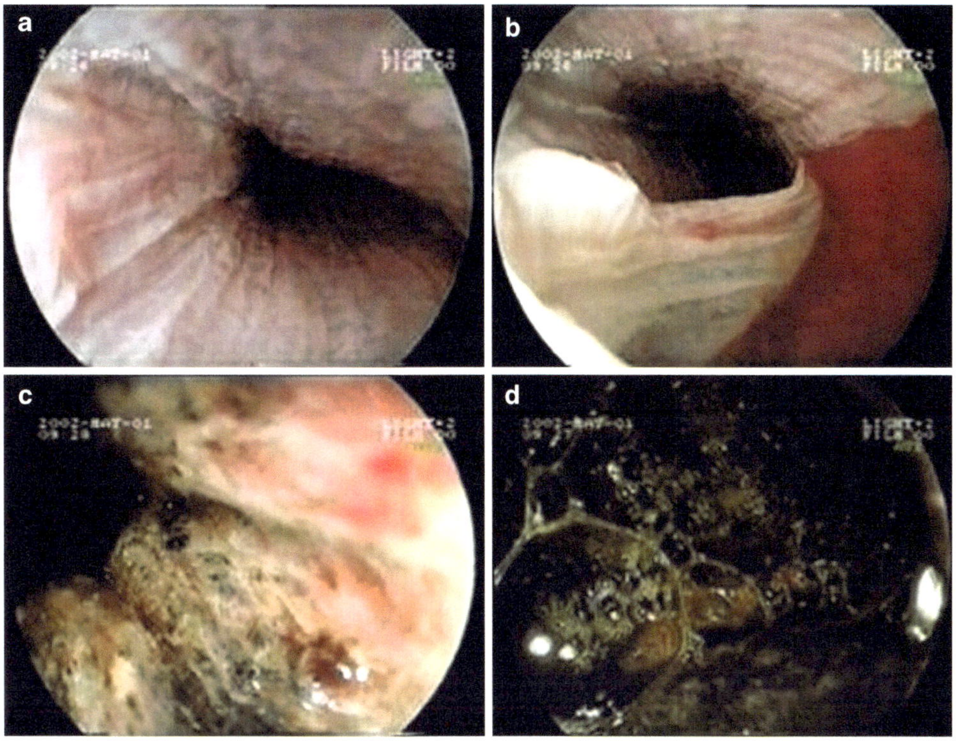

Fig. 3.1 Acute corrosive injury. (**a**, **b**) Inflamed esophageal mucosa covered with eschar. (**c**, **d**) Gastric mucosa

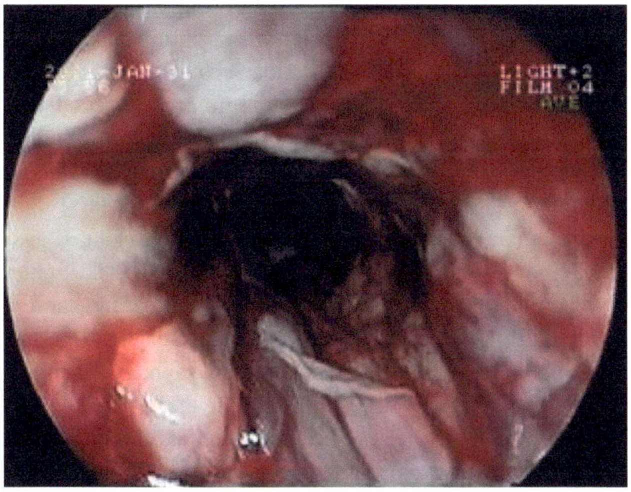

Fig. 3.2 Inflamed esophageal mucosa 2 weeks after injury

Table 3.1 Acute corrosive injury of the esophagus: Zargar endoscopic grading

Grade	Endoscopic findings
1	Erythema and edema
2	(a) Hemorrhage, erosions, blisters, and ulcers with exudate
	(b) Circumferential esophageal ulceration
3	(a) Scattered deep ulcers with discoloration (brown, black, grey)
	(b) Extensive deep ulcers with similar discoloration
4	Esophageal perforation

Table 3.2 CECT grading of acute corrosive injury of the esophagus

Grade	CECT findings
1	Normal-appearing organs
2	Mucosal enhancement with a hypodense wall due to edema Surrounding soft tissue inflammatory changes Enhancement of the outer esophageal wall (target sign)
3	Absence of post-contrast wall enhancement, indicating severe transmural injury

3.3 Management

Management of acute corrosive ingestion mainly emphasizes prompt resuscitation, early detection of complications, nutritional support, and stricture prevention.

3.3.1 Initial Resuscitation

The primary goal of initial resuscitation is to prevent further injury and effectively manage systemic complications. Following basic principles of airway and circulatory management is essential. In cases of laryngeal injury, tracheostomy and mechanical ventilation might be required to secure the airway. Certain procedures, such as placing the patient in a supine position, gastric lavage, and inducing vomiting, are contraindicated because they can worsen esophageal injuries by reexposing tissue to the corrosive substance. Likewise, neutralizing acids with alkalis (and vice versa) is not recommended since the heat produced during the exothermic chemical reaction can intensify tissue damage. Acute-phase treatment focuses on supportive care rather than specific antidotes. Intravenous proton pump inhibitors (PPIs) are frequently given to patients with severe injuries to help reduce additional damage to the gastric mucosa and prevent esophageal injury from gastroesophageal reflux. However, the efficacy of PPIs in this setting is not conclusively established. The use of corticosteroids to prevent stricture formation lacks supporting evidence and is generally not recommended, except in cases of airway compromise. Broad-spectrum antibiotics are not routinely used but should be considered for patients with severe injuries or on systemic steroids. Antibiotics should target both oral and intestinal bacteria, as high-grade injuries can lead to systemic sepsis from the virulent bacteria colonizing the oropharynx and esophagus. Early and precise resuscitation is crucial for improving outcomes in the acute management of corrosive ingestion.

3.3.2 Emergency Surgery

Emergency surgery is required for patients showing signs of transmural necrosis during initial assessment, with the goal of removing all dead tissue. Laparotomy remains the standard procedure, although minimally invasive techniques may be used in specialized high-volume centers. Diagnostic laparoscopy is often performed before laparotomy in patients with suspicious findings. For combined esophageal and gastric injuries, an esophagogastrectomy with cervical esophagostomy is performed through a combined abdominal and cervical approach, utilizing the transhiatal esophageal stripping technique. The lack of mediastinal adhesions during the acute phase, along with corrosive-induced periesophageal edema and thrombosis of perivisceral vessels, makes blunt esophageal stripping easier. In cases involving airway injury or significant mediastinal contamination, a transthoracic approach might be necessary.

Total gastrectomy is indicated for isolated gastric wall necrosis, with delayed reconstruction preferred over immediate oesophagojejunostomy due to the high risk of sepsis and hemodynamic instability in these patients. A partial gastrectomy is avoided because the remaining gastric tissue can continue to necrose, leading to complications. Resection of nearby organs such as the colon, spleen, or pancreas may be necessary if necrosis spreads to these areas. However, extensive surgeries like pancreatoduodenectomy significantly increase morbidity and mortality and are usually avoided. A feeding jejunostomy should be placed during emergency surgery to allow early enteral nutrition and improve the patient's nutritional status for future definitive reconstruction.

3.3.3 Prevention of Stricture Formation

Given the technical challenges of managing corrosive-induced esophagogastric strictures, various strategies have been explored to prevent their formation. Early oral feeding in cases of superficial esophageal injuries may prevent synechiae and stricture formation. Nasogastric tube placement can facilitate enteral feeding and serve as a dilator for potential strictures, especially in high esophageal or pharyngo-esophageal locations. Due to their high cost, limited efficacy, and potential complications, stents are not routinely recommended in these scenarios. Numerous pharmacological agents, including mitomycin C, 5-fluorouracil, vitamin E, octreotide, and interferon-alpha-2b, have been examined in experimental and clinical settings for their potential to prevent strictures. However, none have shown consistent or significant benefits, so their routine use is not supported in clinical practice.

3.4 Corrosive Strictures

3.4.1 Clinical Features

Progressive dysphagia, beginning with solids and eventually advancing to liquids, is characteristic of chronic esophageal stricture caused by fibrosis-induced luminal narrowing. Patients frequently experience regurgitation of food and saliva, which can lead to recurrent cough, aspiration pneumonia, and respiratory problems. Without adequate enteral nutrition, prolonged dysphagia may cause significant weight loss, anemia, and malnutrition. Those with an isolated gastric stricture usually show symptoms of gastric outlet obstruction, such as early satiety, post-meal bloating, nausea, and persistent vomiting. When both esophageal and gastric strictures are present, the more common dysphagia can mask gastric outlet obstruction, highlighting the importance of thoroughly evaluating gastric involvement in all patients with esophageal strictures.

3.4.2 Investigations

In a patient with corrosive esophagogastric stricture, the initial preferred investigation is an oral contrast study to evaluate the location, number, and length of esophageal and gastric strictures. Barium is preferred over water-soluble contrast agents unless esophageal perforation is suspected, as it provides better visualization of the stricture and aids in planning subsequent management. Key features to assess in the contrast study include the upper extent of the esophageal stricture, the length of involvement, the number of strictures, the presence of sacculations, and the presence of a tracheoesophageal fistula. These features indicate a lower likelihood of response to endoscopic dilatation. However, in patients with pharyngeal involvement, a barium study may not accurately determine the extent of the disease. Similarly, it may fail to exclude gastric strictures if the patient cannot ingest enough contrast due to a tight esophageal stricture (Fig. 3.3).

CT of the neck and thorax with air swallow and sagittal/coronal reconstruction is useful when pharyngeal or proximal esophageal strictures prevent adequate evaluation with oral contrast. It provides better visualization of the stricture length and the presence of a patent distal esophageal lumen. If the distal esophagus is open, esophageal reconstruction can be planned lower, leading to improved long-term functional outcomes. Flexible fiberoptic laryngoscopy is an important test to assess upper airway involvement, vocal cord mobility, and the presence of pharyngeal adhesions. Severe airway involvement increases the risk of aspiration and may require long-term airway management, including a permanent tracheostomy.

An upright abdominal X-ray after overnight fasting is a simple yet effective screening tool for assessing coexisting gastric outlet obstruction. A gastric fluid level strongly indicates a gastric stricture with gastric outlet obstruction, which has important implications for surgical planning. Upper gastrointestinal endoscopy is primarily used to evaluate the severity of mucosal inflammation and the feasibility of endoscopic dilation. Endoscopic evaluation helps decide whether serial dilation is an option or if surgical intervention is needed. However, endoscopy should be performed carefully to prevent perforation, especially in long or complex strictures. A hemogram, serum electrolytes, and serum albumin should be checked to evaluate nutritional and hydration status, as patients often experience severe malnutrition and electrolyte imbalances due to chronic dysphagia and poor oral intake.

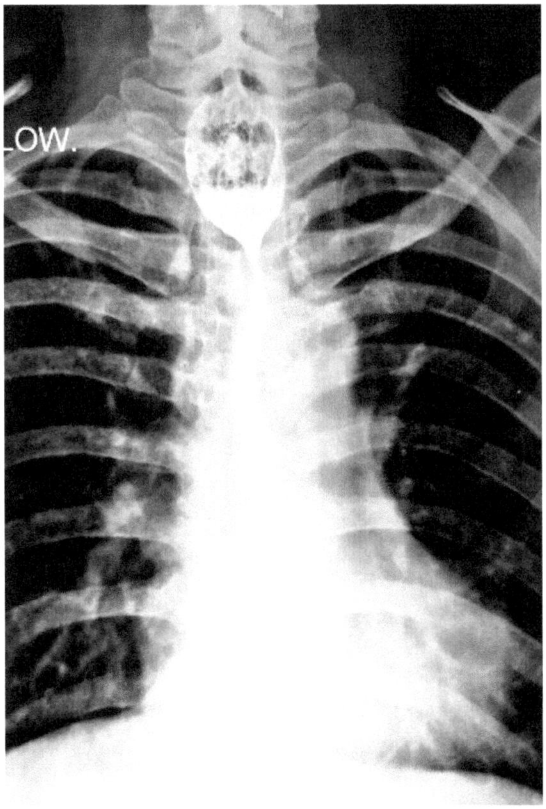

Fig. 3.3 Barium esophagogram showing a long stricture involving the lower cervical and thoracic esophagus

3.5 Management of Esophageal Stricture

3.5.1 Endoscopic Therapy

Strictures are a common complication of corrosive ingestion, usually developing within 2–3 weeks and progressing quickly. Diagnosis is often made through UGI endoscopy. Endoscopic dilation, using either bougie dilators (e.g., Savary-Gilliard) or balloon dilators, is the first treatment for patients with strictures that can be dilated. Bougie dilators offer tactile feedback to the operator, while balloon dilators enable precise dilation under direct visualization. The standard approach involves regular dilations to reach a lumen diameter of 15 mm, providing complete relief from dysphagia. Repeat dilations are done as needed when symptoms recur. Studies from various centers in India show that most patients with suitable strictures experience significant symptom improvement. The procedure generally has an acceptable safety profile, although long-term results and recurrence data are limited. Recurrence rates tend to be higher in corrosive strictures compared to benign peptic strictures. However, recurrence rates in corrosive strictures decrease over time and become similar to those in peptic strictures after 36 months. Some strictures, however, are not suitable for endoscopic dilation and may require surgical intervention in specific cases (Table 3.3).

Table 3.3 Strictures not suitable for endoscopic dilation

Long strictures exceeding 10 cm[a]
Multiple strictures, often defined as more than three strictures in some studies
Irregular strictures with sacculations[a]
Failure of endoscopic dilatation, i.e., requiring more than five unsuccessful sessions
Previous complications of dilatation, such as perforation
Concomitant gastric stricture

[a]High risk of perforation during dilatation

3.5.2 Surgical Management

3.5.2.1 Timing of Reconstruction

Reconstruction should be postponed until the scarring process stabilizes, typically 6–12 months after injury. Attempting reconstruction too soon increases the risk of anastomotic stricture formation. Nutritional optimization is crucial during this period, often requiring a feeding jejunostomy, as long-term nasogastric feeding is poorly tolerated and gastrostomy limits the use of the gastric conduit.

3.5.2.2 Esophageal Resection Versus Bypass

The choice between esophageal resection and bypass remains a topic of debate. Supporters of resection emphasize risks such as malignancy, mucoceles, and rupture of remaining esophageal segments. However, the risk of developing malignancy after corrosive injury is very low. Conversely, bypass surgery avoids the significant risks of morbidity and death associated with esophagectomy, especially in malnourished patients.

3.5.2.3 Choice of Replacement Conduit

Conduits for esophageal replacement include the stomach, colon, and jejunum.

Stomach The stomach is a common esophageal substitute because it is easy to mobilize and requires only one anastomosis. However, in cases of corrosive esophageal stricture, the stomach is often involved in the scarring process, especially after acid ingestion, making it a less preferred choice compared to patients with esophageal cancer. Additionally, functional outcomes with gastric conduits may decrease over time due to complications such as symptomatic reflux, anastomotic stricture, and columnar metaplasia of the remaining squamous epithelium.

Colon The colon offers good vascularity, and its long vascular arcades allow for tension-free transfer with a better luminal match. The choice between the right and left colon for esophageal replacement remains a matter of debate. In conventional right colon esophagocoloplasty, the ileum, ascending colon, and proximal transverse colon are used, with the middle colic artery and vein providing the vascular supply. The ileum is anastomosed to the cervical esophagus. Benefits of right colon esophagocoloplasty include preserving the ileocecal valve, which helps prevent pharyngeal reflux. Additionally, the left colon remains available as a backup conduit if postoperative right colon necrosis occurs. However, the highly variable vascular anatomy of the right colon increases the risk of conduit ischemia. In left colon esophagocoloplasty, the conduit is made from the transverse colon and proximal descending colon, supplied by the ascending branch of the left colic artery. Advantages include more reliable blood supply and the structural suitability of the left colon, which has thicker walls and a consistent lumen. A potential concern is the presence of diverticulosis in the left colon, although this is rare in the Indian population.

A modified technique called mid-colon esophagocoloplasty combines the advantages of both right and left colon approaches. It involves mobilizing the colon from the terminal ileum to the mid-descending colon. The descending colon is divided distal to the left colic vessels, while the terminal ileum is divided approximately 2 cm from the ileocecal valve. The conduit relies on one or two left colic vessels, and the right colic, ileocolic, and often the middle colic pedicles are divided. After mobilizing and ensuring the colon is tension-free in the neck, the unused ileum, cecum, and ascending colon are discarded. A wide, side-to-side esophagocolic anastomosis is performed, reducing the risk of stricture and allowing extra length for potential stoma enlargement if needed. This approach avoids complications from tension and ischemia common with traditional right or left colon interpositions. By mobilizing and positioning the colon before dividing it, the proper conduit length is assured. The technique also prevents ischemic complications, such as cervical salivary fistulas, by excluding potentially ischemic terminal segments from the anastomosis (Fig. 3.4).

Jejunum The jejunum is usually not the first choice for esophageal replacement due to its limited length, which restricts its applicability in many cases. However, supercharged jejunal grafts may be a viable alternative when other conduits are unsuitable or unavailable. These grafts enhance

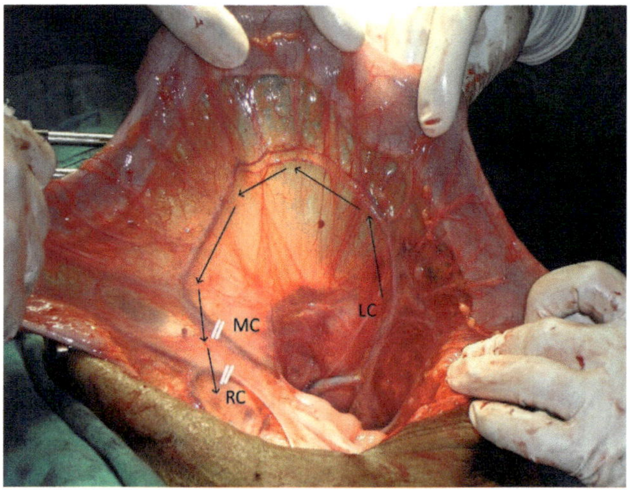

Fig. 3.4 Colonic conduit based on the left colic artery (LC). The middle colic artery (MC) and the right colic artery (RC) are divided proximal to the bifurcation of the main trunks to preserve the vascular arcade (indicated by running arrows). Under transillumination, the arcade is visualized for completeness; the adequacy of blood supply is confirmed by test-clamping the MC and RC

vascular supply through microvascular anastomosis, improving their reliability. Additionally, free jejunal grafts are particularly useful for reconstructing short esophageal defects, such as those resulting from the excision of localized strictures.

3.5.2.4 Routes for Conduit Transfer

Conduits are transferred via:

- Posterior mediastinum: Preferred when the native esophagus has been removed. This provides the shortest route, minimizing vascular compromise.
- Anterior mediastinum (retrosternal): Most commonly used route when the esophagus is left in situ.
- Subcutaneous route (presternal): Seldom used due to poor cosmetic results. It also has drawbacks like a larger conduit size and decreased vascularity. Nonetheless, it may be considered in specific cases, such as patients with a history of mediastinitis or limited mediastinal space.

3.6 Management of Pharyngeal Strictures

Before undertaking a procedure to bypass the thoracic esophageal stricture, it is essential to ensure a patent cervical esophageal segment for proximal anastomosis of the conduit. Any attempt to create a high pharyngo-colic anastomosis is ill-advised due to significant risks of aspiration. Therefore, in cases of high strictures, every effort should be made to perform the anastomosis below the level of the cricopharyngeal sphincter (Table 3.4).

Table 3.4 Classification of pharyngeal strictures and the management strategies

Type	Characteristics	Management strategy
I	Dilatable strictures	Endoscopic dilatation is the first-line treatment
II	Non-dilatable strictures near the laryngeal inlet	Managed with retrograde dilatation via right neck exploration. Once the stricture is adequately dilated, an esophagocoloplasty is performed distal to the treated stricture via a left neck approach along the anterior border of the left sternocleidomastoid. The right-sided esophagostomy typically closes spontaneously in most patients. In the rare event of prolonged patency, the esophagostomy can be surgically closed with interrupted sutures after separating it from the skin
III	Short segment strictures due to granulation tissue	Treated with granulation tissue excision under vision with the help of a direct laryngoscope. Repeated sessions may be required to obtain a stable lumen
IV	Dense strictures with a residual cervical esophagus	Repaired using myocutaneous flaps, such as sternomastoid or pectoralis major flaps. While the pectoralis major flap is a reliable option, it often results in a noticeable scar on the chest wall. Alternatively, the sternomastoid muscle myocutaneous inlay flap may be used for its esthetic advantages. These flaps can serve as definitive treatment for patients with no distal obstruction. However, when a distal obstruction is present, additional interventions such as endoscopic dilatation or esophageal bypass will be necessary to achieve optimal outcomes
V	Pharyngeal strictures with no demonstrable lumen in the cervical esophageal segment	When there is laryngeal involvement requiring a tracheostomy, a pharyngocolic anastomosis above the level of the stricture may be considered. However, in patients with a patent airway, this procedure carries a high risk of aspiration and is generally contraindicated. While adding a tracheostomy may prevent aspiration, it also poses a significant risk of a permanent tracheostomy and inability to swallow, as many patients struggle to regain normal swallowing function with high anastomoses. For these patients, a simpler approach, such as feeding gastrostomy or jejunostomy, often offers a better quality of life than the complications associated with an ill-conceived high pharyngeal anastomosis

Table 3.5 Classification and management guidelines for corrosive gastric strictures

Type	Characteristics	Management
I	Short ring strictures near the pylorus	Limited resection and gastroduodenal reconstruction
II	Strictures extending to the antrum	Distal gastrectomy and gastrojejunostomy. Retrocolic gastrojejunostomy should be avoided as it hinders future coloplasty in patients with combined esophageal stricture.
III	Mid-gastric strictures	Distal gastric resection
IV	Diffuse linitis plastica-like involvement	Total gastrectomy and esophagojejunostomy
V	Gastric strictures with duodenal involvement	Antecolic gastrojejunostomy

3.7 Management of Corrosive Gastric Strictures

Gastric strictures can occur alone but are more often linked with esophageal strictures, making it important to check for gastric involvement in patients with a history of corrosive ingestion. The presence of a gastric stricture greatly influences the approach to managing esophageal strictures. Typically, the extent and type of gastric injury are evaluated using upper gastrointestinal endoscopy and barium swallow imaging. However, in patients with complete dysphagia, these diagnostic methods are not feasible. In such cases, a simple, cost-effective alternative to a CT scan is a plain abdominal X-ray taken after overnight fasting. The appearance of a gastric fluid level on the X-ray strongly indicates gastric outlet obstruction. Although some literature recommend gastrectomy to prevent potential cancer in the scarred stomach, this concern seems exaggerated, as malignancy in a scarred stomach from corrosive injury is extremely rare (Table 3.5).

3.8 Combined Esophageal and Gastric Strictures

When corrosive strictures affect both the esophagus and stomach simultaneously, a single-stage treatment plan can be considered. If the gastric stricture occurs before the esophageal one, a limited gastric resection with gastroduodenal reconstruction may be sufficient initially, postponing esophageal bypass for later if necessary. However, gastric outlet obstruction may develop gradually, weeks or even months after esophageal cicatrization. This delay can occur if mild pyloric stenosis is missed during endoscopic dilatation of the esophageal stricture, which can eventually lead to complete obstruction. Alternatively, subclinical gastric outlet obstruction may remain asymptomatic due to the dysphagia caused by the esophageal stricture, becoming evident only once the patient resumes oral intake after successful esophageal replacement. Such delayed gastric strictures can significantly impact surgical planning, especially when using the stomach as a conduit for esophageal replacement.

For patients with both esophageal and gastric strictures, esophagocoloplasty combined with a gastrojejunostomy distal to the cologastric anastomosis is advised. In cases of esophageal strictures with type IV gastric strictures, colonic bypass with an anastomosis between the distal colon and proximal jejunum is preferred, leaving the stomach intact. This approach avoids the increased morbidity associated with total gastrectomy and esophageal bypass in these vulnerable patients. Delayed gastric outlet obstruction after esophageal bypass often presents as dilation of the conduit and should not be mistaken for cologastric stenosis. Endoscopic confirmation helps establish the diagnosis, and treatment options include distal gastric resection or gastrojejunostomy distal to the cologastric anastomosis. In patients where the stomach has been utilized for esophageal bypass, delayed gastric outlet obstruction presents a complex challenge. Surgical options such as gastric resection or gastroenterostomy are rarely feasible, requiring alternative solutions like jejunal interposition. In select cases, pyloroplasty may be an effective option.

3.9 Role of Minimally Invasive Surgery

Corrosive esophagogastric strictures mainly impact young adults during their most active and productive years, making effective and patient-friendly treatment options essential. Minimally invasive surgery (MIS) provides a promising alternative because of its potential to reduce postoperative complications and promote faster recovery. Despite these benefits, the adoption of MIS for corrosive esophagogastric stricture has been slow, primarily due to technical challenges in evaluating the vascular arcade and avoiding damage to vascular pedicles. Recent advances in laparoscopic and robotic technologies have driven a shift from hybrid methods to fully minimally invasive techniques. Innovations such as indocyanine green fluorescence imaging have enhanced intraoperative safety by enabling the precise assessment of blood vessels and ensuring anastomotic integrity. However, the long-term effectiveness and benefits of these techniques compared to traditional methods need validation through well-designed, large-scale studies with extended follow-up to establish MIS as the standard care for corrosive esophagogastric strictures (Figs. 3.5 and 3.6).

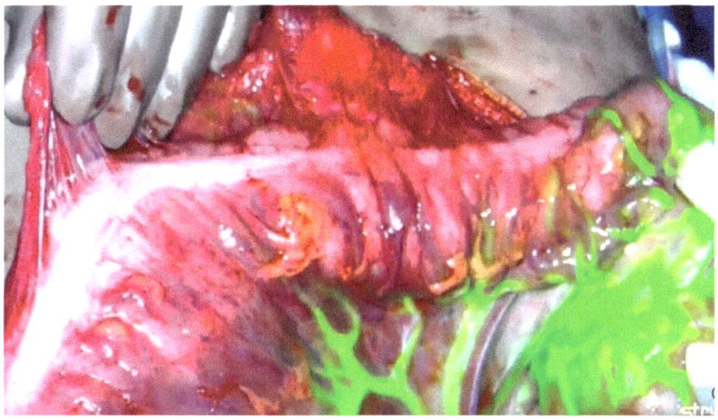

Fig. 3.5 Use of Indocyanine green to assess completeness of vascular arcade

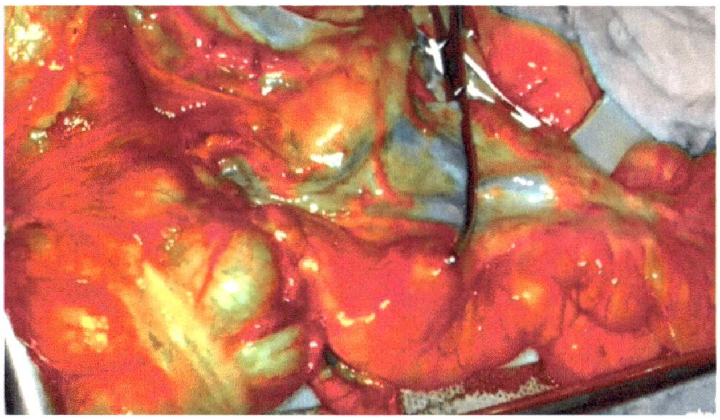

Fig. 3.6 Quantitative estimation of blood flow in the colon (red color indicates good blood flow to the bowel)

Key Points

- Corrosive ingestion is a primary cause of benign esophageal stricture in developing countries, often accidental in children and intentional in adults (typically during suicidal attempts).
- Alkalis cause liquefaction necrosis, frequently affecting the esophagus, while acids induce coagulation necrosis, usually involving the stomach.
- Symptoms vary by severity, ranging from odynophagia, dysphagia, hoarseness, and epigastric pain to severe complications such as perforation and airway compromise.
- Most esophageal or gastric perforations occur within 3–12 days after ingestion, requiring close monitoring during this period.
- Endoscopy is essential for early injury assessment but should be avoided between days 5 and 15 due to perforation risk.
- CECT assists in evaluating transmural damage and complements endoscopy.
- Initial management includes airway protection, avoiding gastric lavage and emesis and providing cautious supportive care with PPIs. Routine use of corticosteroids and antibiotics is not generally recommended.
- Emergency surgery is necessary for transmural necrosis, with procedures such as esophagogastrectomy, total gastrectomy, and feeding jejunostomy to ensure nutrition.
- Stricture Prevention: Early oral feeding and nasogastric tube placement may be beneficial; however, pharmacologic agents like mitomycin C and octreotide have no proven advantages.
- Contrast studies, including barium enema, CT scan, and upper GI endoscopy, help determine the location, length, and suitability for dilation or surgery.
- Surgical reconstruction should be delayed 6–12 months after injury.
- Bypass is preferred over resection due to a lower risk of cancer and decreased morbidity.
- The colon (especially mid-colon) is favored over the stomach or jejunum as a replacement conduit.
- Management of pharyngeal and gastric strictures should be tailored based on the specific stricture type.
- Advanced techniques such as ICG fluorescence imaging improve conduit vascular assessment and the safety of anastomoses.

Selected Reading

1. Ananthakrishnan N, Subbarao KS, Parthasarathy G, Kate V, Kalayarasan R. Long-term results of esophageal bypass for corrosive strictures without esophageal resection using a modified left colon esophagocoloplasty–a report of 105 consecutive patients from a single unit over 30 years. Hepatogastroenterology. 2014;61(132):1033–41.
2. Ananthakrishnan N, Parthasarathy G, Kate V. Chronic corrosive injuries of the stomach—a single unit experience of 109 patients over thirty years. World J Surg. 2010;34:758–64.
3. Ananthakrishnan N, Subba Rao KSVK, Rajendran P. Mid-colon esophagocoloplasty for corrosive esophageal strictures. Aust N Z J Surg. 1993;63:389–95.
4. Ananthakrishnan N, Kate V, Parthasarathy G. Therapeutic options for management of pharyngoesophageal corrosive strictures. J Gastrointest Surg. 2011;15:566–75.
5. Ananthakrishnan N, Parthasarathy G, Maroju NK, Kate V. Sternocleidomastoid muscle myocutaneous flap for corrosive Pharyngo-esophageal strictures. World J Surg. 2007;31:1592–6.
6. Kalayarasan R, Durgesh S. Changing trends in the minimally invasive surgery for corrosive esophagogastric stricture. World J Gastrointest Surg. 2023;15(5):799–811.

Carcinoma Esophagus

4

R. Kalayarasan and Pothugunta Sai Krishna

Abstract

The two main subtypes of esophageal cancer are squamous cell carcinoma (SCC) and adenocarcinoma (EAC), each with distinct epidemiology, risk factors, and tumor biology. Dysphagia and weight loss are the most common presenting symptoms; advanced cases may exhibit aspiration, pain, or upper GI bleeding. Endoscopy with biopsy is the diagnostic gold standard; CT, PET-CT, and EUS are essential for comprehensive staging. Neoadjuvant therapy is standard for locally advanced esophageal cancer. Definitive chemoradiotherapy is the standard for cervical esophageal cancers and a nonsurgical option in patients unfit for surgery, particularly for SCC. Curative surgery remains central for resectable tumors. Choice of procedure depends on the tumor location: McKeown esophagectomy for mid/upper thoracic SCC and Ivor Lewis esophagectomy for distal EAC/GEJ tumors. D3 lymphadenectomy (N1–N3 nodes) is recommended, with a target of ≥15 lymph nodes for accurate staging. Minimally invasive and robotic-assisted esophagectomy (RAMIE) offers equivalent oncologic outcomes with reduced morbidity.

Keywords

Esophageal carcinoma · Dysphagia · Esophagectomy

Esophageal cancer remains a significant global health issue, ranking as the sixth leading cause of cancer-related deaths worldwide. According to the 2020 GLOBOCAN data, about 600,000 new cases were reported globally. The two main histological subtypes are squamous cell carcinoma (SCC) and adenocarcinoma (EAC), with SCC predominating worldwide, especially in high-incidence regions like the so-called 'esophageal cancer belt' stretching from East Asia to parts of Africa. Adenocarcinoma, however, is more common in Western countries, and its incidence is rising in developing nations alongside increasing obesity and gastroesophageal reflux disease (GERD). These two subtypes differ in their anatomical origins—EAC usually develops in the distal esophagus, while SCC arises in the proximal esophagus—and vary significantly in terms of pathogenesis, risk factors, treatment options, and outcomes. Despite advances in multimodal therapy, the overall five-year survival rate for esophageal cancer remains low, around 21%.

4.1 Etiology and Risk Factors

The risk of developing esophageal cancer increases with age and is more common in men (Table 4.1). Lifestyle and environmental exposures are essential factors, and the specific risks differ between SCC and EAC (Fig. 4.1).

Table 4.1 Etiopathogenesis of esophageal cancer

Squamous cell carcinoma	Esophageal adenocarcinoma
Common in the East (carcinoma belt)	Common in the West (Barrett's prevalent zones)
Occurs in the mid and lower thoracic esophagus	Occurs in the distal esophagus and GE junction
Risk factors Smoking (2- to 9-fold increased risk) Alcohol consumption (3-fold increased risk) Achalasia of the cardia (10-fold increased risk) Tylosis (10-fold increased risk) Bloom syndrome, Fanconi anemia Thoracic irradiation	*Risk factors* Obesity (2- to 4-fold increased risk if BMI >30 kg/m^2) Barrett's esophagus and GERD Smoking (2-fold increased risk) Diet low in fiber and high in animal fats Thoracic irradiation

R. Kalayarasan (✉) · P. S. Krishna
Jawaharlal Institute of Post-Graduate Medical Education and Research (JIPMER), Puducherry, India

M. Ibrarullah (ed.), *Recent Concepts in Gastrointestinal (GI) Surgery*, https://doi.org/10.1007/978-981-92-1118-0_4

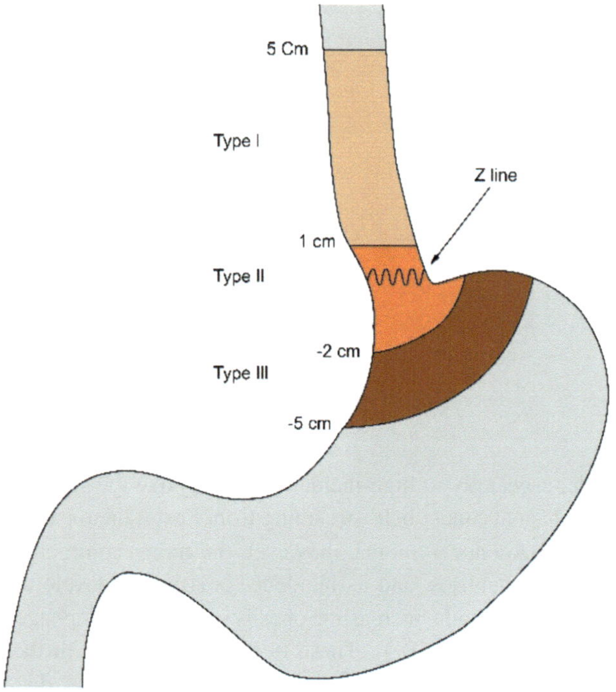

Fig. 4.1 Siewert's classification of GE junction tumor (see Table 4.2 for details)

Table 4.2 Siewert's classification of gastroesophageal (GE) junction tumor

Types	Description
I	Epicenter of the tumor 1–5 cm proximal to the GE junction
II	Epicenter of the tumor 1 cm above and 2 cm below the GE junction
III	Epicenter of the tumor 2–5 cm below the GE junction (Tumor with epicenter below this is considered gastric cancer)

4.2 Clinical Features

Progressive dysphagia, starting with solids and later involving liquids, is the most common clinical presentation of esophageal carcinoma, mainly caused by progressive luminal obstruction from tumor growth. This is often accompanied by significant weight loss, which results from impaired nutritional intake due to dysphagia rather than anorexia. When the tumor affects the cervical or upper thoracic esophagus, it may directly infiltrate the tracheobronchial tree, increasing the risk of recurrent aspiration of esophageal contents. This complication markedly raises the chances of aspiration pneumonia and pulmonary abscess development. Furthermore, tumor extension or compression of nearby mediastinal structures can cause referred upper back pain.

4.3 Investigations (Figs. 4.2, 4.3, and 4.4; Table 4.3)

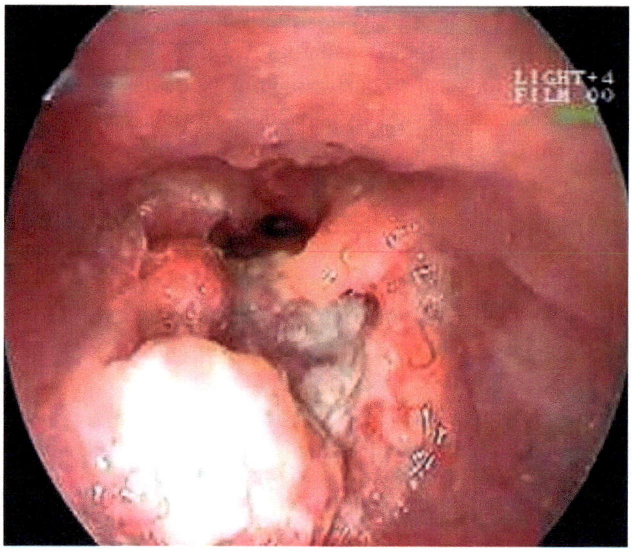

Fig. 4.2 UGI endoscopy showing an ulceroproliferative growth in the esophagus

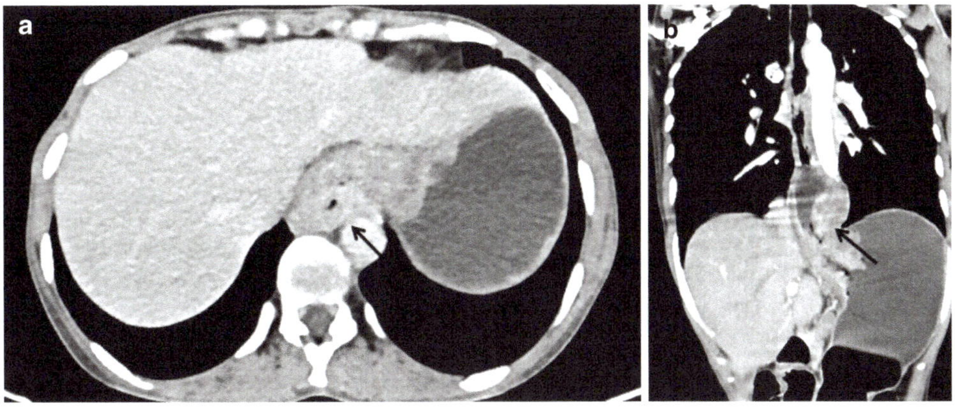

Fig. 4.3 (**a**, **b**) Adenocarcinoma involving the lower third of the esophagus, extending across the GE junction to the stomach. The contact angle with the aorta (**a**) is more than 90° (arrow), indicating a locally advanced tumor

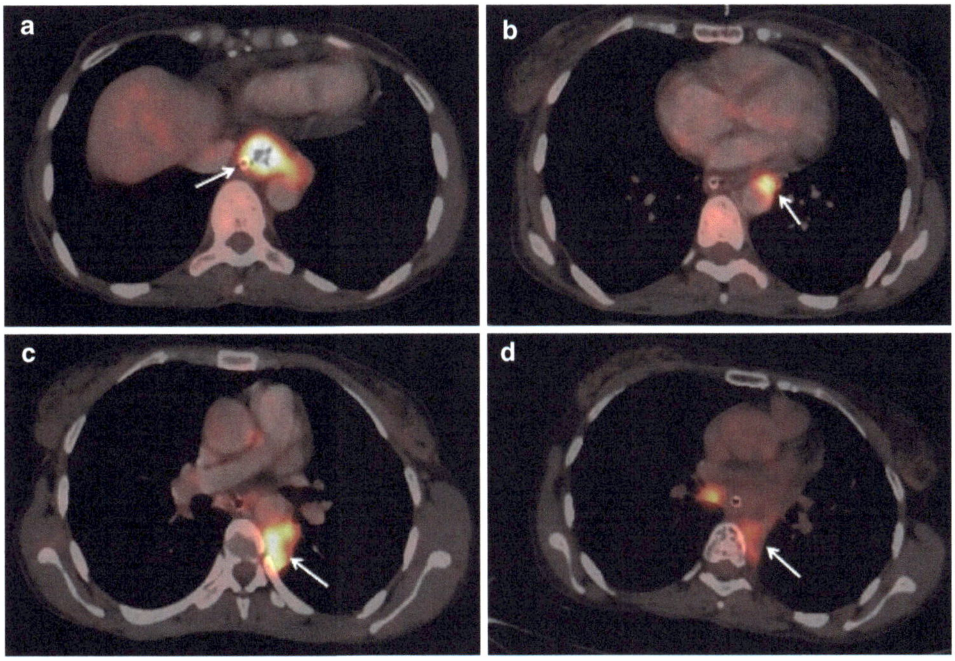

Fig. 4.4 Positron emission tomography (PET-CT) whole body. (**a**) Hypermetabolic region in the distal esophagus (arrow). (**b**) Hypermetabolic region anterior to aorta (arrow). (**c**) Hypermetabolic region (arrow) posterior to aorta. (**d**) Response after chemotherapy (arrow)

Table 4.3 Diagnostic investigations

Investigation	Assessment	Pros	Cons
UGIE	Diagnoses the tumor location, length, and histological subtyping	Mandatory initial investigation Provides a histological diagnosis	Difficult to evaluate constricting growth as the scope cannot be passed beyond
CECT of the neck, chest, and abdomen	Mandatory investigation for staging and assessment of response to therapy Features: Irregular esophageal wall thickening greater than 5 mm Enhancing growth on arterial contrast Hypodense lesions >1 cm (short axis diameter) for abdominal/mediastinal nodes and >0.5 cm for supraclavicular nodes	T stage—specificity for involvement of surrounding structures >90% More than 80% accuracy in revealing aorta involvement (>*90° contact with the aorta is considered locally advanced*) N stage—sensitivity 74% M stage—Metastatic disease evaluation sensitivity up to 80%	Less sensitive (<70%) for response assessment as it does not provide functional activity
EUS	More sensitive for primary tumor (T) and nodal (N) status than cross-sectional imaging T stage is evaluated based on the destruction or expansion of the esophageal wall layers Nodal characteristics— Round hypoechoic lesions with a well-defined border, size >5 mm	T staging—sensitivity 81–92% N status—sensitivity 85% Mandatory in early tumors for planning endoscopic resection or upfront surgery	Observer-dependent investigation; high interobserver variability
PET	Reveals metabolically active tissues—trapping and uptake of FDG (fluorodeoxyglucose) by cancer cells in primary tumors, lymph nodes, and metastases Mandatory investigation for locally advanced disease before commencing neoadjuvant therapy Recommended in patients with suspicion of metastatic disease Follow-up investigation on neoadjuvant therapy with no response or suspicion of progression of disease	Metastatic disease—sensitivity of up to 70% and specificity of 95% Upstages the tumor in 20% of patients	Cannot be applied to PET non-avid tissues such as poorly cohesive, signet cell, and poorly differentiated tumors Poor sensitivity in differentiating tumors from inflammatory tissue
Bronchoscopy	Preferred method for investigating cervical and upper thoracic tumors to assess airway infiltration Features indicative of tracheobronchial involvement—widening of the carina; tumor infiltration or fistulization	Can exclude approximately 18% of patients scheduled for surgery Accuracy of involvement of the respiratory tree—more than 90%	—
Endobronchial ultrasonogram (EBUS)	Signs of trachea or bronchi involvement include disruption of the external hyperechoic layer	High sensitivity for tracheobronchial tree involvement—more than 95%	—

UGIE uppergastrointestinal endoscopy, *CECT* contrast-enhanced computed tomography, *EUS* endoscopic ultrasonography, *PET* positron emission tomography

4.4 Treatment of Esophageal Cancer (Table 4.4)

Neoadjuvant therapy, such as chemotherapy or chemoradiotherapy, is considered the standard of care for locally advanced esophageal carcinoma (LAEC), defined as clinical stage T2 or higher and/or node-positive disease. The main goal of neoadjuvant treatment is to improve resectability, achieve local and regional control, and enhance long-term survival outcomes.

4.4.1 Neoadjuvant Chemotherapy

Early evidence supporting Neoadjuvant chemotherapy (nCT) came from the OE02 trial (2002) and was further confirmed by the MAGIC trial, which involved patients with resectable gastric and GE junction cancers. In the MAGIC study, patients received three cycles of epirubicin, cisplatin, and 5-fluorouracil (ECF) before surgery, followed by three additional postoperative cycles. The five-year overall survival (OS) reached 36%, demonstrating a significant survival benefit compared to surgery alone.

Table 4.4 The management algorithm for SCC and EAC

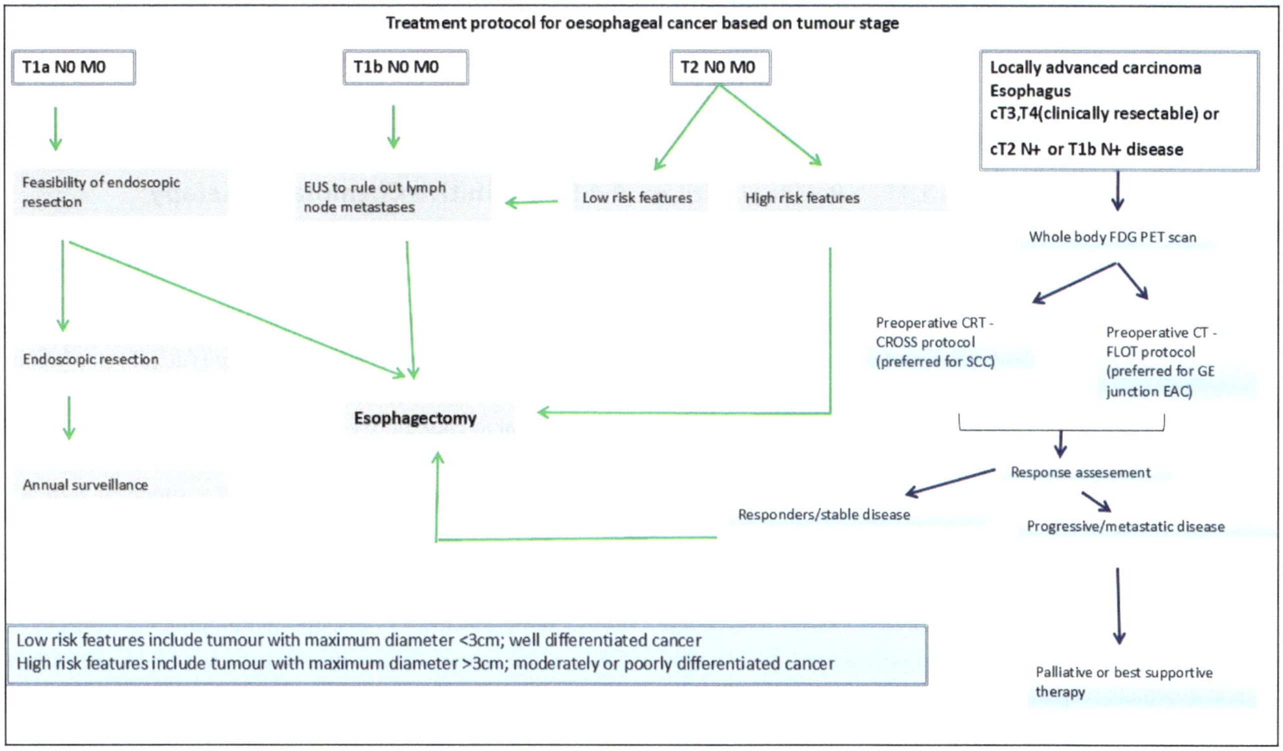

TNM staging—AJCC 8th edition. Note the key differences in treatment strategies based on histological subtype, tumor location, and stage of the disease

Further improvements in perioperative chemotherapy regimens were demonstrated in the FLOT4-AIO trial, where patients with locally advanced GE junction adenocarcinoma received four cycles of FLOT (5-fluorouracil, leucovorin, oxaliplatin, and docetaxel) before surgery and four cycles afterward. This regimen resulted in significant gains in both disease-free survival (DFS) and overall survival (OS), with OS increasing by approximately 15 months. However, it is important to note that these trials primarily involved distal esophageal or GE junction adenocarcinomas and are less applicable to SCC.

For thoracic esophageal squamous cell carcinoma, the JCOG 9907 trial (Japanese Clinical Oncology Group) compared nCT (two cycles of cisplatin and 5-fluorouracil) with the same regimen given postoperatively. Neoadjuvant treatment led to a significantly improved 5-year OS (55% vs 43%), particularly among patients with upper/mid-thoracic SCC and nodal involvement, although progression-free survival was similar between the groups. These trials demonstrated the superiority of nCT over surgery alone in esophageal cancer.

4.4.2 Neoadjuvant Chemoradiotherapy

Neoadjuvant chemoradiotherapy (nCRT) has become widely accepted for LAEC following the landmark CROSS trial. In this phase III study, 366 patients (75% with adenocarcinoma and 25% with SCC) were randomized to receive either nCRT followed by surgery or surgery alone. The nCRT protocol involved 41.4 Gy of radiotherapy combined with weekly carboplatin and paclitaxel. Long-term follow-up revealed a significant survival benefit, with a median OS of 43.2 months in the nCRT group compared to 21.7 months in the surgery-only group. Progression-free survival was also improved (29.9 vs. 17.7 months). Notably, the study reported a 23% pathological complete response (pCR) rate overall, with higher rates in patients with SCC (up to 49%). The NEOCRTEC5010 trial, which focused exclusively on patients with resectable SCC of the esophagus, compared surgery alone to nCRT using vinorelbine, cisplatin, and 40 Gy of radiation. Results showed better outcomes in the nCRT group, with a 3-year OS of 69% versus 59%, median OS of 100 versus 66.5 months, and pCR rates reaching 45%. The CROSS and NEOCRETEC trials demonstrated the superiority of nCRT over surgery alone in esophageal cancer.

4.4.3 Neoadjuvant Chemotherapy Versus Chemoradiotherapy

Studies directly comparing nCT and nCRT are limited. The ESOPEC trial is the largest randomized phase III study on this topic to date. It compared perioperative chemotherapy with the FLOT regimen to nCRT following the CROSS protocol in patients with resectable LAEC. Results showed a clear benefit for the FLOT regimen, with a median progression-free survival (PFS) of 38 months in the FLOT group versus 16 months in the CROSS group ($P = 0.001$). Additionally, the 3-year PFS rates were 51.6% for FLOT and 35.0% for CROSS, while the 5-year PFS rates were 44.4% and 30.9%, respectively. These findings strongly support perioperative chemotherapy with FLOT as the preferred neoadjuvant approach for patients with resectable EAC.

The CMISG1701 trial was a prospective, multicenter, randomized phase III study conducted in China that compared the efficacy and safety of nCT versus nCRT followed by minimally invasive esophagectomy in patients with locally advanced SCC (cT3–T4aN0–1 M0). The study showed that the nCRT arm had a significantly higher pathological complete response rate than the nCT arm, indicating better tumor downstaging potential. However, this improvement in pathological response did not lead to a statistically significant difference in 3-year overall survival between the two groups. These findings suggest that while nCRT may enhance locoregional tumor control, nCT remains a viable and less intensive alternative, especially for patients who may not tolerate radiation well or in settings with limited access to radiotherapy infrastructure.

4.4.4 Adjuvant Therapy

The current standard of care after neoadjuvant therapy and curative surgical resection for esophageal cancer is active surveillance, especially in patients who achieve an R0 resection and have no residual nodal disease. Institutional practices have traditionally guided the role of adjuvant therapy in this setting, as high-quality evidence from randomized controlled trials is lacking. Adjuvant treatment is generally considered for select high-risk patients, particularly those with residual nodal disease or microscopically positive margins (R1/R2 resections) after neoadjuvant therapy.

However, this paradigm has changed with the results of the CheckMate 577 trial, a landmark phase III study showing a significant improvement in DFS and a positive trend in OS with adjuvant nivolumab, a PD-1 immune checkpoint inhibitor. This benefit was seen in patients with resected stage II/III esophageal or gastroesophageal junction cancer who had received nCRT followed by R0 resection but still had residual pathological disease. Based on these results, adjuvant nivolumab has been added to the National Comprehensive Cancer Network (NCCN) guidelines as a recommended option for patients with resected esophageal and gastroesophageal junction cancers who have residual disease after nCRT and surgery.

4.4.5 Definitive Chemoradiotherapy

The increased morbidity associated with surgery after neoadjuvant therapy, along with evidence of complete pathological response in about one-third of patients receiving nCRT, led to considering definitive chemoradiotherapy (dCRT) as a potential nonsurgical treatment option for esophageal cancer. This approach gained popularity, especially among elderly patients and those with significant comorbidities who were deemed unfit for surgery. The earliest evidence supporting dCRT came from a landmark randomized trial published in 1992, which evaluated patients with locally advanced SCC and EAC. Participants received 50 Gy of radiotherapy over 5 weeks with concurrent cisplatin and continuous infusion of 5-FU administered during weeks 1, 5, 8, and 11. The study reported a disease progression rate of 40% and local recurrence in 24% of patients. Despite this, the median overall survival was 8.9 months, and the 5-year overall survival reached 26%, outcomes comparable to those achieved with surgical resection at that time. Based on these findings, the PRODIGE5/ACCORD17 trial, published by Conroy et al. in 2014, randomized 267 patients with locally advanced SCC and EAC to receive either FOLFOX plus radiotherapy or the standard regimen of cisplatin and 5-FU with 50 Gy radiotherapy. Approximately 45% of patients developed progressive disease, with a median overall survival of 20.2 months and a 3-year overall survival of 19.9%, reaffirming the feasibility of dCRT in selected patient populations.

Current evidence supports using dCRT as the standard treatment for cervical esophageal cancers, where surgical resection carries significant risks. It is also an accepted alternative for thoracic SCC in patients who are unfit for surgery, with similar survival outcomes to trimodality therapy (nCRT followed by surgery).

4.5 Surgical Management

Curative surgical resection remains a crucial part of multimodal treatment for locally advanced esophageal cancer, especially in patients with resectable disease and sufficient physiological reserve. While open esophagectomy has been the traditional standard, the advent of minimally invasive techniques, such as thoracoscopic and robotic-assisted procedures, has significantly enhanced surgical outcomes with lower perioperative morbidity.

4.5.1 Principles of Surgical Resection

Surgical management of esophageal cancer aims to achieve:

- Oncologically sound resection with adequate proximal and distal margins.
- Clear circumferential radial margins (CRM).
- Optimal lymphadenectomy, aiming for at least 15 lymph nodes.
- Tension-free anastomosis performed with an appropriate conduit, usually a gastric pull-up.

Early-stage tumors (cTis, cT1a) are generally suitable for endoscopic resection (EMR or ESD). However, in cases with circumferential involvement that carry a risk of stricture formation, esophagectomy remains a valid alternative.

4.5.2 Surgical Approach and Lymphadenectomy

The extent of lymphadenectomy depends on tumor location and stage. Because of the longitudinal submucosal lymphatic network in the esophagus, even early tumors can spread widely through lymphatic pathways. The traditional classification into single, two, or three-field lymphadenectomies is increasingly being replaced by the Japanese classification, which assigns nodal dissection levels as D1–D4, similar to gastric cancer. The 11th edition of the Japanese Classification of Esophageal Cancer provides a detailed map of nodal stations and designates N1–N3 as regional and N4 as distant lymph nodes. A D3 lymphadenectomy (removal of N1–N3 nodes) is generally recommended with curative intent (Table 4.5).

Table 4.5 Japanese Esophageal Society classification of nodal stations for esophageal cancer (11th edition)

11th edition Japanese oesophageal nodal stations			
Cervical nodes (No.)		*Abdominal nodes (No.)*	
100	Superficial cervical	1	Right paracardial
101	Cervical para-oesophageal	2	Left paracardial
102	Deep cervical	3a	Lesser curvature along braches of left gastric artery and right gastric artery
103	Peripharyngeal	3b	
104	Supraclavicular	4	Along greater curvature
Thoracic nodes (No.)		4sa	Along short gastric vessels
105	Upper thoracic para-oesophageal	4sb	Along left gastroepiploic artery
106	Thoracic paratracheal	4d	Along right gastroepiploic artery
Rec	Recurrent laryngeal nerve nodes	5	Suprapyloric nodes
Pre	Pretracheal nodes	6	Infrapyloric nodes
tbL	Tracheao-bronchial nodes	7	Left gastric artery nodes
107	Subcarinal	8a	Anterior common hepatic artery nodes
108	Middle thoracic para-oesophageal	8b	Posterior common hepatic artery nodes
109	Principal bronchial	9	Celiac artery nodes
110	Lower thoracic para-oesophageal	10	Splenic hilar nodes
111	Supradiaphragmatic	11p	Proximal splenic artery nodes
112	Para-aortic nodes	11d	Distal splenic artery nodes
113	Ligamentum arteriosum	12	Nodes in hepato-duodenal ligament
114	Anterior mediastinal		

4.5.3 Choice of Surgical Technique

- McKeown (three-incision) esophagectomy is preferred for mid- and upper thoracic SCC, enabling thorough cervical and mediastinal lymph node removal.
- Ivor Lewis (two-incision) esophagectomy is generally performed for distal esophageal and GE junction adenocarcinoma, allowing for adequate intrathoracic lymphadenectomy.
- Transhiatal esophagectomy, while associated with less pulmonary morbidity, offers limited lymph node clearance and is thus less favored for oncologically complex cases. It is typically reserved for high-risk or frail patients due to its restricted exposure and lower lymph node yield.

4.5.4 Minimally Invasive Esophagectomy

Minimally invasive esophagectomy (MIE) provides benefits such as less pain, fewer pulmonary complications, and quicker recovery.

- The TIME trial found significantly fewer pulmonary complications with thoracoscopic esophagectomy (9% versus 29%) compared to open transthoracic surgery, with similar lymph node yield and survival.
- The MIRO trial, a phase III French multicenter study, demonstrated a 70% reduction in pulmonary complications with hybrid MIE (laparoscopic abdominal phase plus open thoracic phase) compared to fully open surgery.

Robot-assisted minimally invasive esophagectomy (RAMIE) further enhances precision through:

- High-definition 3D visualization.
- Greater articulation and range of motion of instruments.
- Improved surgeon ergonomics.

The ROBOT trial, a randomized comparison of RAMIE versus open esophagectomy, demonstrated:

- Lower surgical and cardiopulmonary complications.
- Reduced blood loss and postoperative pain.
- Faster functional recovery.
- Comparable oncologic outcomes.

4.5.4.1 Patient Positioning in Thoracoscopic Esophagectomy

- Left lateral decubitus position: Familiar anatomy and exposure similar to open surgery; requires single-lung ventilation, which may complicate tracheal retraction.
- Prone position: Offers better ergonomics and improved visualization and avoids single-lung ventilation. Limitations include difficulty with emergent conversion to thoracotomy.
- The semi-prone position combines the ergonomic benefits of prone positioning with easier access for thoracotomy if needed.
- Hybrid positioning with a tilt-adjustable table allows smooth switching between left lateral and prone positions during the procedure.

Bronchial blockers can replace double-lumen tubes for selective lung collapse, thereby decreasing tracheal injury and facilitating easier intubation.

4.5.5 Alternative Approaches

Laparoscopic (mediastinoscopic) esophagectomy, which avoids thoracic entry, is emerging as an option for patients with extensive pleural adhesions or severe pulmonary comorbidities. Although technically demanding, it decreases the risk of thoracic complications (Figs. 4.5 and 4.6).

4.5.6 Minimally Invasive McKeown Esophagectomy

The minimally invasive McKeown esophagectomy is increasingly favored due to its excellent postoperative outcomes and comparable cancer control to open procedures.

4.5.6.1 Thoracic Phase

Typically performed in the prone or semi-prone position, thoracoscopic esophagectomy utilizes four ports, whereas robot-assisted approaches may employ three or four robotic arms. Omitting the fourth arm in patients with short stature can lower costs and reduce the risk of robotic arm collisions.

Key steps include:

The inferior pulmonary ligament is divided. Anterior esophageal mobilization from the pericardium; posterior dissection from the aorta is initially deferred to create working space. Subcarinal lymph node dissection begins on the right side. Careful preservation of the pulmonary branches of the vagus nerve is essential. Division of the azygous vein and right bronchial artery facilitates access to the right recurrent laryngeal nerve (RLN). Dissection proceeds along the right vagus nerve to its branch point near the right subclavian artery. Preserving the left bronchial artery and longitudinal

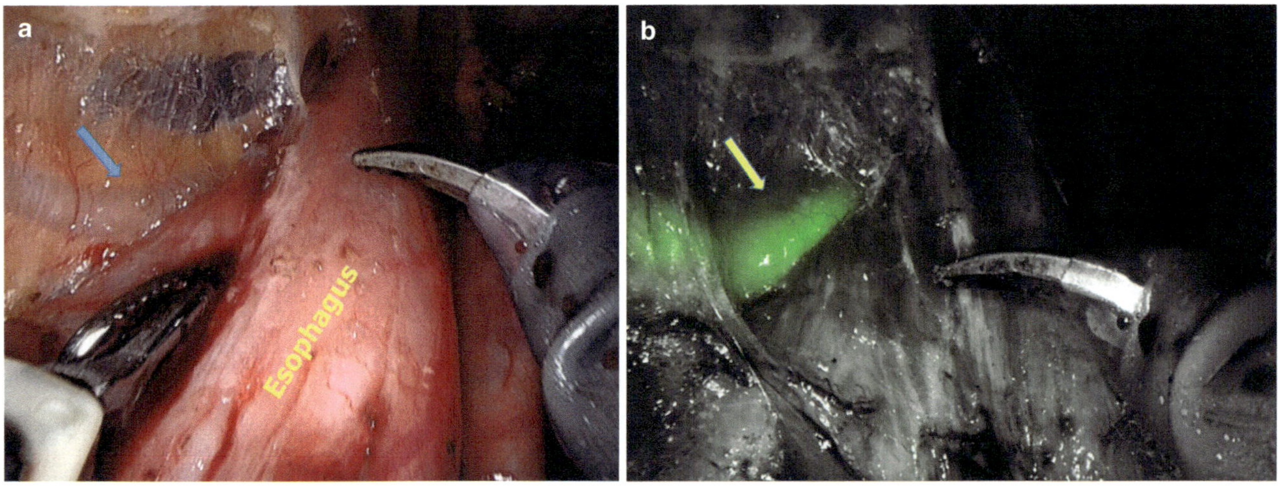

Fig. 4.5 Robotic esophagectomy. Thoracic duct visualization with normal (**a**) and near-infrared light (**b**). Indocyanine green (ICG) fluorescence facilitates thoracic duct identification (arrow)

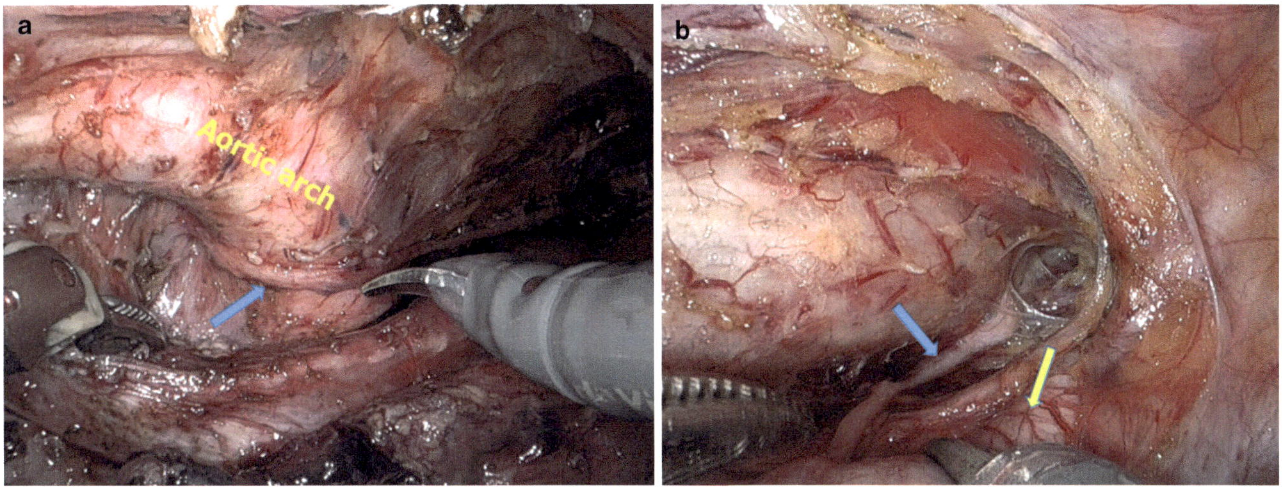

Fig. 4.6 Post-mediastinal lymphadenectomy. (**a**) Left recurrent laryngeal nerve (blue arrow) looping around the arch of the aorta. (**b**) Right recurrent laryngeal nerve (blue arrow) looping around the subclavian artery (yellow arrow)

tracheal arcade is essential to prevent tracheal ischemia. The thoracic duct, usually located between the azygous vein and the aorta, is preserved. Routine thoracic duct ligation is not recommended because it can lead to long-term complications such as chylothorax and possible hepatic dysfunction. Injection of indocyanine green (ICG) into the inguinal nodes or the dorsum of the foot can help with intraoperative visualization. Completion of the left subcarinal and left RLN node dissection concludes the thoracic phase. The left RLN dissection is more technically demanding due to the nerve's longer intrathoracic course. Isolating the nerve during this phase prevents traction injury during the cervical dissection.

4.5.6.2 Abdominal Phase

Performed laparoscopically, the gastrocolic omentum is divided approximately 3 cm away from the gastroepiploic arcade to preserve vascularity. The short gastric vessels are divided cautiously to avoid splenic injury. After abdominal lymphadenectomy and division of the left gastric vessels, a gastric conduit is fashioned. Although the conduit can be formed laparoscopically, many surgeons prefer a mini-laparotomy for specimen retrieval, open conduit creation, and feeding jejunostomy placement if indicated. The conduit diameter is ideally maintained between 3.5 and 4.0 cm. Division along the lesser curvature should begin below the fifth branch of the left gastric artery, as nodal involvement above this level is rare.

4.5.6.3 Anastomotic Techniques and Reconstruction

A tubularized gastric conduit is the most common reconstruction method after esophagectomy. The location of the anastomosis depends on the surgical approach.

- Intrathoracic anastomosis (Ivor Lewis) is associated with a lower leak rate.
- Cervical anastomosis (McKeown) is associated with less severe clinical consequences in the event of a leak.

Both hand-sewn and stapled techniques are used. Meta-analyses show no significant difference in leak rates, though stricture rates may be lower with stapled anastomoses following a leak.

Key Points

- The two main subtypes of esophageal cancer are squamous cell carcinoma (SCC) and adenocarcinoma (EAC), each with distinct epidemiology, risk factors, and tumor biology.
- SCC is associated with tobacco, alcohol, achalasia, and genetic syndromes, while EAC is linked to GERD, Barrett's oesophagus, and obesity.
- Dysphagia and weight loss are the most common presenting symptoms; advanced cases may exhibit aspiration, pain, or upper GI bleeding.
- Endoscopy with biopsy is the diagnostic gold standard; CT, PET-CT, and EUS are essential for comprehensive staging.
- Neoadjuvant therapy is standard for locally advanced esophageal cancer:
- Although nCRT achieves better tumor downstaging, nCT remains a feasible alternative for patients who are unsuitable for radiation. Adjuvant nivolumab enhances DFS in patients with residual disease after nCRT and R0 resection.

(continued)

- Definitive chemoradiotherapy is the standard for cervical esophageal cancers and a nonsurgical option in patients unfit for surgery, particularly for SCC.
- Curative surgery remains central for resectable tumours. Choice of procedure depends on the tumour location: McKeown esophagectomy for mid/upper thoracic SCC and Ivor Lewis esophagectomy for distal EAC/GEJ tumors.
- D3 lymphadenectomy (N1–N3 nodes) is recommended, with a target of ≥15 lymph nodes for accurate staging.
- Minimally invasive and robotic-assisted esophagectomy (RAMIE) offers equivalent oncologic outcomes with reduced morbidity.
- Cervical anastomosis is safer if leaks occur, while intrathoracic anastomosis has a lower leak rate; stapled anastomoses may reduce stricture after leaks.
- With improving outcomes from CRT and endoscopic therapy, surgery in the future will be increasingly reserved for salvage resection or select early-stage disease, emphasizing the need for multidisciplinary, tailored care.

Suggested Reading

1. Sung H, Ferlay J, Siegel RL, et al. Global Cancer Statistics 2020: GLOBOCAN estimates of incidence and mortality worldwide for 36 cancers in 185 countries. CA Cancer J Clin. 2021;71(3):209–49. https://doi.org/10.3322/caac.21660.
2. Lagergren J, Smyth E, Cunningham D, Lagergren P. Oesophageal cancer. Lancet. 2017;390(10110):2383–96. https://doi.org/10.1016/S0140-6736(17)31462-9.
3. Al-Batran SE, Hofheinz RD, Pauligk C, et al. Perioperative chemotherapy with fluorouracil plus leucovorin, oxaliplatin, and docetaxel versus fluorouracil or capecitabine plus cisplatin and epirubicin for locally advanced, resectable gastric or gastro-oesophageal junction adenocarcinoma (FLOT4): a randomized, phase 2/3 trial. Lancet. 2019;393(10184):1948–57. https://doi.org/10.1016/S0140-6736(18)32557-1.
4. Ando N, Kato H, Igaki H, et al. A randomized trial comparing postoperative adjuvant chemotherapy with cisplatin and 5-fluorouracil versus preoperative chemotherapy for localized advanced squamous cell carcinoma of the thoracic esophagus (JCOG9907). Ann Surg Oncol. 2012;19(1):68–74. https://doi.org/10.1245/s10434-011-2043-5.
5. Liu Y, Zhang X, Zhang H, et al. A randomized clinical trial of neoadjuvant chemoradiotherapy versus neoadjuvant chemotherapy followed by minimally invasive esophagectomy for locally advanced esophageal squamous cell carcinoma: the CMISG1701 trial. Ann Surg. 2023;277(3):408–15. https://doi.org/10.1097/SLA.0000000000005625.
6. Ronellenfitsch U, Schwarzbach M, Hofheinz R, et al. Perioperative chemo-versus chemoradiotherapy for resectable esophageal adenocarcinoma: first results of the ESOPEC trial. J Clin Oncol. 2023;41(16_suppl):4004. https://doi.org/10.1200/JCO.2023.41.16_suppl.4004.
7. Herskovic A, Martz K, Al-Sarraf M, et al. Combined chemotherapy and radiotherapy compared with radiotherapy alone in patients with cancer of the esophagus. N Engl J Med. 1992;326(24):1593–8. https://doi.org/10.1056/NEJM199206113262403.
8. Conroy T, Galais MP, Raoul JL, et al. Definitive chemoradiotherapy with FOLFOX versus fluorouracil and cisplatin in patients with oesophageal cancer (PRODIGE5/ACCORD17): a randomized, multicenter, open-label, phase 2/3 trial. Lancet Oncol. 2014;15(3):305–14. https://doi.org/10.1016/S1470-2045(13)70549-0.
9. Mariette C, Meunier B, Peix JL, et al. Hybrid minimally invasive esophagectomy for esophageal cancer. N Engl J Med. 2019;380(2):152–62. https://doi.org/10.1056/NEJMoa1805101.
10. van der Sluis PC, van der Horst S, May AM, et al. Robot-assisted minimally invasive thoracolaparoscopic esophagectomy versus open transthoracic esophagectomy for resectable esophageal cancer: a randomized controlled trial. Ann Surg. 2019;269(4):621–30. https://doi.org/10.1097/SLA.0000000000003093.
11. Sasikumar K, Kalayarasan R, Gnanasekaran S, et al. Minimally invasive oesophagectomy with a total two-field lymphadenectomy after neoadjuvant chemoradiotherapy for locally advanced squamous cell carcinoma of the oesophagus: a prospective study. J Minim Access Surg. 2021;17(1):49–55. https://doi.org/10.4103/jmas.JMAS_242_19.
12. Kalayarasan R, Sai KP. Robotic esophagectomy with function--preserving radical mediastinal lymphadenectomy for esophageal cancer. Ann Gastroenterol Surg. 2024;9(1):12–23. https://doi.org/10.1002/ags3.12862.

Peptic Ulcer Disease

5

Banabihari Mishra and Rupashree Sahoo

Abstract

The primary causes of peptic ulcers are hyperacidity, *Helicobacter pylori*, and NSAIDs. Gastric ulcers are less common than duodenal ulcers; gastric ulcers may be malignant in 5–8%. UGIE is the preferred method for diagnosis and biopsy in cases of gastric ulcer. The treatment for uncomplicated peptic ulcers is mainly medication; surgery is reserved for stubborn ulcers and complications. Gastric antisecretory agents and *H. pylori* eradication therapy are the cornerstones of peptic ulcer management. Common complications of peptic ulcers include bleeding, perforation, and stenosis or outlet obstruction. Posterior duodenal ulcer more commonly bleeds, while anterior duodenal ulcer perforates. The gastroduodenal artery in cases of duodenal ulcer and the left gastric artery in gastric ulcer need to be surgically transfixed if endoscopic management fails. An acid-reducing procedure (vagotomy) must be performed in cases of duodenal ulcer bleeding to prevent recurrence. A perforated peptic ulcer is a surgical emergency. The patient must be adequately resuscitated before surgical intervention. Gastric outlet obstruction is treated by a bypass procedure combined with vagotomy.

Keywords

Peptic ulcer · Chronic duodenal ulcer · Gastric ulcer

Peptic ulcer is defined as a gastroduodenal mucosal erosion that extends through the muscularis mucosa or beyond and is caused by unprotected exposure to gastric acid. The incidence, prevalence, and complications of peptic ulcers have steadily declined over the past few decades, especially in developed countries compared to developing ones. This decline may be due to a better understanding of ulcer pathogenesis, the interaction of host and environmental factors, increased detection rates, the availability of effective antisecretory medications, and the eradication of *Helicobacter pylori* (*H. pylori*) infection. However, despite the decrease in chronic complication rates, the occurrence of acute complications such as bleeding and perforation has largely remained unchanged.

5.1 Pathogenesis

The spectrum of peptic ulcer disease (PUD) includes superficial mucosal erosions, deep chronic penetrating ulcers, perforation, bleeding, cicatrization, and stenosis. The development of peptic ulcers can be linked to mucosal injury caused by gastric acid, which results from an imbalance between the body's defense mechanisms and aggressive factors (Table 5.1).

Table 5.1 Pathogenesis of peptic ulcer

Host defense factors (protective)	Aggressive factors (damaging)
Mucus layer	Hydrochloric acid secretion
Mucosal bicarbonate secretion	Pepsin
Mucosal blood flow	Alcohol abuse
Growth factors	Smoking
Endogenous prostaglandins	Bile reflux Mucosal ischemia Hypoxia Nonsteroidal anti-inflammatory drugs (NSAIDs) *H. pylori* infection

B. Mishra (✉) · R. Sahoo
Srirama Chandra Bhanja Medical College and Hospital, Cuttack, India

M. Ibrarullah (ed.), *Recent Concepts in Gastrointestinal (GI) Surgery*, https://doi.org/10.1007/978-981-92-1118-0_5

5.2 Sites of Peptic Ulcer

Ulcers usually develop over epithelium that is least resistant to gastric acid or at the junction between two different types of epithelia. The likely sites are,

1. Lesser curvature/gastric incisura
2. Prepyloric antrum
3. First part of the duodenum (D1)
4. Gastric metaplasia in duodenum*
5. Gastrojejunostomy stoma*
6. Heterotopic gastric mucosa in the proximal esophagus*
7. Barrett's esophagus*
8. Meckel's diverticulum with ectopic gastric mucosa*

* *Less common sites*

The incidence of chronic duodenal ulcer (DU) has been decreasing in Western, resource-rich countries due to the use of gastric antisecretory agents and *H. pylori* eradication therapy in patients with dyspepsia. The disease remains relatively stable in Eastern European regions, while it is increasing in resource-poor countries, showing an inverse relationship between infection and socioeconomic status. The peak incidence occurs in the older age group. Men are more commonly affected than women, although the difference may not be very significant. Chronic DU is always linked to hyperacidity, whereas gastric ulcer (GU) may be associated with hypo- or normo-acidity. However, in all types of peptic ulcers, acid mainly acts as a cofactor for ulcer development rather than the primary cause. GU is classified based on its location and acid output, which also influence the most likely complications and treatment options.

5.3 Classification of Gastric Ulcer (Table 5.2)

Giant gastric ulcers (>2 cm in diameter) are typically located on the lesser curvature and carry a higher risk of malignancy (10–30%), with the risk increasing with the size of the ulcer.

Table 5.2 Classification, key features, and proposed treatment of gastric ulcer

Type	Incidence	Location	Acid output	Treatment
I	60%	Lesser curvature near incisura	Low to normal	Wedge resection of ulcer/ distal gastrectomy
II	15%	Body of stomach + duodenal ulcer	High	Distal gastrectomy/ truncal vagotomy + drainage
III	20%	Prepyloric	High	Distal gastrectomy/ truncal vagotomy + drainage
IV	<10%	High on the lesser curvature, near the GE junction	Normal	Wedge resection of ulcer + truncal vagotomy + drainage (Csendes procedure)/ distal gastrectomy
V	<5%	Any location associated with long-term NSAID use	Normal	Distal gastrectomy, including the ulcer

5.4 Clinical Features

The most common presenting symptom is epigastric pain. It is well localized, mild to moderate, burning or gnawing in nature, intermittent or episodic, and may be seasonal (spring and fall). Pain is worsened by food in GU but relieved in chronic DU. The periodicity of pain suggests spontaneous ulcer healing. Constant pain indicates deeper ulcer penetration, while pain radiating to the back suggests pancreatic involvement. Diffuse pain throughout the entire abdomen is a sign of perforation into the peritoneal cavity.

5.5 Diagnosis

Upper gastrointestinal endoscopy (UGIE) is the gold standard for diagnosing peptic ulcers. Ulcers located high on the lesser curvature or at the esophagogastric junction may be missed unless carefully examined with retroflexion (J maneuver) of the endoscope. All GU should undergo multiple biopsies and show healing during treatment to exclude malignancy. The anterior wall of D1 is the most common site for chronic DU. Ulcers on the posterior wall, both walls (kissing ulcers), or in the post-bulbar region are not uncommon. The presence of multiple ulcers, especially in very young or very old patients, warrants further investigation to rule out gastrinoma. An ulcer with a clean base typically indicates an uncomplicated DU. Scarring, deformity of the duodenal bulb, and pseudo-diverticula suggest a chronic ulcer. A barium contrast study for diagnosing PUD is considered outdated and is no longer used (Figs. 5.1 and 5.2).

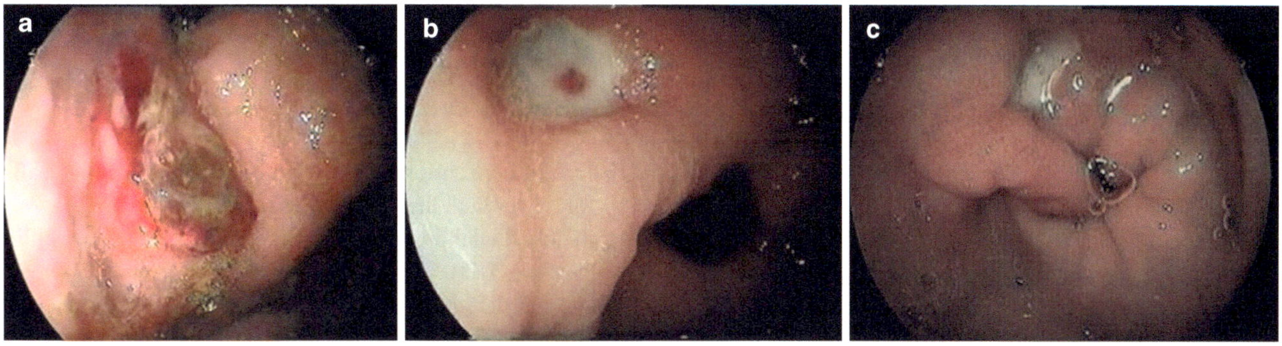

Fig. 5.1 Endoscopic appearance of gastric ulcer, (**a**) Ulcer high on lesser curvature, (**b**) Ulcer on incisura with a flat red spot, (**c**) Prepyloric ulcer

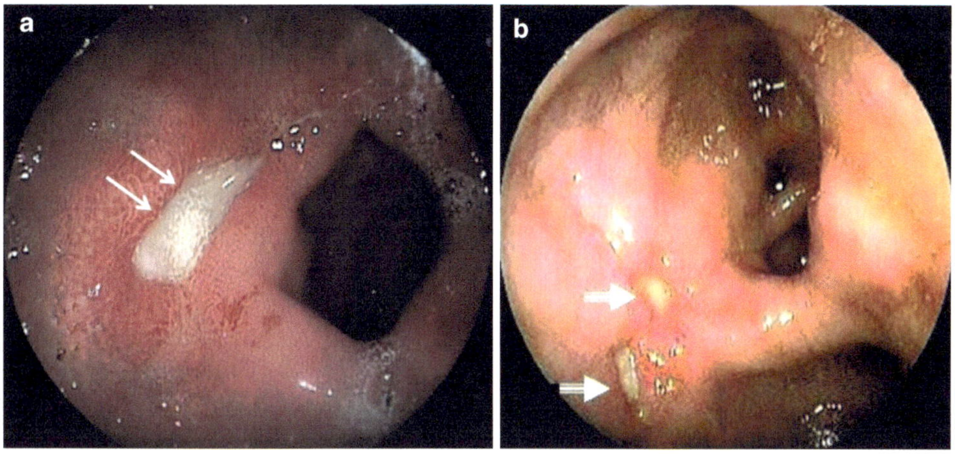

Fig. 5.2 Endoscopic appearance of duodenal ulcer. (**a**) An active ulcer (arrows) on the anterior wall of D1. (**b**) Healing ulcers (arrows) on the anterior wall of the duodenum. Note the deformed bulb and multiple pseudodiverticula, indicating chronic DU

5.6 Treatment

5.6.1 Medical Management

Ulcer healing can be achieved in more than 90–95% of cases with medical management alone. Lifestyle modifications, such as quitting smoking, limiting caffeine and alcohol intake, and avoiding NSAIDs, are essential adjuncts to pharmacotherapy in today's practice.

Pharmacotherapy

Pharmacotherapy is the first line of treatment in PUD.

- *Gastric acid secretion inhibitors:* Proton pump inhibitors (PPIs), such as Omeprazole, Lansoprazole, Dexlansoprazole, Pantoprazole, Rabeprazole, and Esomeprazole, effectively relieve symptoms and promote healing of most benign ulcers within 2 weeks by inducing achlorhydria. PPIs are generally safe with minimal side effects when used long-term and have replaced H2-antagonists (such as cimetidine, Ranitidine, and famotidine) as the preferred treatment options.
- *Gastric acid neutralizers (antacids):* Antacids are more commonly used alongside PPIs for quick symptom relief.
- *Cytoprotective agents:* Sucralfate and colloidal Bismuth subcitrate form a coating that protects the ulcerated mucosa.
- *Eradication of H. pylori*: Approximately 60–80% of chronic DU cases are linked to *H. pylori* infection. Therefore, eradicating the infection along with antisecretory therapy is expected to deliver a long-term cure and reduce the risk of ulcer recurrence. The recommended treatment plan is as follows,

  First-line therapy (14 days)
  The different regimens are

- Bismuth Quadruple Therapy (BQT): PPI (standard dose twice daily) + Metronidazole (250 mg four times daily) + Tetracycline (500 mg four times daily)/ Amoxicillin (1 g twice daily) + Bismuth compound (300 mg four times daily).
- Clarithromycin Triple Therapy: PPI (standard or double dose twice daily) + Clarithromycin (500 mg twice daily) + Amoxicillin (1 g twice daily) or Metronidazole (500 mg twice daily).
- Levofloxacin Triple Therapy: PPI (standard/double dose twice daily) + Amoxicillin (1 g twice daily) + Levofloxacin (500 mg once daily).
- Metronidazole Triple Therapy: PPI (standard or double dose twice daily) + Metronidazole (500 mg twice daily) + Amoxicillin (1 g twice daily).

In cases of clarithromycin resistance, alternative antibiotics such as cefuroxime, rifabutin, furazolidone, or minocycline can be used.

Sequential therapy (10 days):

Days 1–5: PPI (standard or double dose twice daily) + Amoxicillin (1 g twice daily).
Day 6–10: PPI (standard/double dose twice daily) + Clarithromycin (500 mg twice daily) + Tinidazole (500 mg twice daily).

Second line therapy (14 days):

Failure of conventional triple and quadruple therapies calls for newer dual therapy regimens for 10–14 days.
High dose dual therapy: PPI (double dose BD) + Amoxicillin (100 mg TID).
VHA-dual therapy: Vonoprazan (20 mg BD) + Amoxicillin (750 mg QID).

Eradication therapy may be avoided in NSAID-associated ulcers and replaced with potent antisecretory drugs.

Newer drugs, such as potassium-competitive acid blockers (PCABs) like Vonoprazan, bind competitively to the H+/K+ ATPase enzyme and prevent its activation by K+ ions. They are more potent than PPIs, have a faster onset, and a longer duration of action. They are acid-stable (can be taken independently of food, unlike proton pump inhibitors, or PPIs) and are effective in treating peptic ulcers, gastritis, and gastroesophageal reflux disease (GERD).

Probiotics enhance eradication success and remain a focused research area.

Vaccines based on antigens VacA, CagA, UreB, and NAP are currently under trial. Their goal is to boost mucosal immunity by increasing levels of secretory IgA.

5.7 Surgery for Peptic Ulcer (Table 5.3)

The main principle of surgery in PUD is to reduce gastric acid secretion. However, in GU, excising the ulcers or the ulcer-bearing segment of the stomach takes priority, making gastrectomy the preferred method. The surgical approach based on the ulcer's location is shown in Table 5.2 above. In chronic DU, surgery aims to prevent duodenal exposure to acid by decreasing gastric acid secretion and/or diverting acid away from the duodenum. The former is achieved by dividing the vagus nerve and/or removing the gastric antrum. Vagotomy reduces acid output by 50%, while antrectomy eliminates gastrin release.

Table 5.3 Indications for surgery

Nonhealing ulcers
Failure of eradication therapy
Noncompliance with pharmacotherapy
Complications such as bleeding, perforation, and stenosis
Suspicion of malignancy (GU only)

5.8 Vagotomy-Based Procedures

Truncal Vagotomy and Drainage
The anterior and posterior vagus nerves are divided at the lower esophagus, above the origins of the celiac and hepatic branches. It is always combined with a gastric drainage procedure to prevent gastric stasis after motor denervation of the antrum-pyloric segment. The various drainage procedures include Heineke-Mikulicz pyloroplasty, Finney pyloroplasty, Jaboulay gastroduodenostomy, gastrojejunostomy, and antrectomy.

Selective Vagotomy and Drainage
Both vagus nerves are transected distal to the origin of the celiac and hepatic branches, and a gastric drainage procedure is added. This approach is rarely used now due to a high rate of ulcer recurrence and lack of significant benefits compared to truncal vagotomy.

Highly Selective Vagotomy
Highly selective vagotomy (HSV), also called proximal gastric vagotomy (PGV) or parietal cell vagotomy (PCV), involves dividing the anterior and posterior vagal branches while keeping the nerve supply (crow-foot) to the gastric antrum and pylorus intact. Denervation occurs along the lesser curvature, starting from the incisura and extending about 5–6 cm beyond the cardia. No additional drainage procedure is required because maintaining the innervation of the antropyloric region preserves normal motility.

Seromyotomy
Anterior and posterior seromyotomy involve making an incision about 1 cm below and parallel to the lesser curvature, starting from the gastroesophageal junction up to the incisura. Similar to HSV, the seromyotomy effectively divides all vagal fibers entering the stomach from the main trunk. Antral innervation remains intact to preserve its motility. Because antral innervation can be maintained with only anterior innervation, posterior truncal vagotomy is performed for technical simplicity, especially when using a laparoscopic approach.

Table 5.4 Postoperative complications of gastric surgery

Early	Delayed
Bleeding from the anastomotic site	Anastomotic stricture
Anastomotic leak	Postgastrectomy syndromes
Stomal obstruction	Marginal ulcer bleed
Gastric ileus	Gastro-jejuno-colic fistula
Duodenal stump blow-out	Small stomach syndrome
Small bowel obstruction	Remnant carcinoma

5.9 Gastrectomy-Based Procedures

Partial gastrectomy or hemigastrectomy aims to remove the antrum and part of the gastric mucosa responsible for secreting gastrin and acid, respectively. The reconstruction is performed by connecting the gastric remnant to the duodenum (Billroth I) or jejunum (Billroth II, Polya). A posterior penetrating ulcer that is difficult to excise can be left attached to its base and excluded from the resected gastric segment. Once excluded from the stomach, the ulcer will eventually heal.

5.9.1 Gastrojejunostomy

Gastrojejunostomy (GJ) is based on the principles of diverting acid away from the duodenum and simultaneously channeling alkaline bile into the stomach to promote ulcer healing. A very high ulcer recurrence rate (>50%) questions the usefulness of GJ as a 'standalone' procedure for chronic DU (Table 5.4).

5.10 Complications of Peptic Ulcer Disease

- Bleeding
- Perforation
- Stenosis
- Penetration into adjacent viscera
- Malignant transformation

5.10.1 Bleeding

Peptic ulcer bleeding, with an incidence of approximately 40%, is the second most common cause of upper GI hemorrhage, after variceal bleed. 10–15% of PUD cases, mainly in elderly patients with comorbidities, develop bleeding as a

Table 5.5 Forrest classification of peptic ulcer bleeding

Grade	Endoscopic findings	Rebleed risk
Ia	Active, pulsatile bleed	High
Ib	Active, nonpulsatile bleed	High
IIa	Non-bleeding visible vessel	High
IIb	Adherent clot	Intermediate
IIc	Black dot	Low
III	No signs of recent bleeding	Low

complication. Chronic bleeding from the ulcer bed appears as microcytic hypochromic anemia and requires endoscopic evaluation. An acute bleed presenting as hematemesis, melena, or hematochezia is a medical emergency and the leading cause of death in PUD. There is a strong link between NSAID use and *H. pylori* infection, suggesting a synergistic effect. The most common sites of bleeding are the posterior duodenal ulcer and ulcers on the lesser curvature, which involve erosion of the gastroduodenal artery and the left gastric artery, respectively (Table 5.5).

Management of UGI bleeding follows standard protocols involving resuscitation, diagnosis, and treatment. Endoscopy is the most effective tool for both diagnosing and managing UGI bleeding. At this stage, a nasogastric (NG) tube is inserted to help evaluate bleeding severity. Bright red aspirate indicates active, brisk bleeding that requires urgent intervention. The NG tube also aids in evacuating clots that cause antral distension, which stimulates acid secretion. Removing the clot and performing aggressive gastric lavage with room temperature normal saline improve visualization of the bleeding ulcer. Intravenous metoclopramide is also administered before endoscopy for the same purpose. The risk of rebleeding is stratified based on findings from the initial endoscopy, classified by the Forrest system. Early therapeutic endoscopy—using a combination of adrenaline injection, heater probe application, argon coagulation, and hemoclips—successfully controls bleeding in most cases. Continuous high-dose infusion of PPIs combined with endoscopic therapy achieves bleeding control in more than 90% of patients. An *H. pylori* eradication regimen is prescribed to prevent ulcer recurrence and rebleeding. Eradication of the infection reduces the risk of further bleeding and eliminates the need for long-term acid suppression (Fig. 5.3).

5.10.2 Angiography

Selective angiography and transcatheter embolization of the bleeding vessel are indicated if the source of bleeding cannot be identified on endoscopy or if the patient presents with rebleeding after endoscopy.

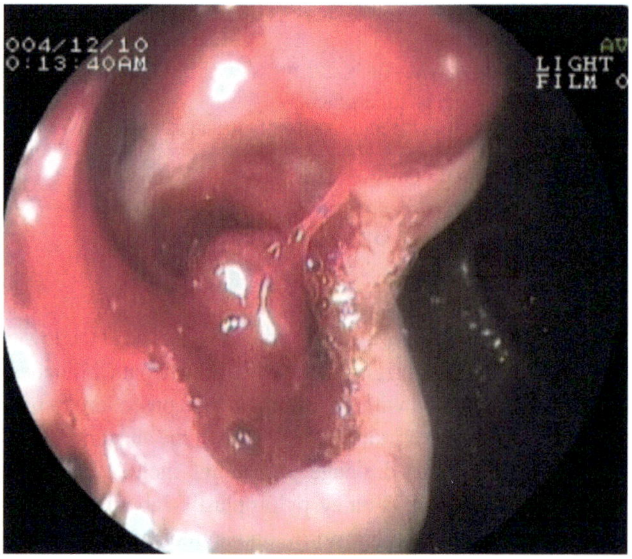

Fig. 5.3 Giant anterior duodenal ulcer covered with fresh clot seen on endoscopy

5.10.3 Surgical Management

Surgery is required in less than 10% of patients with peptic ulcer bleeding.

Indications for Surgery

- Hemodynamic instability: shock and low hemoglobin, blood transfusion of more than 6 units (8–10 units in younger patients).
- Intractable bleeding from a major vessel (gastroduodenal/left gastric artery).
- Failed endoscopy/embolization procedure.
- Recurrent bleeding after two unsuccessful endoscopic attempts.
- Recurrent bleeding with shock.

Relative Indications for Surgery

- Rare blood type/challenging cross-matching.
- Advanced age.
- Bleeding chronic gastric ulcer (suspicion of malignancy).
- Ulcers larger than 2 cm or with Forrest grades Ia, IIa, or IIb often require surgical management to control bleeding.

The basic principles of surgery for peptic ulcer bleeding involve suture transfixation of the ulcer base (bleeding vessel) and adding an acid-reducing procedure such as vagotomy. Bleeding DU, usually on the posterior wall, is exposed by a long pylorotomy. The ulcer base is obliterated by deep transfixation sutures. The superior gastroduodenal artery above and below the duodenum should be transfixed, although this might not be possible if extensive fibrosis surrounds the ulcer-bearing duodenum. The pylorotomy is closed by converting it into a pyloroplasty. Then, bilateral truncal vagotomy is performed. Bleeding GU is treated by making a gastrotomy and transfixing the ulcer base with deep sutures. Afterward, a truncal vagotomy with drainage is performed. However, a stable patient should be managed with a partial gastrectomy, which involves removing the ulcer-bearing part of the stomach (Figs. 5.4 and 5.5).

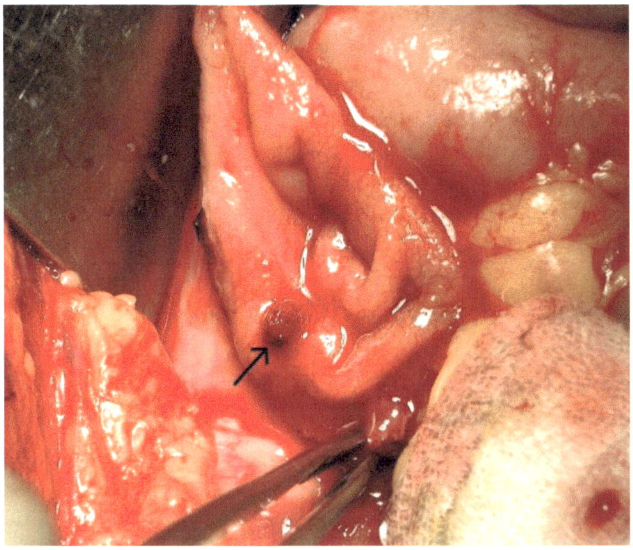

Fig. 5.4 Bleeding posterior duodenal ulcer (arrow) exposed after pylorotomy

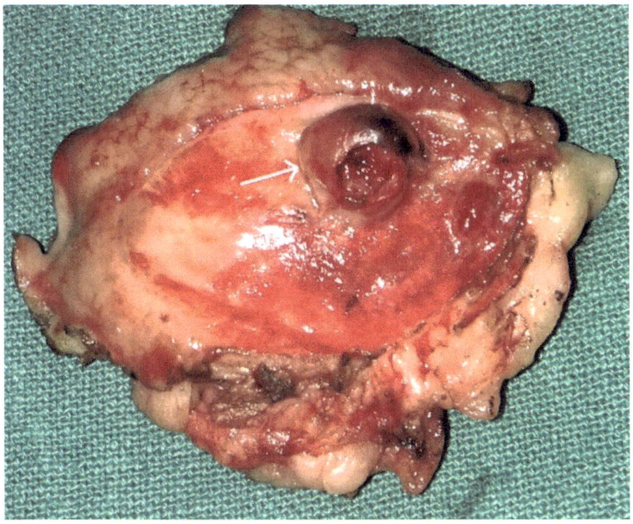

Fig. 5.5 Full-thickness wedge excision of bleeding gastric ulcer. Note the visible vessel (arrow) in the center of the ulcer

5.10.4 Peptic Ulcer Perforation

The incidence of peptic ulcer perforations has remained constant despite a decline in overall peptic ulcer cases recently. There is a slow increase in the age of patients, along with a shift toward more female patients, compared to previous trends where young males have been mainly affected.

Active duodenal ulcers, ulcers with *H. pylori* infection, and the concurrent use of NSAIDs, steroids, alcohol, antimalarials, and smoking are risk factors for perforation. Perforation is more common with anterior ulcers, whereas posterior ulcers are more likely to bleed. Gastric ulcers have a thicker wall and fibrosis and do not perforate unless there is an underlying malignancy or when immunity is compromised.

5.10.5 Clinical Features

About 20% of duodenal ulcer perforations are silent. Typically, most patients present with sudden abdominal pain and signs of peritonitis. The patient may be in any of the three stages of peritonitis.

1. Stage of chemical peritonitis: immediately after perforation, caused by peritoneal irritation from gastric contents.
2. Stage of reaction: up to 6 h after perforation, signs and symptoms decrease as gastric contents are diluted by peritoneal fluid.
3. Stage of bacterial peritonitis: after 6 h, clear signs of peritonitis and sepsis appear.

Occasionally, patients may present with pain in the epigastrium and right iliac fossa (Valentino's syndrome), mimicking acute appendicitis. This is due to the accumulation of inflammatory fluid in the iliac fossa tracking along the right paracolic gutter (Table 5.6).

Table 5.6 Prognostic factors in peptic perforation

Age > 60 years
Delayed presentation (> 24 h)
Delayed surgery (> 24 h)
Comorbidities
Shock on admission
Total leucocyte count >15,000 cells/mm^3
High C-reactive protein (CRP)
Low albumin (< 3 g/dL)
Elevated lactate (> 2 mmol/L)

5.10.6 Investigations

- Hematological and systemic biochemical parameters are influenced by sepsis. Serum amylase may be elevated (typically <1000 IU/L) due to the absorption of duodenal contents from the peritoneal cavity. Amylase levels exceeding 1000 IU/L or more than three times the normal range indicate a diagnosis of acute pancreatitis.
- Erect abdominal X-ray: free gas under the diaphragm is observed in more than 50% of patients.
- CT imaging of the abdomen: It is considered the most accurate method not only for diagnosing duodenal perforation but also for excluding other causes of an acute abdomen.

5.10.7 Treatment

An adequate resuscitation is paramount in minimizing adverse postoperative outcomes in a patient with perforation and peritonitis.

5.10.7.1 Surgery for Perforated Duodenal Ulcer

Despite the traditional midline laparotomy, the laparoscopic approach for perforated duodenal ulcers is now widely accepted. After thoroughly cleaning the peritoneal cavity, the perforation is closed with full-thickness, long-acting, absorbable interrupted sutures, reinforced with an omental patch. The conventional Graham closure of duodenal perforation involves suturing the perforation using only a pedicled omental patch. Alternatively, a mobilized round ligament can also be used instead of the omentum. Very large (>2–3 cm) duodenal perforations may present technical challenges for closure and require careful consideration of alternative techniques (Table 5.7).

Concurrent definitive surgery in peptic perforation should be avoided in a very sick patient. However, it may be considered in a stable patient under the following circumstances,

- Surgery deemed necessary for the ulcer before perforation
- Associated pyloric stenosis
- Concurrent bleeding

Table 5.7 Alternative techniques for giant perforation closure

Omental plugging
Jejunal serosal patch
Suture closure, duodenal (pyloric) exclusion, and gastrojejunostomy
Partial gastrectomy (antrectomy)
Pyloroplasty at the site of perforation
Gastric disconnection/ modified triple tube technique (vagotomy, antrectomy, gastrostomy, lateral duodenostomy)
Feeding jejunostomy should be added to any of the above procedures

5.10.7.2 Surgery for Perforated Gastric Ulcer

A perforated gastric ulcer is treated similarly to the method described above. Additionally, an ulcer biopsy must be performed to rule out malignancy. Alternatively, a wedge excision of the perforated ulcer can be performed for biopsy purposes, followed by closure of the defect with omental reinforcement, known as the Cellan-Jones technique. However, healing can be problematic in inflamed and edematous stomach walls. For stable, fit patients with minimal contamination, partial gastrectomy including the perforated ulcer is often the best option, as it addresses both the risk of incidental malignancy and acid secretion.

Nonoperative management may be considered for stable patients with duodenal ulcer perforation presenting more than 24 h after onset, confirmed by radiological evidence (water-soluble contrast study) of spontaneous ulcer sealing. It is not recommended for gastric ulcer perforations due to the higher risk of re-perforation and complications. Postoperative *H. pylori* eradication therapy and follow-up endoscopy are advised, especially for patients with gastric ulcers.

5.10.8 Gastric-Outlet Obstruction

Cicatrization at the site of a chronic or recurrent ulcer can cause contracture and narrowing of the lumen in 5–8% of patients with peptic ulcer disease. Chronic duodenal ulcers and type II or III gastric ulcers may present with gastric outlet obstruction (GOO). Cicatricial contracture of gastric ulcers can lead to hourglass or teapot deformities, depending on the ulcer's location on the lesser curvature.

5.10.8.1 Clinical Features

- Symptoms of gastric retention include early satiety, postprandial fullness, bloating, and indigestion.
- Retention vomiting several hours after meals.
- Non-bilious gastric contents and undigested food particles in the vomitus.
- Dehydration with metabolic alkalosis.
- Weight loss and malnutrition.
- Epigastric fullness due to dilated stomach; visible gastric peristalsis may be evident on examination of the abdomen.

5.10.8.2 Diagnosis

UGI endoscopy is the preferred investigation not only to diagnose GOO but also to rule out malignancy, which is a much more frequent cause of obstruction. UGIE in the presence of obstruction carries a significant risk of regurgitation, vomiting, and aspiration. Technically, endoscopic examination can be challenging when there is retained fluid and food residue. Therefore, lavage with a wide-bore nasogastric tube is recommended before endoscopy to improve visualization of the pathology.

5.10.8.3 Treatment

Preoperative preparation includes,

- Gastric lavage with a wide-bore nasogastric tube. This not only cleanses the stomach for a clear operative field but also helps it regain its tone and thereby reduces postoperative gastric ileus.
- Correction of chronic dehydration and metabolic alkalosis using intravenous isotonic saline and potassium supplements.
- Endoscopic balloon dilatation and placement of a retrievable self-expandable metal stent (SEMS) across the obstruction may be performed as a temporizing measure in a surgically unfit or nutritionally depleted patient. Bilateral truncal vagotomy and gastrojejunostomy are recommended for chronic duodenal ulcer-related obstruction. Partial gastrectomy with excision of the scarred segment is recommended for GU.

5.10.9 Ulcer Penetration

Gastric ulcers can sometimes penetrate anteriorly into the liver or posteriorly into the pancreas, making them hard to distinguish from cancer. When a posterior duodenal ulcer penetrates into the pancreas, the pain may mimic that of pancreatitis. Penetration into the common bile duct can cause biliary stricture or a choledocho-duodenal fistula. Changes in the pain characteristics and symptoms of biliary obstruction may occur alongside ulcer symptoms. Persistent fistula and biliary symptoms after adequate anti-ulcer treatment require surgical intervention. Removing the fistula is technically challenging due to extensive fibrosis. Often, cholecystectomy and Roux-en-Y hepatico-jejunostomy are needed.

5.10.10 Malignant Transformation

Chronic gastric ulcers may undergo malignant transformation into adenocarcinoma in 5–8%. The characteristic features are

- Ulcer on the greater curvature
- Large and deep ulcers
- Flattening of mucosal folds
- Irregular ulcer margins
- Necrotic slough over the ulcer base
- Everted ulcer edges
- Nodules, ulcers, or mucosal irregularities in the surrounding region

Endoscopic confirmation with multisite biopsy followed by radical gastrectomy is recommended.

Key Points

- The primary causes of peptic ulcers are hyperacidity, *H. pylori*, and NSAIDs.
- Gastric ulcers are less common than duodenal ulcers; gastric ulcers may be malignant in 5–8%.
- UGIE is the preferred method for diagnosis and biopsy in cases of gastric ulcer.
- The treatment for uncomplicated peptic ulcers is mainly medication; surgery is reserved for stubborn ulcers and complications.
- Gastric antisecretory agents and *H. pylori* eradication therapy are the cornerstones of peptic ulcer management.
- Common complications of peptic ulcers include bleeding, perforation, and stenosis or outlet obstruction.
- Posterior duodenal ulcer more commonly bleeds, while anterior duodenal ulcer perforates.
- In more than 90% of cases, bleeding can be managed with pharmacological and endoscopic interventions.
- The gastroduodenal artery in cases of duodenal ulcer and the left gastric artery in gastric ulcer need to be surgically transfixed if endoscopic management fails.
- An acid-reducing procedure (vagotomy) must be performed in cases of duodenal ulcer bleeding to prevent recurrence.
- A perforated peptic ulcer is a surgical emergency. The patient must be adequately resuscitated before surgical intervention.
- Gastric outlet obstruction is treated by a bypass procedure combined with vagotomy.

Selected Reading

1. Kamada T, Satoh K, Itoh T, et al. Evidence-based clinical practice guidelines for peptic ulcer disease. J Gastroenterol. 2021;56(4):303–22. https://doi.org/10.1007/s00535-021-01769-0.
2. Tarasconi A, Coccolini F, Biffl WL, et al. Perforated and bleeding peptic ulcer: WSES guidelines. World J Emerg Surg. 2020;15(1):19. https://doi.org/10.1186/s13017-019-0283-9.
3. Laine L, Barkun AN, Saltzman JR, Martel M, Leontiadis GI. ACG clinical guideline: upper gastrointestinal and ulcer bleeding. Am J Gastroenterol. 2021;116:899–917. https://doi.org/10.14309/ajg.0000000000001245.
4. William DC, Colin WH, Steven FM, et al. ACG clinical guideline: treatment of helicobacter pylori infection. Am J Gastroenterol. 2024;119(90):1730–53. https://doi.org/10.14309/ajg.0000000000002968.

6 Early Gastric Cancer: Diagnosis and Management

Sonmoon Mohapatra and Ashutosh Mohapatra

Abstract

EGC is defined as carcinoma confined to the mucosa or submucosa, irrespective of lymph node status. Helicobacter pylori infection is the principal driver of gastric carcinogenesis, initiating the Correa cascade of gastritis, atrophy, intestinal metaplasia, dysplasia, and carcinoma. High-definition endoscopes and magnifying NBI enhance the ability to recognize subtle mucosal abnormalities. Key diagnostic indicators of EGC include focal color changes (reddish or whitish) and surface change on white light imaging, as well as the presence of a demarcation line with irregular microvascular and microsurface patterns within it on magnifying NBI (VS classification). The treatment strategy for EGC is determined by three main factors: depth of invasion, lateral extension, and tumor subtype. Successful endoscopic resection depends on multimodal evaluation and strict adherence to well-defined selection criteria.

Keywords

Early Gastric cancer · Gastric intestinal metaplasia · Low-grade dysplasia · High-grade dysplasia · Endoscopic submucosal dissection

Gastric cancer (GC) remains a significant global health issue, ranking as the fifth most common cancer and the fourth leading cause of cancer-related deaths worldwide. Asia bears the heaviest burden, with India reporting the third-highest number of new cases after China and Japan, and the second-highest mortality after China. In East Asia, population-based screening has proven effective: Japan and Korea have implemented nationwide endoscopic programs that significantly improve survival rates, while China has launched regional initiatives in high-incidence areas.

The success of such programs relies not only on access but also on high-quality endoscopy. Missed lesions continue to be a concern; one Japanese study found that over 75% of superficial neoplasia had been missed during previous endoscopies. This underscores the importance of structured training, standardized protocols, and increased vigilance to recognize subtle mucosal changes characteristic of early gastric cancer (EGC).

In India, where formal screening programs are lacking, a prospective study found that EGC accounts for 25% of all GC cases, indicating that early disease is not rare in routine practice. However, reliable detection remains technically challenging, especially where endoscopists lack training in advanced diagnostic techniques. Conversely, countries with established screening systems and standardized training, like Japan, achieve higher early detection rates and better outcomes. This chapter offers an overview of current best practices in evaluating, diagnosing, and managing early gastric cancer, with a focus on advances in endoscopic detection and treatment methods.

6.1 Gastric Cancer: Pathogenesis and Risk Factors

Most GCs are sporadic; however, 1%–3% occur in individuals with a family history, especially those with hereditary diffuse GC. Most sporadic GCs develop through a multistep process involving chronic inflammation, mucosal changes, and molecular alterations, collectively known as the Correa cascade. This pathway usually begins with Helicobacter pylori infection, progressing from chronic gastritis to chronic atrophic gastritis (CAG), gastric intestinal metaplasia (GIM), dysplasia, and finally invasive adenocarcinoma. H. pylori is linked to 75%–89% of non-cardia GCs, making it the leading infectious cause. Its role might be underestimated because the infection often clears in advanced CAG; thus, patients

S. Mohapatra · A. Mohapatra (✉)
Sai Institute of Gastroenterology and Liver Sciences, Bhubaneswar, India

M. Ibrarullah (ed.), *Recent Concepts in Gastrointestinal (GI) Surgery*, https://doi.org/10.1007/978-981-92-1118-0_6

with a history of H. pylori should be considered at increased risk. Epstein–Barr virus accounts for up to 9% of gastric adenocarcinomas and represents a distinct molecular subtype, though it does not cause recognizable precursor lesions on endoscopy.

Environmental factors—including high salt intake, nitrosamines, smoking, and alcohol—worsen mucosal injury and speed up carcinogenesis. Host factors such as age, sex, and comorbidities also affect progression: people over 45 years old, males, and smokers have higher risks of CAG, GIM, and cancer transformation. Pernicious anemia is another known risk factor, with a meta-analysis showing a relative risk of 6.8 (95% CI, 2.6–18.1). Both CAG and GIM are more common in those with a family history of GC. At the same time, ethnicity and geographic background further influence risk progression rates, which are higher in East Asian populations and among immigrants from high-incidence areas. Incomplete GIM, though not always subtyped in pathology practice, may suggest a particularly high risk of malignant progression.

On a molecular level, gastric carcinogenesis involves a cumulative process of genetic and epigenetic changes, including TP53 mutations, microsatellite instability, promoter hypermethylation, and amplification of oncogenes such as HER2, MET, and FGFR2. Loss of E-cadherin (CDH1) is a hallmark of diffuse-type GC, promoting early infiltration and metastasis.

According to Lauren's classification, intestinal-type GC (50%–60% of cases) follows the Correa pathway, is strongly linked to infectious and environmental exposures, and is more common in older men and high-incidence regions. In contrast, diffuse-type GC (30%–40% of cases) arises de novo, often in younger patients, is associated with CDH1 germline mutations in familial cases, and has a more aggressive course with poorer therapeutic response.

Together, these pathways highlight that gastric carcinogenesis involves a complex interplay of infectious, environmental, genetic, and host-related factors. Identifying high-risk groups and precursor conditions is vital for targeted surveillance, early detection, and prevention strategies.

6.2 Early Gastric Cancer: Definition

Early gastric cancer is defined as a lesion limited to the mucosa or submucosa, regardless of lymph node involvement. However, pathological diagnostic criteria vary between Japan and Western countries. In Western practice, invasion beyond the lamina propria is usually required to diagnose carcinoma, whereas in Japan, significant cytological atypia alone is enough, regardless of invasion depth. The Vienna classification was introduced to unify these differences. Nonetheless, discrepancies remain: lesions classified as high-grade adenoma or dysplasia (Vienna category 4.1) in the West are often diagnosed as carcinoma in Japan, and many of these are later confirmed as cancer after endoscopic resection.

6.3 Prerequisite for Detection of Early Gastric Cancer (Fig. 6.1)

6.3.1 Training

Proficiency in esophagogastroduodenoscopy (EGD) requires more than just completing the procedure—it involves a systematic, careful examination and precise interpretation of mucosal findings. Structured training, especially over 2 years, significantly improves detection, while shorter targeted courses and web-based modules also provide benefits. Mentorship and direct feedback further enhance diagnostic accuracy.

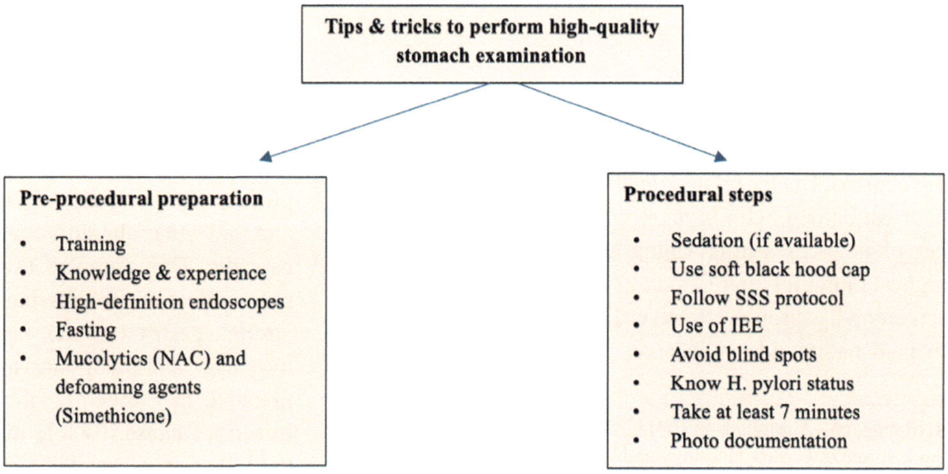

Fig. 6.1 Basic requirements for achieving a high-quality stomach examination. NAC N-acetylcysteine, IEE Image-enhanced endoscopy

6.3.2 Knowledge and Experience

Effective detection requires a solid foundation in disease understanding and ongoing hands-on practice. Endoscopists must recognize background risk features such as H. pylori-associated gastritis, atrophy, or intestinal metaplasia. If the mucosa appears normal, cancer is less likely, while magnified endoscopy can help confirm risk changes and identify subtle neoplasia. When an abnormality is detected on white-light imaging (WLI), it should first be classified macroscopically using the Paris system, then further examined with chromoendoscopy or narrow-band imaging (NBI), and finally assessed with optical or digital magnification to define lesion borders, surface, and vascular patterns. Equally important is a clear understanding of the normal mucosal appearance in the esophagus and stomach, which allows recognition of subtle abnormalities indicative of early disease.

6.3.3 Equipment

High-definition gastroscopes with water-jet function, image-enhanced modes (e.g., NBI/LCI), and optical magnification are recommended for detailed inspection of the upper GI tract. Third-generation NBI systems (e.g., GIF-XZ1200, up to 125×) offer optimal magnification for evaluating micro-surface and microvascular patterns, with manual zoom levers providing precise adjustments. High-magnification NBI enhances diagnostic accuracy for delineating EGC compared to conventional or low-magnification imaging. The use of a soft black hood (e.g., MAJ-1989, Olympus) is strongly recommended, as it maintains an optimal focal distance, reduces glare and reflection, and minimizes mucosal trauma during close inspection.

6.3.4 Mucosal preparation

Mucus and foam can obscure mucosal details and increase the risk of missing important lesions. Proper gastric distension and thorough rinsing are crucial for detecting subtle abnormalities during EGD. Premedication to improve visualization may include defoaming agents (simethicone), mucolytics (N-acetylcysteine), proteolytic enzymes (pronase), and antispasmodics such as cimetropium bromide, scopolamine, or hyoscine N-butyl bromide. Although simethicone and N-acetylcysteine improve mucosal clarity and reduce the need for repeated washes, current evidence does not confirm an increase in neoplasia detection rates. Antispasmodics reduce peristalsis, but their effect on detection remains inconsistent. Standardized mucosal visualization scales may help enhance quality assurance.

6.3.5 Avoiding blind spots

Using systematic mapping with full insufflation, thorough cleansing, and complete visualization of all stomach regions is crucial. Protocols like the Systematic Screening for the Stomach (SSS), which employs 22 sequential images, have significantly boosted detection rates.

6.3.6 Examination time

Longer observation times are linked to higher detection rates of gastric neoplasia. In one study, procedures lasting less than 7 min found no cases of early gastric cancer, while those with a mean duration of 7 min or more identified four lesions (0.9%). However, although guidelines highlight the importance of thorough inspection, they do not specify a minimum duration. These findings indicate that setting minimum time thresholds may be crucial for detection, but more research is needed to determine the best cutoffs and to see if benefits level off after a certain point.

6.3.7 Use of image-enhanced endoscopy (IEE)

EGC can be missed on WLI, especially when obscured by chronic inflammation. The reported sensitivity of WLI for detecting GIM, dysplasia, and EGC is modest, with a range of 29%–59.1%, 51%–74%, and 48%–72%, respectively. In contrast, IEE or NBI improves the detection of gastric atrophy and GIM, helps map GIM severity, and facilitates the endoscopic diagnosis of H. pylori infection. Dye-based chromoendoscopy with indigo carmine enhances mucosal irregularities and shows a pooled sensitivity and specificity of 90% and 82% for detecting EGC and precancerous lesions, respectively. NBI alone may produce dark images due to weak light in the gastric lumen, although newer systems have improved brightness. Recent studies suggest that, compared with WLI, NBI does not significantly increase EGC detection but improves the positive predictive value of diagnosis. Magnifying endoscopy with NBI (ME-NBI) has greatly advanced lesion characterization, with diagnostic accuracy, sensitivity, and specificity reported at 98.1%, 85.7%, and 99.4%, respectively. However, ME-NBI has limitations in identifying undifferentiated adenocarcinoma and fundic gland-type adenocarcinoma, which often spread laterally in deeper mucosa without superficial exposure.

6.4 Detection and Diagnosis of Early Gastric Cancer

The detection of EGC requires a systematic, step-by-step approach starting with WLI, then NBI, and finally magnifying endoscopy (ME) or M-NBI. Accurate diagnosis relies on three key components: (1) recognizing normal gastric mucosa and distinguishing it from high-risk backgrounds such as CAG or GIM, (2) identifying areas suspicious for malignancy, and (3) using image-enhanced endoscopy (IEE) for detailed characterization to differentiate neoplastic from non-neoplastic changes.

6.4.1 Normal Gastric Mucosa

Fundic and pyloric mucosae exhibit distinct M-NBI features. Diagnosis relies on the assessment of vessel (V) and surface (S) patterns. The vascular (V) component includes the subepithelial capillary network (SECN), collecting venules (CV), and microvessels (MV)—the latter describing vessels that cannot be clearly categorized as capillaries or venules in pathological conditions. The surface (S) component consists of the marginal crypt epithelium (MCE), crypt openings (CO), and intervening areas between crypts.

Fundic gland mucosa The surface epithelium appears as oval or round white belt-like structures. The SECN forms polygonal closed loops that interconnect to create a regular honeycomb pattern, which then converges into a starfish-like, cyan-colored CV. These venules produce the "regular arrangement of collecting venules" (RAC), a highly reliable marker of *H. pylori*-negative mucosa, with reported sensitivity of 93.8% and specificity of 96.2%.

Pyloric gland mucosa The surface epithelium displays a ridged pattern with a white belt-like MCE or 'white zone.' The vascular pattern consists of dark brown, coil-shaped, open loops, while CVs are rarely seen because they are situated deeper within the mucosa.

6.4.2 High-risk background mucosa

At the time of scope insertion, the endoscopist should carefully evaluate the background mucosa for features associated with *H. pylori* gastritis, atrophy, or intestinal metaplasia. While a detailed description of ME findings in these preneoplastic conditions is beyond the scope of this chapter, a few practical points are noteworthy. First, when the mucosa appears normal, the probability of cancer is low. Second, the presence of RAC (Fig. 6.2a, b) is a strong predictor of *H. pylori*-negative normal mucosa, with sensitivity and specificity values of 93.8% and 96.2%, respectively. Third, in pathological conditions, the appearance of a light blue crest (LBC) or white opaque substance (WOS) can serve as objective markers of intestinal metaplasia (Fig. 6.3). Importantly, WOS may obscure the subepithelial microvascular pattern but can itself serve as an alternative marker of EGC.

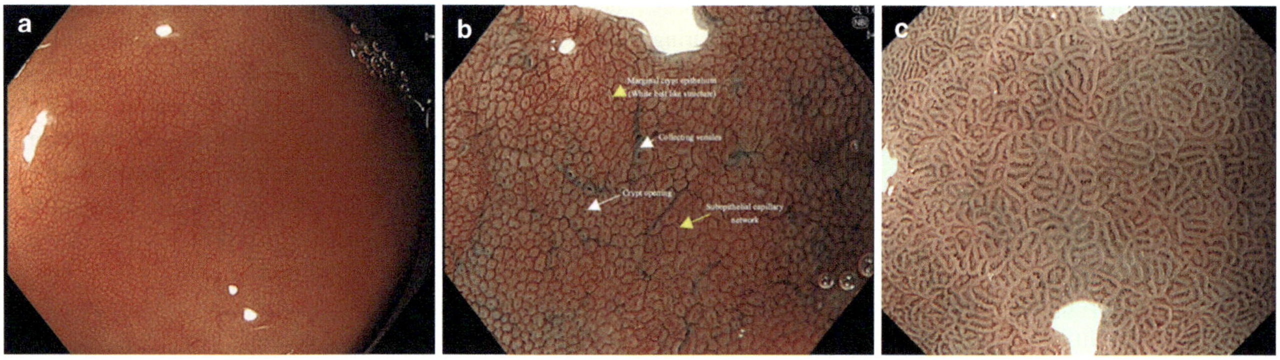

Fig. 6.2 (**a**) White-light endoscopy showing normal gastric body mucosa with a regular arrangement of collecting venules that look like minute red points. (**b**) Narrow-band imaging with magnification of the fundic gland mucosa demonstrating key anatomical landmarks, including the marginal crypt epithelium (white belt-like structure), crypt openings, subepithelial capillary network (honeycomb-like pattern), and collecting venules (starfish-like configuration). (**c**) Magnified view of normal pyloric gland mucosa, showing ridge-like surface epithelium and coiled subepithelial capillary networks

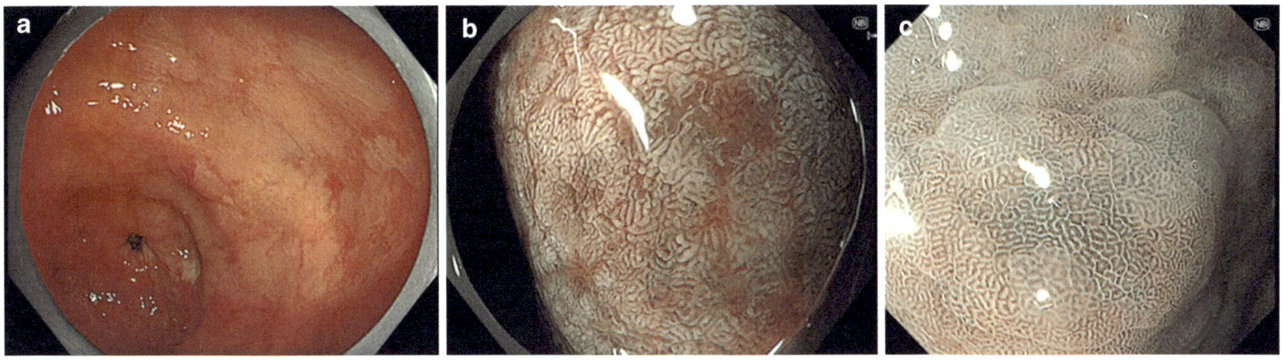

Fig. 6.3 High-risk background mucosa: (**a**) White-light endoscopy showing patchy, pale mucosa with loss of normal gastric folds. (**b**) Magnified NBI highlighting the white opaque substance (WOS) and regular microsurface pattern, with additional markers suggestive of GIM. The WOS obscures the underlying microvascular pattern, making the assessment of EGC more challenging. (**c**) NBI with magnification demonstrating a ridge/villous pattern and light-blue crest, characteristic of GIM

6.4.3 Detecting suspicious lesions

The first step is learning to identify subtle suspicious changes. The two main signs are surface irregularities and color changes. Surface irregularities can appear as small protrusions, slight elevations or depressions, or unevenness of the mucosal surface. Even very small lesions may look like erosive gastritis, making them hard to spot, but these subtle signs can often indicate early cancer. Color changes, such as localized redness or pallor within a well-demarcated area, are also important and often suggest gastritis-like cancer. Other indicators include sudden changes in vascular or mucosal patterns, thickened or irregular folds, and spontaneous bleeding. Carefully tracing the background vascular pattern can reveal areas where vessels are abruptly interrupted at the margin of a lesion—a helpful clue for early detection.

Accurate recognition of macroscopic morphology is essential for diagnosis. The traditional Japanese classification of advanced gastric carcinoma by Borrmann identifies four types: type 1 (polypoid), type 2 (circumscribed excavated), type 3 (ulcerated), and type 4 (diffusely infiltrating). Early gastric cancer was later designated as type 0, with further subdivisions into 0-I (protruded), 0-II (superficial), and 0-III (excavated). Type 0-II lesions are categorized as 0-IIa (slightly elevated), 0-IIb (flat), and 0-IIc (slightly depressed), with 0-IIc being the most common form. Mixed morphologies are common, and when present, the dominant type is recorded first (e.g., 0-IIc+IIa). The Paris classification, introduced in 2003, standardized superficial gastrointestinal lesions worldwide, distinguishing type 0-I from 0-IIa by a 2.5 mm height threshold and defining sm1 versus sm2 invasion based on a submucosal depth of 500 μm. Pure type 0-III lesions are rare, making up less than 1% of EGCs. To simplify routine clinical use, the GUP system has been proposed, grouping lesions into three practical categories: gastritis-like (G; including gastritis versus superficial cancers such as 0-IIa, IIb, IIc), ulcerative (U; peptic ulcer versus superficial cancers with ulceration, including 0-III), and polypoid (P; benign polyp versus polypoid cancers, 0-I). This simplified approach has gained acceptance, providing a practical framework for endoscopists in real-world practice.

6.4.4 Lesion characterization with ME (VS classification)

The vessel plus surface (VS) classification, proposed by Yao et al., is an established system for distinguishing cancerous from noncancerous gastric lesions. It is based on two key features: (1) a clear demarcation line (DL) between cancerous and noncancerous mucosa, and (2) irregular microvascular (MV) and/or microsurface (MS) patterns within the DL. The DL is defined by an abrupt change in MV or MS patterns between lesion and non-lesion areas (Fig. 6.4).

Regular patterns: MV networks appear as polygonal or open-looped structures with uniform morphology, symmetrical distribution, and orderly arrangement. Similarly, regular MS patterns show curved, oval, or circular MCE with homogeneity and symmetry.

Irregular patterns: MV become tortuous, branched, or bizarrely shaped with heterogeneity and asymmetry. MS pat-

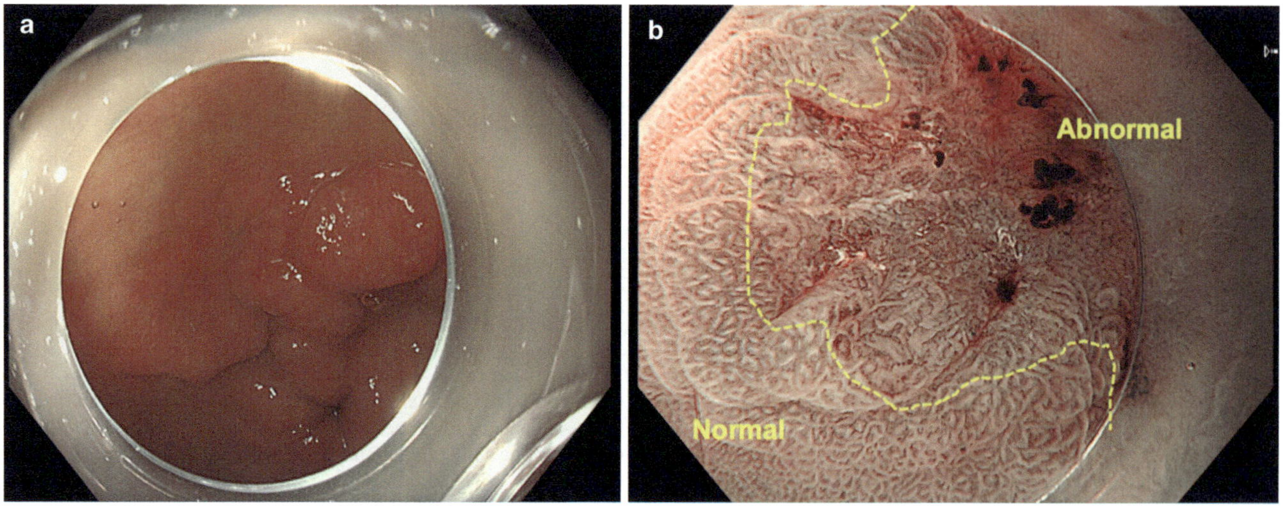

Fig. 6.4 (**a**) An approximately 4 cm superficially elevated, nodular, reddish lesion observed on the anterior wall and lesser curvature of the prepyloric region. (**b**) Magnified NBI demonstrating a distinct demarcation line (yellow dashed line) with irregular microvascular and microsurface patterns, features strongly indicative of EGC

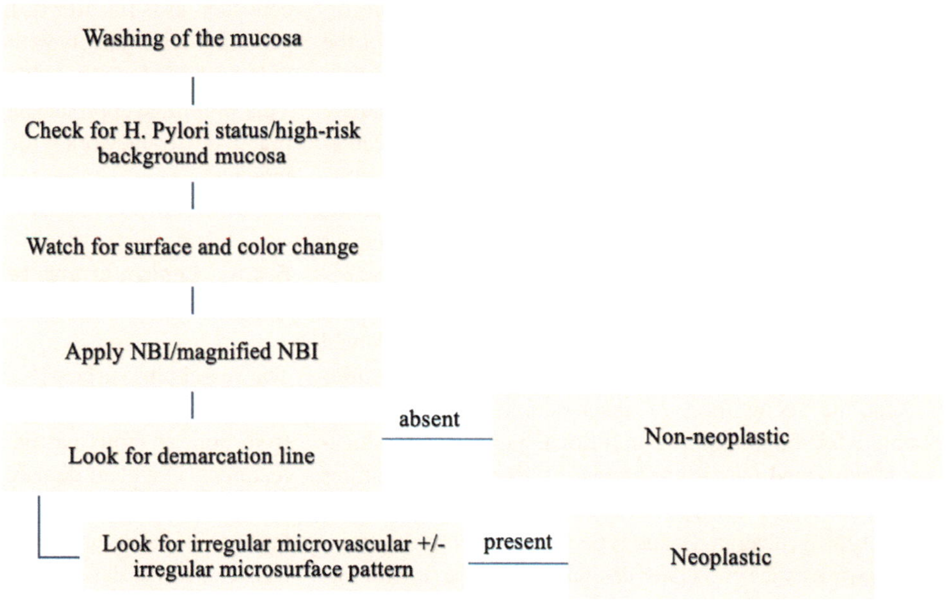

Fig. 6.5 Essential steps for the detection of early gastric cancer

terns appear distorted, characterized by irregular curved, oval, circular, or villous structures, which are also heterogeneous and asymmetrical.

While the VS system is highly effective for identifying most EGCs, some limitations exist. Flat or slightly depressed lesions with mild discoloration (often pale yellow) may show an indistinct DL, a feature often linked to undifferentiated EGC with subepithelial spread. In such cases, the true cancer extent may exceed that suggested by NBI-ME, necessitating biopsies of both the lesion and surrounding mucosa for accurate diagnosis (Fig. 6.5).

6.5 Management of Early Gastric Cancer

Over the past two decades, treatment of EGC has shifted toward minimally invasive endoscopic approaches, supported by advances in imaging, resection techniques, and strong outcome data from East Asia. Among these, endoscopic submucosal dissection (ESD) is preferred because it achieves higher en bloc resection rates than EMR and is endorsed by both Japanese and Western guidelines. Comparative studies and meta-analyses show that, compared with gastrectomy, ESD offers similar long-term survival with shorter hospital stays and fewer complications. However, it carries a slightly higher risk of local or metachronous recurrence, which is usually manageable through surveillance and retreatment. Consequently, endoscopic resection is now considered the standard of care for selected EGC cases, combining the potential for cure with organ preservation and reduced morbidity.

6.5.1 Indications of Endoscopic Resection

The absolute indications for endoscopic resection of gastric dysplasia and invasive cancer include the following:

- Visible low-grade dysplasia
- High-grade dysplasia
- Well to moderately differentiated-type intramucosal adenocarcinomas, irrespective of size and without ulcerations
- Well to moderately differentiated-type intramucosal adenocarcinomas, <3 cm in size if ulceration is present
- Well to moderately differentiated-type submucosal (SM) adenocarcinomas, <3 cm size, with superficial SM1 invasion (<500 micron SM invasion as measured in a vertical line from the deepest fiber of muscularis mucosae)
- Poorly differentiated intramucosal adenocarcinoma ≤2 cm in size

6.5.2 Curability Criteria After Endoscopic Resection

The concept of "curative resection" (eCura) incorporates histologic assessment of en bloc resection, tumor size, depth of invasion, histologic type, lymphovascular invasion, and margin status (Table 6.1). Patients fulfilling eCuraA or eCuraB criteria can be managed with surveillance alone, whereas eCuraC (non-curative) cases warrant additional surgical resection or close follow-up depending on surgical risk (Table 6.2 and Fig. 6.6).

Table 6.1 Curative resection (eCura) classification summary

Category	Criteria	Management implications
eCuraA	En bloc endoscopic resection with (i) Differentiated-type IMCA, UL0, HM0, VM0, Ly0, V0 irrespective of size (ii) Undifferentiated-type IMCA ≤2 cm, UL0, HM0, VM0, Ly0, V0 (iii) Differentiated-type IMCA ≤3 cm, UL1, HM0, VM0, Ly0, V0	Curative—surveillance only
eCuraB	En bloc, differentiated type ≤3 cm, pT1b1 (SM1 <500 μm), HM0/VM0, Ly0, V0	Curative—surveillance only, though long-term evidence is limited
eCuraC-1	Differentiated-type lesions otherwise meeting A or B, but not resected en bloc or HM+	High risk of residual disease—consider additional surgery, repeat ESD, or close follow-up
eCuraC-2	All other lesions not fulfilling A or B criteria (e.g., undifferentiated >2 cm, deeper invasion, LVI+)	Non-curative—surgery with lymphadenectomy recommended

IMCA Intramucosal cancers, *UL0* No ulceration, *UL1* Presence of ulceration, *HM0* Negative horizontal margin, *VM0* Negative vertical margin, *Ly0* No lymphatic invasion, *V0* No venous invasion

Table 6.2 Risk of lymph node metastasis in non-curative resections

Risk group	Total points	Observed risk of LNM (%)	Management recommendation
Low risk	0–1	≈2–3	Close surveillance may be acceptable
Intermediate risk	2–3	≈6–7	Additional surgery is generally recommended
High risk	4–7	≈22–23	Surgery with lymphadenectomy strongly recommended

Note: The following points are assigned for a non-curative endoscopic resection: 3 points for lymphatic invasion (Ly+), and 1 point each for the following factors: tumor size over 30 mm, submucosal invasion of 500 μm or more (SM2), positive vertical margin (VM+), and venous invasion (V+)

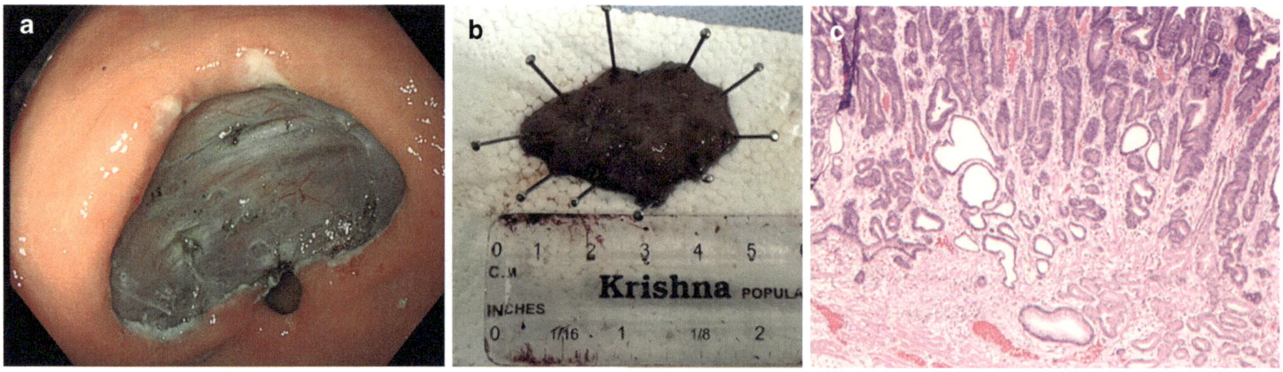

Fig. 6.6 (**a**) The lesion depicted in Fig. 6.4 was successfully resected en bloc using endoscopic submucosal dissection (ESD). (**b**) The excised specimen measured approximately 5 × 3 cm. (**c**) Final histopathological examination showed a well-differentiated adenocarcinoma (G1), measuring 2.6 cm, confined to the lamina propria with extension into the muscularis mucosa (pT1a), with negative horizontal and vertical margins (HM0, VM0), and no evidence of lymphovascular invasion (Ly0, V0). These findings fulfill the criteria for curative resection (eCura A)

Key Points

- Gastric cancer remains a significant global health burden, and patient outcomes are strongly determined by the stage at diagnosis.
- EGC is defined as carcinoma confined to the mucosa or submucosa, irrespective of lymph node status.
- While the majority of gastric cancers are sporadic, 1–3% occur in the context of hereditary predisposition, such as CDH1 mutation in hereditary diffuse gastric cancer.
- Helicobacter pylori infection is the principal driver of gastric carcinogenesis, initiating the Correa cascade of gastritis, atrophy, intestinal metaplasia, dysplasia, and carcinoma.
- Accurate EGC detection requires structured training, adequate inspection time (≥7 min), careful mucosal preparation, and systematic mapping of the stomach to avoid blind spots.
- High-definition endoscopes and magnifying NBI enhance the ability to recognize subtle mucosal abnormalities.
- Key diagnostic indicators of EGC include focal color changes (reddish or whitish) and surface change on white light imaging, as well as the presence of a demarcation line with irregular microvascular and microsurface patterns within it on magnifying NBI (VS classification).
- Comparative studies demonstrate that endoscopic resection achieves survival outcomes equivalent to surgery, with the advantage of lower morbidity and organ preservation.
- The treatment strategy for EGC is determined by three main factors: depth of invasion, lateral extension, and tumor subtype.
- Successful endoscopic resection depends on multimodal evaluation and strict adherence to well-defined selection criteria.
- The eCura system stratifies endoscopic resections into curative (A and B) and non-curative (C1 and C2) categories, guiding the need for additional surgical treatment.
- Long-term surveillance is essential following endoscopic resection, and future advances are expected to include artificial intelligence-assisted diagnosis and standardized global training programs.

Selected Reading

1. Yao K. The endoscopic diagnosis of early gastric cancer. Ann Gastroenterol. 2013;26:11–22.
2. Yao K, Uedo N, Kamada T, et al. Guidelines for endoscopic diagnosis of early gastric cancer. Dig Endosc. 2020;32:663–98.
3. The Paris endoscopic classification of superficial neoplastic lesions: esophagus, stomach, and colon: November 30 to December 1, 2002. Gastrointest Endosc. 2003;58:S3–43.
4. Ono H, Yao K, Fujishiro M, et al. Guidelines for endoscopic submucosal dissection and endoscopic mucosal resection for early gastric cancer (second edition). Dig Endosc. 2021;33:4–20.
5. Mohapatra A, Mohapatra S, Mahawar S, et al. Endoscopic diagnosis and prevalence of early gastric cancer in India: a prospective study. DEN Open. 2024;4:e309.

Gastric Cancer

7

Mahesh Thombare, Vidyachandra Gandhi,
and Nikhil Jillawar

Abstract

Gastric cancer has an incidence of 5.6 per 100,000 people, making it the sixth most common cancer and the second leading cause of cancer death worldwide. Surgery is the main curative treatment for gastric cancer, with the goal of achieving an R0 resection. D2 lymphadenectomy is the standard procedure for resectable cancers, providing optimal oncologic outcomes with manageable morbidity. Surgery has a limited but evolving role in advanced disease, especially after a good response to neoadjuvant chemotherapy; R0 resection enhances survival in selected patients with limited metastases (e.g., solitary liver metastasis, para-aortic LN involvement).

Keywords

Gastric cancer · Stomach cancer · Gastrectomy

Gastric cancer (GC) has an incidence of 5.6 per 100,000 people, making it the sixth most common cancer and the second leading cause of cancer death worldwide, according to GLOBOCAN (WHO). It occurs twice as often in males and typically affects older men in their 70s. The highest rates are reported in East Asia, Eastern Europe, and Central and South America. Japan has the highest national incidence, with improved survival rates since screening programs began in the 1970s. Recently, there has been an increase in cases among younger American men, linked to obesity and high salt intake. Asia reports the highest global incidence and mortality, with rates of 15.8 new cases and 11 deaths per 100,000 in men and 7.0 and 4.9 per 100,000 in women.

There has been a decline in distal (antral) gastric cancer and a rise in proximal cancers in developed countries, due to obesity, Helicobacter pylori infection, and dietary factors. Over 90% of GC cases are sporadic, about 10% have familial clustering, and 1–3% are caused by inherited cancer syndromes.

7.1 Risk Factors

Helicobacter pylori and other infections: H. pylori is a gram-negative, spiral-shaped, urease-producing bacterium that inhabits the gastric lining and is a confirmed carcinogenic factor in gastric cancer (GC), especially non-cardia types (making up over 90% of cases). It changes the gastric environment, leading to chronic gastritis, atrophy, intestinal metaplasia, dysplasia, and eventually, intestinal-type GC. Recent studies indicate that eradicating H. pylori reduces the incidence and mortality rates of GC.

Other bacteria involved in gastric cancer (GC) include Mycoplasma hyorhinis (from pork), which promotes GC through WNT pathway activation. Fusobacterium nucleatum (from oral sources) contributes to diffuse-type GC by causing inflammation and immune evasion. After H. pylori eradication, overgrowth of Propionibacterium acnes, Streptococcus anginosus, and Prevotella melaninogenica may also promote cancer development via local inflammation.

Epstein-Barr Virus (EBV): EBV is associated with 8.77% of gastric cancer cases, primarily in the cardia and corpus, as well as in remnant gastric cancers. It promotes tumor growth by increasing pro-inflammatory and anti-apoptotic genes.

Dietary Factors: High salt intake (e.g., >16 g/day in Japan), salted or smoked meats (nitrates), red meat, and low fruit consumption increase GC risk. Ascorbic acid from fruits neutralizes N-nitroso compounds. Smoking introduces similar carcinogens and raises the risk for both cardia and non-cardia GC. Folate and cobalamin deficiency, alcohol (via

M. Thombare (✉) · N. Jillawar
D Y Patil Medical College, Hospital and Research Centre, Pune, India

V. Gandhi
Ruby Hall Clinic, Pune, India

M. Ibrarullah (ed.), *Recent Concepts in Gastrointestinal (GI) Surgery*, https://doi.org/10.1007/978-981-92-1118-0_7

mucosal injury, acetaldehyde, CYP2E1 induction), and obesity (especially for cardia GC) are additional risk factors.

Hereditary Risk and Cancer Genetics: Hereditary GC accounts for 1–3% of cases. Hereditary diffuse gastric cancer (HDGC), caused by germline CDH1 mutation, usually presents with diffuse signet-ring cell carcinoma and a higher risk of lobular breast cancer. Prophylactic gastrectomy and mastectomy are recommended before age 30. Other conditions linked to GC include Peutz-Jeghers syndrome, juvenile polyposis, Lynch syndrome, familial adenomatous polyposis (FAP), Li-Fraumeni syndrome, and Gastric adenocarcinoma and proximal polyposis of the stomach (GAPPS). FAP often involves proximal gastric polyps; Li-Fraumeni (p53 mutation) increases the risk of GC and other cancers. Lynch syndrome predisposes individuals to intestinal-type GC.

Gastric Polyps: Most are benign. Hyperplastic, fundic gland, and inflammatory polyps have a low risk of becoming cancerous. Adenomatous polyps are considered precancerous. FAP-related fundic gland polyps can involve the entire stomach, whereas sporadic ones are usually limited to the fundus. Larger or multiple polyps should be biopsied or removed endoscopically. Sessile, larger than 2 cm, or invasive polyps need surgical removal. Hyperplastic polyps shrink in 80% of cases after H. pylori eradication.

Proton Pump Inhibitors (PPIs): Although still speculative, the risk of gastric cancer related to PPIs is associated with H. pylori and hypochlorhydria-induced dysbiosis, especially the overgrowth of Streptococcus species. More research is needed.

Other Risk Factors: GC risk increases with obesity, smoking, abdominal radiation, and heavy alcohol use.

7.2 Premalignant Conditions

Atrophic Gastritis: It is categorized into two types: environmental, caused by H. pylori, and autoimmune, which is often associated with pernicious anemia. The environmental type affects the gastric corpus and is closely associated with GC, while the autoimmune type involves the fundus and corpus but has a lower GC risk. The risk increases with H. pylori infection, especially strains carrying the cytotoxin A gene, as well as with advancing age and environmental factors like high salt intake, processed meats, and smoking, which promote H. pylori-related inflammation.

Intestinal metaplasia: This condition involves a progression from atrophic gastritis, where the gastric epithelium is replaced by intestinal-type mucosa. Type I (complete) includes goblet cells, sialomucins, and a brush border; Types II and III (incomplete) have a higher risk of becoming cancerous. It can lead to low-grade and high-grade dysplasia. Low-grade dysplasia regresses in 60% of cases. In contrast, high-grade dysplasia rarely regresses and has a 40-fold increased risk of gastric cancer, with an annual incidence of 6% over 5 years compared to 0.6% in mild cases.

Peptic ulcer: Gastric ulcers are linked to a tenfold increased risk of GC, whereas duodenal ulcers do not exhibit this association.

Previous gastrectomy: GC risk increases over the long term after gastrectomy for both benign and malignant reasons, likely due to bacterial overgrowth and bile reflux. As the need for surgery decreases because of PPIs and H. pylori eradication, the incidence of GC after gastrectomy is expected to decline.

Ménétrier's disease: Although rare, it has an 8.9% GC risk. Its exact cause remains unknown.

7.3 Classifications of Gastric Cancer

7.3.1 Classification by Depth

- Early GC (EGC): Confined to mucosa/submucosa (T1), with a 5-year survival rate exceeding 90%.
- Advanced GC (AGC): Invades muscularis propria or beyond (T2–T4); 5-year survival rate is 7–27% (Table 7.1).

7.3.2 Borrmann Classification (Macroscopic)

- Type I: Polypoid
- Type II: Ulcerated with raised margin
- Type III: Ulcerated, infiltrating base
- Type IV: Diffusely infiltrative (Linitis plastica)

Table 7.1 Lauren classification

Feature	Intestinal	Diffuse
Differentiation	Well differentiated	Poorly differentiated
Location	Atrophic gastritis/ metaplasia	Normal mucosa
Age/sex	Older, M > F	Younger, M = F
Etiology	Environmental	Genetic
Histology	Glandular	Signet ring cells
Spread	Hematogenous, late	Peritoneal, early
Prognosis	Better	Poor
Genetics	MSI, p53/p16↓	CDH1↓, p53/p16↓

7.3.3 Molecular Classifications

(a) TCGA—The Cancer Genome Atlas (2014)
- EBV+ (9%): PIK3CA mut., PD-L1↑
- MSI-H (22%): Best prognosis
- Genomically Stable (20%): CDH1, RHOA mutations
- CIN (50%): TP53 mut., RTK amplifications

(b) ACRG—Asian Cancer Research Group (2015)
- MSI (23%)—Best outcome
- MSS/EMT (15%)—Worst, peritoneal spread
- MSS/TP53—(36%)—Common
- MSS/TP53+ (26%)—Better prognosis

7.3.4 WHO Histologic Subtypes (2010)

- Papillary, tubular, mucinous adenocarcinoma
- Poorly cohesive (e.g., SRCC)
- Rare types: hepatoid, lymphoepithelioma-like, SCC

7.3.5 Paris Classification (Macroscopic, for EGC)

- Type 0-I: Protruded
- Type 0-II: Flat (IIa: elevated, IIb: flat, IIc: depressed)
- Type 0-III: Excavated
- Type 0-IIc/0-III suggests deeper invasion

7.4 Clinical Presentation

Symptoms of early gastric cancer (EGC) are often absent or nonspecific, such as dyspepsia or mild gastritis. Advanced gastric cancer (AGC) manifests with symptoms like anorexia, early satiety, epigastric pain, weight loss, vomiting (due to gastric outlet obstruction in distal tumors), dysphagia or regurgitation (associated with tumors at the gastroesophageal junction), anemia, hematemesis, melena, and abdominal distension caused by ascites. During examination, findings may include Virchow's node (left supraclavicular), Irish node (left axillary), Sister Mary Joseph nodule (periumbilical), or a palpable epigastric mass, which may indicate large antral or omental deposits. A per-rectal exam can identify Blumer's shelf (rectal deposits) or Kruckenberg tumors (bilateral ovarian metastases).

7.5 Screening and Surveillance

Screening aims for early GC detection to improve survival. Countries with high incidence rates, such as Japan, South Korea, and Chile, implement routine surveillance. High-risk groups include individuals with adenomas, multiple gastric polyps, pernicious anemia, and FAP. In hereditary diffuse GC (HDGC), screening is limited because lesions are often submucosal. White light endoscopy (WLI) remains the primary screening method.

7.6 Staging Systems

The AJCC 8th edition TNM staging is the current global standard and aligns with the 15th Japanese GC classification. Unlike previous versions, AJCC 8th no longer considers nodal location for staging, but it still plays a role in determining the type of lymphadenectomy (D1 vs D2) according to Japanese guidelines.

7.7 Management

Upper Gastrointestinal Endoscopy (UGIE): Endoscopy confirms tumor location, diagnosis, histology (via biopsy), and presence of atrophic gastritis. It also treats bleeding and gastric outlet obstruction. At least 6–8 biopsies are required for an accurate diagnosis.

Endoscopic Ultrasound (EUS): EUS assesses depth (T stage) and lymph node (LN) involvement. Metastatic LNs appear hypoechoic, round, sharply defined, and larger than 10 mm. EUS-guided fine needle aspiration (FNA) confirms nodal disease. Depth invasion on EUS and the corresponding T stage are as follows: fourth layer = T2; expanded subserosa = T3; breached fifth layer = T4a; involvement of adjacent organ or vessel = T4b. The sensitivity and specificity for distinguishing T1/T2 from T3/T4 lesions are approximately 80% and 90%, respectively. Operator dependence remains a limitation (Figs. 7.1, 7.2, 7.3, and 7.4).

Computed tomography (CT): CT scans of the thorax and abdomen evaluate locoregional disease. CT often underestimates the T stage; accuracy improves with multiplanar reconstruction. EUS is more dependable for T staging but less precise for nodal or distant spread. The accuracy of LN staging (CT/EUS) is about 75–79%. Enlarged lymph nodes may result from inflammation, whereas metastasis can occur in normal-sized nodes.

Positron Emission Tomography (PET-CT): Intestinal-type gastric adenocarcinoma is more FDG-avid than diffuse-type gastric adenocarcinoma, which enhances the detection of distant metastases. PET-CT alters management in 3–29% of patients by upstaging the disease. Peritoneal disease is missed in approximately 8–19% of cases.

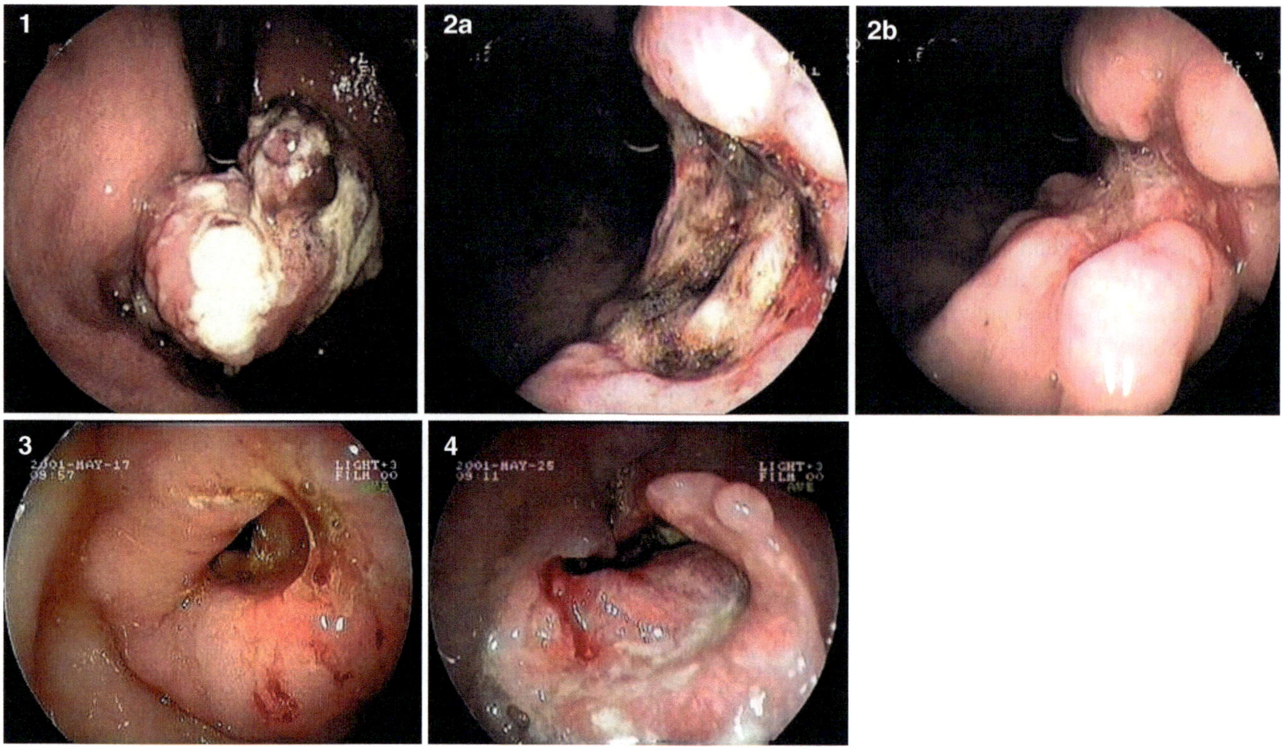

Figs. 7.1, 7.2, 7.3 and 7.4 Endoscopic images of GC. (1): Polypoidal tumor just below GEJ, (2**a**, **b**): Ulcerated tumor involving lesser curve and incisura, (3): Nodular prepyloric tumor, (4): Ulcerated prepyloric tumor

Fibroblast Activation Protein Inhibitor (FAPI)-PET: [^{68}Ga] FAPI-04 PET MRI/CT surpasses [^{18}F] FDG-PET in detecting primary tumors (100% vs 84%), nodal metastases (82% vs 67%), and peritoneal metastases (100% vs 44.7%); higher uptake occurs due to fibroblast-rich lymph node structures (Fig. 7.5).

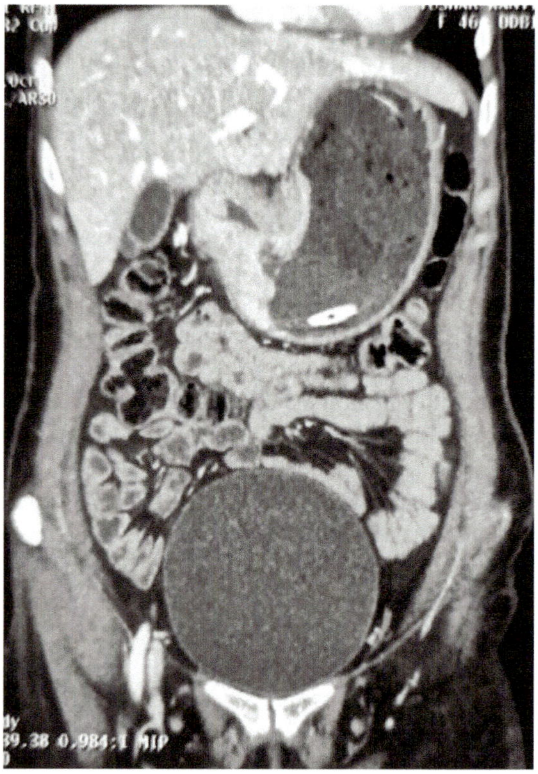

Fig. 7.5 Coronal image of CT scan showing antral tumor

Staging Laparoscopy (SL): SL helps prevent unnecessary laparotomies by detecting hidden peritoneal metastases (PM). Despite imaging, 20–30% of T2+ cases still have undetected PM. SL offers 90% sensitivity and can alter treatment plans in 6–60% of cases. It is endorsed by NCCN, ESMO, SAGES, and guidelines from Japan and Italy. SAGES recommends against using SL in cases with obstructive, bleeding, or perforated gastric cancer that require urgent palliative surgery, as well as in early gastric cancer (T1–2) or after major abdominal surgery. The Japanese Gastric Cancer Association suggests SL for advanced gastric cancer with a high risk of PM, including Linitis plastica, Borrmann types III–IV, poorly differentiated tumors, and nodal disease seen on CT.

Peritoneal cytology (PC): During SL, 150 mL of saline is injected into the hepatorenal and splenic recesses, and 200 mL into the paracolic gutters and pelvis for cytology. Positive PC is a poor prognostic marker and predicts recurrence after surgery.

7.8 Surgical Management

Surgery for GC aims to remove the primary tumor with a wide margin and perform lymphadenectomy to ensure no microscopic residual tumor, achieving an R0 resection. A positive resection margin is an independent predictor of poor prognosis. About 16% of patients have a positive resection margin, which can lead to local recurrence. According to Japanese and Chinese guidelines for intestinal-type gastric cancer, a 3 cm macroscopic negative margin is recommended. For diffuse or signet ring cell cancer, a macroscopic negative margin of at least 5 cm should be achieved. The extent of gastrectomy depends on the tumor's location, infiltration of adjacent organs, tumor size, and lymph node status (Table 7.2).

D1 resection involves removing only perigastric lymph nodes (LN 1-7). D2 dissection adds the hepatic, left gastric, celiac, and splenic nodes to D1 (LN 1-12a). D3 dissection further includes the porta hepatis and periaortic nodes (LN 1-16). The debate between D1 and D2 gastrectomy is now mostly settled; D2 gastrectomy is the current gold standard for gastric cancer resection. Routine distal pancreatectomy and splenectomy, which contribute to the high morbidity of D2 gastrectomy, are no longer routinely performed. Adjacent organ removal is only indicated if it results in an R0 resection. The extent of the proximal resection margin remains controversial. The NCCN guidelines recommend achieving negative resection margins with at least 16 lymph nodes in the specimen for proper pathological staging. Long-term follow-up from Dutch and Italian studies over 15 years has confirmed that D2 lymph node dissection is associated with significantly improved disease-specific survival, a lower risk of gastric cancer-related death, and reduced locoregional recurrence compared to D1. The standard surgical procedure for gastric cancer with positive nodes at T2-T4a stages is distal or total gastrectomy with D2 lymph node dissection. Patients with pancreatic or splenic invasion should undergo total gastrectomy. When an adequate resection margin is present, subtotal gastrectomy or distal gastrectomy can replace total gastrectomy for distal gastric cancer (Table 7.3).

In contrast to earlier recommendations, station 10 LNs are no longer part of standard resection for GC. The recent Japanese Gastric Cancer Guidelines recommend excision of station 10 LNs in patients with locally advanced gastric cancer invading the greater curvature or when the tumor is more than 5 cm in dimension. The 3-year overall survival of the D2+ LN 10 was better than the D2 group. The distal gastrectomy described in Japanese guidelines includes the distal two-thirds of the stomach and differs from that of a four-fifth subtotal gastrectomy performed in Europe. In patients with duodenal infiltration, the station 13 LNs are not considered distant metastases according to Japanese guidelines. Routine excision of para-aortic LNs is not recommended (Table 7.4).

Table 7.2 LN stations in Fig. 7.6

No	Definition
1	Right paracardiac LNs
2	Left paracardiac LNs
3a	Lesser curvature LNs along the branches of the LGA
3b	Lesser curvature LNs along the second branch and distal part of the RGA
4sa	Left greater curvature LNs along the SGA
4sb	Left greater curvature LNs along the left GEA
4d	Left greater curvature LNs along the second branch and distal part of the right GEA
5	Suprapyloric LNs along the first branch and proximal part of the RGA
6	Infrapyloric LNs along the first branch and proximal part of the right GEA
7	LNs along the trunk of LGA between its root and the origin of its ascending branch
8a	Anterosuperior LNs along the CHA
8p	Posterior LNs along the CHA
9	Celiac artery LNs
10	Splenic hilar LNs
11p	Proximal splenic artery LNs
11d	Distal splenic artery LNs
12a	Hepatoduodenal ligaments LNs along the PHA
12p	Hepatoduodenal ligaments LNs along the PV
12b	Hepatoduodenal ligaments LNs along the CBD
13	LNs at the posterior aspect of the pancreatic head
14	LNs at the root of the mesentery
15	LNs in the mesocolon of the transverse colon
16	Para-aortic LNs

LGA left gastric artery, *RGA* right gastric artery, *SGA* short gastric artery, *GEA* gastroepiploic artery, *CHA* common hepatic artery, *PHA* proper hepatic artery, *PV* portal vein, *CBD* common bile duct

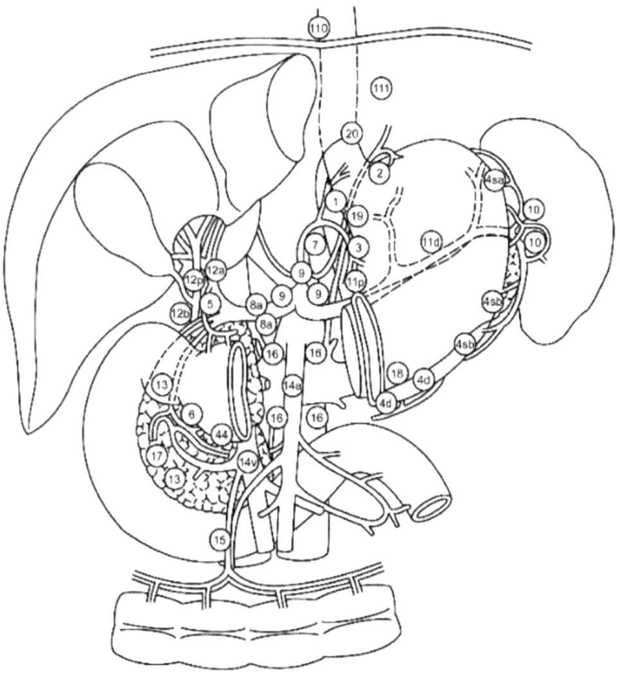

Fig. 7.6 Lymph node (LN) stations in gastric cancer

Table 7.3 Extent of LN dissection corresponding with the gastrectomy

Gastrectomy type	Extent of LN dissection
Total gastrectomy	D0: lymphadenectomy less than D1 D1: LN 1–7 D1 +: D1 + LN 8a, 9, 11p D2: D1 + LN 8a, 9, 11p, 11d, 12a For tumors invading the esophagus, resection of Nos. 19, 20, and 110 should be added to D2
Distal gastrectomy	D0: lymphadenectomy less than D1 D1: LN 1, 3, 4sb, 4d, 5, 6, 7 D1+: D1 + LN 8a, 9 D2: D1 + LN 8a, 9, 11p, 12a
Pylorus-preserving gastrectomy	D0: lymphadenectomy less than D1 D1: LN 1, 3, 4sb, 4d, 6, 7 D1+: D1 + LN8a, 9
Proximal gastrectomy	D0: lymphadenectomy less than D1 D1: LN 1, 2, 3a, 4sa, 4sb, 7 D1+: D1 + LN 8a, 9, 11p D2: D1 + LN 8a, 9, 11p, 11d

Table 7.4 Indications for extended lymphadenectomy

Indication	LN stations
Proximal gastric cancer invading the greater curvature, with or without splenectomy	10
Cancer of the distal stomach with metastasis to infrapyloric LN (LN-6)	14v
Cancer invading the duodenum	13
After neoadjuvant chemotherapy for extensive LN involvement	16

7.9 Treatment of Proximal Gastric Cancer

The Japan Esophageal Society (JES) and the Japanese Gastric Cancer Association (JGCA) joint committee use the Nishi classification for gastroesophageal junction (GEJ) cancer, while Western countries prefer the Siewert classification. The Siewert classification considers type I GEJ cancers as thoracic cancers and type III GEJ cancers as gastric cancers. Although the treatment for type II cancer is not standardized in either the Siewert or Nishi classifications, JES and JGCA report that the incidence of lymph node (LN) positivity varies with the extent of esophageal invasion. If the invasion is less than 2 cm, the likelihood of mediastinal LN involvement is low; if it is between 2 and 4 cm, the involvement of lower mediastinal LN (110) is higher, while upper and middle mediastinal LN involvement remains low; and if the invasion exceeds 4 cm, the incidence of upper and middle mediastinal LN involvement is high. Options for resection of the esophagus and stomach include proximal gastrectomy with or without lower esophageal resection, total gastrectomy with or without lower esophageal resection, or esophageal resection with proximal gastric resection. For esophageal invasion less than 4 cm, transhiatal esophageal resection is also an option. Even for tumors smaller than 2 cm, LN 110 attached to the esophagus needs to be removed to achieve an adequate resection margin (Table 7.5).

Role of Omentectomy: For T3-T4 lesions, complete removal of the omentum is recommended, while for T1-T2

Table 7.5 Algorithm of the surgical approach and LN dissection for GEJ tumor

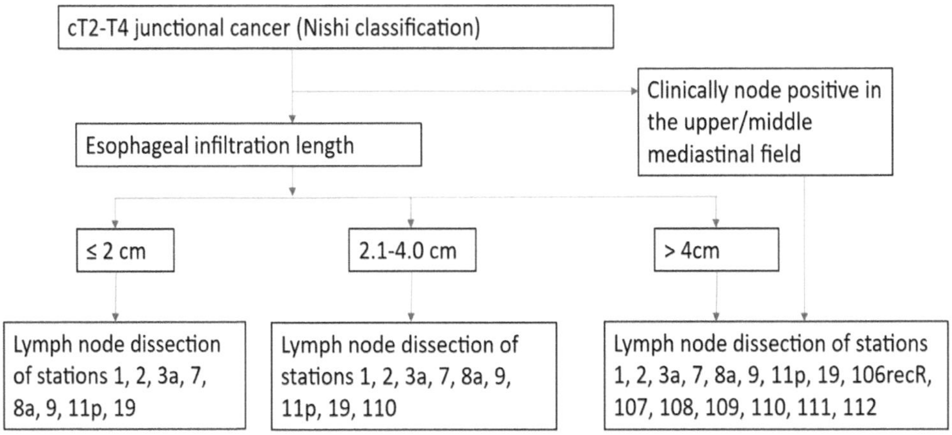

lesions, the omentum is divided 3 cm away from the gastroepiploic arcade. Removal of the omental bursa does not provide additional survival benefits.

7.10 Surgery for Advanced Disease

For advanced GC, conversion gastrectomy is weakly recommended if chemotherapy effectively reduces tumor size or stage and R0 resection is possible. The Phase 2 Arbeitsgemeinschaft Internistische Onkologie (AIO) FLOT3 trial and the CONVO-GC-1 trial showed improved median overall survival with R0 resection. Simultaneous removal of the primary tumor and synchronous liver metastasis may also provide a survival benefit. Meta-analysis suggests that patients with unilobar liver metastases, fewer than three metastases, and tumors smaller than 5 cm are good candidates for metastasectomy.

7.11 Locally Advanced Gastric Cancer

Locally advanced gastric cancer (LAGC) is characterized by gastric cancer with infiltration of adjacent organs, extensive lymphadenopathy, or para-aortic lymphadenopathy. Patients with LAGC who achieve R0 resection tend to have better outcomes than those receiving palliative resection. Neoadjuvant therapy aims to increase the resectability rate with curative intent, whereas adjuvant treatments are intended to decrease the risk of recurrence. Neoadjuvant treatments are administered and intensified in relatively fit patients.

7.12 First-Line Chemotherapy for Unresectable Advanced or Recurrent Gastric Cancer

Human epidermal growth factor receptor-2 (HER2) testing is strongly recommended in this case. In Japan, a combination of S-1 and cisplatin (SP) is the standard treatment. Outside Japan, capecitabine and cisplatin (XP) are commonly used. Other recommended regimens include capecitabine and oxaliplatin (CapeOX), S-1 plus oxaliplatin (SOX), and a combination of 5FU/levofloxacin calcium with oxaliplatin (FOLFOX) (Table 7.6).

Table 7.6 Chemotherapy regimens

First line	Second line	Third line	Fourth line
HER2(−) SOX +/− Nivolumab CapeOX +/− Nivolumab FOLFOX +/− Nivolumab S-1 +/− CDDP Cape +/− CDDP	*MSI high* Pembrolizumab Weekly PTX + RAM	*HER2 (−)* Nivolumab FTD/TPI IRI	Consider a treatment that switches treatments at appropriate times for unused drugs among the candidate drugs up to third-line therapy
HER2(+) Cape + CDDP + T-mab S-1 + CDDP + T-mab CapeOX + T-mab SOX + T-mab	*Non-MSI-high* Weekly PTX + RAM	*HER2 (+)* T-Dxd	

CDDP Cis-Diaminedichloro Platinum, *FTD* Trifluridine, *IRI* Irinotecan, *PTX* Paclitaxel, *RAM* Ramucirumab, *S-1* Tegafur/5-Cholro 2,4-Dihydroxypyridine/Potassium Oxonate, *T-mab* Trastuzumab, *TPI* Tiriracil, *T-Dxd* Trastuzumab + Deruxtecan

7.13 Conditionally Recommended Regimens

In West perioperative chemotherapy, the FLOT regimen, which includes fluorouracil plus leucovorin, oxaliplatin, and docetaxel, is currently the standard. In East Asian countries, D2 gastrectomy followed by adjuvant chemotherapy with S-1 or capecitabine plus oxaliplatin is the current standard of care. In Japan, S-1 plus cisplatin is recommended for bulky N disease with non-scirrhous gastric cancer. Phase 3 PRODIGY and RESOLVE studies have shown survival benefits of adding neoadjuvant chemotherapy to surgery, followed by adjuvant chemotherapy, compared to upfront surgery followed by adjuvant chemotherapy in Asian patients. Adjuvant treatment intensification in the JACCRO-GC07 study, which involved adding docetaxel to S-1, resulted in improved 3-year relapse-free survival in patients with stage III tumors. The addition of oxaliplatin to S-1 in the ARTIST2 study led to prolonged disease-free survival in patients with stage II or III lymph node-positive tumors. In the same study, adding radiation therapy to oxaliplatin plus S-1 did not improve disease-free survival compared to chemotherapy alone. The diagnostic approach before neoadjuvant chemotherapy is not standardized and should include an FDG PET scan, EUS, and possibly diagnostic laparoscopy (Table 7.7).

Adding immunotherapy agents like pembrolizumab, atezolizumab, and durvalumab to the perioperative FLOT regimen has increased the rate of pathological complete response (pCR); however, their ability to extend event-free survival still needs to be confirmed. Post-neoadjuvant therapy and post-resection staging (ypStage) have demonstrated that tumor involvement of the lymph nodes (ypN+) is independently linked to a worse outcome. A high tumor burden, indicated by T stage or N2–3 stage, serves as a poor prognostic indicator.

The PRODIGY study has correlated (post hoc analysis) clinical stage (cStage) with post-neoadjuvant stage (ypStage) and formed three groups (Table 7.8).

7.13.1 Immunotherapy

Immune checkpoint inhibitors (ICI) enhance pathologic complete response (pCR), but their effect on survival remains unclear. Tumors with high PD-L1 expression (≥1%) tend to have better outcomes with nivolumab plus chemotherapy. ICI is effective for MSI-high tumors, and neoadjuvant immunotherapy is an option for MSI-high locally advanced gastric cancer (LAGC). The role of adjuvant immunotherapy is still being studied. Nivolumab combined with chemotherapy (CapeOX, FOLFOX, SOX) proves more effective than chemotherapy alone. Dual ICI in MSI-high gastric cancer showed a 58% pCR rate in the GERCOR NEONIPIGA Phase II trial. Future research will compare dual ICI versus ICI plus chemotherapy in MSI-high gastric cancer.

Table 7.7 Results of neoadjuvant stage III trials in Asia

	PRODIGY	RESOLVE	JCOG0501
Target population	cT2/3 N + or cT4N-any	cT4aN + or cT4bNany	Borrmann type 4 or large (≥8 cm) type 3
Treatment	3 cycles of neoadjuvant DOS followed by surgery and adjuvant S-1	3 cycles of neoadjuvant SOX and 5 cycles postoperative SOX followed by 3 cycles of S-1	2 cycles of neoadjuvant SP and adjuvant S-1
Control	Adjuvant S-1	Adjuvant S-1	Adjuvant S-1
R0 resection rate	95% (vs. 84%)	93% (vs. 87%)	80.6% (vs. 66.6%)
pCR rate	10%	5.6%	2%
3-year PFS (DFS)	66.3% (vs. 60.2%)	59.4% (vs. 51.1%)	47.7% (vs. 47.7%)
OS	63.8% (vs. 54.6%) at 8 years	60.0% (vs. 52.1%) at 5 years	60.9% (vs. 62.4%) at 3 years

DOS docetaxel, oxaliplatin, and S-1, *SOX* S-1 plus oxaliplatin, *SP* S-1 plus cisplatin, *CAPOX* capecitabine plus oxaliplatin, *PFS* progression-free survival, *DFS* disease-free survival, *OS* overall survival, *pCR* pathological complete response, *HR* hazard ratio, *CI* confidence interval

Table 7.8 PRODIGY study results (Kim HD, Gastric Cancer, 2024)

	cStage	ypStage	5 year PFS	Surveillance
Group I	II	0/1	95%	Adjuvant therapy may not be required
Group II	Remaining pts		77%	
Group III	III	III	31%	Need to have adjuvant therapy optimization
	IIIC	II	Poor outcomes	

7.13.2 Adjuvant Chemotherapy

Adjuvant chemotherapy is recommended for patients who undergo surgery without prior neoadjuvant therapy and have pT3-pT4 or pN+ disease. Its goal is to decrease recurrence risk by eliminating residual cancer cells. The ACTS-GC trial (2006) in Japan showed that S-1 was more effective than no chemotherapy. For pStage II-III gastric cancer, regimens like CapeOX (CLASSIC trial), S-1 plus docetaxel (JACCRO GC 07 trial), and S-1 plus oxaliplatin (SOX) (ARTIST2 trial) have demonstrated improved disease-free survival (DFS) compared to S-1 alone. For stage-IV gastric cancer with curative resection, adjuvant chemotherapy is weakly recommended due to limited evidence.

7.13.3 Adjuvant Chemoradiotherapy

The INT0116 trial (USA) demonstrated that adjuvant chemoradiotherapy combined with chemotherapy is more effective than surveillance alone. The ARTIST trial (South Korea) found no significant differences in OS or DFS between chemoradiotherapy alone and chemoradiotherapy plus chemotherapy. Subgroup analysis revealed DFS benefits for chemoradiotherapy in patients with positive lymph nodes (LNs). The CRITICS trial (Netherlands) did not find survival benefits from adding radiotherapy to chemotherapy. An analysis from the National Cancer Database showed benefits of adjuvant chemoradiotherapy in patients with positive LNs and lymphovascular invasion. Overall, chemoradiotherapy offers advantages for a small subset of patients.

7.14 Palliative Therapy

More than 50% of patients with GC are diagnosed at an advanced or metastatic stage. The median survival for these patients is 3–5 months. Palliative therapy is recommended for them. The complications and available treatment options are detailed in Tables 7.9, 7.10, and 7.11, Figs. 7.7 and 7.8.

Table 7.9 Complications of GC and palliative therapeutic options

Complication	Endoscopy	RT	Surgery	Chemotherapy/medication/ other
Bleeding	Endoscopic therapy: argon plasma coagulator, forceps coagulation	External radiotherapy	Palliative resection	To shrink the tumor angioembolization
Nausea, vomiting	Evaluate the cause Pyloric stenting Venting gastrostomy	To shrink the tumor	Palliative bypass/gastrectomy	Antiemetics CT to shrink the tumor.
Tumor perforation	–	–	Omental patch closure/ palliative gastrectomy	–

Table 7.10 The algorithm of gastric cancer treatment recommended by the Japanese Gastric Cancer Association (JGCA)

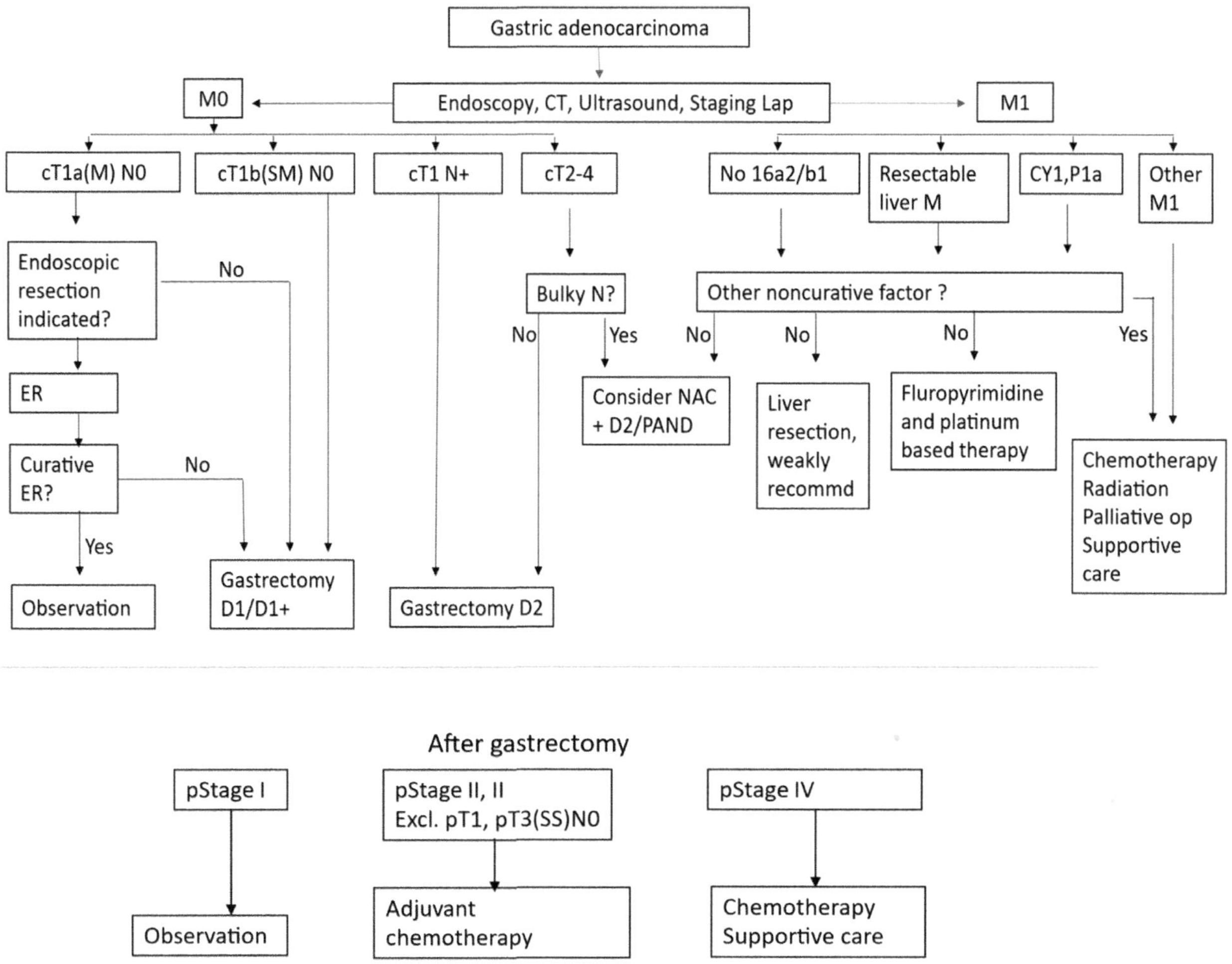

Table 7.11 Five-year overall survival (OS) and disease-specific survival (DSS) for location, stage, and resection type

	5 year OS (%)	5 year DSS (%)
Location		
Upper third	65.4	75
Middle third	79	86
Lower third	70	80
Stage (TNM, AJCC 5th edition)		
Stage IA	91	99
Stage IB	83	93
Stage II	69	79
Stage IIIA	49	58
Stage IIIB	32	38
Stage IV	17	21
Type of surgery		
Distal gastrectomy	77	85
Total gastrectomy	54	62
Proximal gastrectomy	82	92
Pylorus-preserving gastrectomy	93	98
Combined resection		
Yes	59	68
No	77	85
Extent of resection		
D1	68	78
D1 + α (LN station 7)	76	86
D1 + β (LN station 7, 8, and 9)	84	91
D2	70	77
D3	47	54

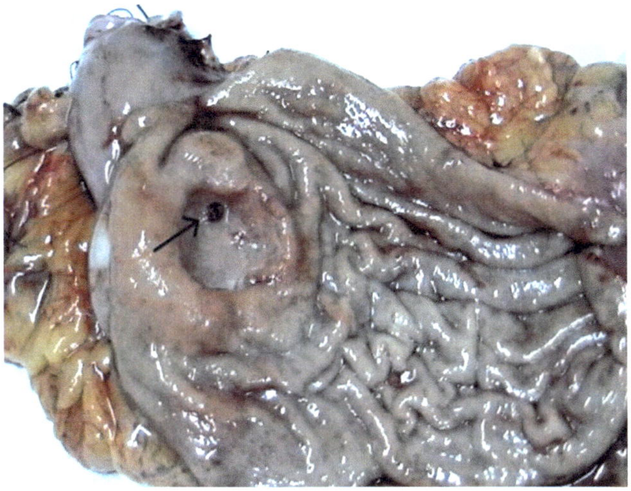

Fig. 7.7 Distal gastrectomy for bleeding malignant ulcer. Note antral ulcer with elevated margin and visible vessel (arrow) at the base

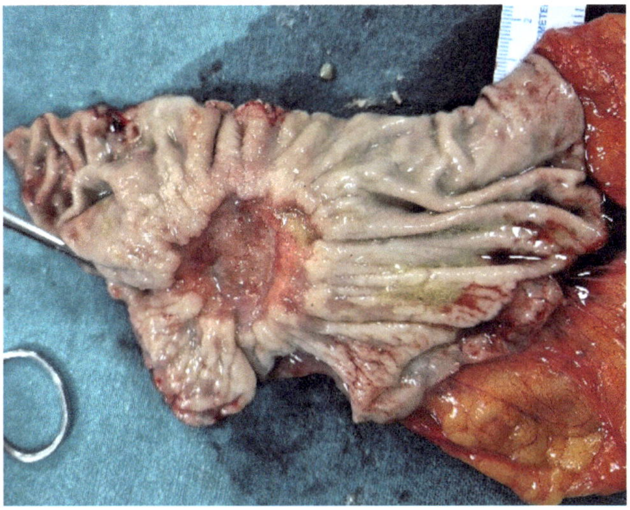

Fig. 7.8 Malignant ulcer in the antrum

Key Points

- Surgery is the main curative treatment for gastric cancer, with the goal of achieving an R0 resection.
- D2 lymphadenectomy is the standard procedure for resectable cancers, providing optimal oncologic outcomes with manageable morbidity.
- Surgery has a limited but evolving role in advanced disease, especially after a good response to neoadjuvant chemotherapy; R0 resection enhances survival in selected patients with limited metastases (e.g., solitary liver metastasis, para-aortic LN involvement).
- Conversion therapy is cautiously recommended after chemotherapy when R0 resection becomes possible, supported by trials like FLOT3 and CONVO-GC-1.
- For LAGC, multivisceral resection may be necessary to achieve R0 status, although it raises morbidity; neoadjuvant therapy enhances resectability and outcomes.
- Perioperative FLOT chemotherapy is the standard in the West, while East Asia prefers D2 surgery followed by S-1 or CapeOX; trials like PRODIGY and RESOLVE support neoadjuvant strategies.
- Immunotherapy (e.g., nivolumab, pembrolizumab) benefits MSI-high and PD-L1+ tumors, especially when combined with chemotherapy; ongoing trials evaluate its effect on survival.
- Postoperative surveillance and adjuvant therapy are crucial in ypN+ or pT3–pT4 cases, while palliative care focuses on managing symptoms and using targeted therapies and chemotherapy to prolong median survival.

Selected Readings

1. Japanese Gastric Cancer Association. Japanese gastric cancer treatment guidelines 2021 (6th edition). Gastric Cancer. 2023;26:1–25.
2. Nakamura T, Hojo Y, Kumamoto T, Kurahashi Y, Ishida Y, Shinohara H. History of the lymph node numbering system in the Japanese Classification of Gastric Carcinoma since 1962. Surg Today. 2022;52:1515–23.
3. Beyer K. Surgery matters: progress in surgical management of gastric cancer. Curr Treat Options in Oncol. 2023;24:108–29.
4. Li GZ, Wang J. The evolution of treatment for resectable gastric cancer. Clin Surg Oncol. 2023;2(1):100008.
5. Morgan AD, Seely KD, Hagenstein LD, Florey GM, Small JM. Bacterial involvement in progression and metastasis of adenocarcinoma of the stomach. Cancers (Basel). 2022;14:4886.

Part II

Small Bowel

Small Bowel Diverticulum

8

Kaushik Bhattacharya

Abstract

A true diverticulum involves all layers of the intestinal wall, while a false diverticulum only includes mucosal and submucosal layers herniating through weak spots in the intestinal wall. Small bowel diverticula are usually asymptomatic and are often found incidentally during laparotomy. Meckel's diverticulum is a true diverticulum, present in 2% of the population. Complications of Meckel's diverticulum include gastrointestinal bleeding (due to ectopic gastric tissue), intussusception, diverticulitis (which can mimic appendicitis), and small bowel obstruction. The Technetium-99 m Pertechnetate Scan (Meckel's Scan) is used to detect ectopic gastric mucosa in cases of bleeding. Wedge excision or segmental excision is recommended for symptomatic Meckel's diverticulum.

Keywords

Jejunal diverticulum · Meckel's diverticulum

The occurrence of small bowel diverticula is relatively uncommon compared to the colon. With a prevalence ranging from 0.3% to 2.3% in the general population, it is distributed as shown in the table below (Table 8.1).

Table 8.1 Distribution of small bowel diverticula

Site	Incidence (%)
Duodenum	05–10
Jejunum	60–70
Jejuno-ileal	20–30
Terminal ileum (Meckel's)	02–04

8.1 Classification and Etiopathogenesis

Congenital (True) Diverticulum: A true diverticulum includes all layers of the intestinal wall. Meckel's diverticulum is considered congenital, caused by the incomplete closure of the vitello-intestinal duct during embryonic development.

Acquired (False) Diverticulum: It occurs when the mucosal and submucosal layers herniate through weak spots in the intestinal wall, such as where mesenteric vessels penetrate the small bowel. Although the exact cause of small bowel diverticulum remains unknown, potential predisposing factors include,

- Peristalsis abnormalities and intestinal spasms
- Intestinal dyskinesia
- High segmental intraluminal pressures

The conditions associated with intestinal diverticula are,

- A diet that is low in fiber and high in red meat
- Obesity
- Age >60 years
- Systemic sclerosis
- Visceral myopathy
- Visceral neuropathy
- Medications, such as nonsteroidal anti-inflammatory drugs, opiates, and steroids (Fig. 8.1)

K. Bhattacharya (✉)
Mata Gujri Memorial Medical College and LSK Hospital,
Kishanganj, Bihar, India

M. Ibrarullah (ed.), *Recent Concepts in Gastrointestinal (GI) Surgery*, https://doi.org/10.1007/978-981-92-1118-0_8

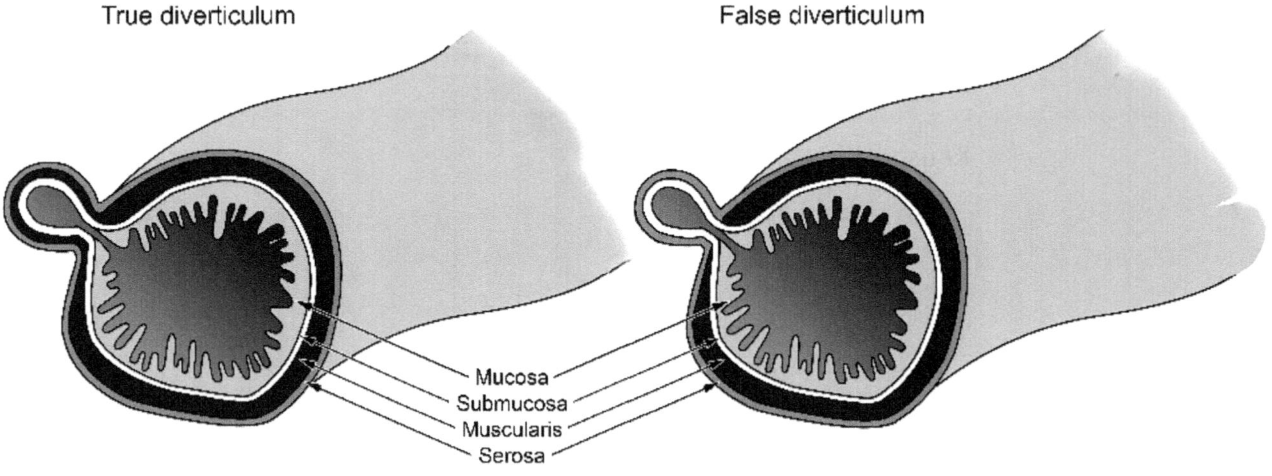

Fig. 8.1 True versus acquired diverticulum

8.2 Clinical Presentation

Small bowel diverticula are often found incidentally during imaging or laparotomy. Uncomplicated diverticula may lead to nonspecific abdominal pain, bloating, or changes in bowel habits.

8.2.1 Complications

- More than two-thirds of duodenal diverticula are located around the ampulla of Vater. These can lead to biliary dyskinesia, dilation of the common bile duct, biliary stone formation, and recurrent pancreatitis.
- Diverticulitis (20–40%): Inflammation, mass, or abscess formation presenting with abdominal pain, fever, and localized tenderness.
- Perforation and peritonitis (5–10%).
- Bleeding (10–20%): it may present with occult bleeding and anemia or intermittent to massive lower gastrointestinal bleeding.
- Obstruction (10–20%): Mechanical obstruction results from diverticular inflammation or adhesions.
- Fistula formation: Enterocutaneous fistula and entero-enteric fistula result from recurrent inflammation.
- Malabsorption syndrome: Caused by bacterial overgrowth in diverticula, presenting with diarrhea, flatulence, and weight loss.

8.3 Diagnosis

Juxta-ampullary diverticula are identified using a side-viewing endoscope during diagnostic or therapeutic procedures for biliary or pancreatic conditions.

Investigations are needed for symptomatic or complicated intestinal diverticula. Contrast-enhanced CT scan of the abdomen and CT enteroclysis help diagnose diverticula and detect any inflammatory mass with or without perforation.

Magnetic resonance enterography/enteroclysis (MRE) imaging of intestinal diverticulitis typically reveals the presence of multiple diverticula, as well as asymmetric, focal mesenteric, and mural inflammation.

A double-contrast barium meal and enteroclysis help diagnose intestinal diverticula but are contraindicated in cases of acute diverticulitis or perforation.

Double balloon enteroscopy, angiography, and bleeding scan are helpful in cases of lower GI bleeding (Figs. 8.2 and 8.3).

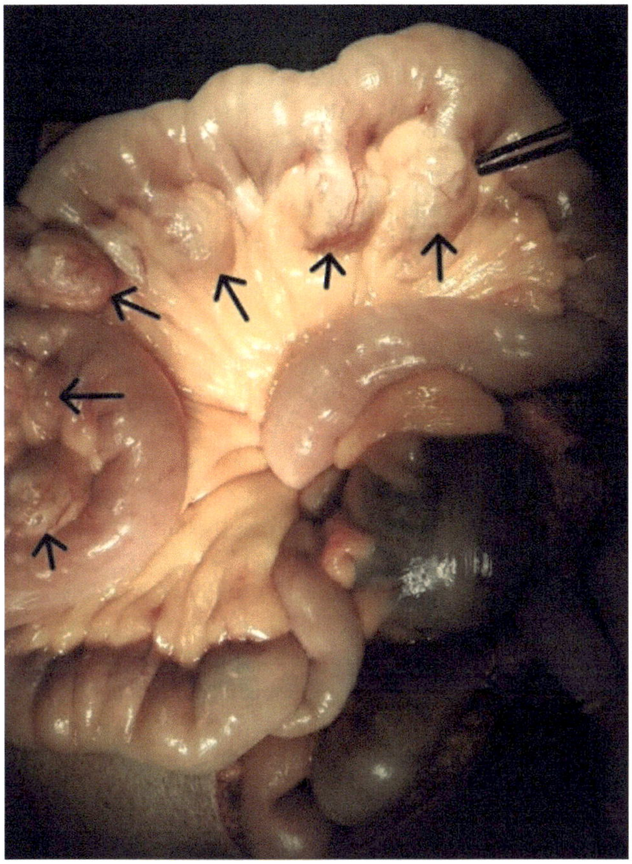

Fig. 8.2 Multiple jejunal diverticula found on the mesenteric border (arrows)

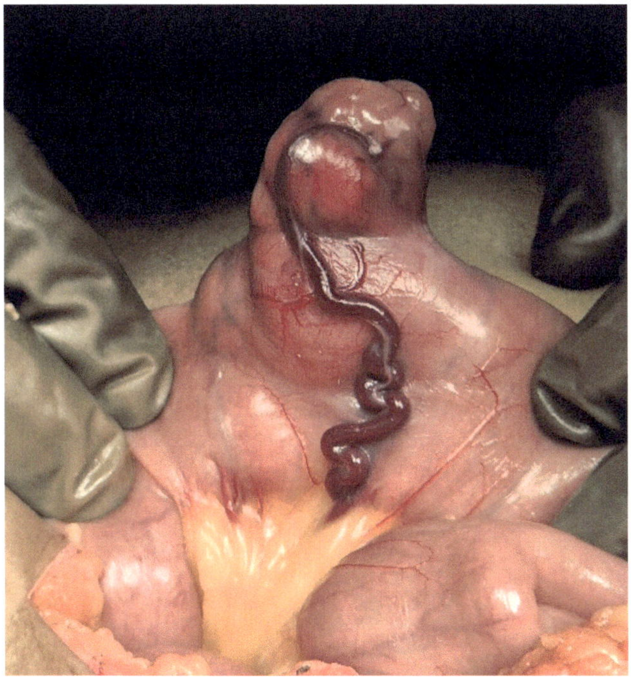

Fig. 8.3 Incidental detection of Meckel's diverticulum during laparotomy

8.4 Treatment

Nonspecific symptoms like flatulence, abdominal bloating, or cramps are managed conservatively with antispasmodics, GI prokinetics, and antiflatulent medications.

Acute diverticulitis is managed with complete bowel rest, intravenous fluids, and broad-spectrum antibiotics.

Perforation and peritonitis require emergency laparotomy. Simple closure of perforation and diverticulopexy can be done by inverting the diverticulum and approximating the intestinal wall. A segmental excision of the intestine and repair might be necessary for a severely inflamed and thickened segment.

GI bleeding poses a major challenge in locating the problematic diverticulum. Intraoperative enteroscopy can be helpful. When the diverticulum cannot be identified, resection and anastomosis of the most diverticulum-bearing segment of the intestine are recommended. However, for widespread disease, diverticulopexy of all visible diverticula, though tedious and meticulous, is advised. The neck of the diverticulum is dissected all around along the mesenteric border, carefully separating the mesenteric fat and tiny blood vessels. A purse-string suture around the neck near the intestinal muscular wall closes off the diverticulum and any blood vessels within its wall. Small diverticula can be carefully dissected from the mesentery and inverted using a purse-string or interrupted sutures to approximate the intestinal wall.

Entero-cutaneous or entero-enteric fistulas require excision and repair of the involved segment.

8.5 Meckel's Diverticulum

Meckel's diverticulum is a true diverticulum of the small intestine caused by incomplete obliteration of the vitello-intestinal duct. It is located in the distal ileum, about 60–100 cm from the ileocecal valve, and may contain ectopic gastric mucosa that secretes acid. Long diverticula (height-to-diameter ratio >2) have ectopic tissue at the body and tip, while short diverticula have ectopic tissue distributed throughout, including the base (Table 8.2).

Table 8.2 Meckel's diverticulum, the 'rule of 2'

Occurs in 2% of the population
Male-to-female ratio 2:1
Located approximately 2 feet from the ileocecal junction
Typically, 2 inches long
Mucosa may contain 2 types of ectopic tissue (gastric or pancreatic)

8.6 Clinical Presentation

Meckel's diverticulum is usually asymptomatic and often discovered incidentally during laparotomy. The complication rate is about 4%, including gastrointestinal bleeding (due to ectopic gastric tissue) in 25–50%, intussusception in 10%, diverticulitis mimicking appendicitis in 10–20%, and small bowel obstruction in 10–40% of symptomatic cases. Intestinal obstruction typically results from intussusception, volvulus, a mesodiverticular band, or adhesions around the diverticulum, and rarely from stricture or perforation. Fewer than 1% of cases may develop benign tumors, such as leiomyomas, or malignant tumors like carcinoid, adenocarcinoma, or sarcoma within the diverticulum.

8.7 Diagnosis

Diagnostic tests are required for symptomatic cases of Meckel's diverticulum. The investigations employed are,

- Technetium-99 m Pertechnetate Scan (Meckel's Scan): Used especially in patients with lower GI bleeding. A positive scan confirms the presence of ectopic gastric mucosa in the diverticulum, causing ulceration and bleeding.
- CT or MRI enterography.
- Diagnostic laparoscopy.

8.8 Management

Indications for surgery in Meckel's diverticulum are,

- Symptomatic or presenting with complications
- Diverticulum >2 cm/narrow base /thick wall
- Presence of ectopic tissue (e.g., gastric, pancreatic)
- Children (<18 years)*
- Adults with high-risk features (e.g., family history of cancer)*

**Relative indications of surgery*

Conservative treatment is recommended for incidentally discovered Meckel's diverticulum unless the indications listed above are present. Diverticulectomy may be considered for a long diverticulum, making sure the intestinal lumen is not compromised after its excision. Wedge excision or segmental excision is advised for a symptomatic diverticulum. When performing wedge excision for bleeding, the excised margin and the intestinal mucosa should be inspected for any ulcer or bleeding point, as these often occur at the junction of normal and ectopic gastric mucosa.

Key Points

- The jejunum is the most common site for small bowel diverticula.
- A true diverticulum involves all layers of the intestinal wall, while a false diverticulum only includes mucosal and submucosal layers herniating through weak spots in the intestinal wall.
- Small bowel diverticula are usually asymptomatic and are often found incidentally during laparotomy.
- They may experience complications such as diverticulitis, bleeding, perforation, and peritonitis.
- Meckel's diverticulum is a true diverticulum, present in 2% of the population.
- Complications of Meckel's diverticulum include gastrointestinal bleeding (due to ectopic gastric tissue), intussusception, diverticulitis (which can mimic appendicitis), and small bowel obstruction.
- The Technetium-99 m Pertechnetate Scan (Meckel's Scan) is used to detect ectopic gastric mucosa in cases of bleeding.
- Wedge excision or segmental excision is recommended for symptomatic Meckel's diverticulum.
- When found incidentally, it should be removed if it is long, has a thick wall, or has a narrow base.

Selected Reading

1. Sagar J, Kumar V, Shah DK. Meckel's diverticulum: a systematic review. J R Soc Med. 2006;99(10):501–5. https://doi.org/10.1258/jrsm.99.10.501.
2. Lequet J, Menahem B, Alves A, Fohlen A, Mulliri A. Meckel's diverticulum in the adult. J Visc Surg. 2017;154:253–9.

Gastrointestinal Stromal Tumors

9

Keng Xin Yi, Shao Qian Lian, Sean Siwei Li, and Vishal G. Shelat

Abstract

Gastrointestinal stromal tumors (GISTs) are the most common mesenchymal tumors of the GI tract. GISTs most often present with upper gastrointestinal bleeding, anemia, or abdominal pain, but small tumors may be asymptomatic. Diagnosis depends on a combination of imaging techniques (CT, MRI, PET, EUS), histopathology, immunohistochemistry (for CD117, CD34, DOG1), and molecular genetic testing to identify specific mutations and guide treatment. Complete surgical removal with clear margins (R0 resection) is the standard treatment for localized GIST. Adjuvant imatinib therapy for 3 years is recommended for high-risk localized GIST patients with sensitive driver mutations (excluding PDGFRA exon 18 D842V). Imatinib is the standard first-line treatment for unresectable or metastatic GIST; sunitinib is the standard second-line therapy. The most important prognostic factors for GIST are mitotic rate, tumor size, and tumor location; tumor rupture is an adverse prognostic factor.

Keywords

GIST · Stromal tumor

Gastrointestinal Stromal Tumors (GISTs) are the most common mesenchymal tumors of the gastrointestinal (GI) tract. These subepithelial tumors originate from the interstitial cells of Cajal in the intramuscular layer of the bowel wall. Most GISTs develop in the stomach (about 60%) and the small intestine (around 35%), but they can also be found in the esophagus, colon, rectum, omentum, and mesentery.

The term "GIST" was introduced by Mazur and Clark in 1983, identifying the origin of these tumors as the interstitial cells of Cajal. It wasn't until 1998 that Hirota and colleagues linked c-KIT (receptor tyrosine-protein kinase) mutations, present in most GISTs, to their development. Before 2000, GISTs were often misclassified as other GI soft tissue tumors, such as leiomyomas, leiomyosarcomas, or schwannomas. Research indicates that individuals with GISTs are at a higher risk of developing other cancers, such as colorectal, pancreatic, and breast cancer.

9.1 Epidemiology

GISTs comprise about 1–2% of all GI tumors, with an annual incidence of 10–15 cases per million people. Their incidence increases with age, with a median diagnosis age of 60–65 years worldwide. They are rare in individuals under 40 and are often linked to specific genetic syndromes (see "Associated Syndromes"). GISTs show a slight male predominance, with a global male-to-female ratio of about 1.2:1, rising to 1.5:1 in Asia. Most GISTs occur sporadically, without a family history. Rare familial cases are often associated with KIT or platelet-derived growth factor receptor alpha (PDGFRA) gene mutations. PDGFRA mutations are more common in East Asian populations than in Western populations, influencing treatment outcomes, as PDGFRA-mutated GISTs respond differently to therapies like Imatinib.

9.2 Pathogenesis

Most GISTs test positive for CD-117 (c-KIT) and PDGFRA mutations. About 70–80% of GISTs have KIT mutations, while 10–15% have PDGFRA mutations. Gain-of-function mutations in these genes activate downstream signalling pathways, specifically the RAS/RAF/MAPK and PI3K/

K. X. Yi · S. Q. Lian · S. S. Li
Lee Kong Chain School of Medicine, Nanyang Technological University, Singapore, Singapore

V. G. Shelat (✉)
Department of General Surgery, Surgical Science Training Centre, Tan Tock Seng Hospital, Singapore, Singapore

M. Ibrarullah (ed.), *Recent Concepts in Gastrointestinal (GI) Surgery*, https://doi.org/10.1007/978-981-92-1118-0_9

AKT/mTOR pathways, leading to uncontrolled growth signalling and tumor development. Mutations can occur sporadically or be inherited. Notably, Neurofibromin 1 (NF1) inhibits the RAS/RAF/MEK/MAPK pathway, acting as a tumor suppressor gene in GISTs, which is why patients with Neurofibromatosis Type 1 are at high risk of developing GISTs.

In cases where there is no KIT or PDGFRA mutation, succinate dehydrogenase (SDH) deficiency is the next most common cause of GIST development. SDH deficiency causes succinate to build up, which triggers abnormal DNA methylation and increases HIF1-alpha levels. This promotes GIST development through faulty growth signalling, involving DNA methylation, and promotes unchecked cell proliferation and angiogenesis through the upregulation of HIF1-alpha.

In rare cases, GIST tumors can develop without mutations in KIT, PDGFRA, or deficiencies in the SDH signalling pathway. These tumors are called wild-type GISTs, and their development occurs independently of the RAS/RAF/MAPK and PI3K/AKT/mTOR pathways.

9.3 Clinical Presentation

Clinical presentations of GISTs vary widely and depend on the tumor's location, size, and whether it is primary or metastatic. Smaller tumors may be asymptomatic and are often discovered incidentally during other imaging procedures such as CT scans, endoscopy, or surgery. The clinical presentation of GIST is usually related to larger size or complications within the tumor. Nonspecific symptoms include anorexia, weight loss, abdominal pain, distention, or a palpable mass. GI bleeding is the most common complication in luminal GISTs regardless of the site. Bleeding may be severe and result from mucosal ulceration at the tumor's apex. Other organ-specific symptoms are listed in Table 9.1 below.

Metastatic disease (10–20% of patients), often involving the liver, omentum, or peritoneum, may lead to abdominal pain, bowel obstruction, or lymphatic involvement. In rare cases, the tumor may metastasize to abdominal lymph nodes, regions outside the abdominal cavity, or the lungs. Advanced GISTs may cause severe hypoglycemia and hypothyroidism.

Table 9.1 Summary of symptoms based on location of GIST

Primary tumor	Incidence (%)	Symptoms
Esophagus	01	GI bleeding, dysphagia, vomiting
Stomach	64	GI bleeding, abdominal pain, dyspepsia, vomiting Obstruct the pylorus or duodenum by a pedunculated tumor
Small intestine	30	Obstructive jaundice (duodenum), GI bleeding, abdominal pain, intestinal obstruction
Colon/ rectum	05	Constipation, GI bleeding, bowel obstruction, urinary hesitancy in men

9.4 Diagnosis

Diagnosis of GISTs depends on clinical, radiological, histopathological, immunohistochemical, and molecular genetic features. The tumor can be biopsied, such as with a CT-guided biopsy, for a definitive diagnosis. Histopathology and immunohistochemistry should be performed on biopsy samples to confirm the diagnosis of GIST and its subtype.

9.4.1 Imaging Techniques

Computed Tomography (CT) Scan: Contrast-enhanced CT is the primary imaging modality for diagnosing and staging GIST, effectively evaluating tumor size, location, extent, and liver or peritoneal metastases. GIST usually appears as well-defined, enhancing masses; larger lesions may show central necrosis or cavitation. While small GISTs demonstrate uniform enhancement, their nonspecific features and rarity often lead to initial misdiagnoses (e.g., pancreatic cancer, esophageal cancer, and lymphoma). A well-defined exophytic gastric mass may raise suspicion (Fig. 9.1).

Magnetic Resonance Imaging (MRI): On MRI, GISTs appear as low signal intensity on T1-weighted images and high signal intensity on T2-weighted images, with increased signal after gadolinium contrast is administered. Its superior soft tissue contrast makes it effective for detecting tumors in the rectum and assessing liver metastases. MRI also provides valuable quantitative metrics, including the apparent diffusion coefficient (ADC) and degree of enhancement, which can help monitor treatment response.

Positron Emission Tomography (PET): 18F-fluorodeoxyglucose (FDG) PET can help classify histopathological risk and monitor treatment response to TKIs. FDG-PET has high sensitivity and specificity for restaging, but false-positive results may occur due to concurrent inflammatory issues, especially after surgery. A decrease in FDG uptake indicates an effective therapeutic response.

Endoscopic Ultrasonography (EUS): EUS offers more detailed imaging of the tumor. For tumors smaller than 2 cm, EUS reveals homogeneous hypoechoic masses with smooth margins originating from the muscularis propria. A lobulated margin may suggest malignancy. However, distinguishing GISTs from other submucosal tumors can be difficult due to overlapping EUS features.

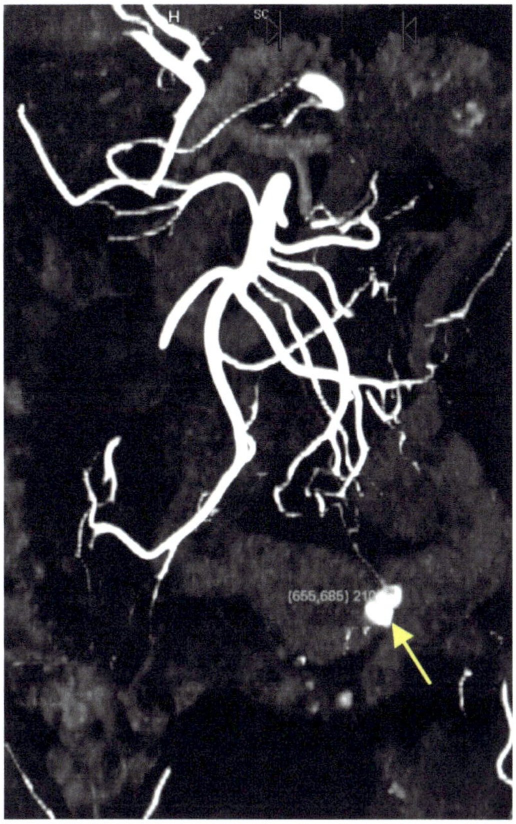

Fig. 9.1 CT angiography showing a well-enhancing small bowel GIST (arrow)

Histopathology: A comprehensive diagnosis of GIST requires a biopsy, ideally using both formalin-fixed paraffin-embedded (FFPE) and fresh-frozen tissue samples for histopathological and molecular genetic analyses. Microscopically, GIST tumor cells can exhibit three different morphological types.

- Spindle cell type (70%): The most common type, consisting of elongated nuclei, eosinophilic cytoplasm in a syncytial pattern
- Epithelioid type (20–25%): Round or polygonal cells with clear to eosinophilic cytoplasm in sheets or nests, seen more often in tumors with *PDGFRA* mutations and a higher tendency for pleomorphism than the spindle type
- Mixed type (10%): Features of both spindle and epithelioid cells

Immunohistochemistry (IHC): Immunohistochemical staining is essential for confirming a GIST diagnosis. KIT (CD117) is the most sensitive and specific marker for GIST, detected in about 95% of tumors. CD34 is expressed in 60–70% of GISTs. Although less specific, it remains valuable in the diagnostic panel. GISTs located in the esophagus and rectum are mostly CD34-positive (95–100%). Smooth muscle actin (SMA) is positive in approximately 30% and is linked to a better prognosis in gastric and small intestinal GISTs. DOG1 (Discovered on GIST-1) is highly sensitive and specific for GIST, including some KIT-negative cases. It is particularly useful in PDGFRA-mutant GISTs, which may not express KIT. Positivity for Desmin and S100 protein is uncommon.

Molecular genetic testing is essential for confirming the diagnosis and guiding treatment options, especially for patients considered for targeted therapies with TKIs like Imatinib. Testing typically involves identifying mutations in the KIT or PDGFRA genes. GISTs without mutations in KIT or PDGFRA are classified as wild-type and may harbor other genetic changes such as BRAF or NF1 mutations. These tumors often respond less well to TKI therapy.

9.5 Fletcher's and Miettinen's Classifications

Fletcher's and Miettinen's classifications provide risk stratification models based on tumor size, location, and mitotic activity. These classifications assist in predicting the malignant potential of GISTs. Fletcher Classification (2002) classifies GISTs into risk groups according to tumor size and mitotic figures, which refers to the number of mitotic cells per 50 high-power fields (HPF).

- Very low risk: Tumor size less than 2 cm and fewer than 5 mitotic figures.
- Low-risk: Tumors with a size of 2–5 cm and fewer than 5 mitotic figures.
- Intermediate-risk: Tumor size less than 5 cm or 6–10 mitotic figures; or size 5–10 cm with fewer than 5 mitotic figures.
- High risk: Tumor larger than 5 cm, more than 5 mitotic figures, or any size with over 10 mitotic figures.

Miettinen's Classification (2006) offers a more precise risk stratification by considering tumor size, mitotic rate, and the anatomical site of GIST. Risk levels—very low, low, intermediate, and high—are assigned based on how these factors interact. For example, small tumors (<2 cm) with a low mitotic rate (<5/50 HPF) are classified as very low risk regardless of location. However, larger tumors in specific areas, such as a 5–10 cm tumor in the rectum, would be categorized as higher risk even with a lower mitotic count.

9.6 Management

Optimal GIST management requires a team approach involving a multidisciplinary group, including pathologists, radiologists, surgeons, medical oncologists, gastroenterologists, and nuclear medicine specialists, to ensure comprehensive patient care. Treatment decisions are guided by the European Society of Medical Oncology (ESMO) Scale for Clinical Actionability of Molecular Targets (ESCAT) and the ESMO-Magnitude of Clinical Benefit Scale (ESMO-MCBS), which provide a structured framework to evaluate the clinical utility and benefits of available therapies. Treatment plans are personalized based on specific molecular markers (KIT, PDGFRA, NTRK, BRAF, SDH) identified through genetic testing. Surgical removal aims for complete tumor excision with clear margins. For unresectable GISTs, preoperative Imatinib can facilitate subsequent surgical removal, aligning with risk assessment and tumor characteristics.

9.6.1 Pharmacological Treatment

GISTs are highly resistant to conventional cytotoxic chemotherapy, probably because of their increased expression of P-glycoprotein and MRP1, which are cellular efflux pumps that prevent these agents from achieving effective intracellular concentrations.

Tyrosine Kinase Inhibitors (TKIs) are highly effective in treating GISTs. By selectively blocking abnormal signaling pathways associated with GIST development, TKIs can cause rapid tumor shrinkage and are used when surgery is not feasible (e.g., very large tumors, hard-to-reach tumors that are borderline resectable, metastatic disease). Imatinib is the first-line treatment for GISTs with KIT or PDGFRA mutations but is usually avoided in wild-type GISTs (SDH-deficient or NF1-related) due to high resistance rates. Avapritinib is the first-line therapy for PDGFRA D842V mutations. Sunitinib, Regorafenib, and Ripretinib are second-line options for KIT/PDGFRA-mutant GISTs. The use of TKIs can cause potential side effects like fluid retention and pancreatitis, which require monitoring.

Preoperative Imatinib therapy can facilitate surgical resection, potentially reducing intraoperative bleeding and rupture risks, especially in cases with borderline resectable disease. Resection decisions after TKI treatment should consider the possible benefits, such as delaying disease progression and lowering complications, versus the risks linked with additional surgery. For treating advanced and metastatic GISTs, initial therapy starts with Imatinib 400 mg daily, following an assessment of the tumor's mutation status. Dosage and follow-up treatment options, like Avapritinib or other TKIs or clinical trials, are tailored based on whether the tumor has KIT, PDGFRA, or wild-type mutations, and whether the disease is symptomatic or rapidly progressing. For KIT and PDGFRA wild-type GIST, Sunitinib and Regorafenib are options, along with participation in clinical research.

Response to treatment is typically assessed using serial imaging. Traditional response criteria (Response Evaluation Criteria in Solid Tumors (RECIST)) may not fully capture the response to targeted therapy in GIST. Alternatively, Choi criteria, which consider changes in tumor density (Hounsfield units on CT scans) along with size reduction, often give a more accurate picture of the response to targeted therapy. It addresses the limitations of RECIST in evaluating GIST response because of the often irregular shape and heterogeneous nature of these tumors.

For advanced GISTs that cannot be removed surgically, continuous therapy is recommended until the disease progresses or for life if it remains stable. This is because stopping Imatinib treatment often leads to rapid disease progression in most patients with advanced GISTs.

9.6.2 Surgical Treatment

Surgical resection remains the primary treatment for GIST. For tumors smaller than 2 cm with five or fewer mitotic figures per 50 HPF, endoscopic monitoring may suffice due to their slow growth and low metastatic risk. Surgery aims for complete gross resection with an intact pseudocapsule and clear microscopic margins. Minimally invasive methods, such as laparoscopy and robotic-assisted surgery, offer benefits like reduced morbidity and quicker recovery. However, their application is limited by tumor size, location, and the surgeon's experience, with open surgery still favored for large or complex tumors. Wide excision is usually unnecessary because GISTs are typically well-encapsulated and minimally invasive. Lymphadenectomy is generally not needed unless dealing with SDH-deficient GISTs or enlarged lymph nodes. Neoadjuvant Imatinib may shrink unresectable tumors to enable subsequent removal.

Contrary to earlier beliefs, R1 resection (microscopic involvement) in GIST is not a significant independent risk factor for recurrence unless accompanied by tumor rupture. Tumor rupture, not R1 margins, is the primary driver of recurrence in GIST. The 2021 ESMO guidelines no longer recommend routine re-excision after R1 resection in the absence of tumor rupture. The main goal of GIST resection is R0 (complete removal with clear margins), but the surgeon should weigh the potential morbidity and benefits based on each patient's situation. Intraoperative tumor rupture is a serious complication during GIST surgery, potentially increasing the risk of recurrence. To reduce this risk, meticulous surgical technique, careful handling of the tumor, and measures to prevent spillage are essential (Figs. 9.2, 9.3, and 9.4).

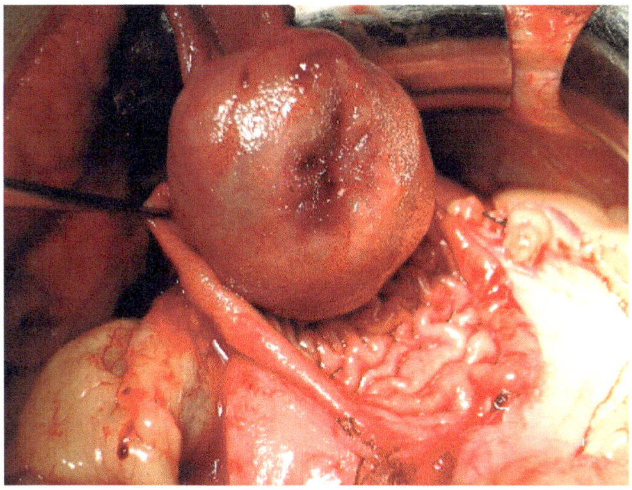

Fig. 9.2 Gastric submucosal GIST with a central ulceration

9.6.3 Palliative Treatment

Since most GISTs are potentially curable with surgery and respond well to TKIs like Imatinib, palliative measures are rarely needed. In very rare cases, radiation therapy may be used for patients with painful metastasis or unresectable bleeding tumors. Complete removal of metastatic lesions, when possible, improves outcomes in Imatinib-responsive patients. In advanced GIST, cytoreductive surgery might help manage symptoms such as unresectable bleeding or obstruction, or be considered in cases with a complete response to systemic therapy and limited residual disease. However, the decision to perform cytoreductive surgery should be carefully assessed based on patient factors, tumor burden, and surgical feasibility.

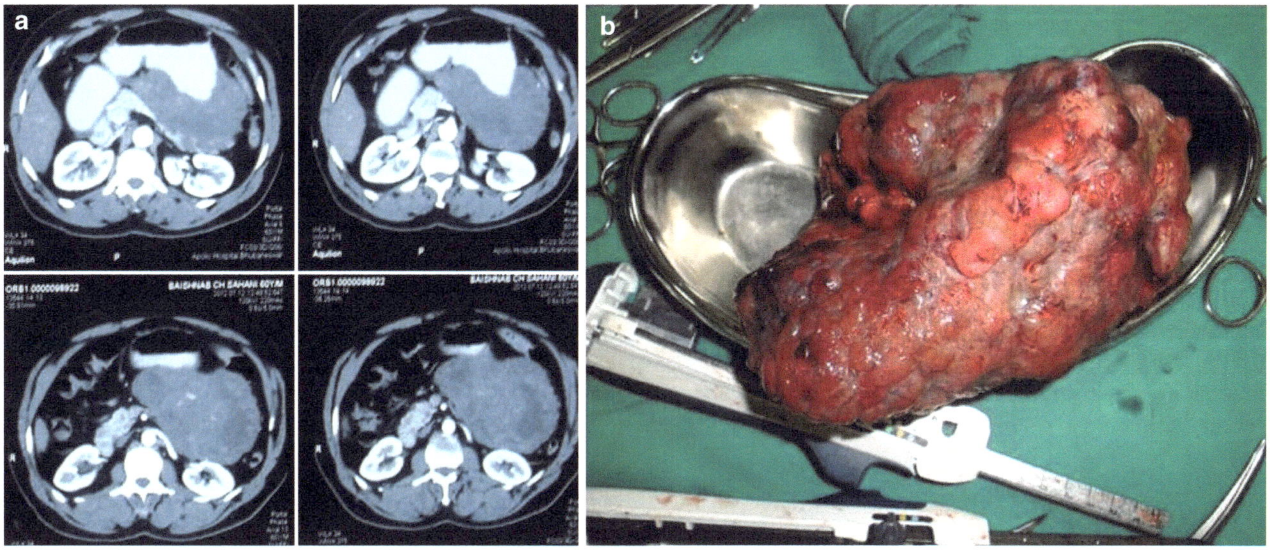

Fig. 9.3 (**a**) Large subserosal pedunculated gastric GIST on CT scan, (**b**) Same tumor after removal

Fig. 9.4 (**a**) CT scan showing small bowel GIST (arrow) (**b**) Segment of the intestine containing the tumor

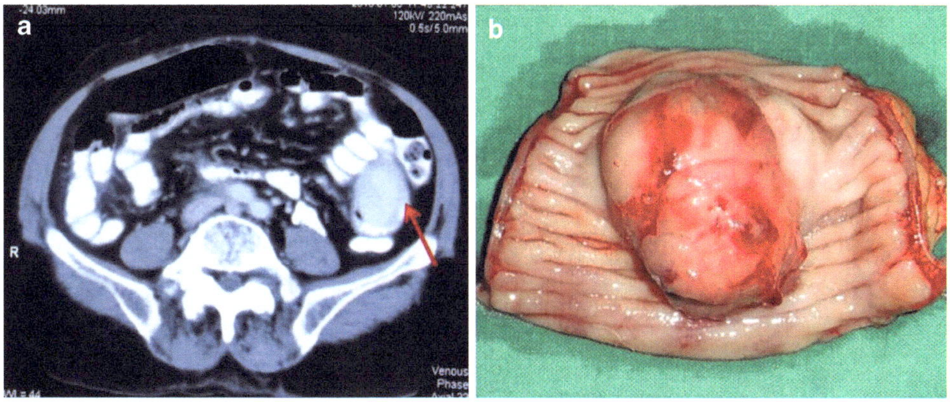

9.7 Follow-Up and Surveillance

Post-treatment surveillance protocols differ among institutions but often include routine imaging (CT/MRI) and clinical assessments, tailored to individual tumor characteristics and recurrence risk. Risk stratification models (National Institutes of Health [NIH], Armed Forces Institute of Pathology [AFIP], Joensuu, Memorial Sloan Kettering Cancer Center [MSKCC] nomogram) assist in predicting the chance of recurrence. These models consider factors like tumor size, mitotic rate, location, and rupture status.

Response evaluation should go beyond simply measuring tumor size; it also includes assessing density changes on imaging, FDG-PET uptake, and the absence of progression. For completely resected GISTs, the National Comprehensive Cancer Network (NCCN) guidelines recommend follow-up with medical history, physical examinations, and CT scans every 3–6 months for the first 5 years, then annually afterward. For locally advanced or metastatic GISTs on Imatinib, follow-up involves medical history, physical examinations, full blood counts, serum phosphate levels, and CT scans every 3–6 months.

ESMO guidelines emphasize the importance of risk stratification. Patients on adjuvant Imatinib undergo CT/MRI scans every 3–6 months during the first 3 years, then every 3 months for the following 2 years, and finally every 6–12 months for the next 8 years. For low-risk tumors, the benefit of elective surveillance with scans every 6–12 months over 5 years remains uncertain. Those with very low-risk tumors only need a single CT scan 2 years after treatment. Routine follow-up is not recommended in these cases.

9.8 Prognosis

Prognosis in GIST depends on various factors, including tumor size, location, mitotic rate, and genetic mutations. The location of the GIST (gastric vs. small bowel) is correlated with specific genetic mutations and influences prognosis (Table 9.2).

Table 9.2 Prognosis based on specific genetic mutation

Genetic mutation	Prognosis
KIT exon 8	Better response to Imatinib as they are found upstream to the Imatinib target site
KIT exon 9	Unfavorable prognosis, requiring high-dose Imatinib
KIT exon 11	These tumors often have high mitotic counts and a high risk of recurrence, but are sensitive to Imatinib
KIT exon 13	Often more aggressive in gastric than intestinal GISTs, they can be resistant to Imatinib but respond to Sunitinib
KIT exon 17	Higher resistance rates to Imatinib
PDGFRA exon 14	It also has a better prognosis and is sensitive to Imatinib
PDGFRA exon 18	Low mitotic count and favorable prognosis. There may be resistance to most TKIs, but patients may respond to Avapritinib
PDGFRA D842V substitution (exon 18)	Confers resistance to Imatinib and Sunitinib. May require alternative TKIs like Dasatinib and Crenolanib

9.9 Associated Syndromes

While most GISTs are sporadic, certain syndromes predispose individuals to developing GISTs due to specific molecular defects. Recognizing these syndromes through genotyping can aid in planning diagnostic, prognostic, and treatment strategies. These syndromes should be considered whenever there are multiple GISTs or associated signs (Table 9.3).

Table 9.3 Summary of syndromes associated with GISTs

	KIT-mutant syndrome	PDGFRA-mutant syndrome	NF1-associated GISTs	Syndromic SDH-deficient GISTs
Location	4q12	4q12	17q11.2	1p36.13 1q23.3 5p15.33 11q23.1
Inheritance pattern	Autosomal dominant	Autosomal dominant	Autosomal dominant	Autosomal dominant
Epidemiology	Male: Female 1:1	Male: Female 4:11	Mean age of diagnosis: 49 years Makes up 1.5% of all GISTs	5% of all GISTs
Typical location of GIST	Entire GI tract	–	Intestines Occasionally in the stomach	Stomach (particularly the antrum)
Typical histopathology	Spindle/ Epithelioid/ Mixed cytology	Epithelioid	Spindle/ Epithelioid/ Mixed cytology	Epithelioid
Typical Immuno-histochemistry	*CD117+* *DOG1+*	*DOG1+* *CD117+/–*	*CD117+*	*DOG1+* *CD34+* *CD117+*
Associated symptoms/signs	Hyperpigmentation Diffuse ICCH[3] Hypopigmentation Melanomas	Inflammatory fibroid polyps GI lipomas Large hands	ICCH Gastrointestinal motility disorders Neuroendocrine tumors	Carney's triad Carney-Stratakis Syndrome[5]
Penetrance	High penetrance	High penetrance	Incidence of 1 in 3000 births	Complete penetrance Variable expression
Complications/ prognosis	More likely to suffer from frequent and severe gut occlusion/hemorrhage (present with more tumors)	May require alternative TKIs, Dasatinib and Crenolanib	Mostly indolent (≤15–20% are aggressive) Respond poorly to Imatinib (should never be treated with adjuvant Imatinib)	Typically, indolent Frequent relapses even after radical surgery due to high rates of lymph vascular invasion (≤50%) and LN metastasis (≤10%) TKIs like Imatinib and Sunitinib are only partially effective.

ICCH Interstitial cells of Cajal Hyperplasia, *Carney's Triad* Paragangliomas, GISTs, Pulmonary chondromas, *Carney-Stratakis Syndrome* Paragangliomas and GISTs without pulmonary chondromas, *TKI* Tyrosine Kinase Inhibitors, *LN* Lymph node

Key Points

- Gastrointestinal stromal tumors (GISTs) are the most common mesenchymal tumors of the GI tract. Most arise sporadically.
- GISTs most often present with upper gastrointestinal bleeding, anemia, or abdominal pain, but small tumors may be asymptomatic.
- Diagnosis depends on a combination of imaging techniques (CT, MRI, PET, EUS), histopathology, immunohistochemistry (for CD117, CD34, DOG1), and molecular genetic testing to identify specific mutations and guide treatment.
- Complete surgical removal with clear margins (R0 resection) is the standard treatment for localized GIST.
- Adjuvant imatinib therapy for 3 years is recommended for high-risk localized GIST patients with sensitive driver mutations (excluding PDGFRA exon 18 D842V).
- Imatinib is the standard first-line treatment for unresectable or metastatic GIST; sunitinib is the standard second-line therapy.
- Ripretinib and Avapritinib are used later in the disease course for specific mutations and may require special access or funding.
- The most important prognostic factors for GIST are mitotic rate, tumor size, and tumor location; tumor rupture is an adverse prognostic factor.
- Regular follow-up is essential, though optimal schedules remain unclear, particularly for low-risk patients, and should be tailored to the patient's risk stratification.

Selected Reading

1. Li J, Khajoueinejad N, Sarpel U. Surgical management of gastric gastrointestinal stromal tumors. Surg Clin North Am. 2025;105(1):109–24. https://doi.org/10.1016/j.suc.2024.06.009.
2. Judson I, Jones RL, Wong NACS, et al. Gastrointestinal stromal tumour (GIST): British sarcoma group clinical practice guidelines. Br J Cancer. 2024. https://doi.org/10.1038/s41416-024-02672-0.
3. Blay JY, Hindi N, Bollard J, et al. SELNET clinical practice guidelines for soft tissue sarcoma and GIST. Cancer Treat Rev. 2022;102:102312. https://doi.org/10.1016/j.ctrv.2021.102312. Epub 2021 Nov 14. Erratum in: Cancer Treat Rev. 2023; 115:102523. https://doi.org/10.1016/j.ctrv.2023.102523.
4. Brinch CM, Aggerholm-Pedersen N, Hogdall E, et al. Medical oncological treatment for patients with gastrointestinal stromal tumor (GIST) - a systematic review. Crit Rev Oncol Hematol. 2022;172:103650. https://doi.org/10.1016/j.critrevonc.2022.103650.

Short Bowel Syndrome

10

Laxminarayan Mohanty and Mohammad Ibrarullah

Abstract

Short bowel syndrome (SBS) occurs when less than 200 cm of small intestine remains in adults or less than 25% of the intestine in children. The three phases of SBS are the acute phase (up to 4 weeks), the adaptive phase (1–2 years), and the maintenance phase (beyond 2 years). Malnutrition, diarrhea, nephrolithiasis, and gallstone formation are some of the key complications of SBS. Small bowel transplant is the most definitive procedure for SBS, often performed along with liver transplantation for liver failure.

Keywords

Short bowel syndrome · Intestinal failure · Small bowel transplant

Short bowel syndrome (SBS) in adults occurs when less than 200 cm of small intestine is present, leading to symptoms caused by rapid intestinal transit and malabsorption of fluids and nutrients. To prevent permanent dependence on parenteral nutrition, the remaining small bowel should be over 100 cm if the colon is absent or over 60 cm if a fully functioning colon remains. In children, SBS is diagnosed when less than 25% of the expected small bowel for their age is present (Table 10.1).

Table 10.1 Etiology

	Adults	Children
Loss of intestinal length from extensive or multiple resections	Mesenteric ischemia Trauma Malignancies Crohn's disease	Congenital atresia, Necrotizing enterocolitis Malrotation of the gut
Loss of functional length of bowel	Radiation enteritis	Sprue Congenital villous atrophy

10.1 Pathophysiology

The normal length of the small intestine from the duodenojejunal (DJ) flexure is about 20 feet, which is approximately 600–670 cm. Around nine liters of fluid (including saliva, gastric, pancreatic, and biliary secretions) pass through the small bowel every 24 h, of which seven liters are absorbed in the small intestine and the remaining two liters from the large intestine. The absorption of water, various nutrients, vitamins, and minerals occurs at different preferential sites in the gastrointestinal (GI) tract, with most occurring in the proximal bowel, and vitamin B12 and bile salts being absorbed in the terminal ileum (Table 10.2).

The clinical presentation of SBS results from loss of intestinal absorptive surfaces, faster intestinal transit, loss of the ileocecal valve, and loss of various GI hormones. Anatomically, SBS is categorized into three types.

Type 1: Removal of part of the jejunum, the entire ileum, and part of the colon, followed by an end jejunostomy.

Type 2: Part of the jejunum, along with the entire ileum, is removed, followed by a jejuno-colic anastomosis.

L. Mohanty (✉)
Srirama Chandra Bhanja Medical College and Hospital, Cuttack, India

M. Ibrarullah
Department of Surgical Gastroenterology, Apollo Hospitals, Bhubaneswar, Odisha, India

M. Ibrarullah (ed.), *Recent Concepts in Gastrointestinal (GI) Surgery*, https://doi.org/10.1007/978-981-92-1118-0_10

Table 10.2 Mediators and absorption of nutrients from various sites in the GI tract

Site	Humoral and neural mediators	Nutrients absorbed
Stomach	Gastrin	
Duodenum and proximal jejunum	Cholecystokinin Secretin Glucose-dependent Insulinotropic polypeptide Vasoactive intestinal polypeptide	Proteins, fats, sugars, iron, folate, calcium, and water-soluble vitamins
Jejunum and proximal ileum	Neurotensin	Proteins, fats, sugars, lactose, calcium, and water-soluble vitamins
Distal ileum	Peptide YY, Glucagon-like peptide 1 and 2	Bile salts, fat-soluble vitamins, and vitamin B12
Colon		Amino acids and carbohydrates

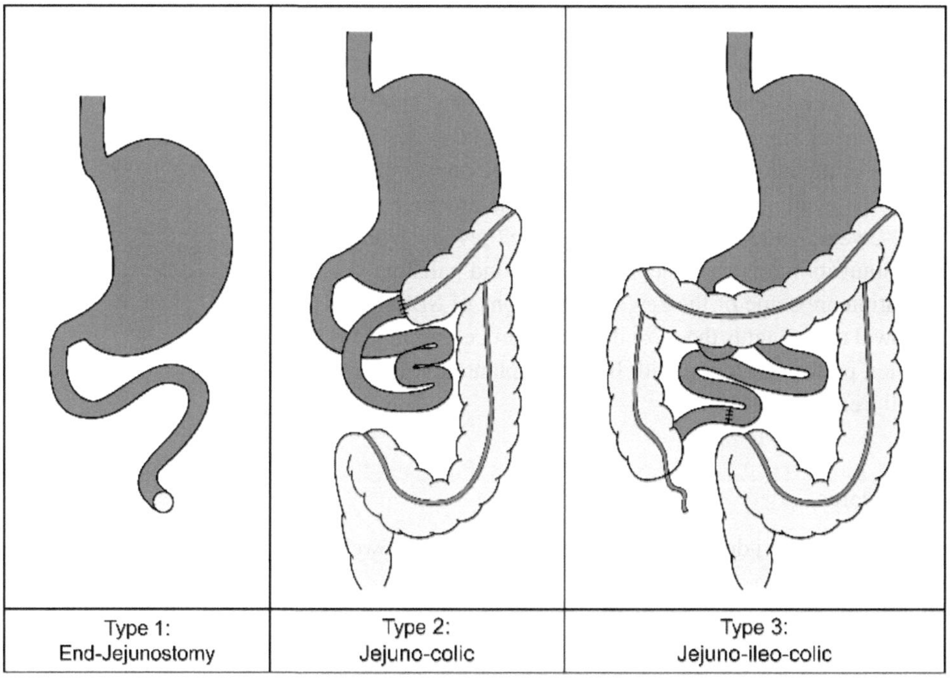

Fig. 10.1 Types of short bowel

Type 3: Large segment of jejunum removed, followed by jejuno-ileal anastomosis (Fig. 10.1).

SBS, in its evolution, passes through three stages:

- Acute phase (up to 4 weeks)
- Adaptive phase (1–2 years)
- Maintenance phase (beyond 2 years)

The *acute phase* is marked by diarrhea, malabsorption, water and electrolyte loss, and gastric hypersecretion caused by the loss of gastric inhibitory hormones secreted from the terminal ileum. Increased gastric acid also worsens diarrhea.

During the *adaptive phase*, the body compensates for losses by increasing absorption through mucosal hyperplasia, which includes the formation of additional villi and crypts, as well as the differentiation of specialized cells. Additionally, the intestinal wall elongates. Functional adaptation involves the hyperfermentation of undigested carbohydrates by colonic bacteria, producing short-chain fatty acids that are absorbed in the colon and used as an energy source. There is also a delay in intestinal transit time, which increases contact with the luminal surface. This phase heavily relies on the presence of nutrients in the lumen (with glutamine being especially important), as they speed up the process; thus, enteral nutrition is encouraged. If this adaptive phase does not occur, chronic intestinal failure develops.

During the *maintenance phase*, nutrition is managed through various specialized diets supported by multiple pharmacological agents.

10.2 Clinical Features

The clinical presentation is specific to malabsorption and water-electrolyte imbalance, which manifest as diarrhea, malnutrition, weight loss, steatorrhea, dehydration, and signs of various vitamin and micronutrient deficiencies, as well as certain forms of renal insufficiency. It also depends on particular short-term and long-term complications that may develop over time.

10.3 Investigations

Management of SBS requires regular monitoring of serum electrolytes, micronutrients, and nutritional parameters, including serum albumin, vitamin D, and B12, as well as liver and kidney function tests. Serum citrulline levels increase proportionally to the mass of enterocytes. A higher level is currently used to predict the successful withdrawal of total parenteral nutrition (TPN).

10.4 Management

It is crucial to know the length of the remaining bowel rather than the length that was resected. Therefore, the surgeon must document the length of the remaining unstretched small bowel, measured along the antimesenteric border from the duodenojejunal (DJ) flexure to the tip of the end-jejunostomy, or the point of colonic anastomosis or ileocecal (IC) junction, depending on the case. The operation note should also indicate whether the IC valve is intact and functional (not bypassed). The status of the end-jejunostomy is the most challenging, whereas retention of small bowel with an intact IC valve is the most favorable case for management.

Management of the acute phase includes fluid, electrolyte, and nutritional supplementation, as well as control of diarrhea. TPN should be initiated to meet nutritional requirements at this stage. Oral dietary supplements are initiated gradually in the adaptive phase and should culminate in full oral intake during the maintenance phase.

10.4.1 Fluid, Electrolytes, and Micronutrient Management

Enteric fluid loss in SBS can be significant, leading to chronic dehydration. Electrolyte loss presents as hyponatremia, hypokalemia, hypomagnesemia, and hypocalcemia. Therefore, regular monitoring is essential to ensure a urine output of at least 1 L per day and a urinary sodium concentration above 20 mEq/L. Levels of fat-soluble vitamins should be checked periodically and supplemented as needed. Additionally, periodic assessments of bone density, serum calcium, phosphorus, magnesium, vitamin D (25-hydroxyvitamin D), parathyroid hormone levels, and the presence of metabolic acidosis are recommended. Serum levels of iron, zinc, and other trace elements such as selenium, copper, and chromium should also be monitored and supplemented as necessary.

10.4.2 Parenteral Nutrition

TPN is an integral part of SBS, especially in the initial stage. The weaning process from TPN should be completed within 2 years; however, some patients may require up to 5 years to complete it. For long-term use, a tunnelled central venous catheter is preferred over a peripherally inserted central catheter or a port. The amount and content of the parenteral infusion should correspond to the patient's calorie needs, hydration status (assessed through urine and stoma output), serum electrolyte levels, and micronutrient requirements. Additional requirements are determined by the patient's nutritional assessment and lab results.

10.4.3 Enteral Fluid and Nutrition

Patients with excised or bypassed colon and end-jejunostomy are known as 'net secretors' because their stoma output usually exceeds their oral intake. For those with a jejunal length of less than 100 cm, the stoma output can reach up to 4 L in 24 h. Therefore, careful monitoring is necessary to ensure sufficient oral intake. Hypotonic or hypertonic fluids such as water, tea, coffee, or fruit juices should be avoided as they can increase stoma output. A balanced solution containing glucose and electrolytes is the ideal fluid for 'net secretors'.

A hyperphagic diet, meaning 50% more than the usual requirement, is recommended to offset losses caused by malabsorption. The dietary composition varies between patients with an end jejunostomy and those with an intact colon. For the latter group, a high-carbohydrate (60%) and low-fat (20%) diet is suggested. This type of diet helps reduce fecal calorie loss, improve overall energy absorption, and decrease absorption of calcium, magnesium, and oxalate. Conversely, fat restriction is not recommended for patients with jejunostomy, and their diet should include additional fat. Tube feeding with formula may be considered primarily for individuals who cannot or do not wish to take oral feeds, or as a supplement to oral intake.

Table 10.3 Management of short-term and long-term complications of SBS

Complications	Etiopathogenesis	Prevention/management
Diarrhea	Malabsorption Intestinal hurry Gastric hypersecretion Bacterial overgrowth	Dietary modifications Balanced oral fluid Antimotility agents PPI Luminal antibiotics
Acute kidney injury Nephrolithiasis Oxaluria	Dehydration Undigested fatty acid binds with calcium; oxalate remains free and gets absorbed.	Adequate hydration Low-fat, low-oxalate diet, potassium citrate, and calcium carbonate supplementation
Cholestatic or steatotic liver diseases Cirrhosis Cholelithiasis	TPN Bacterial overgrowth Loss of bile salts, bile stasis due to prolonged fasting	Restrict intravenous lipid infusion to <1 g/kg/d Use a non-soybean-based lipid emulsion Encourage oral/enteral intake Treat sepsis or small intestinal bacterial overgrowth Prophylactic cholecystectomy
Osteoporosis Osteopenia Osteomalacia	Calcium, magnesium, and vitamin D deficiency Metabolic acidosis	Periodic assessment of bone mineral density Correct metabolic acidosis Treat osteoporosis
Encephalopathy Altered mental status Slurred speech Ataxia	D-lactic acidosis resulting from the fermentation of undigested sugars in the colon	Carbohydrate restriction Luminal antibiotics Correction of acidosis

10.4.4 Pharmacological Intervention

Proton pump inhibitors (PPIs): Massive small bowel resection leads to increased levels of gastrin and acid secretion. PPIs are used to counter the adverse effects of gastric hyperacidity, such as diarrhea, peptic ulcers, and pancreatic malabsorption. However, prolonged use of PPIs may worsen intestinal bacterial overgrowth. Therefore, PPIs should be used sparingly beyond 12 months unless a clear benefit is demonstrated.

Antimotility agents: Loperamide in high doses (up to 32 mg/day), codeine, and clonidine are recommended to slow intestinal transit and control diarrhea. However, prolonged use of these drugs may cause bowel dilation and worsen bacterial overgrowth and diarrhea.

Somatostatin analogue: Recommended selectively in patients with large-volume diarrhea and unmanageable fluid and electrolyte loss, it is known to suppress pancreatic secretion and exacerbate malabsorption.

Glucagon-like Peptide-2 (GLP-2) is secreted by L cells in the distal ileum and proximal colon and has enterotrophic effects. Teduglutide, its synthetic analogue, is administered subcutaneously and has shown a promising impact on intestinal absorption, leading to the subsequent withdrawal of parenteral nutrition. Due to its trophic effect on the mucosa, Teduglutide is contraindicated in patients with GI polyps or a recent history or presence of malignancy anywhere in the body (Table 10.3).

10.5 Surgical Management

Surgical options in SBS are limited and are typically reserved for patients who cannot achieve their nutritional goals despite optimal dietary therapy. The surgical procedures can be classified into four categories.

- Restoration of the unused bowel
- Delaying intestinal transit
- Reconstruction: lengthening and tapering procedures
- Small bowel transplant

Restoration of bowel continuity should be carried out once the patient's overall condition and nutritional status are optimized. This procedure converts type 1 to type 2 or 3 category SBS, providing additional surface area for nutrient absorption.

Delaying intestinal transit by creating valves or inserting a reversed segment of bowel has been suggested as a possible solution. However, the limited availability of sufficient bowel length restricts the use of such procedures.

Reconstructive surgery to increase bowel length is only suitable for dilated bowel loops (>4 cm in diameter). These dilated loops are prone to stasis and bacterial overgrowth. The lengthening and tapering procedures aim to reduce the intestinal lumen, sacrificing lumen size to gain additional bowel length and function. The various such procedures are,

- Longitudinal intestinal lengthening and tapering (LILT), also known as the Bianchi procedure
- Serial Transverse Enteroplasty (STEP)

- Spiral Intestinal Lengthening & Tapering (SILT) (Figs. 10.2 and 10.3)

In LILT, the dilated small bowel is split vertically into two halves. The blood vessels in the mesentery are carefully isolated to supply each half of the bowel segment. The segments are then closed and joined end-to-end, adding length to the small bowel. In STEP, the dilated bowel is sequentially incised in a stepladder fashion to increase its length.

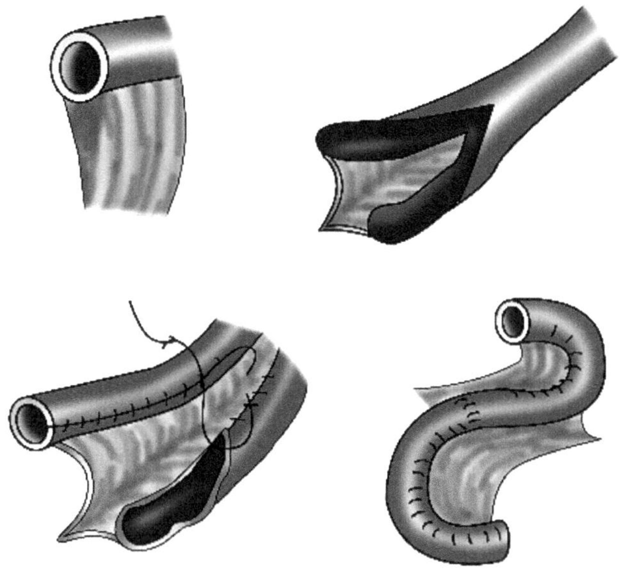

Fig. 10.2 Longitudinal intestinal lengthening and tapering (LILT)

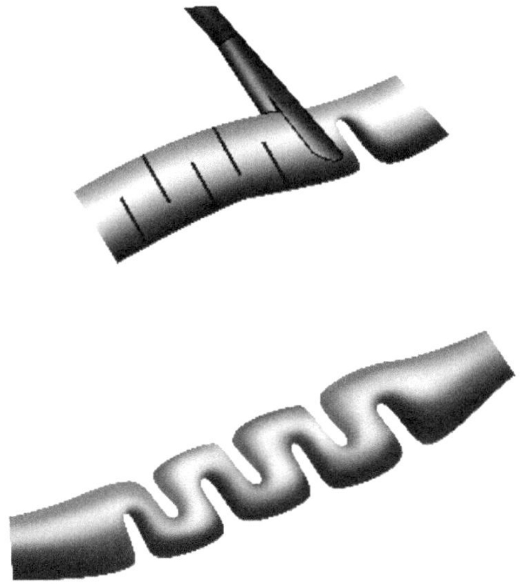

Fig. 10.3 Serial transverse enteroplasty (STEP)

10.5.1 Small Bowel Transplant

Small bowel transplant is considered the most definitive answer to the problems of SBS. Its indications are,

- Intestinal failure
  Permanent parenteral nutrition dependency.
- Parenteral nutrition failure
  - Progressive intestinal failure-associated liver diseases (IAFLD)
  - Impending liver failure/ established liver disease with cirrhosis
  - Recurrent central venous catheter-related sepsis
    Thrombosis of two of the six major central access veins
- Impairment of growth & development in children
- Severe dehydration with refractory electrolyte changes

Almost half of the patients requiring a small bowel transplant are also candidates for a simultaneous liver transplant, suggesting a tendency on the part of the treating physician to delay referral. The subpar results of combined procedures should be a reason to consider early referral for small bowel transplants. With a 5-year survival rate exceeding 65%, as reported by leading transplant centers worldwide, this procedure has proven highly successful.

Key Points

- Short bowel syndrome (SBS) occurs when less than 200 cm of small intestine remains in adults or less than 25% of the intestine in children.
- Depending on the extent of bowel loss, SBS is categorized into three types: (1) Part of the jejunum, the entire ileum, and part of the colon are removed, followed by an end jejunostomy. (2) Part of the jejunum, along with the entire ileum, is removed, followed by a jejuno-colic anastomosis. (3) A large segment of the jejunum is removed, followed by a jejuno-ileal anastomosis.
- The three phases of SBS are the acute phase (up to 4 weeks), the adaptive phase (1–2 years), and the maintenance phase (beyond 2 years).
- Fluid and electrolyte management and TPN are priorities during the acute phase. Oral feeds are introduced and gradually increased in the adaptive phase. The maintenance phase is marked by full acceptance of oral feeds and discontinuation of parenteral nutrition.

(continued)

- Malnutrition, diarrhea, nephrolithiasis, and gallstone formation are some of the key complications of SBS.
- Corrective surgical procedures like LILT, STEP, and SILT have a limited role in increasing intestinal length.
- Small bowel transplant is the most definitive procedure for SBS, often performed along with liver transplantation for liver failure.
- Intestinal failure and parenteral nutrition failure are the two primary indications for transplant.
- Small bowel transplant has a 5-year success rate of more than 65%.

Selected Reading

1. Nightingale J, Woodward JM. Guidelines for management of patients with a short bowel. Gut. 2006;55(Suppl IV):iv1–2. https://doi.org/10.1136/gut.2006.091108.
2. Wall E. An overview of short bowel syndrome management: adherence, adaptation and practical recommendations. J Acad Nutr Diet. 2013;113:1200–8.
3. Tappenden KA. Pathophysiology of short bowel syndrome: considerations of resected and residual anatomy. JPEN J Parenter Enteral Nutr. 2014;38(1 suppl):14S–22S.
4. Iyer K, DiBaise JK, Rubio-Tapi A. AGA Clinical practice update on management of short bowel syndrome: expert review. Clin Gastroenterol Hepatol. 2022;20:2185–94.

11 Small Bowel Transplantation: An Overview

Soumen Roy

Abstract

Small bowel transplant is the most effective salvage procedure for intestinal failure occurring due to various causes. The isolated small bowel graft comprises the entire length of the jejunum and ileum based on the SMA and SMV. In the recipient, the GI continuity is established by jejuno-jejunostomy proximally; the distal bowel is brought out as a Bishop-Koop ileostomy, loop, or end ileostomy. In multivisceral transplant, the liver, along with intact hilar structures, the small bowel, and the pancreas allograft, is harvested en bloc. Segment of the aorta in continuity to the CA and SMA is used for the arterial supply. The venous drainage is connected to the hepatic veins/donor vena cava. For immunosuppression, induction agents, such as Basiliximab, Lemtuzumab, or Rituximab, are used for T-cell depletion, administered before the transplant if possible, along with steroids on the day of surgery. Afterwards, Tacrolimus and Mycophenolate mofetil (MMF) are started on POD 1 and adjusted as needed. Rejection, acute or chronic, is the most common postoperative complication.

Keywords

Small bowel transplant · Intestinal failure

Small bowel transplantation represents a significant advance in treating patients with irreversible intestinal failure (IF). It occurs when the small intestine cannot absorb enough nutrients and fluids to sustain life, often requiring long-term parenteral nutrition (PN). Although PN can sustain life, it is also associated with many complications that can greatly affect a patient's quality of life and even survival. Despite being a complex and technically demanding procedure, small bowel transplantation offers the potential for nutritional independence and improved quality of life for carefully selected patients with IF. A 2022 study reports that about 1 in 50,000 people in India have chronic IF. The prevalence of short bowel syndrome (SBS), a common cause of IF, is estimated at 24.5 cases per million people annually.

11.1 Intestinal Failure

To fully understand the role of small bowel transplantation, it is essential to understand the pathophysiology and management of IF. IF can result from various causes, such as:

1. *Short Bowel Syndrome*: SBS results from surgical resection of a significant portion of the small intestine due to conditions like necrotizing enterocolitis (most common in pediatrics), volvulus, or trauma.
2. *Intestinal Dysmotility*: Impaired intestinal motility due to conditions such as chronic intestinal (pan-intestinal) pseudo-obstruction, which disrupts normal propulsion of intestinal contents.
3. *Mucosal Diseases*: Inflammatory conditions, such as Crohn's disease or radiation enteritis, cause damage to the intestinal lining and impair absorption.
4. *Congenital Anomalies*: Conditions such as gastroschisis or intestinal atresia, resulting in an insufficient length or function of the small intestine (Table 11.1).

S. Roy (✉)
Apollo Hospitals, Bhubaneswar, India

M. Ibrarullah (ed.), *Recent Concepts in Gastrointestinal (GI) Surgery*, https://doi.org/10.1007/978-981-92-1118-0_11

Table 11.1 Classification of intestinal failure

Type	Nature	Common causes	Characteristics
1	Acute onset	Resection, infections, or trauma	Often temporary Resolves with appropriate medical treatment Does not usually require long-term intervention
2	Prolonged but reversible	Resection, trauma	Need for extended hospital care and parenteral nutrition support Recovery can take weeks to months
3	Chronic	Crohn's disease, radiation enteritis, trauma, necrotizing enterocolitis, and intestinal atresia	Requires ongoing medical care and lifelong total parenteral nutrition

11.2 Indications for Small Bowel Transplantation

Small bowel transplantation is reserved for patients with irreversible IF who have developed severe, life-threatening complications related to PN or underlying intestinal disease. The decision to proceed with transplantation requires careful evaluation by a multidisciplinary team. Specific indications include:

Intestinal failure-associated liver disease (IFALD): This is one of the primary indications, as ongoing liver damage can result in cirrhosis and liver failure, significantly reducing the patient's long-term survival.

Loss of venous access: When central venous access is exhausted and no alternative routes are possible, transplantation becomes a necessary option.

Recurrent catheter-associated bloodstream infections (CRBSI): Frequent CRBSIs despite optimal catheter care and antibiotic therapy can severely impact patient health. Fungal infections are especially concerning.

Unreconstructable gastrointestinal tract: When the native intestine cannot be surgically repaired or reconstructed, transplantation may be the only viable option.

Complete porto-mesenteric thrombosis: Thrombosis of the major veins draining the intestine can lead to IF and make the patient a candidate for transplantation.

Tumors involving the root of the mesentery: Certain slow-growing tumors, like desmoids or neuroendocrine tumors, may necessitate en bloc resection of the intestine and surrounding structures, requiring transplantation.

Frozen abdomen: Severe intra-abdominal adhesions can prevent access to the intestines and hinder their function, potentially requiring a transplant.

11.3 Patient Selection

A multidisciplinary team comprising a surgeon, gastroenterologist, hepatologist, infectious disease specialist, nutritionist, and psychosocial support staff is involved in the evaluation of the patients. This includes,

- Comprehensive medical history and physical examination: Evaluation of the patient's overall health and identification of any comorbidities.
- Nutritional assessment: Assessment of the patient's current nutritional status, PN needs, and potential for enteral feeding.
- Gastrointestinal evaluation: Imaging studies, endoscopy, and motility studies to assess the extent and nature of the IF.
- Infectious disease evaluation: Screening for active infections and assessing the risk of opportunistic infections.
- Psychosocial assessment: Evaluation of the patient's and family's understanding of the transplantation process, adherence potential, and coping mechanisms.

11.4 Contraindications to Small Bowel Transplantation

Certain conditions may preclude a patient from undergoing small bowel transplantation:

Active systemic infection: Uncontrolled infection raises the risk of post-transplant complications.

Uncontrolled malignancy: Active cancer may recur or worsen quickly after transplantation because of immunosuppression.

Severe cardiac or pulmonary disease: Patients with serious cardiovascular or respiratory issues may not tolerate surgery and immunosuppression.

Active substance abuse: Substance abuse can cause noncompliance with medication and necessary lifestyle changes.

Significant psychosocial instability: Lack of adequate support or mental health issues can hinder post-transplant care.

Irreversible neurological damage: Severe neurological impairment may limit the benefits of transplantation.

11.5 Types of Small Bowel Transplantation

The type of transplant depends on the extent of IF and the involvement of other organs (Table 11.2).

Table 11.2 Types of small bowel transplants

Isolated Intestinal Transplant	Transplantation of the small intestine alone. This is performed when the liver and other abdominal organs are functioning adequately.
Combined liver-intestinal transplant[a]	Simultaneous transplantation of the liver and small intestine. This is indicated when the patient has IFALD or other significant liver disease.
Multivisceral transplant[a]	Encompasses transplantation of multiple abdominal organs, including the stomach, duodenum, pancreas, small intestine, and liver (or some combination thereof). This is reserved for complex cases involving extensive abdominal disease.

[a]Cadaveric Transplant

11.6 Operative Technique (*Basic Steps*)

11.6.1 Cadaveric Transplantation

11.6.1.1 Donor Operation

Dissection of the supra-celiac and infrarenal aorta and identification of the aortic take-off of the celiac axis and superior mesenteric artery (SMA) are performed, followed by dissection of the superior mesenteric vein (SMV), splenic vein (SV), and portal vein (PV). Next, the aorta is cross-clamped, and an aortic flush with University of Wisconsin (UW) solution is conducted.

Isolated intestinal procurement without pancreas procurement: The SMA is included with the bowel graft on an aortic Carrel patch, the SV is ligated near its junction with the PV, the SMV is dissected free as done in Whipple's procedure, and the PV is divided halfway between the superior border of the pancreas and the liver.

Intestinal procurement with simultaneous pancreas procurement: The usual steps are dissection of the proximal SMA and identification of the take-off of the inferior pancreatico-duodenal artery (IPDA), division of the SMA distal to this take-off, and division of the SMV proximal to its junction with the PV. The intestinal graft type decides the level of visceral transection and its vascular anatomy as follows:

Small bowel alone-grafts: The intestine is divided just proximal to the ileocecal valve

Small bowel-colon graft: A short segment of ascending and proximal transverse colon (with the right and middle colic artery) is procured (the inclusion of the ileocecal valve with the graft may aggravate the delayed transit time frequently observed in small bowel grafts)

Stomach-bowel graft: The left gastric artery on an aortic Carrel-patch must be procured

11.6.1.2 Recipient Operation

The graft can be drained systemically into the infrarenal vena cava (IVC) or into the portal system via the superior mesenteric vein (SMV). Arterial revascularization is usually achieved by creating an arterial anastomosis to the infrarenal abdominal aorta. After the proximal anastomosis between the graft and the recipient's gastrointestinal (GI) tract, the distal graft ileum is exteriorized, and intestinal continuity is restored by creating a Bishop Koop ileostomy (to facilitate easy endoscopic access for graft monitoring and biopsies).

11.6.2 Living Donor Transplantation

11.6.2.1 Donor Operation

After preoperative angiography analysis, a segment of the ileum approximately 150–200 cm long is isolated on a vascular pedicle consisting of the ileocolic artery (ICA) and vein. The donor retains the ileocecal valve and the distal 20–25 cm of the ileum, supplied by the right colic artery (RCA), for absorption of vitamin B12 and other nutrients. The ICA and vein are dissected at their respective origins, which are at the level of vascular transection from the superior mesenteric artery and vein. The graft is flushed ex situ with UW solution. Intestinal continuity in the donor is restored by creating an ileo-ileal anastomosis.

11.6.2.2 Recipient Operation

Vascular anastomosis is performed in an end-to-side manner between the ICA and the vein, with the recipient's infrarenal aorta and IVC, respectively. Intestinal continuity in the recipient is restored as previously described.

11.6.3 Combined Liver-Intestinal Transplantation

11.6.3.1 Donor Operation

Vascular dissection is similar to that in isolated small bowel retrieval. The common bile duct is divided. After an in situ flush with UW solution and transection of the inferior vena cava above the kidneys and diaphragm, as well as proximal and distal small bowel transection, the bowel-liver graft is procured as a single unit. This includes a 10 cm supraceliac aortic segment in continuity with an aortic Carrel patch containing the celiac axis (CA) and SMA. Combined bowel-liver procurement precludes the simultaneous procurement of a whole pancreas graft. However, procurement of the distal pancreas (body and tail, supplied by the splenic artery and vein) for a segmental pancreatic transplant remains possible. The distal end of the aortic segment is oversewn.

11.6.3.2 Recipient Operation

Hepatectomy and liver transplantation are done in the conventional manner. Flushing of the bowel-liver graft is done with UW/RL solution before removal of the caval vascular clamps. Intestinal reconstruction is performed as described above. Direct anastomosis between donor and recipient CBD or a Roux-Y-choledocho-enterostomy is performed if the distal CBD end is unavailable (Figs. 11.1 and 11.2).

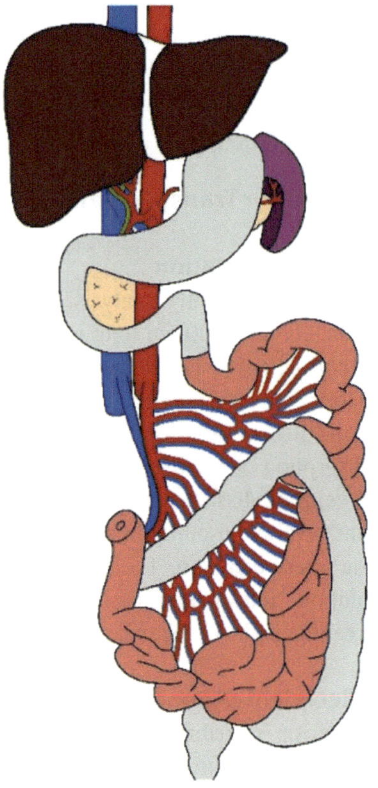

Fig. 11.1 The isolated small bowel graft comprising the entire length of the jejunum and ileum based on SMA and SMV. In the recipient, the GI continuity is established by jejuno-jejunostomy proximally; the distal bowel is brought out as a Bishop-Koop ileostomy, loop, or end ileostomy

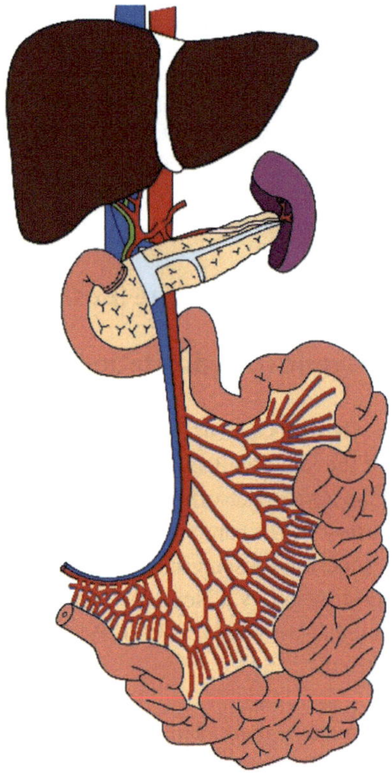

Fig. 11.2 Multivisceral transplant. The liver, along with intact hilar structures, the small bowel, and the pancreas allograft, is harvested en bloc. A segment of the aorta, in continuity with the CA and SMA, is used for arterial supply. The venous drainage is connected to the hepatic veins/donor vena cava. Alternatively, the thoracic aortic conduit is attached to the infrarenal or suprarenal aorta, and the caval anastomosis is done either as standard caval replacement or piggyback fashion. The bowel continuity is established by a jejuno-jejunostomy proximally and an ileo-colic anastomosis distally

11.7 Post-transplant Management

Immunosuppression: Lifelong immunosuppression is crucial to prevent rejection. Protocols vary between centers. Induction agents such as Basiliximab, Alemtuzumab, or Rituximab, used for T-cell depletion, are administered before transplant, if possible, along with steroids on the day of surgery. Afterward, Tacrolimus and Mycophenolate mofetil (MMF) are started on POD 1 and adjusted as needed.

Rejection Monitoring: Regular endoscopic biopsies from the intestinal stoma site are performed to detect early rejection. These biopsies are graded according to standardized criteria.

Prevention of Infection: Prophylactic antibiotics and antifungal agents are given for 2 weeks, and antivirals are administered for 6 months to reduce the risk of infections.

Nutritional Support: A contrast study is performed on POD 7 to rule out anastomotic leak. Enteral nutrition is initiated orally or via a feeding tube. The feed should be of low osmolarity to prevent diarrhea. Ideally, it should contain medium-chain triglycerides (which are absorbed even in the initial absence of lymphatic drainage), small peptides, and glutamine (to stimulate enterocytes). A shortened intestinal transit time is common after small bowel transplantation and can be managed pharmacologically.

Fluid and Electrolyte Management: Careful monitoring and replacement of fluids and electrolytes are crucial to prevent dehydration and electrolyte imbalances.

11.8 Complications

- *Rejection: the most common complication*. It can be acute (occurring within the first few months) or chronic (developing over a more extended period). Antibody-mediated rejection is increasingly recognized.
- *Infection*: Infection is a significant cause of morbidity and mortality due to immunosuppression. Common infections include bacterial, viral (CMV, EBV), and fungal infections.
- *Sepsis*: Can arise from infections or other sources and lead to multi-organ failure.
- *Renal Dysfunction*: Calcineurin inhibitors (Tacrolimus) can cause nephrotoxicity.
- *Post-transplant Lymphoproliferative Disorder (PTLD)*: A type of lymphoma associated with EBV infection.
- *Graft*-versus-*Host Disease (GVHD)*: Can occur in multivisceral transplants involving lymphoid tissue.
- *Thrombosis*: Blood clots can form in the transplanted vessels, leading to graft ischemia.
- *Anastomotic Leaks:* Anastomotic leaks can occur at bowel anastomosis sites.

Key Points

- Small bowel transplant is the most effective salvage procedure for intestinal failure occurring due to various causes.
- The various types of small bowel transplantations are isolated intestinal transplant, combined liver-intestinal transplant, and multivisceral transplant.
- The isolated small bowel graft comprising the entire length of the jejunum and ileum based on SMA and SMV. In the recipient, the GI continuity is established by jejuno-jejunostomy proximally; the distal bowel is brought out as a Bishop-Koop ileostomy, loop, or end ileostomy.
- In multivisceral transplant, the liver, along with intact hilar structures, the small bowel, and the pancreas allograft, is harvested en bloc. Segment of the aorta in continuity to the CA and SMA is used for the arterial supply. The venous drainage is connected to the hepatic veins/donor vena cava.
- For immunosuppression, induction agents such as Basiliximab, Alemtuzumab, or Rituximab are used for T-cell depletion, administered before the transplant if possible, along with steroids on the day of surgery. Afterwards, Tacrolimus and Mycophenolate mofetil (MMF) are started on POD 1 and adjusted as needed.
- Rejection, acute or chronic, is the most common postoperative complication.

Selected Reading

1. Sudan D. The current state of intestine transplantation: indications, techniques, outcomes and challenges. Am J Transplant. 2014;14:1976–84.
2. Gürkan A. Advances in small bowel transplantation. Turk J Surg. 2017;33:135–41.
3. Canovai E, Hlaing HH, Sharkey L. Small bowel transplantation – the latest developments. Medicine. 2024;52:186–92.

Part III

Colon, Rectum, and Anal Canal

Inflammatory Bowel Disease

12

Rajesh Panwar and Peush Sahni

Abstract

Ulcerative Colitis (UC) is a continuous mucosal inflammation that begins at the anorectal junction and extends proximally to involve the colon. The inflammation is characteristically limited to the mucosal layer. Crohn's Disease (CD) is characterized by transmural inflammation that can affect any segment of the GI tract from mouth to anus, with skip areas of normal tissue between diseased segments. Failure of medical treatment, both in emergency and elective situations, is an indication for surgery. Non-remitting acute fulminant colitis, toxic megacolon, colonic perforation, and massive lower GI bleeding are indications for emergency surgery. Staged restorative proctocolectomy (J pouch ileoanal anastomosis) is the surgical procedure of choice for UC. Treatment of CD is essentially medical; surgery is more often palliative. Surgery in CD is indicated for failure of medical treatment to achieve remission or to treat complications like stricture, fistulae, or lower GI bleeding.

Keywords

IBD · Crohn's disease · Ulcerative colitis

Inflammatory Bowel Disease (IBD) refers to a group of chronic, immune-mediated disorders characterized by inflammation of the gastrointestinal (GI) tract. IBD is an idiopathic, relapsing and remitting condition that affects different parts of the GI tract with varying depths and patterns of inflammation. The two most common forms are Ulcerative Colitis (UC) and Crohn's Disease (CD). UC is a continuous mucosal inflammation that begins at the anorectal junction and extends proximally to involve the colon. The inflammation is characteristically limited to the mucosal layer. In contrast, CD is characterized by transmural inflammation that can affect any segment of the GI tract from mouth to anus, with skip areas of normal tissue between diseased segments. The clinical features of UC and CD are distinct and therefore need to be described separately. However, it is important to remember that classic UC and CD represent the two ends of the disease spectrum. Patients with features that overlap both conditions fall somewhere in between, making it difficult to classify them as either UC or CD. In fact, there is a group of patients in whom it is impossible to distinguish between UC and CD even after histopathological examination of a subtotal colectomy specimen. These patients are labeled as having indeterminate colitis. During follow-up, patients with indeterminate colitis may evolve toward either end of the spectrum, leading to classification as either UC or CD.

12.1 Pathogenesis

IBD results from a complex and poorly understood interaction of genetic, environmental, and clinical factors. Although monogenic IBD caused by a single gene defect has been documented, it is rare and primarily affects children. It is now understood that adult IBD is polygenic. IBD occurs more frequently in first-degree relatives of affected patients, with a relative risk as high as 20 compared to the general population. CD is believed to have a higher genetic predisposition compared to UC. Developed countries, northern latitude locations, higher socioeconomic status, urbanization, and improved hygiene are associated with a higher incidence of IBD. The typical age of onset is between 15 and 30 years, with a smaller peak occurring between 50 and 80 years. The incidence is higher among White and Jewish populations compared to Hispanics and Black populations. Although the incidence of IBD in India is rising, it remains lower than in Western countries. Additional risk factors for IBD are listed in Table 12.1.

R. Panwar
Department of GI Surgery & Liver Transplantation, All India Institute of Medical Sciences, New Delhi, India

P. Sahni (✉)
Centre for Liver and Biliary Sciences, Max Super Speciality Hospital, Saket, New Delhi, India

M. Ibrarullah (ed.), *Recent Concepts in Gastrointestinal (GI) Surgery*, https://doi.org/10.1007/978-981-92-1118-0_12

Table 12.1 Risk factors for inflammatory bowel disease

Risk factor	Incidence of ulcerative colitis	Incidence of Crohn's disease
Smoking	Same or decreases	Increases
Physical activity	Same	Decreases
High fiber diet	Same	Decreases
Increased dietary fat	Increases	Increases
Vitamin D	Probably decreases	Decreases
Omega-3 fatty acids	Probably decreases	Decreases
Appendectomy	Decreases	Same or increases

12.2 Ulcerative Colitis

UC is a chronic, idiopathic, inflammatory disease of the colon characterized by continuous mucosal inflammation that starts in the rectum and extends proximally in a continuous pattern. It is a major subtype of IBD and mainly affects the mucosa and submucosa of the colon. UC follows a relapsing and remitting clinical course and significantly impacts quality of life.

12.3 Clinical Presentation and Diagnosis

The main symptom of UC is diarrhea with mucus and/or blood in stools. Patients usually have increased stool frequency with urgency and tenesmus due to the rectal involvement. The symptoms develop and progress gradually. However, a small number of patients may begin with severe symptoms. A number of other diseases such as infectious colitis, CD, and some other forms of colitis (radiation-induced, drug-related, diversion colitis, etc.) may have a similar presentation and may need to be ruled out before the diagnosis of UC is established.

The diagnosis of UC should be considered in a patient with

- Chronic diarrhea of more than 4 weeks duration
- Active inflammation on endoscopy
- Chronic inflammation on biopsy

Besides the bowel symptoms, patients with UC may also have some extraintestinal manifestations (EIM). These may be present at the time of initial presentation or may develop later in the course of disease. Most of these EIM follow the course of colitis; however, primary sclerosing cholangitis, ankylosing spondylitis, and uveitis may follow a disease course independent of the colonic disease (Table 12.2).

UC is a risk factor for colorectal cancer. The risk is related to disease severity as well as disease duration and is two to three times as compared to the general population. Patients with UC require regular screening especially after 10–15 years of disease onset depending on the disease severity.

Table 12.2 Common extraintestinal manifestations of ulcerative colitis

System	Manifestations
Musculoskeletal	Arthralgia, peripheral arthritis, ankylosing spondylitis
Hepatobiliary	Primary sclerosing cholangitis
Skin	Erythema nodosum, pyoderma gangrenosum
Eye	Uveitis, episcleritis

A full-length colonoscopy is necessary to evaluate the extent and severity of inflammation. Visualization of the terminal ileum is also important to identify features of CD, which is always a differential diagnosis. Contiguous involvement of the terminal ileum, known as backwash ileitis, may also be observed in UC with severe pan-colitis. While a complete endoscopic evaluation is essential, it should be avoided during the acute stage. However, a gentle, flexible sigmoidoscopy with minimal insufflation is usually possible even during an acute episode. This procedure also permits the collection of biopsy specimens for histopathological examination, as well as to look for infections such as cytomegalovirus (CMV). Endoscopic findings include loss of mucosal vascular pattern, erythema, mucosal edema, granularity, erosions, friability, spontaneous bleeding, ulcerations, and pseudopolyps. These mucosal changes typically start at the anorectal junction and extend continuously to the proximal extent of the disease (Fig. 12.1).

The biopsy findings in UC include cryptitis, crypt abscesses, crypt branching, mucin depletion, and paneth cell metaplasia. There's increased cellularity in the lamina propria, with basal plasmacytosis and basal lymphoid aggregates. None of these features is pathognomonic, but having two or more of them is highly indicative of UC.

Several laboratory tests are typically performed to either rule out other differential diagnoses or assess the disease stage, which can help guide treatment. Stool testing for Clostridium difficile toxin, stool culture for Escherichia coli, Shigella, Salmonella, Campylobacter, and other bacteria, as well as stool microscopy for ova and parasites, should be conducted.

A complete blood count, serum electrolytes, serum albumin, erythrocyte sedimentation rate (ESR), and C-reactive protein (CRP) levels are essential blood tests that help evalu-

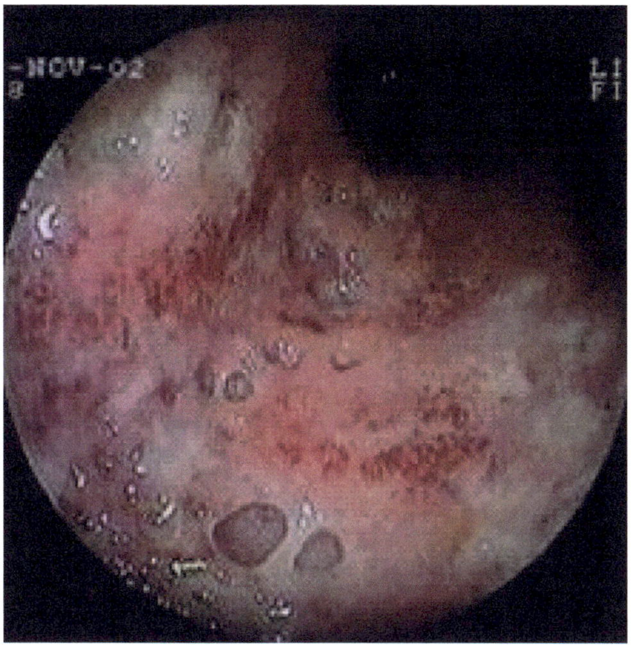

Fig. 12.1 Colonoscopic appearance of severe ulcerative colitis. Note diffuse ulcerations and mucosal destruction

ate the severity of UC. Fecal calprotectin, a noninvasive test, is also useful for assessing disease severity.

Radiological investigations are generally not needed for diagnosis but can be useful in guiding treatment for severe cases. A dilated colon (>5.5 cm) on an abdominal radiograph with signs of toxicity suggests toxic megacolon. An abdominal CT scan may be necessary in emergencies or if malignancy is suspected.

12.4 Management

The management of UC depends on the severity of the disease. The Montreal classification is used to categorize UC based on the extent and disease severity to guide the choice of treatment (Table 12.3).

The Mayo score is also widely used to assess the severity of UC. It includes four parameters: stool frequency, rectal bleeding, endoscopic appearance of the colon, and physician's global assessment. Each parameter is graded on a scale of 0–3, with higher scores indicating more severe disease. The total Mayo score, ranging from 0 to 12, reflects the overall disease activity.

The goals of medical therapy in UC are to induce remission during the acute phase and to maintain remission afterward. Several medications have been proven effective in treating UC, and in fact, most patients with UC respond well to medical management (Tables 12.4 and 12.5).

Table 12.3 Montreal classification

Extent of the disease	
E1: Ulcerative proctitis	Inflammation limited to the rectum
E2: Left-sided colitis	Involvement up to the splenic flexure
E3: Pancolitis	Extends beyond the splenic flexure
Severity	
Mild	<4 stools/day ± blood, no systemic toxicity
Moderate	>4 stools/day, minimal systemic disturbance
Severe:	>6 bloody stools/day, systemic toxicity (fever, tachycardia, anemia, elevated ESR)
Fulminant	>10 stools/day, bleeding, abdominal distension, transfusion requirement

Table 12.4 Pharmacotherapy for ulcerative colitis

Drug class	Examples	Mechanism of action	Role
Aminosalicylates (5-ASA)	Mesalamine, Sulfasalazine, Olsalazine, Balsalazide	Inhibit cyclo-oxygenase (COX) and lipoxygenase pathways; reduce mucosal inflammation	First-line for mild to moderate UC; both induction and maintenance
Corticosteroids	Prednisone, Budesonide MMX, Hydrocortisone, Methylprednisolone	Inhibit inflammatory cytokines (IL-1, TNF-α) Broad immunosuppressive effect	Induction of remission in moderate–severe disease; not for maintenance
Immunomodulators	Azathioprine, 6-Mercaptopurine	Inhibit purine synthesis; reduce lymphocyte proliferation	Maintenance of remission; steroid-sparing agent
Calcineurin inhibitors	Cyclosporine, Tacrolimus	Inhibit T-cell activation via calcineurin blockade	Used in severe, steroid-refractory UC; bridge to biologics or surgery
Antitumor necrosis factor (TNF) agents	Infliximab, Adalimumab	Neutralize TNF-α, a pro-inflammatory cytokine	For moderate–severe UC; induction and maintenance, especially in refractory cases
Anti-integrin agents	Vedolizumab	Blocks lymphocyte gut migration via α4β7 integrin inhibition	Moderate–severe UC; gut-specific biologic
Anti-IL-12/23 agents	Ustekinumab	Inhibits IL-12 and IL-23 signaling pathways (Th1/Th17 suppression)	Effective in moderate–severe UC, especially after anti-TNF failure
JAK inhibitors	Tofacitinib, Upadacitinib	Inhibits the JAK-STAT pathway, reducing cytokine signaling	Oral small molecule; moderate–severe UC, anti-TNF refractory
S1P receptor modulators	Ozanimod	Sequesters lymphocytes in lymph nodes; reduces gut infiltration	Emerging oral option for moderate-to-severe UC
Topical agents	Mesalamine enema/suppository, Hydrocortisone enema	Local anti-inflammatory action on rectal/sigmoid mucosa	Essentially for distal UC (proctitis), often combined with oral 5-ASA

Table 12.5 Medical management of ulcerative colitis

Disease extent	Induction	Maintenance
Mild to moderate proctitis or proctosigmoiditis	First line: Topical mesalamine Alternate: Topical corticosteroids Add oral mesalamine if topical therapy is ineffective Oral corticosteroids only if no response to oral mesalamine + Topical therapy	Topical or oral mesalamine
Mild to moderate left-sided colitis or pancolitis	Oral + Topical mesalamine Oral mesalamine + Topical steroids Oral corticosteroids only if no response to oral mesalamine + Topical therapy Nfliximab/Tofacitinib for steroid-refractory disease	Topical and oral mesalamine
Moderate to severe disease	Oral corticosteroids Infliximab Vedolizumab Ustekinumab Tofacitinib	Azathioprine Infliximab +/−Azathioprine Vedolizumab Ustekinumab Tofacitinib

12.5 Management of Acute Severe Ulcerative Colitis (ASUC)

ASUC is a life-threatening condition characterized by severe bloody diarrhea and signs of systemic inflammation. Truelove and Witt's criteria are useful to diagnose ASUC as well as to monitor the response to therapy (Table 12.6).

Patients with ASUC are typically treated with high-dose intravenous glucocorticoids. Intravenous hydrocortisone is given at 100 mg every 8 h, and patients are closely monitored for any signs of deterioration. Supportive care includes fluid and electrolyte management, nutritional support, and blood transfusions to maintain hemoglobin levels above 7 g/dL. Enteral nutrition is preferred for those who can tolerate oral intake, while patients unable to do so may require parenteral nutrition. Because UC is a prothrombotic state, pharmacological prophylaxis for venous thromboembolism is recommended, but its advantages should be balanced against the increased risk of bleeding.

Some patients have a more fulminant disease course with fever, tachycardia, and leukocytosis. This clinical presentation, along with a dilated colon (>5.5 cm) on an abdominal radiograph, is called toxic megacolon. Toxic megacolon is initially treated with intravenous steroids, but surgery should be considered promptly if the patient does not improve within 48–72 h.

Most patients with ASUC respond to treatment within 3–5 days. They begin to feel better, and stool frequency decreases with little or no blood in the stools. The steroids are switched to oral (60 mg prednisone) and continued until 2 weeks after the symptoms resolve. After that, steroids are gradually tapered at a rate of 5–10 mg per week until reaching a dose of 20 mg/day, then reduced by 2.5 mg per week until stopping. These patients also require either infliximab and/or thiopurine as maintenance therapy.

Approximately 30% of patients with ASUC do not respond to intravenous steroids. These patients may be offered surgery or rescue medical therapy. The options for rescue therapy include infliximab, cyclosporine, or tacrolimus. Patients who respond to rescue therapy will require maintenance therapy based on the rescue drug used for induction. Those who received infliximab can continue it as maintenance, while patients who received cyclosporine or tacrolimus are placed on thiopurine maintenance. Patients who do not respond to rescue therapy will need surgery.

Table 12.6 Truelove and Witts' criteria for ASUC

Parameter	Mild	Moderate	Severe
Stools per day	≤4	4–6	≥6 with blood
Blood in stool	No or small amounts	Moderate	Visible blood
Temperature (°C)	Normal	≤37.8	>37.8
Heart rate (beats/min)	Normal	≤90	>90
Hemoglobin (g/dL)	>11	10.5–11	<10.5
ESR (mm/hr)	Normal or mildly raised	20–30	>30
Systemic toxicity	None	Minimal	Present
CRP (mg/L)	<10	10–30	>30

12.6 Surgical Management

Although most patients with UC can be managed medically, some will ultimately require surgery. Since the disease process in UC is confined to the large bowel, total colectomy is considered a curative treatment. Restorative total proctocolectomy (TPC) with ileal pouch-anal anastomosis (IPAA) is regarded as the standard of care for UC and can be performed as three-stage, two-stage, or single-stage procedures. The choice of procedure depends on the clinical situation. TPC with a permanent end ileostomy also remains a reasonable option for patients who are of advanced age, have poor sphincter function, or have malignancy of the mid to lower rectum (Table 12.7).

Table 12.7 Surgical strategies for restorative total proctocolectomy

Procedure	First stage	Second stage	Third stage	Indications
Three-stage	Subtotal colectomy + end ileostomy	Completion proctectomy + IPAA + loop ileostomy	Ileostomy closure	Emergency
Two-stage	Total proctocolectomy + IPAA + loop ileostomy	Ileostomy closure	–	Elective
Modified two-stage	Subtotal colectomy + end ileostomy	Completion proctectomy + IPAA	–	Emergency
One stage	Total proctocolectomy + IPAA	–	–	Elective (in selected patients)

IPAA Ileal Pouch Anal Anastomosis

12.7 Emergency Surgery

The most common clinical situation leading to emergency surgery is ASUC that does not respond to 5 days of intravenous corticosteroids. As previously discussed, there is also an option of medical rescue therapy with infliximab, cyclosporine, or tacrolimus in this scenario. Failure of rescue medical therapy would be a definitive indication for surgery. It has been observed that delaying surgery in medical refractory ASUC beyond 5–7 days from the start of intravenous steroids increases the risk of morbidity and mortality. Other indications for emergency surgery include fulminant colitis or toxic megacolon not responding to medical management, severe bleeding or perforation, and peritonitis.

Patients of UC who require emergency surgery are often in poor health. Prolonged use of corticosteroids and other immunosuppressants, combined with malnutrition, significantly increases their risk of complications such as wound infection, sepsis, and anastomotic failure. In this situation, emergency subtotal colectomy with end ileostomy is the preferred option. Subtotal colectomy is well-suited for emergencies because it can be performed quickly and does not require pelvic dissection or anastomosis. The procedure can be done via open or minimally invasive techniques, depending on the patient's condition, the surgical team's expertise, and available equipment. It involves mobilizing the entire colon from the cecum to the rectosigmoid junction. The ileocolic, right colic, middle colic, left colic, and sigmoid vessels are ligated and divided towards the colon side, unlike colectomy for malignancy, which involves ligating vessels at their origin. A core colectomy is an alternative that involves dividing the colonic mesentery very close to the colon without ligating specific vessels. The superior rectal vessels are preserved, and pelvic dissection is strictly avoided. The ileum is divided near the ileocecal junction, and the colon is divided at the level of the sacral promontory using a stapling device, after which the specimen is removed (Figs. 12.2 and 12.3). The ileal end is brought out as an end ileostomy in the right iliac fossa. The rectal stump is oversewn with nonabsorbable monofilament sutures, leaving long suture ends for easy identification of the rectal stump during the second stage. A Malecot's catheter or soft drain may be inserted per anus into the rectum and left for 2–3 days to drain blood and mucus. If the rectal tissue is friable or unable to hold sutures, the rectal stump may also be brought out as a mucus fistula.

Most patients with ASUC improve after a subtotal colectomy. However, the risk of complications is high, especially in patients operated on for issues like perforation with peritonitis or toxic megacolon. Common postoperative complications include wound infection, stoma-related problems, and rectal stump bleeding. Most of these can be managed conservatively, but some patients may need reoperation for wound dehiscence, stoma retraction, or persistent bleeding from the remaining rectum.

Intravenous corticosteroids are maintained at the same dose for the first 48–72 h after surgery, while other immunosuppressants are discontinued. Afterwards, the intravenous corticosteroids are transitioned to oral prednisone and gradually tapered before stopping. Patients may also use topical mesalamine or steroids to manage the disease in the remaining rectum. The histopathology of the resected specimen further confirms the diagnosis of ulcerative colitis, especially in patients with a short disease history.

Patients are typically allowed to recover for about 6 months following a subtotal colectomy. This period helps patients recover from the effects of corticosteroids and other

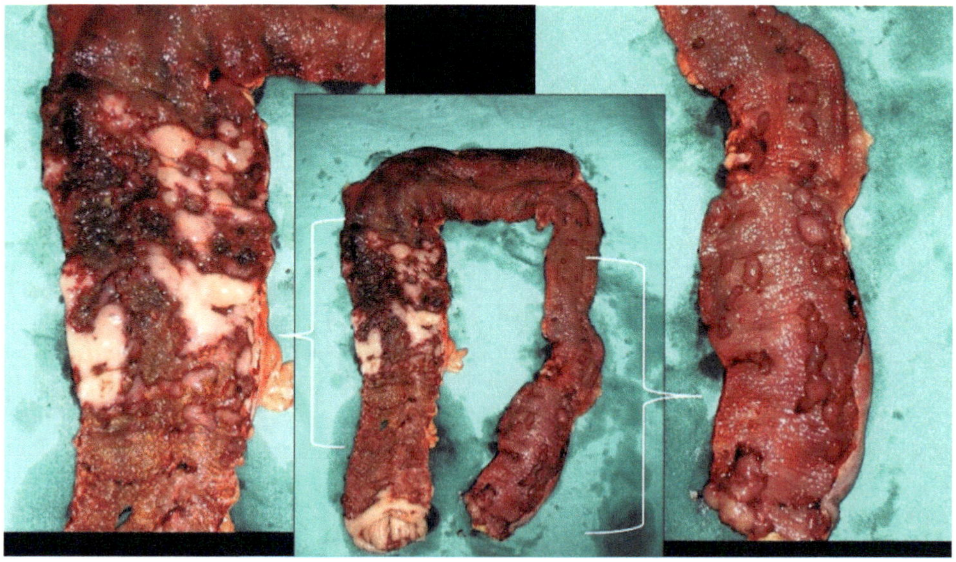

Fig. 12.2 Total colectomy for fulminant colitis and perforation. Note the mucosal destruction and thinning of the right colon and ulcerated mucosa and pseudopolyps in the left colon

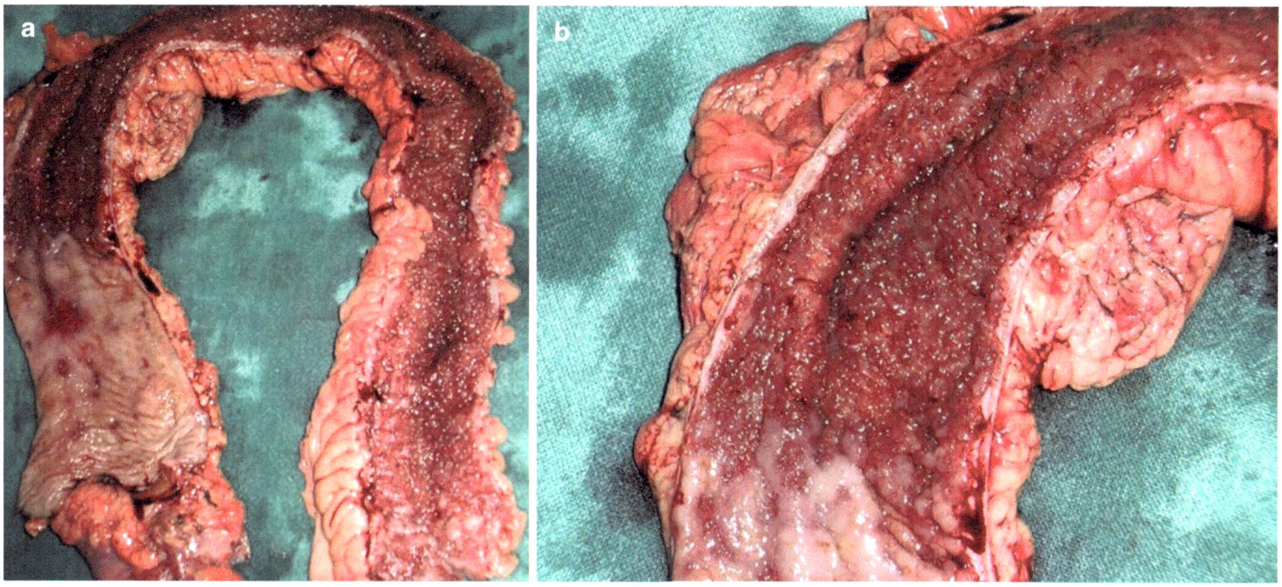

Fig. 12.3 (**a**) Colectomy specimen showing extensive mucosal disease. (**b**) Close-up view of mucosa showing pseudopolyps

immunosuppressants and also improves their nutritional status. At this stage, patients are offered the second-stage procedure, which includes a completion proctectomy and IPAA, performed either through an open or minimally invasive approach. The initial entry into the abdomen may be challenging due to adhesions from previous surgery. These adhesions are usually more severe in patients who experienced wound dehiscence, rectal stump blow-out, or other intra-abdominal complications and tend to be less severe if the STC was performed minimally invasively. The entry should be performed carefully to avoid inadvertent bowel injury. Limited adhesiolysis is carried out to separate the small bowel from the anterior abdominal wall and pelvic structures.

The rectal stump is identified using the long sutures left from previous surgery. Both ureters are also identified before beginning dissection. The rectal mesentery is incised near the rectal wall, and the superior rectal vessels are doubly ligated and divided. Dissection is strictly kept close to the rectal wall (perimuscular dissection) to prevent autonomic nerve injury. The rectum is circumferentially mobilized till 4–5 cm from the anal verge. The rectum is divided using a stapler, and the specimen is taken out.

The ileostomy is taken down, and adhesiolysis is completed. The small bowel mesentery is mobilized up to the duodeno-jejunal (DJ) flexure. The tip of the prospective pouch should reach the rectal stump without tension. Kocher's maneuver, transverse peritoneal incisions along the superior mesenteric vessels, creation of a mesenteric window, and high ligation of the ileocolic pedicle are options to increase the reach of the pouch. Once reach is confirmed, a J pouch is created by folding the distal 15 cm of ileum on itself. Although other pouch configurations such as S pouch and W pouch have been described, they are rarely used. A J pouch is easy to construct using a stapling device, has less bulk, and offers comparable or better results than other configurations. An enterotomy at the tip allows serial firing of a linear stapler to form the pouch and to insert the anvil of a circular stapler. The anvil is secured with a purse-string suture. A 29 mm circular stapler is generally used for creating the ileal pouch-anal anastomosis. The circular stapler is inserted through the anal opening, and the trocar is advanced so that it pierces slightly posterior to the rectal staple line. The trocar is matched with the anvil, and the stapler is closed to bring it into the firing range. The orientation of the pouch should be confirmed before firing the stapler to avoid angulation or rotation. The stapler is then fired to complete the anastomosis. The proximal and distal 'donuts' are inspected for integrity and completeness. The pouch is distended with air to check for leaks (Fig. 12.4). A drain is usually placed behind the pouch, and a diverting loop ileostomy is often added. The ileostomy is typically reversed around 3 months later after confirming the IPAA's integrity with a distal loopogram.

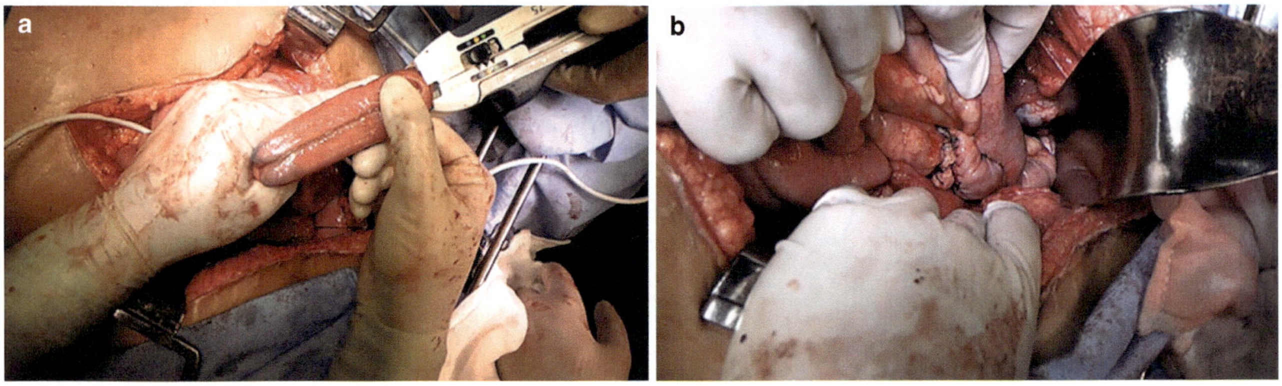

Fig. 12.4 (**a**) Creation of J pouch with the help of linear stapler, (**b**) A completed pouch anal anastomosis

12.8 Elective Surgery

The elective indications for surgery in UC include medical refractory disease, patient preference, intolerance to medical treatment due to adverse effects, and the development of dysplasia or cancer. Limited affordability of prolonged and expensive medical therapy is another reason for surgery in UC in India. Patients with non-neoplastic indications for elective surgery may undergo a two-stage or, less commonly, a one-stage procedure if they are well preserved. However, a three-stage or modified two-stage procedure should be considered if patients are on high-dose steroids or immunosuppressants.

The management of patients with colitic-carcinoma depends on the stage and location. A subtotal colectomy is a reasonable procedure if the cancer is located in the colon. The IPAA may be created in these patients later, after completing any adjuvant treatment. Patients with rectal cancer should be offered neoadjuvant therapy. After neoadjuvant treatment, young patients with cancer of the upper or middle rectum may be offered a restorative TPC with IPAA and loop ileostomy. Patients with cancer of the lower rectum, advanced age, and poor sphincter function are best treated with TPC and a permanent end-ileostomy. Patients with high-grade dysplasia in the rectum who wish to preserve anal function should undergo TPC with mucosectomy, a hand-sewn IPAA, and loop ileostomy.

12.8.1 Complications of IPAA

12.8.1.1 Early Postoperative Complications

Malnourished patients and patients on high-dose steroids and other immunosuppressants are at much higher risk for early postoperative complications.

- Anastomotic leak and pelvic sepsis: The long staple line of IPAA presents a significant risk for anastomotic leaks. A diverting ileostomy is often added to the pouch procedure to protect this long staple line of IPAA. While a diverting ileostomy may not completely prevent an anastomotic leak, it helps reduce the risk of pelvic sepsis if a leak occurs. Patients may present with fever, abdominal pain, leucocytosis, or frank peritonitis. A CT scan with rectal contrast can reveal a collection or contrast leak. Conservative treatment with antibiotics and percutaneous drainage of the collection often suffices for patients with a diverting ileostomy. Patients without a diverting ileostomy are at a much higher risk for pelvic sepsis and typically require surgical exploration, lavage, drainage, and fecal diversion. Pelvic sepsis increases the long-term risk of pelvic fibrosis and pouch failure.
- Wound infection is another common complication, managed with local wound care and antibiotics. Patients on high-dose steroids are at risk for wound dehiscence and might need reoperation.
- Bleeding from the staple line or pouch mucosa is usually self-limited but may require endoscopic cauterization in some cases.
- Bladder dysfunction and urinary retention can happen due to accidental injury to pelvic nerves during posterior and lateral rectal dissection.

12.8.1.2 Late Complications

- Small bowel obstruction is a common complication that can occur early after surgery or later during follow-up. The most frequent cause is postoperative adhesions, which lead to partial obstruction. Most patients improve with conservative treatment. Those who do not respond to conservative management require surgical exploration and adhesiolysis. Patients with complete bowel obstruction, due to an acute kink or internal herniation, need early surgery to prevent bowel strangulation.
- Pouchitis is a common long-term complication of pouch surgery in patients with UC. Its cause is unknown but may be linked to bacterial overgrowth or immune dysregulation. Symptoms include diarrhea, urgency, abdominal

cramps, rectal bleeding, and low-grade fever. Diagnosis usually involves pouchoscopy with biopsy. Acute pouchitis is usually treated with antibiotics like metronidazole or ciprofloxacin. Chronic pouchitis is challenging to treat. Treatment options include probiotics, rotating antibiotics, budesonide enemas, or even biologics for refractory cases.

- Strictures: Anastomotic strictures may develop at the ileal pouch-anal anastomosis. These strictures usually respond to digital or endoscopic dilation. Ischemic strictures develop due to poor blood supply and ischemic necrosis around the IPAA. These strictures can be difficult to dilate and might require surgical intervention.
- Fistula and sinus formation: Pouch-vaginal, pouch-perineal, pouch-enteric fistulae, and blind-ending sinus tracts are often caused by anastomotic leaks and pelvic sepsis, or if Crohn's disease is misdiagnosed as ulcerative colitis. Pouch-vaginal fistula may also develop if the posterior vaginal wall is accidentally included in the circular stapler or suture. The management depends on the location, size, and severity. Small fistulae may heal spontaneously with conservative treatment such as antibiotics, drainage of collections, or seton placement, while larger fistulae often require surgical repair.
- Pouch dysfunction: These patients experience chronic symptoms such as frequent stools, incontinence, urgency, and seepage. Causes include poor pouch compliance due to fibrosis after pelvic sepsis, injury to the sphincter complex, or chronic pouchitis. Some of these patients eventually develop pouch failure over time.
- Pouch failure is defined as the inability to maintain pouch function, which may require pouch revision, excision, or permanent diversion. The most common causes of pouch failure include refractory pouchitis, pelvic sepsis, fistulae, poor function, and misdiagnosed CD. Pouch failure occurs in 5%–10% of patients over a long period and often necessitates pouch revision or a permanent ileostomy.

12.8.1.3 Functional and Quality of Life Issues

Most patients with UC who undergo IPAA report an improvement in quality of life. Initially, stool frequency is high but gradually decreases as the pouch function improves during the first year. Patients may also experience urgency and fecal incontinence, which tend to improve over time. Most patients achieve a stool frequency of 5–6 times during the day and 1–2 times at night, with occasional incontinence. Males may experience sexual dysfunction, such as erectile or ejaculatory issues, due to pelvic nerve injury. Females are at risk of infertility after IPAA because of tubal adhesions resulting from pelvic dissection. If possible, pouch surgery may be delayed until their family is complete. A laparoscopic approach is associated with fewer adhesions and may reduce the risk of infertility.

12.9 Crohn's Disease

Crohn's disease is a chronic, idiopathic, inflammatory bowel disease (IBD) that can affect any part of the gastrointestinal (GI) tract from the mouth to the anus. Unlike ulcerative colitis (UC), which is limited to the colon and involves only the mucosal layer, Crohn's disease involves transmural inflammation of the bowel, leading to complications such as fistulas, strictures, and abscesses. The cause is multifactorial, involving a complex interaction of genetic susceptibility, immune dysregulation, environmental factors, and changes in gut microbiota.

The most frequently affected area is the terminal ileum and proximal colon, although isolated involvement of the small bowel, colon, perianal region, or upper GI tract can also occur. Small bowel involvement is observed in up to 80% of patients, while colonic involvement occurs in about half of the cases. Approximately 50% of patients have isolated small bowel involvement, and isolated colonic involvement is seen in around 20%. Unlike UC, the rectum is typically spared, but involvement of the anal canal and perianal region is quite common.

The clinical presentation of CD is variable, depending on the location and severity of inflammation. It can range from subtle symptoms to severe complications.

12.9.1 Gastrointestinal Symptoms

- Crampy abdominal pain is the most common symptom.
- Chronic non-bloody diarrhea.
- Weight loss: Due to anorexia, malabsorption, and chronic inflammation.
- Anemia: Due to chronic GI blood loss, malabsorption, malnutrition.
- Growth failure: usually seen in children with CD.
- Fever: Low-grade, especially during active disease or abscess formation.
- Perianal disease: Includes fissures, fistulas, and abscesses. Present in up to 40% of patients.
- Obstructive symptoms: Crampy pain, bloating, and vomiting due to strictures.
- Intra-abdominal abscess formation: Psoas abscess, ileocecal phlegmon, or interbowel collections.
- Fistulae.
  - Enteroenteric: Usually asymptomatic or may present as a palpable mass
  - Enterovesical: Recurrent urinary tract infections, pneumaturia
  - Enterovaginal: Passage of wind or feces per vagina
  Enterocutaneous: Usually forms after percutaneous drainage of an intra-abdominal abscess

12.9.2 Extraintestinal Manifestations (EIMs)

- Musculoskeletal: Arthralgia, ankylosing spondylitis
- Dermatologic: Erythema nodosum, pyoderma gangrenosum
- Ocular: Uveitis, episcleritis
- Hepatobiliary: Primary sclerosing cholangitis (less common in CD than UC)
- Renal: Nephrolithiasis (oxalate stones) and hydronephrosis

12.10 Diagnosis

The diagnosis of CD relies on clinical suspicion supported by a combination of endoscopic, radiological, histological, and laboratory findings. There is no single diagnostic test, and intestinal tuberculosis is always included in the differential diagnosis. In fact, many patients with CD are initially diagnosed and treated as tuberculosis.

12.10.1 Laboratory Tests

- Complete blood count (CBC): Anemia (iron or B12 deficiency), leukocytosis.
- C-reactive protein/ESR: Markers of systemic inflammation.
- Fecal calprotectin: Sensitive marker of intestinal inflammation.
- Stool tests: To rule out infections.

12.10.2 Endoscopy

A full-length colonoscopy with intubation of the ileocecal valve and evaluation of the terminal ileum is the most useful initial test. Typical endoscopic findings in CD include aphthous ulcers, deep serpiginous ulcers, cobblestone appearance, and stricture formation. Unlike UC, skip lesions with normal intervening bowel segments are a common finding. Biopsies from the lesions show transmural acute and chronic inflammation, crypt distortion, and crypt abscesses. Noncaseating granulomas are suggestive of CD but are seen in only 30% of patients.

Upper GI endoscopy is helpful for patients suspected of having esophageal, gastric, or duodenal involvement.

12.10.3 Imaging

Abdominal radiograph and ultrasonography are routinely done but are usually nonspecific. As compared to UC, cross-sectional imaging has a much more important role in the diagnostic evaluation of patients with CD. A CT enterography provides a detailed assessment of intra-abdominal organs, including the portions of small bowel that are difficult to reach via endoscopy (Figs. 12.5 and 12.6). The typical findings include

- Asymmetric thickening of the bowel wall, which is usually multifocal
- Long segment strictures showing luminal compromise with upstream bowel dilatation
  - Inflammatory: wall enhancement, ulcerations, and bowel wall edema
  - Fibrotic: little or no inflammation
- Penetrating disease
  - Intra-abdominal abscesses
  - Internal fistulae: Entero-enteric, entero-sigmoid, or entero-vesical
- Mesenteric involvement
  - Creeping fat
  - Lymphadenopathy
  - Engorged vasa recta: Comb sign

Magnetic resonance (MR) enterography has better resolution and provides information similar to CT enterography. MR enterography avoids radiation and thus is preferred in young patients. MR enterography is also preferred when serial imaging is required to assess the treatment response.

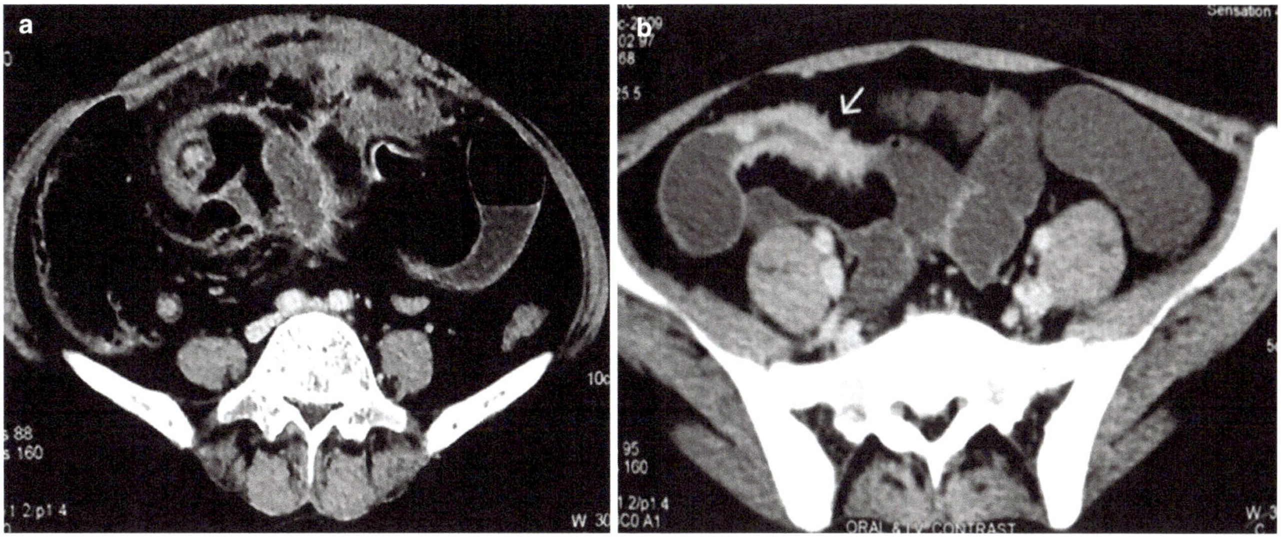

Fig. 12.5 CT Enterography picture showing (**a**) penetrating Crohn's disease, (**b**) stricturing Crohn's disease

Fig. 12.6 (**a**) CECT showing thickened cecum (arrows), (**b**) limited right hemicolectomy in the same patient. Note the ulcers and cobblestone mucosa in the cecum and ascending colon

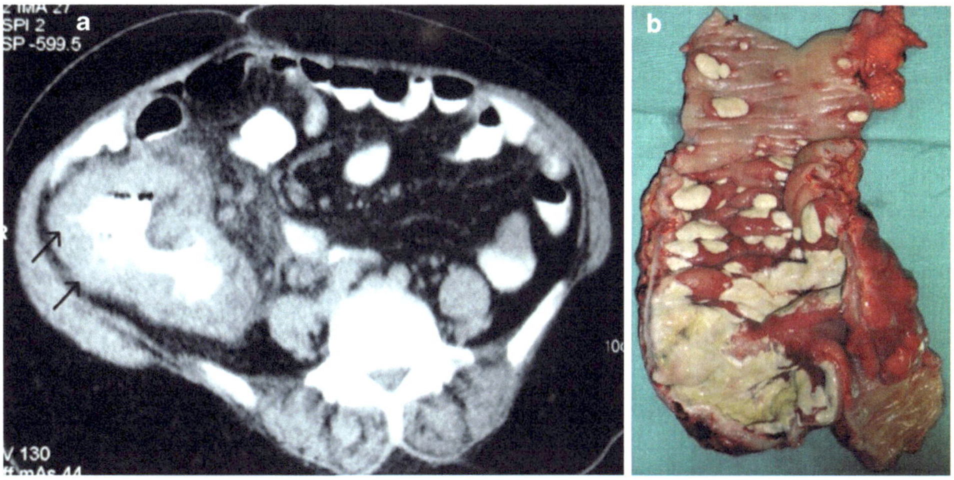

12.11 Classification (Table 12.8)

Table 12.8 The Vienna classification for Crohn's disease

Age	
A1	Diagnosis at or before 40 years of age
A2	Diagnosis after 40 years of age
Location	
L1	Terminal ileum
L2	Colon
L3	Ileocolon
L4	Upper gastrointestinal tract
Behavior	
B1	Non-stricturing, non-penetrating (inflammatory)
B2	Stricturing (narrowing of the intestine)
B3	Penetrating (abnormal connections or fistulas between the intestine and other organs)

12.12 Management

Medical therapy is the treatment of choice in most patients with CD. The goals of treatment are

- Induction of clinical and endoscopic remission
- Maintain long-term remission
- Minimize corticosteroid dependence
- Prevent complications like strictures, fistulas, and abscesses
- Improve nutritional status
- Enhance quality of life

Factors that influence the choice of treatment include disease severity, location, behavior, and presence of complications. There are two broad strategies for the medical management of CD.

- The step-up approach advocates using less potent medicines (5-ASA, corticosteroids, antibiotics), which have mild adverse effects initially, and switching to more potent but more toxic medicines (biologics, immunomodulators) only if the initial treatment fails. This method is used for mild disease.
- A top-down approach that advocates using more potent drugs early on may be helpful for patients with severe disease.

12.13 Surgical Management

Unlike UC, surgery for CD is mostly palliative as the disease can recur anywhere in the GI tract. Still, almost half of the patients with CD require surgery during their lifetime (Table 12.9).

More recently, laparoscopic resection is considered an equivalent treatment to medical therapy with biologics for limited ileocaecal disease that does not respond to initial medical treatment (corticosteroids, 5-ASA, antibiotics).

Choice of surgical procedure in CD depends on the disease phenotype.

12.13.1 Small Bowel and/or Ileocecal Disease

Penetrating/fistulizing disease is usually managed medically and surgery is only considered for managing complications such as intra-abdominal sepsis, fistulae, abscess formation, or free perforation. Role of surgery is limited to drainage of abscess, resection of the diseased segment (only if small segment is involved), peritoneal lavage, and creation of a stoma. Bowel anastomosis is usually avoided due to significant risk of anastomotic leak. Entero-enteral fistulae do not require any specific treatment. Entero-vesical, entero-vaginal, and entero-sigmoid fistula may be dismantled if there is limited involvement. The small bowel portion requires resection while the secondary organs, i.e., urinary bladder, vagina, and even sigmoid colon (if not involved in the disease process), may be primarily repaired. In case there is extensive inflammation, a diverting stoma is done and aggressive medical therapy is administered to control the disease process, and the definitive surgery for internal fistulae is undertaken at a later date (Figs. 12.7 and 12.8).

Table 12.9 Indications for surgery in Crohn's disease

Emergency surgery	Elective surgery
Acute intestinal obstruction	Failure of medical therapy
Perforation	Subacute intestinal obstruction
Massive GI bleeding	Malignancy
Ruptured abscess	
Entero-vesical fistulae	

12.13.1.1 Stricturing Disease

Inflammatory strictures are managed medically, and surgery is reserved for emergency situations or when the disease is localized to the ileocecal region. Fibrotic strictures, if accessible, can be treated with endoscopic dilation. Surgery is considered for strictures that cannot be reached or do not respond to endoscopic dilation. Focal strictures with limited bowel involvement are treated through resection and anastomosis (Figs. 12.9, 12.10 and 12.11). Stricturoplasty should be considered for patients with multifocal disease, as multiple resections pose a risk of short bowel syndrome. Avoid stricturoplasty if any of the following factors are present:

- Inflammatory mass/abscess
- Perforation
- Thick and unyielding bowel wall
- Suspicion of malignancy
- Active bleeding
- Severe malnutrition

Surgery for CD is largely considered palliative, and patients face a risk of disease recurrence after the procedure. The endoscopic recurrence rate can be as high as 80% within approximately 1 year after surgery. However, clinical recurrence occurs at a rate of 10%–15% annually. Recurrent disease is essentially managed with medical therapy, and the indications for surgery are the same as for a primary case. Around 35% of patients require a second surgery within 10 years of the initial procedure. Specific surgical techniques and strategies have been described to decrease the recurrence of CD after surgery.

- Technique of anastomosis.
  - Side-to-side stapled anastomosis as compared to end-to-end handsewn anastomosis.

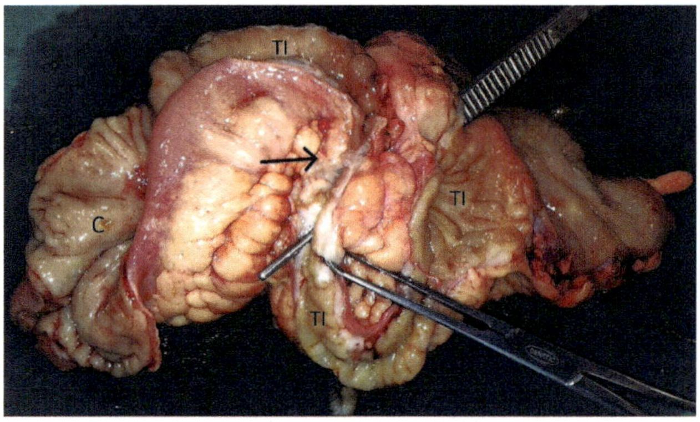

Fig. 12.7 Diseased terminal ileum (TI), stricture (arrow), and ileo-ileal fistula (forceps across the fistula). Cecum (C) is also involved

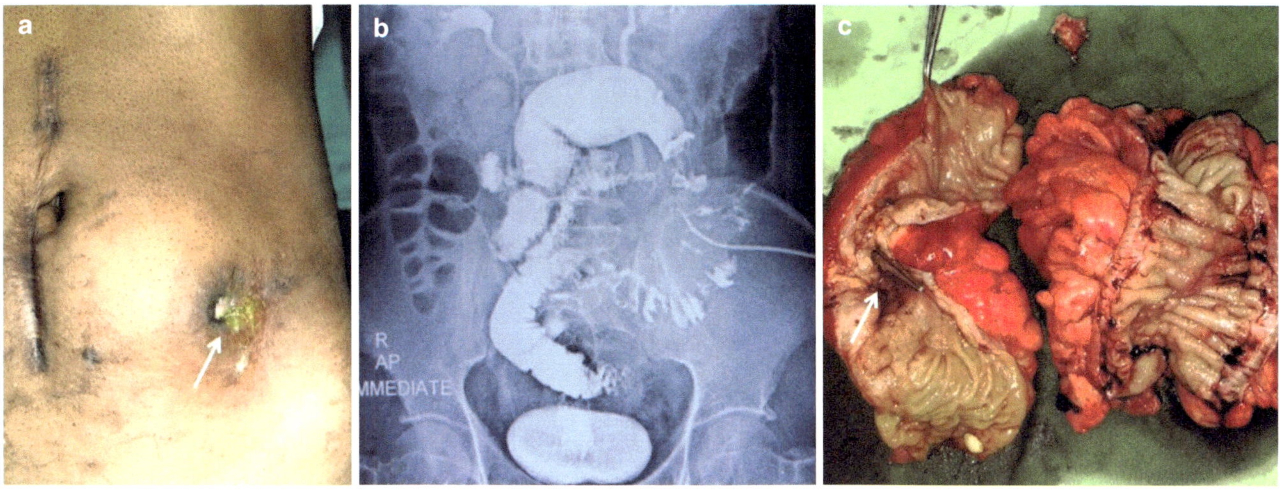

Fig. 12.8 (**a**) Enterocutaneous fistula (arrow) and an inflammatory mass on the left abdomen. The patient had undergone an exploratory laparotomy for intestinal obstruction and mistakenly received antituberculosis treatment for what later proved to be a case of Crohn's disease. (**b**) Opacification of the small bowel and colon on fistulogram confirmed it to be a complex ileo-colo-cutaneous fistula. (**c**) Resected diseased segment of the small bowel and colon. Note the site of stricture (arrow) is also the site of fistula (hemostat across the opening)

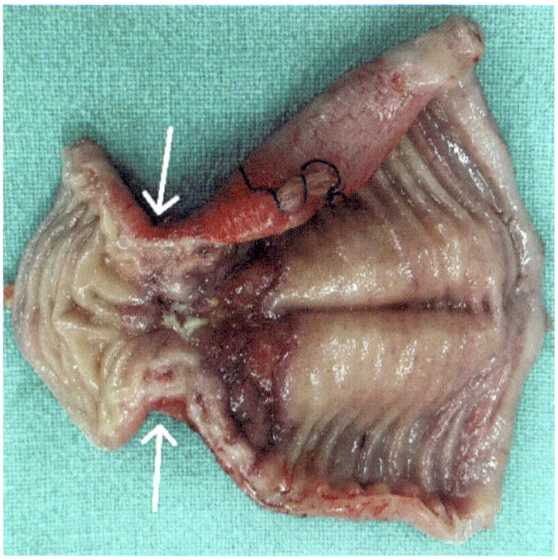

Fig. 12.9 A localized stricture (arrows) in the ileum, treated by segmental excision. Such short stricture is unusual in Crohn's disease

  - Kono-S anastomosis: Handsewn, functional end-to-end anastomosis that completely excludes the mesentery.
- Inclusion of mesentery in the ileocolic resection.
- Wider resection to achieve a histologically negative margin.

12.13.1.2 Isolated Colonic Disease

- Surgery is necessary if medical therapy fails, there is large bowel obstruction due to stricture, or high-grade dysplasia or malignancy develops.
- Focal colonic involvement: Segmental colectomy.
- Diffuse colonic involvement with rectal sparing: Subtotal colectomy with ileorectal anastomosis, usually performed in two stages.

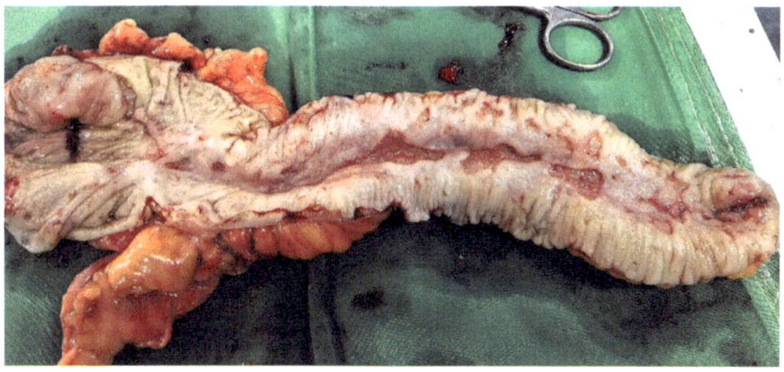

Fig. 12.10 Long-segment involvement of the terminal ileum. Note the serpiginous ulcers in the mesenteric border of the intestine

- Isolated rectal involvement: Total proctectomy with end colostomy.
- Colonic as well as rectal involvement: Total proctocolectomy with end ileostomy.

12.13.1.3 Perianal Disease

The goals of surgery for perianal disease in the presence of active infection or inflammation are

- Drainage of abscess
- Placement of non-cutting setons
- Diversion of fecal stream, usually by loop ileostomy

Definitive surgery for perianal disease is only considered when the luminal disease is in remission and local infection has been controlled. Options for definitive treatment include

- Simple fistulotomy for low fistulae
- Video-assisted anal fistula treatment (VAAFT)
- Advancement flap
- Local injection of mesenchymal stem cells

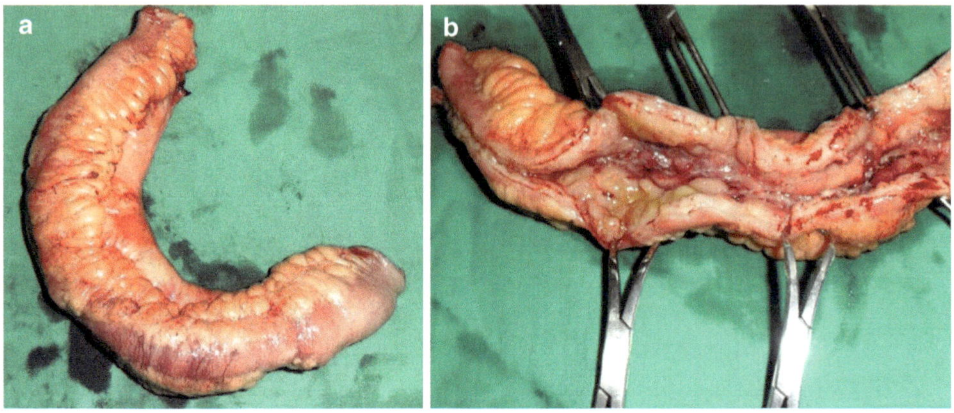

Fig. 12.11 (**a**) Segmental excision of the diseased small intestine. Note the mesenteric creeping, a typical intraoperative finding in Crohn's disease. (**b**) Opened specimen showing serpiginous ulcers along the mesenteric border of the intestine

Key Points

- Ulcerative Colitis (UC) is a continuous mucosal inflammation that begins at the anorectal junction and extends proximally to involve the colon. The inflammation is characteristically limited to the mucosal layer.
- Crohn's Disease (CD) is characterized by transmural inflammation that can affect any segment of the GI tract from mouth to anus, with skip areas of normal tissue between diseased segments.
- UC is suspected in patients presenting with chronic diarrhea of more than 4 weeks duration, confirmed on colonoscopic findings of active inflammation or chronic inflammation on biopsy.
- Extraintestinal manifestations of UC may involve skin, eye, musculoskeletal, or hepatobiliary systems.
- The development of colorectal cancer is directly proportional to the duration of the disease.
- Failure of medical treatment, both in emergency and elective situations, is an indication for surgery.
- Non-remitting acute fulminant colitis, toxic megacolon, colonic perforation, and massive lower GI bleeding are indications for emergency surgery.
- Staged restorative proctocolectomy (J pouch ileoanal anastomosis) is the surgical procedure of choice for UC.
- Treatment of CD is essentially medical; surgery is more often palliative.
- Surgery in CD is indicated for failure of medical treatment to achieve remission or to treat complications like stricture, fistulae, or lower GI bleeding.
- Conservative techniques such as stricturoplasty, bypass, or limited resection should be practiced as the disease is known to recur and may require further surgery in the future.

Selected Reading

1. Nguyen GC, et al. American Gastroenterological Association Institute guideline on the management of Crohn's disease after surgical resection. Gastroenterology. 2017;152(1):271–5.
2. Angriman I, et al. A systematic review of segmental vs subtotal colectomy and subtotal colectomy vs total proctocolectomy for colonic Crohn's disease. Color Dis. 2017;19(8):e279–87.
3. Anto VP, Dawes AJ, Vrees M, et al. Surgical management of inflammatory bowel disease. R I Med J. 2022;105(10):25–30.
4. Cai Z, Cail Z, Wang S, et al. Treatment of inflammatory bowel disease: a comprehensive review. Front Med. 2021;8. https://doi.org/10.3389/fmed.2021.765474.
5. Eskazan T, Hatemi I. Surgical treatment in inflammatory bowel disease. J Enterocolitis. 2025;4(Suppl 1):S81–6.

Prolapse Rectum

13

Manash Ranjan Sahoo and Vikeerna Bharti

Abstract

Rectal prolapse occurs because of failure in the anatomical support system, chronic constipation, or neuromuscular dysfunction. Laparoscopic rectopexy is currently the most popular surgical procedure for rectal prolapse because of minimal morbidity and low recurrence rates.

Keywords

Rectal prolapse

The rectum is supported by a combination of muscular, fascial, and ligamentous structures that keep it in place within the pelvis and prevent descent during periods of increased intra-abdominal pressure (Table 13.1).

Table 13.1 Anatomical support of the rectum

Muscular support (pelvic diaphragm)	The levator ani muscles (puborectalis, pubococcygeus, and iliococcygeus) form the primary muscular support of the rectum.
Fascial support	Denonvilliers' fascia: Provides anterior support by separating the rectum from adjacent structures (e.g., prostate in men, vagina in women). Waldeyer's fascia: Provides posterior support, anchoring the rectum to the sacral promontory.
Ligamentous support	The lateral ligaments of the rectum provide lateral support to help stabilize the rectum.

13.1 Pathophysiology of Rectal Prolapse

Rectal prolapse occurs when the standard support mechanisms of the rectum and pelvic floor fail. It is caused by dysfunction in the muscular, fascial, and neurological components that maintain rectal support.

Key contributors to rectal prolapse include:

- Pelvic floor muscle weakness, especially in the levator ani muscles (puborectalis and pubococcygeus).
- Loss of the anorectal angle, which normally provides resistance to prolapse during increased intra-abdominal pressure.
- Failure of fascia and ligaments, such as weakening of Denonvilliers' and Waldeyer's fascia.
- Chronic intra-abdominal pressure, often caused by constipation and chronic straining.
- Neuromuscular dysfunction, including damage to the pudendal nerve, affects sphincter control and can lead to fecal incontinence.

M. R. Sahoo (✉) · V. Bharti
All India Institute of Medical Sciences, Bhubaneswar, India

M. Ibrarullah (ed.), *Recent Concepts in Gastrointestinal (GI) Surgery*, https://doi.org/10.1007/978-981-92-1118-0_13

13.2 Clinical Presentation

Symptoms of rectal prolapse can be categorized based on the extent of the prolapse (external or internal) and associated conditions, such as pelvic floor dysfunction.

13.2.1 External Rectal Prolapse

Visible prolapse during defecation.

Pain or discomfort, especially while standing or during bowel movements.

Mucus discharge, leading to perianal irritation.

Bleeding due to ulceration of the prolapsed mucosa.

Fecal incontinence, caused by weakening or stretching of the anal sphincter complex and/or nerve damage, is noted in 50%–75% of cases.

13.2.2 Internal Rectal Prolapse (Intussusception)

Incomplete evacuation or the sensation of incomplete defecation.

Obstructed defecation syndrome: Difficulty in passing stool despite the urge, requiring excessive straining or manual assistance.

Chronic constipation: Associated with internal prolapse, leading to infrequent bowel movements and hard stools.

Patients may experience significant psychological distress, social embarrassment, and depression due to incontinence and the visible nature of prolapse.

13.3 Investigations

A combination of clinical examinations and specialized investigations is necessary not only to diagnose rectal prolapse but also to identify the precipitating factors.

- *Clinical Examination*
  Visual inspection and digital rectal exam (DRE) are often used to assess the presence and severity of prolapse.
  Proctoscopy can help identify internal prolapse or associated inflammation.
- *Imaging*
  Defecography (dynamic radiographic assessment during defecation) confirms prolapse and evaluates pelvic floor disorders.
  Magnetic resonance (MR) defecography provides detailed imaging of pelvic structures and associated prolapses.
- *Functional Tests*
  Anorectal manometry assesses sphincter function and rectal sensitivity.
  The balloon expulsion test evaluates defecation mechanics.

13.4 Management of Rectal Prolapse

While conservative management plays a role in symptom control, especially for internal prolapse or unfit patients, surgery remains the definitive treatment for full-thickness rectal prolapse.

13.4.1 Conservative Management

Conservative treatments are usually recommended for patients with early-stage prolapse, internal prolapse (intussusception), or those at high risk for surgery. The aim is to relieve symptoms, prevent further progression, and enhance bowel function without directly correcting the underlying anatomical defect.

13.4.1.1 Dietary and Lifestyle Modifications

A key strategy in conservative management involves addressing factors that contribute to chronic straining and constipation, which are primary causes of worsening prolapse.

High fiber diet: Increasing dietary fiber intake (25–30 grams per day) is essential for improving stool bulk and softness, aiding in easier bowel movements. Common sources include fruits, vegetables, whole grains, and fiber supplements such as psyllium husk and methylcellulose.

Adequate hydration: Patients should drink at least 6–8 glasses of water daily to prevent dehydration and hard stool formation.

Regular bowel habits: Establishing consistent bowel routines and avoiding prolonged straining on the toilet can reduce intra-abdominal pressure. Using a stool to elevate the feet while defecating can help straighten the anorectal angle, making bowel movements easier.

13.4.2 Pharmacological Management

For patients with constipation or diarrhea, medications can help normalize bowel habits, reducing straining and the risk of prolapse worsening.

Stool Softeners: Docusate sodium is often prescribed to soften stool and prevent straining.
Osmotic laxatives: Polyethylene glycol (PEG), lactulose, or magnesium hydroxide draw water into the colon, softening stools and encouraging more regular bowel movements.
Antidiarrheal medications: Loperamide may be used for patients with diarrhea, as excessive bowel movements and loose stools can worsen prolapse.

13.4.3 Pelvic Floor Rehabilitation

For patients with mild or internal prolapse, pelvic floor exercises (such as Kegel exercises) and biofeedback therapy can strengthen the pelvic floor and improve coordination, which may reduce symptoms and slow disease progression.

Kegel exercises: Focus on strengthening the pelvic floor muscles, especially the levator ani muscles, through repeated contractions.
Biofeedback therapy: A technique that helps patients learn to control their pelvic floor muscles using sensory feedback. This is especially helpful for those with pelvic floor dyssynergia (impaired coordination of pelvic muscles during defecation).

13.4.4 Manual Reduction and Skin Care

Manual Reduction: For patients with external rectal prolapse, manual reduction involves gently pushing the prolapsed tissue back into place, usually after defecation.
Perineal Care: Mucus discharge from prolapsed tissue can cause perineal irritation, pruritus ani, and skin breakdown. Proper cleansing with mild soap and the application of barrier creams (such as zinc oxide or petroleum jelly) can protect the skin and prevent infection.

13.4.5 Observation and Monitoring

Patients with mild or asymptomatic prolapse, especially elderly or frail individuals, may benefit from regular monitoring. This involves consistent evaluations to track prolapse progression and identify any new complications.

13.4.6 Surgical Management

Surgery is the definitive treatment for full-thickness rectal prolapse. The choice of procedure depends on several factors, including the patient's age, comorbidities, presence of associated conditions (e.g., constipation, fecal incontinence), and the surgeon's expertise. Surgical approaches are broadly classified into abdominal and perineal procedures, with laparoscopic rectopexy being the preferred option for most patients due to its minimally invasive nature and excellent long-term outcomes.

13.4.6.1 Abdominal Procedures

Abdominal procedures are favored for younger, healthier patients because of their lower recurrence rates and superior long-term results.

Laparoscopic Rectopexy

Laparoscopic rectopexy is emerging as the most preferred abdominal procedure for rectal prolapse. The dissection begins by opening the peritoneum on the right side of the rectum with a harmonic scalpel. Care is taken to identify and protect the right ureter and the autonomic nerves, especially the nervi erigentes. The rectum is carefully dissected free from the presacral fascia in the so-called "holy plane of Heald," which enables nerve-sparing dissection and prevents injury to the parasympathetic nerves. The dissection continues on the left side after identifying the left ureter, followed by anterior dissection downward until the pelvic floor is reached. *Suture rectopexy* involves fixing the rectum directly to the sacral promontory using nonabsorbable sutures. This approach is particularly suitable for patients without significant constipation. The peritoneum is then reapproximated over the rectum to cover the sutures and restore normal anatomy. In *mesh rectopexy*, a synthetic mesh, such as polypropylene, is used to secure the rectum to the sacrum. This method offers additional support and is often recommended for patients with weakened pelvic tissues or recurrent prolapse. After mobilizing the rectum, a polypropylene mesh is placed behind it, sutured to the presacral fascia posteriorly, and covers about two-thirds of the rectal circumference, sparing its anterior surface. The mesh is then reperitonealized, completing the operation similarly to suture rectopexy.

Oral liquids are started on the second postoperative day, followed by a gradual transition to a normal diet as tolerated. Stool softeners are given for 2 weeks after surgery to prevent straining during bowel movements.

Laparoscopic Ventral Mesh Rectopexy (LVMR)

LVMR is a minimally invasive option indicated for patients with concurrent pelvic organ prolapse (e.g., cystocele or enterocele). The procedure involves anterior mobilization of the rectum and placement of a mesh without disrupting its posterior and lateral supports. A strip of synthetic mesh is sutured to the anterior rectal wall and anchored to the sacral promontory.

Resection Rectopexy

Resection rectopexy is indicated in patients with a redundant sigmoid colon and/or severe constipation. The redundant sigmoid colon is resected, and the remaining colon is anastomosed to the rectum, followed by rectal fixation to the sacral promontory.

13.4.6.2 Perineal Procedures

Perineal procedures are preferred for elderly or high-risk patients who might not tolerate major abdominal surgery. These procedures are less invasive but tend to have higher recurrence rates compared to abdominal approaches.

Altemeier's Procedure (Perineal Rectosigmoidectomy)

Altemeier's procedure involves removing the prolapsed rectum and part of the sigmoid colon through the perineum. The prolapsed rectum is exteriorized, and a full-thickness resection is performed. The remaining rectum is pulled down, and a colorectal anastomosis is created. Recurrence rates are higher after this procedure, and there is also a risk of fecal incontinence, especially in patients with preexisting sphincter dysfunction.

Delorme's Procedure

Delorme's procedure is used for short-segment prolapse. It involves a circumferential incision and stripping the mucosa from the prolapsed rectum, followed by plication of the muscle layer to reinforce and shorten the rectum. This procedure is technically simpler but has higher recurrence rates compared to abdominal approaches.

13.4.6.3 Postoperative Complications

Constipation, particularly if tension on the rectum is excessive.

Fecal incontinence can occur due to damage to the sphincter complex or nerve injury.

Mesh-related complications: These include infection and mesh erosion.

Recurrence Rates: Abdominal procedures have lower recurrence rates (2%–10%) compared to perineal procedures (10%–30%).

Key Points

- Rectal prolapse usually occurs because of failure in the anatomical support system, chronic constipation, or neuromuscular dysfunction.
- Management of rectal prolapse involves not only diagnosis but also identification of the precipitating factors.
- Surgical rectopexy offers the most definitive form of treatment that can be performed either by abdominal or perineal approach.
- Laparoscopic rectopexy is currently the most popular surgical procedure for rectal prolapse because of minimal morbidity and low recurrence rates.
- Perineal approach for rectal prolapse has a limited acceptance because of a high recurrence rate.

Selected Reading

1. Bordeianou L, Paquette I, Johnson E, et al. Clinical practice guidelines for the treatment of rectal prolapse. Dis Colon Rectum. 2017;60:1121–31.
2. Oruc M, Erol T. Current diagnostic tools and treatment modalities for rectal prolapse. World J Clin Cases. 2023;11(16):3680–93. https://doi.org/10.12998/wjcc.v11.i16.3680.

Benign and Malignant Tumors of the Colon

14

Ritu Thakur and Ajit Kumar

Abstract

Haggitt classification describes the structure of an adenomatous polyp that has undergone neoplastic changes: up to level 2 infiltration, polyps can be treated by local excision (endoscopic polypectomy), whereas level 3 and 4 require formal surgical removal in the form of segmental colectomy. Infiltration in sessile polyps more often reaches level 4. Proctocolectomy is recommended for all individuals with FAP because of its universal malignant potential. Colorectal cancer (CRC) is the most common GI malignancy that occurs as a result of a disturbed balance between oncogene and tumor suppressor gene. Astler-Coller modifications of Dukes staging and TNM staging are commonly used for colon cancer. Colonoscopy and CECT are standard investigations required for preoperative diagnosis as well as staging of the disease. Segmental excision of the colon for cancer is based on the lymphovascular pedicle. Indications for chemotherapy in colorectal cancer include all patients with T3 lesions, positive lymph nodes, major vein involvement, signet cell carcinoma, or elevated preoperative CEA levels. Patients with isolated liver or lung metastases can undergo surgery for both the primary and metastatic lesions, as resection often achieves reasonable disease control.

Keywords

Carcinoma colon · Colonic adenoma

Colonic tumors consist of a heterogeneous spectrum of benign and malignant conditions, ranging from symptomless benign polyps to malignant obstructive growths. The majority of colorectal malignancies are believed to arise from benign adenomatous polyps that undergo malignant changes over time.

14.1 Polyp

Polyps are characterized by their morphology and internal structure. They are histologically diverse and can appear as isolated growths, occur in small clusters, or be part of a polyposis syndrome.

14.1.1 Inflammatory Polyps

Inflammatory polyps, also known as pseudopolyps, are commonly observed in individuals with inflammatory bowel disease (IBD), especially in ulcerative colitis. These polyps are linked to surrounding dysplasia, which increases the risk of colorectal cancer. Symptoms of inflammatory polyps often resemble those of IBD. Diagnosis is usually confirmed by colonoscopy, which shows characteristic features of IBD. Although inflammatory polyps are considered benign, their presence in IBD patients requires careful monitoring and management due to the associated risks and symptoms.

14.1.2 Hamartomatous Polyps

Hamartomatous polyps are benign growths characterized by an abnormal mixture of native cell types and tissues. Diagnosis involves reviewing personal and family medical history, performing a colonoscopic assessment, and analyzing biopsy samples. These polyps are often associated with various genetic syndromes, including Peutz–Jeghers syndrome (PJS), Cowden syndrome (CS), juvenile polyposis syndrome (JPS), Bannayan-Riley-Ruvalcaba syndrome, and Cronkhite-Canada syndrome. Although hamartomatous polyps are usually considered noncancerous, the development of malignancy from an adenomatous component within the polyp requires regular surveillance.

R. Thakur (✉) · A. Kumar
All India Institute of Medical Sciences, Rishikesh, India

M. Ibrarullah (ed.), *Recent Concepts in Gastrointestinal (GI) Surgery*, https://doi.org/10.1007/978-981-92-1118-0_14

14.1.3 Sessile Serrated Lesions

These are a diverse group of polyps with varying potential for malignancy. They include hyperplastic polyps, traditional serrated adenomas, and sessile serrated polyps. Primarily found in the right colon, these lesions can be difficult to detect during colonoscopy due to their flat appearance. Malignant transformation in these polyps occurs through the "serrated pathway," which is different from the adenoma-carcinoma sequence.

14.1.4 Hyperplastic and Metaplastic Polyps

Hyperplastic and metaplastic polyps are the most common types of colorectal polyps, characterized by their pathogenesis, which involves reduced epithelial cell turnover leading to the accumulation of goblet cells. Generally, these polyps are not considered precancerous and tend to occur in individuals during their sixth or seventh decade of life. However, recent studies have shown that certain subtypes may have malignant potential. Specifically, sessile serrated lesions and hyperplastic polyps larger than 10 mm can harbor mutations in the KRAS or BRAF genes. These mutations can cause gene methylation, promoting malignancy through the so-called "serrated pathway." Because of this potential for malignant transformation, it is recommended that these polyps be removed and monitored with surveillance colonoscopy to detect any signs of progression or cancer.

14.1.5 Adenomatous Polyps

Adenomatous polyps have a very high potential to develop into malignant tumors. The risk of cancer from these polyps depends on their histology, shape, and size. There are three main types of adenomatous polyps: tubular, villous, and tubulovillous. The likelihood of cancer increases with the number and size of the polyps, with nearly one-third of large adenomas (over 3 cm) showing invasive cancer. Villous adenomas are especially concerning because they are more likely to become malignant than tubular adenomas. Additionally, sessile polyps carry a higher risk than pedunculated ones due to their flat shape, which can make detection and removal more difficult. Villous polyps in the rectum may produce mucus rich in bicarbonate and sodium, potentially leading to hyponatremia, metabolic acidosis, and hypoalbuminemia.

14.2 Haggitt Classification of Colonic Polyps

Haggitt classification describes the structure of an adenomatous polyp that has undergone neoplastic changes. Management strategies are determined based on the level of infiltration (Fig. 14.1 and Table 14.1)

Pedunculated polyps with level 1 and 2 invasions can be removed endoscopically. In cases of level 3 invasion, the resection margins and submucosa should be examined for signs of infiltration. A formal surgical resection is advised if the margin is positive or if there is level 4 invasion. Tumor invasion in the case of a sessile polyp often extends to level 4 unless detected very early.

Various techniques, such as hot or cold snare polypectomy, can be used for smaller polyps. For larger or thicker polyps, a submucosal injection might be necessary to lift the polyp before resection. If the polyp does not elevate after injection, malignancy is suspected, and the site should be tattooed for later identification. Biopsy is avoided if endoscopic mucosal resection or submucosal dissection is planned to reduce the risk of perforation during the latter procedure (Figs. 14.2 and 14.3).

14.2.1 Polyp Surveillance

Even after successful removal of polyps, there remains a risk of developing new ones, though the chances of subsequent colorectal cancer are low. The necessity and frequency of follow-up colonoscopy are influenced by several factors, including the morphology, size, and number of polyps, the patient's age and comorbidities, family history of colorectal cancer, and the thoroughness of the initial colonoscopy. According to the guidelines of the British Society of Gastroenterology, high-risk patients who require follow-up colonoscopy include those with two or more premalignant polyps, one of which must be an advanced colorectal polyp (defined as a serrated polyp $\geq$10 mm or any polyp with dysplasia), as well as individuals with five or more premalignant polyps.

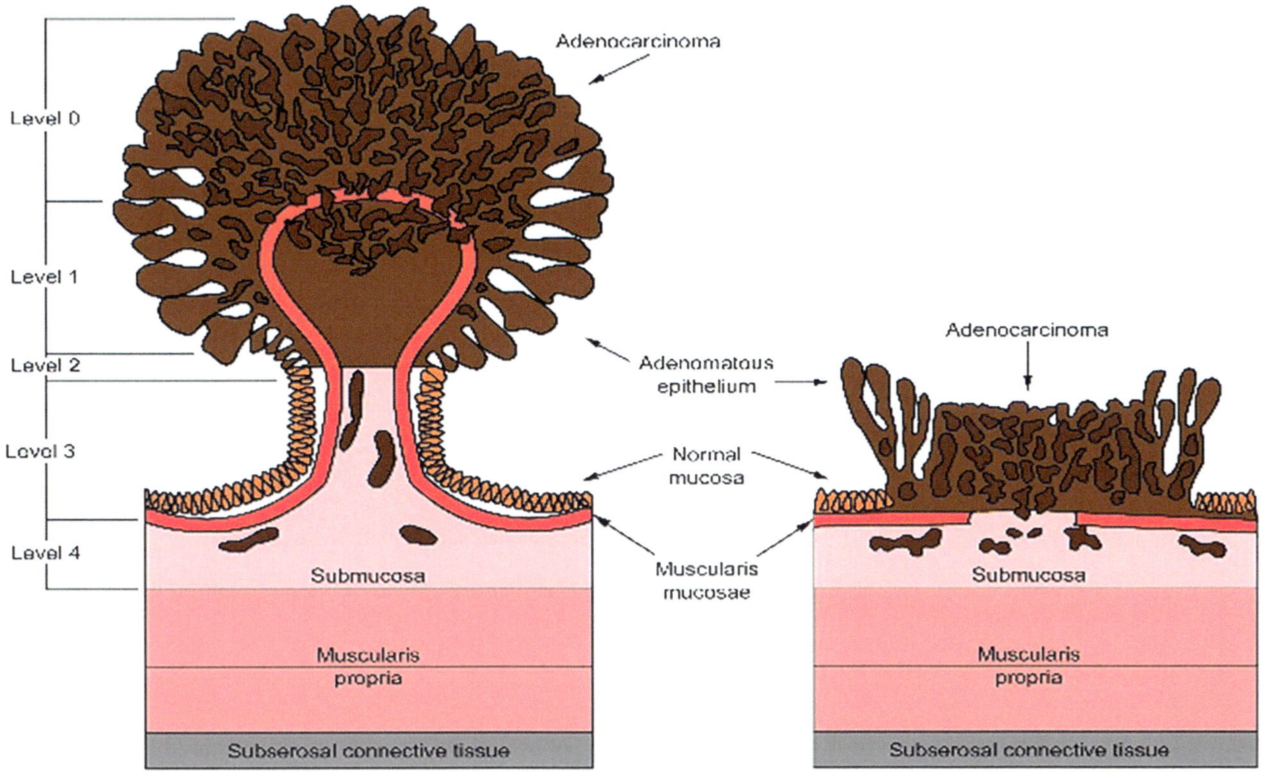

Fig. 14.1 Haggitt classification of the morphology of an adenomatous polyp that has undergone neoplastic change

Table 14.1 Haggitt classification (details in the above figure)

Level	Extent of the tumor invasion
0	Noninvasive (Severe dysplasia)
1	Invading through the muscularis mucosa, but limited to the head of the polyp
2	Invading the neck of the polyp
3	Invading the stalk of the polyp
4	Invading the submucosa below the stalk of the polyp

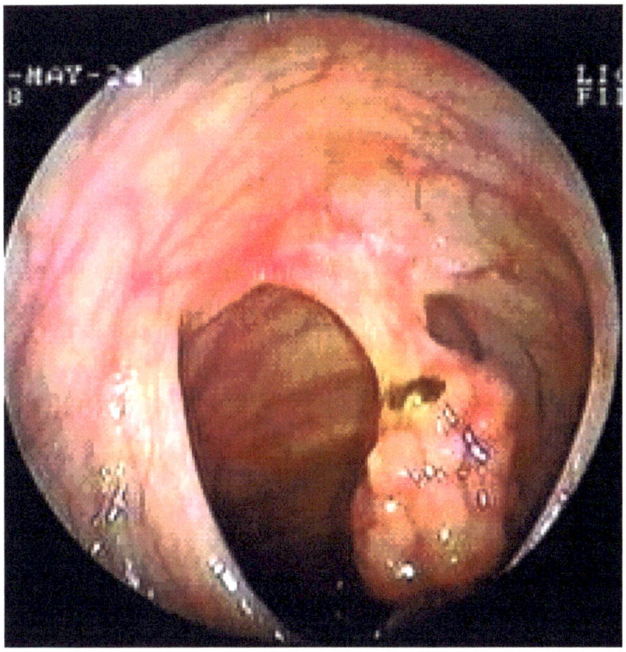

Fig. 14.2 A pedunculated polyp seen on colonoscopy

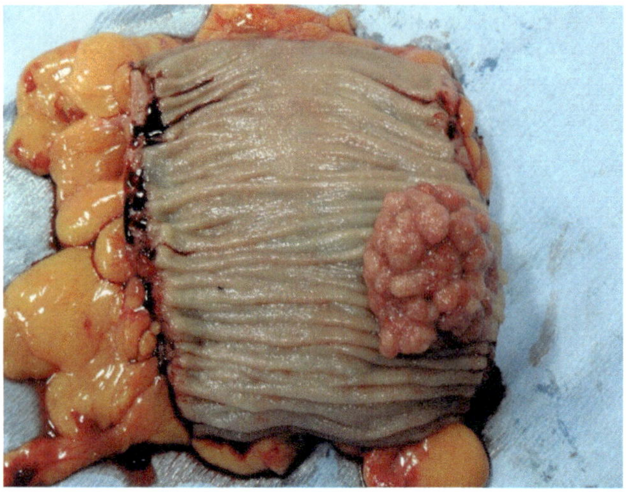

Fig. 14.3 A sessile polyp (villous adenoma) in the descending colon

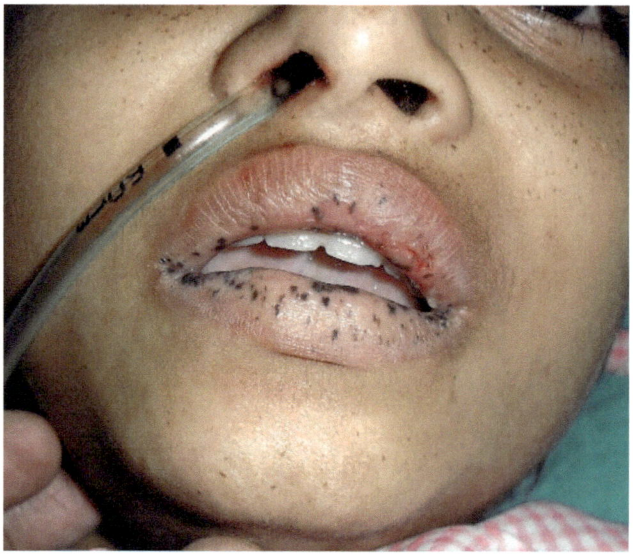

Fig. 14.4 Pigmentation of the lips in a young girl with Peutz-Jeghers polyps

14.3 Syndromes Associated with Polyps

14.3.1 Juvenile Polyposis Syndrome

Juvenile Polyposis Syndrome is a genetic disorder caused by a mutation in the SMAD4 gene. This syndrome features multiple polyps in the gastrointestinal (GI) tract, usually ranging from three to as many as 100. These polyps appear in various areas of the GI tract, most often in the colon and rectum. The condition is inherited in an autosomal dominant manner, meaning an affected person has a 50% chance of passing the mutated gene to their children. A significant concern with juvenile polyposis is the significantly increased risk of developing colorectal cancer at a younger age than the general population. Because of this higher cancer risk, people diagnosed with the syndrome need regular surveillance and management to check for polyp formation and possible malignant transformation.

14.3.2 Peutz-Jeghers Syndrome

Peutz-Jeghers Syndrome is a genetic disorder that typically becomes evident during adolescence, usually between the ages of 10 and 15. This syndrome is linked to mutations in the STK-11/LKB1 gene on chromosome 19 and follows an autosomal dominant inheritance pattern, meaning that an affected parent can pass the condition to their children. Individuals with Peutz-Jeghers Syndrome develop multiple hamartomatous polyps throughout their GI tract, most often in the small intestine, which display a distinctive arborizing pattern under microscopic examination. A key clinical feature of this syndrome is perioral melanosis, characterized by pigmented lesions around the mouth that may also appear on other mucosal surfaces. Patients frequently experience complications such as bowel obstruction caused by intussusception. Additionally, Peutz-Jeghers Syndrome is associated with a substantially increased risk of several cancers, including a 100-fold higher risk for pancreatic cancer. Other concerning cancers include periampullary, thyroid, and colorectal cancers. This heightened cancer risk underscores the importance of regular screening and monitoring for affected individuals (Fig. 14.4).

14.3.3 Cowden Syndrome

Cowden Syndrome is a genetic disorder caused by mutations in the PTEN gene, which is located on chromosome 10. It is inherited in an autosomal dominant manner, meaning that only one copy of the mutated gene is sufficient to increase the risk of developing the associated features. People with Cowden syndrome typically present with multiple GI polyps, which are notable for being nonmalignant. This sets them apart from polyps seen in other syndromes that have a higher risk of malignant transformation. In addition to GI symptoms, affected individuals often show various skin lesions, including lipomas and ganglioneuromas. A key concern with Cowden syndrome is the increased risk of certain cancers. Those with the condition face a higher chance of developing thyroid, breast, and uterine cancers. This increased risk highlights the importance of regular screening and monitoring for potential cancerous changes.

14.3.4 Bannayan-Riley-Ruvalcaba Syndrome

Bannayan-Riley-Ruvalcaba Syndrome is a genetic disorder marked by multiple benign GI polyps. It is linked to mutations in the PTEN gene, similar to Cowden syndrome. Besides GI symptoms, individuals with this syndrome may show other features such as macrocephaly, hypothyroidism, and penile pigmentation. Treatment primarily involves monitoring for polyps and managing endocrine disorders, such as thyroid function, to improve overall health and quality of life for those affected.

14.3.5 Cronkhite-Canada Syndrome

Cronkhite-Canada Syndrome is a rare disorder characterized by the presence of multiple benign polyps in the GI tract. These polyps are associated with significant complications, including rectal bleeding and anemia due to blood loss and nutrient deficiencies. In addition to the GI symptoms, individuals with this syndrome often exhibit signs of ectodermal dysplasia, which manifests as hair loss (alopecia) and brittle nails (koilonychia). The exact cause of Cronkhite-Canada Syndrome remains unclear, although it is thought to involve an autoimmune mechanism. Diagnosis consists of a combination of clinical assessment, colonoscopy, and histological analysis of the polyps.

Polyposis syndromes can be categorized into several types: familial adenomatous polyposis (FAP), attenuated familial adenomatous polyposis (AFAP), MUTYH-associated polyposis (MAP), and NTHL1-associated polyposis (NAP).

14.3.6 Familial Adenomatous Polyposis Syndrome

Familial adenomatous polyposis (FAP) is defined by the presence of over 100 colorectal adenomas and is also marked by the occurrence of duodenal adenomas and various extraintestinal features. More than 80% of cases occur in individuals with a positive family history. In contrast, the remaining cases result from new mutations in the adenomatous polyposis coli (APC) gene located on the long arm of chromosome 5. FAP is inherited in an autosomal dominant pattern, affecting men and women equally (Figs. 14.5 and 14.6). Those with an APC gene mutation have a lifetime risk of colorectal cancer that nears 100%. Up to 50% of individuals with FAP display congenital hypertrophy of the retinal pigment epithelium (CHRPE), which can serve as a screening tool for affected families when genetic testing is not available. Variants of FAP include (Table 14.2):

(a) Gardner syndrome, characterized by the presence of sebaceous cysts, osteomas, and desmoid tumors.
(b) Turcot Syndrome, which is associated with central nervous system tumors, such as glioblastoma, and is inherited in an autosomal recessive pattern.

14.3.7 Treatment

The primary goal of surgery in FAP is to prevent the development of colorectal cancer. Surgical options include restorative proctocolectomy with ileal pouch–anal anastomosis

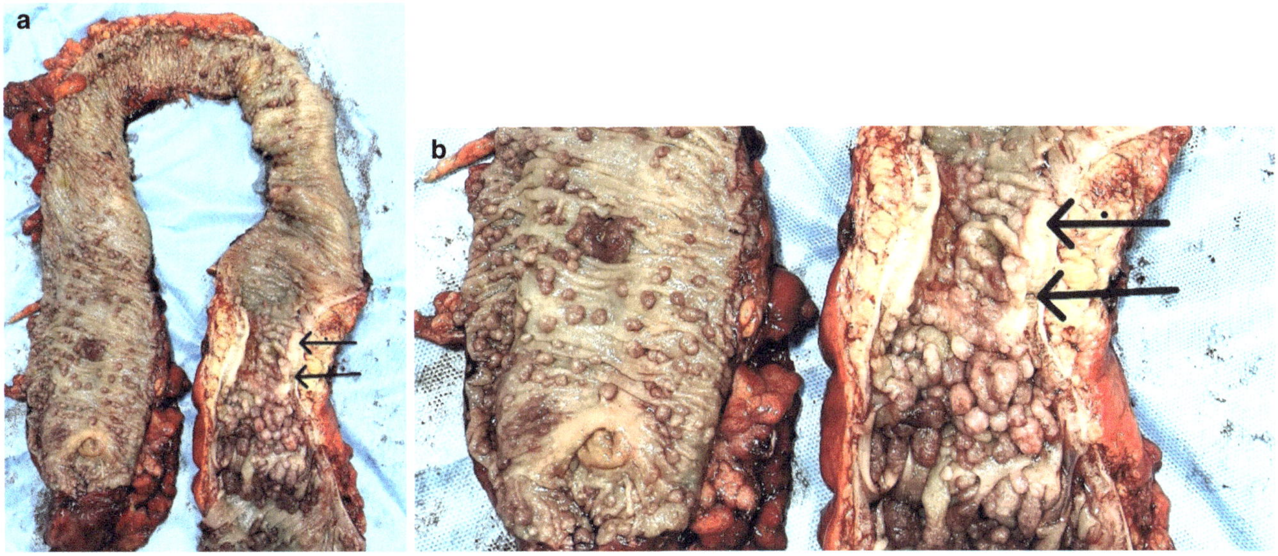

Fig. 14.5 (**a**) Polyps evenly distributed in the entire colon. Malignant transformation of the polyps is seen in the sigmoid colon (arrows). (**b**) Magnified view

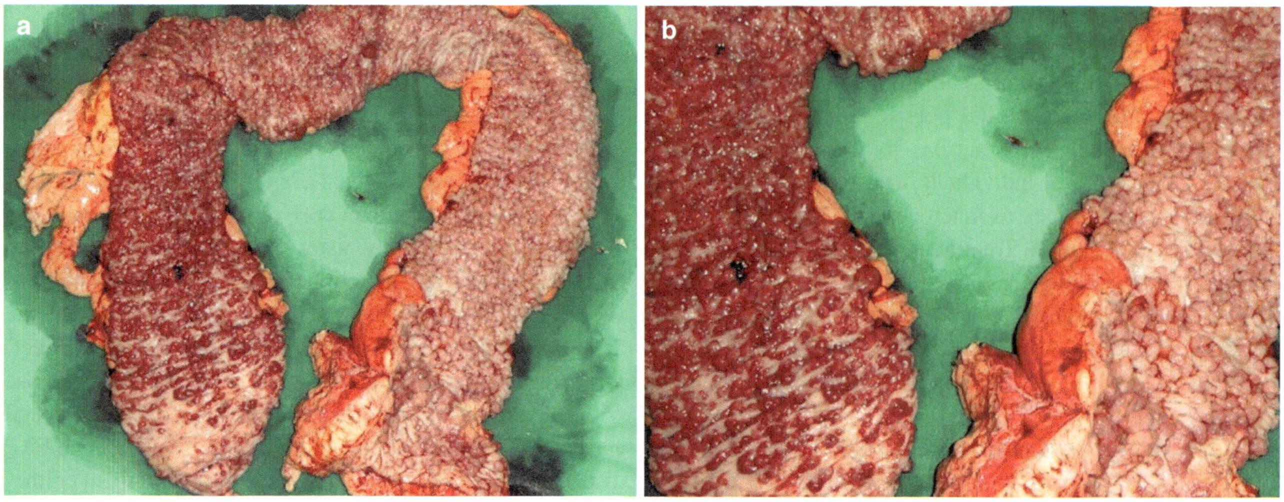

Fig. 14.6 Familial adenomatous polyposis. (**a**) Total colectomy specimen showing the entire colonic mucosa carpeted with tiny sessile polyps. (**b**) Close-up view

Table 14.2 Extracolonic manifestations of FAP

Ectodermal derivatives	Endodermal derivatives	Mesodermal derivatives
Epidermoid cysts	Adenomas and carcinomas of the duodenal ampulla, stomach, small intestine, thyroid, and biliary tree	Desmoid tumors
Pilomatrixoma	Gastric fundic gland polyps	Osteomas
Congenital hypertrophy of the retinal pigment epithelium (CHRPE)	Hepatoblastoma	Dental problems
	Brain tumors	

(IPAA), colectomy with ileorectal anastomosis (IRA), and total proctocolectomy with end-ileostomy.

Restorative proctocolectomy with IPAA removes the entire colon and rectum without needing a permanent stoma. However, there is about a 10% risk of pouch failure. When a stapled anastomosis is performed, endoscopic surveillance is crucial because malignant changes can occur in the "rectal cuff," which is the small strip of rectal mucosa between the pouch and the dentate line. Some experts recommend complete mucosectomy of this residual cuff along with a transanal anastomosis, although this may result in poorer functional outcomes. For patients with relatively limited rectal involvement (fewer than 20 polyps), total colectomy and IRA may be a viable option. Regular endoscopic surveillance of the rectum is necessary, as up to 10% of patients may eventually develop invasive malignancy. In attenuated familial adenomatous polyposis (AFAP), patients may consider rectal preservation surgery, understanding that their cancer risk is lower (around 2%), but still present. Proctocolectomy with ileostomy is recommended for patients with poor anal sphincter function, those who have already developed rectal cancer, or those seeking a definitive single-stage procedure.

14.3.8 Postoperative Surveillance

Given the ongoing risk of cancer, it is vital to perform regular lifelong endoscopic surveillance of the residual rectum and the pouch. Endoscopy is also essential for detecting upper gastrointestinal tumors, especially those near the duodenal ampulla, which requires the use of a side-viewing duodenoscope. Despite these surveillance efforts, life expectancy may still be reduced due to the risk of extracolonic cancers and complications from desmoid tumors.

A first-degree relative of a patient with FAP should undergo genetic counseling followed by genetic testing. If a mutation in the APC gene is identified, screening should start at age 10 with annual sigmoidoscopies. If polyps are found, surgery is recommended, as polyps usually develop between the ages of 13 and 15. If no polyps are found by age 18, the individual is unlikely to develop any, and the risk of cancer becomes similar to that in the general population.

14.3.8.1 MUTYH-Associated Polyposis

MUTYH-Associated Polyposis (MAP) appears similar to FAP but follows an autosomal recessive inheritance pattern. A MUTYH gene mutation increases the likelihood of developing multiple colonic polyps and raises the risk of colorectal cancer by three to six times, depending on the specific mutation. A colonoscopy every 2 years is recommended, and surgery may be needed if endoscopic removal of the polyps is inadequate.

14.3.8.2 NTHL1 Tumor Syndrome

This is a rare autosomal recessive disorder that causes colorectal polyposis and a high risk of colorectal cancer. Polyps in this condition can be adenomatous, hyperplastic, or sessile serrated. The treatment approach is similar to that of MAP.

14.3.8.3 Lynch Syndrome (Hereditary Nonpolyposis Colorectal Cancer—HNPCC)

Lynch syndrome, formerly known as hereditary nonpolyposis colorectal cancer (HNPCC), greatly increases the risk of several cancers, especially those of the colon, endometrium, ovary, stomach, and urinary tract. It is inherited in an autosomal dominant pattern and results from mutations in one of the DNA mismatch repair genes (MLH1, MSH2, MSH6, PMS2). These mutations disrupt the function of MMR proteins, leading to microsatellite instability (MSI) and accelerating the progression from adenomas to carcinomas. Individuals with Lynch syndrome tend to develop colorectal polyps at a younger age (before age 50), and these polyps rapidly transform into cancer. Women with Lynch syndrome face a 30–50% lifetime risk of developing endometrial cancer (Fig. 14.7).

14.3.8.4 Diagnosis

Historically, Lynch syndrome was diagnosed based on family cancer history using the Amsterdam and Bethesda criteria. Recent advances in immunohistochemistry now enable the detection of MMR proteins or MSI in colorectal tumors, leading to subsequent genetic testing.

Amsterdam II Criteria

- Three or more family members with a Lynch syndrome-related cancer (such as colorectal, endometrial, small bowel, ureter, or renal pelvis), with at least one being a first-degree relative of the other two.
- Two or more successive generations affected.
- At least one tumor diagnosed before age 50.
- FAP excluded.
- Tumors confirmed by pathological examination.

The Revised Bethesda Guidelines

- Colorectal cancer diagnosed in a patient younger than 50 years.
- Presence of synchronous, metachronous colorectal, or other HNPCC-associated tumors, regardless of age.
- Colorectal cancer with the MSI-H histology diagnosed in a patient younger than 60 years.
- Colorectal cancer diagnosed in one or more first-degree relatives with an HNPCC-related tumor, with one of the cancers diagnosed before age 50.
- Colorectal cancer diagnosed in two or more first- or second-degree relatives with HNPCC-related tumors, regardless of age.

14.3.9 Screening and Management

For individuals who are carriers of MLH1 and MSH2 mutations, it is recommended to begin biennial endoscopic surveillance starting at age 25. In contrast, those who carry MSH6 mutations should initiate screening at age 35.

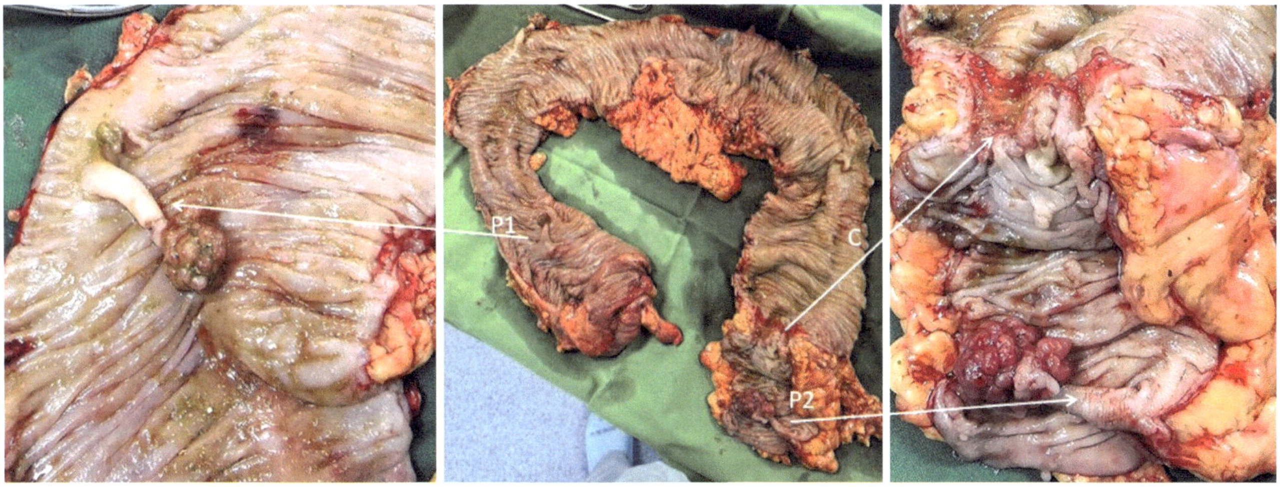

Fig. 14.7 Total colectomy specimen showing two pedunculated polyps (P1 and P2) in the ascending and sigmoid colon, respectively. Infiltrating carcinoma (C) in the descending colon

Individuals carrying PMS2 mutations are advised to undergo screening every five years, starting at age 35. In cases where polyps cannot be adequately managed through endoscopic procedures or in individuals diagnosed with cancer, an extended colectomy is suggested.

14.4 Colorectal Cancer

14.4.1 Epidemiology

Colorectal cancer (CRC) is the most common GI malignancy, ranking fourth in both incidence and mortality among cancers in the United States. Worldwide, CRC accounts for approximately 1.2 million new cases each year, representing 10% of all cancer diagnoses. The incidence of colorectal cancer is notably higher in developed countries. The risk of developing CRC increases with age, particularly after age 40. The average age at diagnosis is between 70 and 75 years.

14.4.2 Geographic Variation

CRC incidence and mortality rates are highest in developed nations. However, a downward trend has been reported in recent times in countries like the U.S., accompanied by improvements in 5-year survival rates.

14.4.3 Emigration Patterns

Migration studies have shown that individuals from low-incidence regions who move to high-incidence areas adopt the CRC risk of their new country within a generation. This change highlights the influence of environmental factors, such as diet and lifestyle, on CRC risk.

14.4.4 Socioeconomic Factors

The incidence of CRC is notably higher among economically affluent populations due to lifestyle factors like a diet high in fats and red meat, as well as sedentary habits. These behaviors contribute to obesity, which is a major risk factor for cancer development.

14.4.5 Anatomic Factors

Recent observations reveal a shift in the distribution of CRC from the distal (left) colon to the proximal (right) colon. Several factors, including increased lifespan, the presence of different luminal carcinogens, and genetic predispositions, may drive this change. A complex interplay of these factors collectively contributes to the development and distribution of colorectal cancer in the population.

14.4.6 Risk Factors, Prevention, and Screening

CRC presents a complex challenge, with its causes primarily involving several genetic and environmental risk factors. To better understand these risks, people can be grouped into three main categories. First, those at average risk are individuals who lack a significant family history or known genetic predispositions to CRC. Second, individuals in the increased risk group have a family history of colorectal cancer or adenomatous polyps, which increases their chances of developing the disease. Third, the high-risk group includes those with hereditary syndromes such as FAP or Lynch syndrome, as well as individuals with specific bowel diseases. Interestingly, most cases of colorectal cancer are sporadic and not directly linked to hereditary syndromes. Additionally, lifestyle choices common in Western societies, like dietary habits and levels of physical activity, significantly influence CRC risk. This complexity underscores the important interaction between genetic factors and lifestyle in shaping an individual's risk profile for colorectal cancer.

14.4.7 Etiology

14.4.7.1 Genetic

A family history of CRC significantly raises lifetime risk. The degree of risk depends on the number of affected relatives and their age of onset. First-degree relatives of CRC patients have double the risk of developing the disease, especially if the relative has been diagnosed before age 60 (Table 14.3).

14.4.7.2 Environmental Factors

Several environmental factors contribute to CRC risk. Diet plays a vital role, with high calorie intake and obesity linked to increased CRC risk, especially among men. Eating red

Table 14.3 Lifetime risk in an individual related to the index CRC patient

Relationship	Risk
Not related	1: 50
One relative affected	1: 17
One first-degree relative and one second-degree relative affected	1: 12
One relative aged <45 years affected	1:10
Two first-degree relatives affected	1: 6
Dominant pedigree	1: 2

meat, compared to white meat, is considered a strong risk factor. Conversely, a high-fiber diet is believed to provide protective benefits against CRC by reducing fecal carcinogens and accelerating transit time in the colon. Additionally, consuming fruits and vegetables, especially raw, green, and cruciferous types, has been associated with a lower CRC risk. Physical activity is another key factor; a sedentary lifestyle raises the risk of CRC, particularly colon cancer. In contrast, regular exercise has been shown to decrease the risk of recurrence and cancer-related death. Beyond these main factors, other elements also influence CRC risk. Alcohol consumption, although only weakly linked to overall CRC, is associated with a higher risk of rectal cancer, especially in men who drink heavily. Smoking is also a significant risk factor; individuals who smoke for over 20 pack-years have a greatly increased risk of developing large adenomas and CRC. The relationship between type 2 diabetes and CRC is complex, often affected by other lifestyle factors like obesity and smoking. Nonetheless, a known link exists between the two. Finally, the regular use of nonsteroidal anti-inflammatory drugs (NSAIDs), such as aspirin, has been linked to lower rates of CRC and adenomas, suggesting a potential protective effect against the disease. This intricate interplay of diet, lifestyle, and medication factors highlights the multifaceted nature of colorectal cancer risk.

14.4.7.3 Cholecystectomy and Bile Acids

Evidence from both experimental and epidemiological research suggests that bile acids may act as cocarcinogens or tumor promoters. These acids can cause hyperproliferation of the intestinal mucosa through various intracellular pathways. Patients who have had their gallbladders removed face a slightly increased risk of developing proximal colon cancer. However, other unknown factors in their bile could be more influential than the surgery alone.

14.4.7.4 Smoking and Alcohol Consumption

Smoking modestly raises the risk of colorectal cancer. Data indicate a dose-response link between the number of pack-years smoked and the likelihood of developing adenomatous polyps or CRC. Similarly, heavy alcohol use has been associated with an increased risk of colon cancer, especially in men.

14.4.7.5 Inflammatory Bowel Disease

Chronic inflammatory bowel disease (IBD) is a major risk factor for colorectal cancer, with the risk increasing with both the duration and extent of the disease. In cases of ulcerative colitis, the risk of developing colorectal cancer rises from about 3% during the first decade to between 10% and 20% in the second decade. Likewise, patients with Crohn's disease affecting the colon also face a higher risk of colorectal cancer; however, this risk is generally lower than that in patients with ulcerative colitis.

14.4.7.6 Adenomatous Polyps

Adenomatous polyps are considered premalignant. Individuals with a personal or family history of adenomatous polyps or CRC are at increased risk of developing colon cancer in the future. The risk of developing metachronous primary cancer ranges from 1.5 to 3% in the first 5 years after surgery.

14.4.7.7 Abdomino-Pelvic Radiation

Patients who received abdomino-pelvic radiation therapy in early childhood or as adults are at high risk of developing GI malignancies, particularly CRC. The magnitude of this risk is similar to that of patients with a family history of colonic adenoma. Currently, there is no clear consensus on the optimal timing to begin screening.

14.5 Pathogenesis

Colorectal carcinogenesis is a complex, multistep process involving multiple genetic changes. A balance between oncogenes, which drive cell growth, and tumor suppressor genes, which prevent excessive proliferation, is essential for maintaining normal cell function. Disruptions in this balance lead to the development and spread of malignant cells.

14.5.1 Adenoma–Carcinoma Sequence

Vogelstein and colleagues established the adenoma-carcinoma sequence in 1988. This model illustrates how a sequence of biological processes and genetic alterations contributes to the development of colorectal cancer. Key genes involved include APC, which is mutated in over 60% of adenomas and carcinomas and plays a role in cell adhesion and communication. The intracellular signal transduction gene K-ras is altered in larger adenomas and carcinomas, promoting cell division. One tumor suppressor gene whose deletion facilitates the development of malignancy is the DCC (deleted in colon cancer) gene. A late event in carcinogenesis, the p53 gene is one of the most frequently altered genes in human cancers. It is rarely found in adenomas but is associated with invasive colon cancers (Table 14.4).

Approximately 80% of colorectal cancers develop through the loss of heterozygosity (LOH) pathway, which

Table 14.4 Fearon-Vogelstein Model of adenoma carcinoma sequence

Normal epithelium → *initiation by 5q loss APC gene* → **Dysplasia** → *DNA methylation* → **Early adenoma** → *12p activation K ras* → **Intermediate adenoma** → *18q loss DCC* → **Late adenoma** → *action by 17p loss p53* → **Carcinoma**

APC, K-ras, DCC, and P53 are oncogenes that convert normal cells to cancerous cells

involves mutations in the APC gene (as seen in FAP), K-ras mutations, loss of DCC, and p53 mutations. This pathway is microsatellite stable (MSS) and is associated with a poorer prognosis than other pathways. In contrast, 20% of colorectal cancers arise via the Replication Error Repair (RER) pathway, which is linked to microsatellite instability (MSI) caused by defective DNA repair mechanisms. These cancers are generally located on the right side of the colon and tend to have a better prognosis.

14.5.2 Pathology

Colorectal cancers are primarily adenocarcinomas that arise in different parts of the colon. The rectum (40%) and sigmoid colon (20%) account for most cases, followed by the cecum (12–15%). Approximately 5% of cases involve multiple synchronous cancers.

Types of lesions in colorectal cancer include annular strictures, which are more common in the left colon and can cause obstruction. Tubular strictures are usually found at the rectosigmoid junction, appearing as narrowed segments of the bowel. Ulcerative lesions primarily occur in the ascending colon and cecum, often characterized by mucosal ulceration. Additionally, proliferative growths are more frequent on the right side of the colon, presenting as raised lesions that may block the bowel or cause symptoms related to tumor growth.

14.6 Clinical Presentation

Carcinomas in the cecum and hepatic flexure of the colon often present as palpable masses during physical examinations. Tumors in the rectum can be detected through a digital rectal exam, making these areas especially accessible for early detection. Anemia is a common finding, particularly with cecal cancers, which may result from chronic blood loss caused by tumor ulceration. This anemia often serves as a key sign in diagnosis. Abdominal pain can be dull and aching or colicky if there is an obstruction.

Changes in bowel habits are another important sign of colorectal cancer. Recent-onset constipation, alternating with episodes of diarrhea, can serve as an early warning sign, especially in patients with no previous history of such issues. Obstruction is more common with constrictive lesions on the left side of the colon, causing symptoms like lower abdominal distension and, in advanced stages, visible peristalsis. This left-sided obstruction can eventually become complete, requiring urgent medical treatment.

In early cases, symptoms can be easily overlooked and may include changes in bowel habits such as diarrhea, general malaise, weakness (often due to anemia), and occasional rectal bleeding, which is frequently mistaken for hemorrhoids or other conditions. In late cases, symptoms may include obstruction, perforation, intussusception (with tumors on the right side), abdominal masses, and liver metastases. Metastasis is seen in approximately 5–10% of patients at diagnosis, with the liver being a common site of spread, especially in cases of mucoid adenocarcinomas. Additionally, patients may present with ascites as a sign of advanced disease (Table 14.5).

Table 14.5 Carcinoma right vs left colon

Features	Right colon	Left colon
Incidence	About 10–20%	About 60–70% (including rectum)
Sex predilection	More common in women	More common in men
Pathology	Ulcerative/ proliferative lesion	Stricturous lesion
Bleeding	Occult blood in stools	Bleeding per-rectum
Abdominal discomfort	Dyspeptic symptoms	Constipation and obstruction
Detection method	Colonoscopy	Flexible sigmoidoscopy
Complication	Obstruction—Less common	Obstruction, perforation, pericolic abscess—Common

14.7 Staging/Classification of Colorectal Cancer

Several classifications and staging systems are used for colorectal cancer, though not all are commonly employed in clinical practice. The most important ones include:

14.7.1 Dukes Staging

Stage A: Cancer invades but does not breach the muscularis propria.
Stage B: Cancer breaches the muscularis propria.
Stage C: Lymph nodes are involved.
Stage D: Metastatic disease (not a part of original staging).

14.7.2 Astler-Coller Modification of Dukes' Staging

Stage A: Limited to the mucosa.
Stage B1: Extends into the muscularis propria.
Stage B2: Involves the entire bowel wall.
Stage B3: Extends into adjacent organs.
Stage C1: B1 + Positive lymph nodes.

Stage C2: B2 + Positive lymph nodes.
Stage C3: B3 + Positive lymph nodes.
Stage D: Presence of distant metastasis.

TNM Staging: (as per AJCC eighth edition).

14.8 Investigations

A complete blood count (CBC) often shows low hemoglobin (Hb) levels, which is a common finding in the disease. The occult blood test is used as a screening tool for CRC. A double-contrast barium enema, rarely performed today, can detect filling defects or the characteristic apple-core deformities associated with tumors. Flexible sigmoidoscopy allows for examination of the lower part of the colon (up to 60 cm) and is usually done in an outpatient setting, especially for patients with rectal bleeding. Colonoscopy is essential for taking biopsies and ruling out synchronous malignancies, which occur in about 5% of CRC cases. Virtual colonoscopy is another diagnostic option that can detect polyps larger than 6 mm; however, it does not allow for biopsies during the procedure. Ultrasound is often the initial test for identifying colonic masses, liver metastases, and ascites, with ultrasound-guided biopsy available for more advanced cases. After colonoscopy, a CT scan is the preferred imaging method for assessing tumor location, evaluating the involvement of adjacent structures, and detecting metastases. Magnetic resonance imaging can be an alternative to CT scan, although it is the imaging modality of choice for rectal cancer.

14.8.1 Carcinoembryonic Antigen (CEA)

Carcinoembryonic Antigen (CEA) is a surface glycoprotein produced by colorectal epithelium, and its levels are elevated in colorectal cancer. A CEA level of 0–4 mg/ml is considered normal. CEA is cleared by the liver, so its half-life may be prolonged in cases of cholestasis or hepatic dysfunction. It is also elevated in other GI malignancies such as gastric and pancreatic cancers, as well as in noncancerous conditions like colorectal polyps, peptic ulcers, and ulcerative colitis. Conversely, a normal CEA level can be observed in poorly differentiated colorectal cancers. CEA levels are directly proportional to the degree of tumor differentiation and the stage of the disease. Very high CEA levels may indicate metastatic disease. Normalization of CEA after surgery suggests R0 resection, and a subsequent increase indicates disease recurrence.

14.8.2 PET Scan

Routine PET scans are not advised for the initial management of colorectal cancer. However, they are useful in follow-up cases and when dealing with recurrent malignancies where CEA levels are increasing, and the source of the rise needs investigation (Figs. 14.8 and 14.9). PET scans are also recommended whenever a metastasectomy is performed (Tables 14.6 and 14.7)

14.8.3 Postoperative Chemotherapy

Indications for chemotherapy in colorectal cancer include all patients with T3 lesions, positive lymph nodes, major vein involvement, signet cell carcinoma, or elevated preoperative CEA levels. A common regimen for these patients is FOLFOX, which includes 5-fluorouracil (5-FU), leucovorin, and oxaliplatin. Alternatively, oral Capecitabine can be used as a substitute for intravenous 5-FU.

In cases of liver metastases, oxaliplatin is recommended in chemotherapy regimens to help downsize these tumors. However, one of the notable side effects of oxaliplatin is

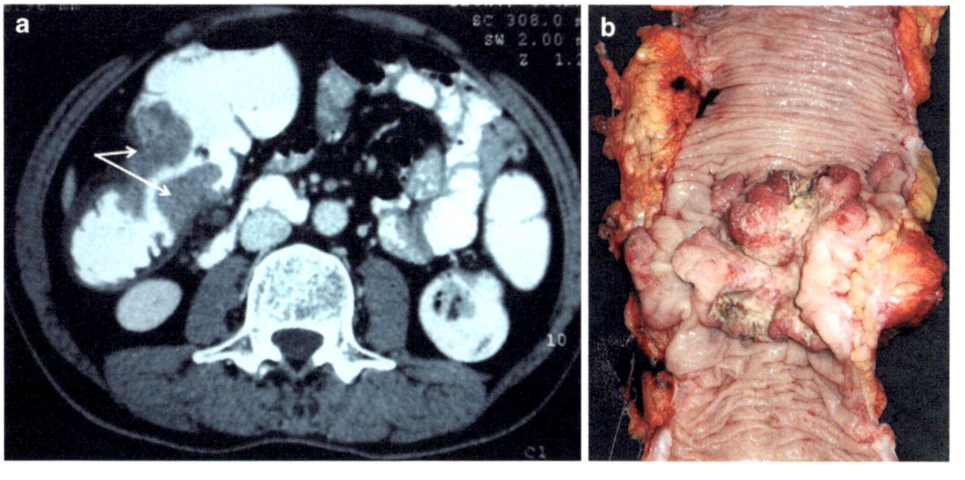

Fig. 14.8 (**a**) Contrast-enhanced CT scan showing a malignant tumor (arrows) in the ascending colon. Note the typical 'apple-core' deformity. (**b**) Right hemicolectomy specimen showing the same tumor

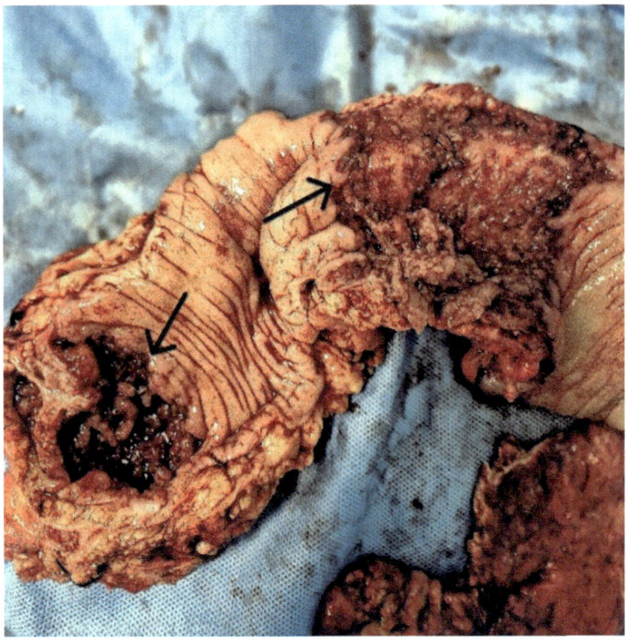

Fig. 14.9 Resected colon showing synchronous malignancies (arrows), involving the cecum and the proximal transverse colon, respectively

Table 14.6 Adverse prognostic factors in colorectal cancer

Patient factor	Molecular markers
Young age	Mutations in BRAF or KRAS
Male sex	Deficiency in the MMR protein Expression or MSI-H tumor status
Obesity	Amplification of the HER2 oncogene or overexpression of its protein
Presentation	*Tumor histology*
Tumor in the right colon	Advanced TNM stage
Obstruction and/or perforation	Poor differentiation
High CEA level	Lympho-vascular and perineural invasion
	Mucinous tumor
	Lymph node involvement
	Tumor budding on the invasive front
	Positive resection margin

peripheral neuropathy, which can impact patients' quality of life during treatment.

14.8.4 Postoperative Radiotherapy

Routine radiotherapy is not effective for adenocarcinoma of the colon. However, it may be indicated for inoperable tumors infiltrating soft tissues or for recurrent tumors.

Table 14.7 Summary of the surgical resections based on the lympho-vascular pedicle in CRC

Site of Tumor	Procedure	Part of the Bowel Resected	Lympho-vascular pedicle
Caecum or ascending colon	Right hemicolectomy	Terminal ileum to mid transverse colon	ICA, RCA, right branch of MCA
Hepatic flexure or transverse colon	Extended right hemicolectomy	Terminal ileum to descending colon	ICA, RCA, MCA
Splenic flexure	Extended left hemicolectomy	Hepatic flexure to rectosigmoid	MCA, LCA, IMA
Descending colon	Left hemicolectomy	Splenic flexure to sigmoid	IMA, left branch of MCA
Sigmoid colon	Sigmoid colectomy	Part of the descending colon and sigmoid colon	IMA

ICA Ileocolic artery, *RCA* Right colic artery, *MCA* Middle colic artery, *LCA* Left colic artery, *IMA* Inferior mesenteric artery

14.8.5 Metastatic Disease Without Obstruction

Patients with isolated liver or lung metastases can undergo surgery for both the primary and metastatic lesions, as resection often achieves reasonable disease control. Neoadjuvant therapy with 5-FU or Capecitabine, combined with radiation therapy (45–50 Gy), is used for large tumors involving the abdominal wall or pelvis. Surgery is considered 6–8 weeks after treatment, once the tumor has reached maximum response. Further adjuvant therapy may be administered based on the pathology report.

New agents for treating colorectal cancer have significantly improved treatment options and patient outcomes. Bevacizumab is a monoclonal antibody that targets vascular endothelial growth factor (VEGF), a key factor in angiogenesis—the process by which new blood vessels form, supplying tumors with essential nutrients and oxygen. By blocking VEGF, bevacizumab effectively slows down tumor growth and progression.

Cetuximab is another monoclonal antibody used in colorectal cancer treatment, specifically targeting the epidermal growth factor receptor (EGFR). By blocking EGFR, cetuximab interrupts downstream signaling pathways that promote cell growth and survival, leading to decreased tumor growth. The use of these new agents has opened up new treatment options, especially for patients with advanced or refractory disease, and has been incorporated into various combination therapies to increase effectiveness and improve patient survival rates.

14.8.6 Screening

The Fecal Occult Blood Test (FOBT) is a traditional screening test for colorectal cancers.. Despite the possibility of false positives, this test has the potential to lower mortality from colorectal cancer by 20% to 30%. Flexible sigmoidoscopy (FS) is recommended at age 60, since this can reduce the mortality from distal colorectal cancer by 60%. In the United States, screening is suggested every 5 years. If a distal adenoma is discovered, a colonoscopy is recommended because proximal adenomas are not uncommon. Virtual colonscopy can be considered but is less popular due to its high cost and complexity; it uses CT scans to create images of the colon but does not allow for biopsies,which limits its clinical utility.

14.8.7 Follow-up

The role of surveillance and follow-up after definitive therapy is to detect recurrence early and screen for second primary cancers. Intense surveillance is necessary for resected stage II and beyond, which includes:

History and physical examination: Every 3–6 months for the first 3 years, then every 6 months during the fourth and fifth years, and yearly thereafter.

CEA: Serum CEA level assessment is recommended at baseline, then every 3–6 months for up to 2 years, and then every 6 months for a total of 5 years.

Colonoscopy: All patients require a full-length colonoscopy either preoperatively or postoperatively. Those who have not undergone a full-length colonoscopy in the preoperative setting due to a non-negotiable obstructing growth should have a colonoscopy at 3–6 months after resection, while others are advised to have a full-length colonoscopy at 1 year post-resection. Repeat colonoscopies are recommended every 3 years, followed by every 5 years thereafter.

Key Points

- All types of colonic polyps carry malignant potential, with adenoma being the most concerning.
- Haggitt classification describes the structure of an adenomatous polyp that has undergone neoplastic changes: up to level 2 infiltration, polyps can be treated by local excision (endoscopic polypectomy), whereas level 3 and 4 require formal surgical removal in the form of segmental colectomy. Infiltration in sessile polyps more often reaches level 4.
- High-risk patients who require follow-up colonoscopy include those with two or more premalignant polyps, one of which must be an advanced colorectal polyp (defined as a serrated polyp ≥10 mm or any polyp with dysplasia), as well as individuals with five or more premalignant polyps.
- A first-degree relative of a patient with FAP should undergo genetic counseling followed by genetic testing. If a mutation in the APC gene is identified, screening should start at age 10 with annual sigmoidoscopies.
- Proctocolectomy is recommended for all individuals with FAP because of its universal malignant potential.
- Lynch syndrome, previously known as hereditary non-polyposis colorectal cancer (HNPCC), is linked to an increased risk of several cancers, especially those of the colon, endometrium, ovary, stomach, and urinary tract.
- Colorectal cancer (CRC) is the most common GI malignancy that occurs as a result of a disturbed balance between oncogene and tumor suppressor gene.
- Proliferative growth is more common in the right colon, whereas stricturous growth occurs more often in the left colon.
- Astler-Coller modification of Dukes staging and TNM staging are commonly used for colon cancer.
- Colonoscopy and CECT are standard investigations required for preoperative diagnosis as well as staging of the disease.
- CEA is an important prognostic marker of CRC; it is also helpful for postoperative surveillance to detect early recurrence of the disease.
- In addition to patient factors, presentation, and tumor histology, molecular markers are now considered important for prognostication of CRC.
- Segmental excision of the colon for cancer is based on the lymphovascular pedicle.
- Indications for chemotherapy in colorectal cancer include all patients with T3 lesions, positive lymph nodes, major vein involvement, signet cell carcinoma, or elevated preoperative CEA levels.
- Patients with isolated liver or lung metastases can undergo surgery for both the primary and metastatic lesions, as resection often achieves reasonable disease control.

Imaging For the evaluation of abdominal and pelvic disease, contrast-enhanced computed tomography of the chest, abdomen, and pelvis is recommended every 6–12 months for up to 5 years in patients with stage II disease who have high-risk factors and beyond.

Selected Reading

1. Moreno CC, Mittal PK, Sullivan PS, et al. Colorectal cancer initial diagnosis: screening colonoscopy, diagnostic colonoscopy, or emergent surgery, and tumor stage and size at initial presentation. Clin Colorectal Cancer. 2016;15:67–73.
2. Rutter MD, East J, Rees CJ, et al. British Society of Gastroenterology/Association of Coloproctology of Great Britain and Ireland/Public Health England post-polypectomy and postcolorectal cancer resection surveillance guidelines. Gut. 2020;69:201–23.
3. Morgan E, Arnold M, Gini A, et al. Global burden of colorectal cancer in 2020 and 2040: incidence and mortality estimates from GLOBOCAN. Gut. 2023;72:338–44.
4. Eng C, Yoshino T, Ruíz-García E, et al. Colorectal cancer. Lancet. 2024;404:294–310.
5. Cotan HT, Emilescu RA, Iaciu CI, et al. Prognostic and predictive determinants of colorectal cancer: a comprehensive review. Cancers. 2024;16:3928. https://doi.org/10.3390/cancers16233928.

Carcinoma Rectum

15

Rajesh S. Shinde, Monika Pohekar, and Shailesh V. Shrikhande

Abstract

Common presentation symptoms are bleeding per rectum, altered bowel habits, loss of weight, and appetite. The work-up of the patient with rectal cancer involves tumor markers (CEA, CA-19.9), colonoscopy, MRI-pelvis for local staging, and CECT and PET-CT for metastatic staging. The management of rectal cancer is a multimodality approach with radiation, surgery, and chemotherapy. The treatment of rectal cancer is tailored according to the location of the tumor, T stage, nodal status, and metastatic status. Total mesorectal excision is the procedure of choice for resectable cancer.

Keywords

Cancer rectum · Anterior resection

Colorectal cancer ranks as the third most common cancer worldwide and the second leading cause of cancer-related deaths. GLOBOCAN 2022 reported that more than 1.9 million new cases of colorectal cancer were diagnosed globally in 2022, with over 900,000 deaths attributed to the disease. In India, colorectal cancer is the most frequently diagnosed gastrointestinal cancer, with an incidence of approximately 6.7 cases per 100,000 people. The management of rectal cancer has significantly advanced in recent years. This progress has been driven by the integrated use of all treatment options, including surgery, chemotherapy, and radiotherapy, which are combined in various ways to optimize oncological outcomes.

R. S. Shinde (✉) · M. Pohekar · S. V. Shrikhande
Tata Memorial Hospital, Mumbai, India

15.1 Surgical Anatomy

The rectum measures 12–15 cm in length. The recto-sigmoid junction is identified by the transition from the sigmoid colon to the rectum and is characterized by the fusion of the taenia coli of the sigmoid colon, forming the circumferential longitudinal muscle of the rectum. This transition occurs anatomically at the level of the sacral promontory. The rectum follows the sacral curve and terminates at the anorectal junction. It is divided into three segments based on the distance from the anal verge: lower rectum (0–5 cm), mid-rectum (5–10 cm), and upper rectum (10–15 cm). The upper rectum is covered anteriorly and laterally by peritoneal reflection, while the mid-rectum is covered only anteriorly. The lower third of the rectum has no peritoneal covering. The rectum has three lateral curvatures: the upper and lower curvatures are convex to the right, while the middle curvature is convex to the left. These curves are marked by transverse semilunar folds, also known as the valves of Houston. The upper and lower valves fold to the right, and the middle valve folds to the left. The middle fold corresponds to the anterior peritoneal reflection (Figs. 15.1 and 15.2).

Artery Supply

The upper rectum is supplied by the superior rectal artery, also called the superior hemorrhoidal artery, which is a terminal branch of the inferior mesenteric artery. The main blood supply to the rectum comes from this artery. The middle rectal artery, a branch of the anterior division of the internal iliac artery, is present in about 20% of cases and shows significant variation in size and presence. The inferior rectal artery, a branch of the internal pudendal artery—another branch of the anterior division of the internal iliac artery—supplies the lower rectum and anal canal.

Venous Drainage

The venous drainage of the rectum mirrors its arterial supply. The superior rectal vein drains into the inferior mesenteric vein, which in turn drains into the splenic vein and eventu-

M. Ibrarullah (ed.), *Recent Concepts in Gastrointestinal (GI) Surgery*, https://doi.org/10.1007/978-981-92-1118-0_15

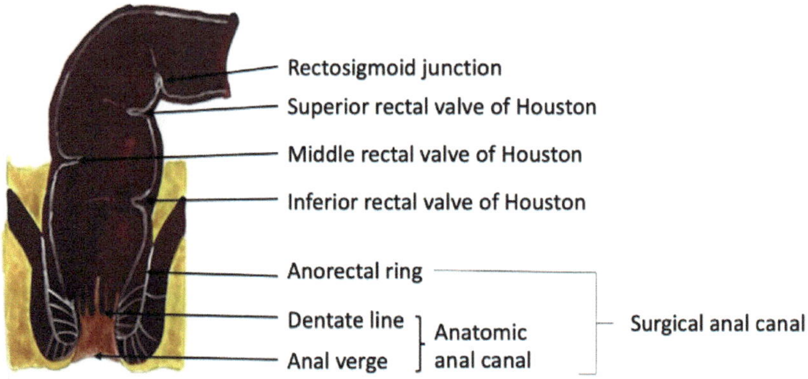

Fig. 15.1 Surgical anatomy of the rectum

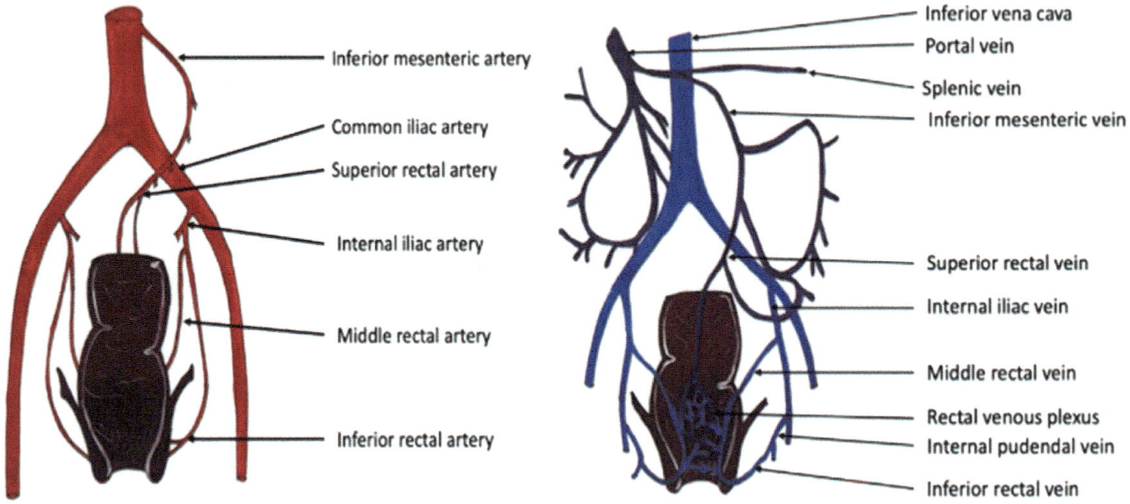

Fig. 15.2 Arterial supply and venous drainage of the rectum

ally into the portal system. The middle rectal vein and inferior rectal vein drain into the internal iliac vein.

Lymphatic Drainage

The lymphatic drainage of the rectum also follows arterial anatomy. The lymphatics from the upper and middle rectum drain into the inferior mesenteric nodes. The lymphatics from the lower rectum drain both superiorly into the inferior mesenteric nodes and laterally into the internal iliac nodes.

Nerve Supply

The rectum receives both sympathetic and parasympathetic innervation. Sympathetic nerves originate from L1-3, form the inferior mesenteric plexus, and travel through the superior hypogastric plexus, which is located in front of the aortic bifurcation. They descend as hypogastric nerves to join the pelvic plexus. The hypogastric nerves follow the sacral promontory, approximately 1 cm lateral to the midline and 2 cm medial to the ureters, then descend into the pelvis behind the superior rectal artery. Parasympathetic nerves, or nervi erigentes, arise from S2-4 and join the hypogastric nerves anterior and lateral to the rectum to form the inferior hypogastric plexus or pelvic plexus, which ultimately forms the periprostatic plexus. The pelvic plexus is attached to the lateral pelvic walls and is next to the lateral stalks of the rectum. The sympathetic hypogastric nerves function to carry semen from the seminal vesicles to the posterior prostatic urethra. The urinary bladder gets both sympathetic and parasympathetic nerve supplies. The pelvic plexus surrounds and supplies nerves to the prostate, urethra, seminal vesicles, urinary bladder, pelvic floor muscles, and cavernous bodies. The cavernous nerves that control erectile function run along the anterolateral aspect of Denonvilliers fascia.

The complication rate of bladder and sexual dysfunction after rectal surgery is about 45%. The type of dysfunction depends on the extent of nerve injury. Therefore, understanding the complex autonomic nerve supply of the rectum and pelvic organs is crucial to reduce genitourinary complications. Injury to the hypogastric nerves at the sacral promontory causes sympathetic dysfunction, which can lead to retrograde ejaculation, increased urinary frequency, nocturia, and incontinence. Damage to the mixed sympathetic and

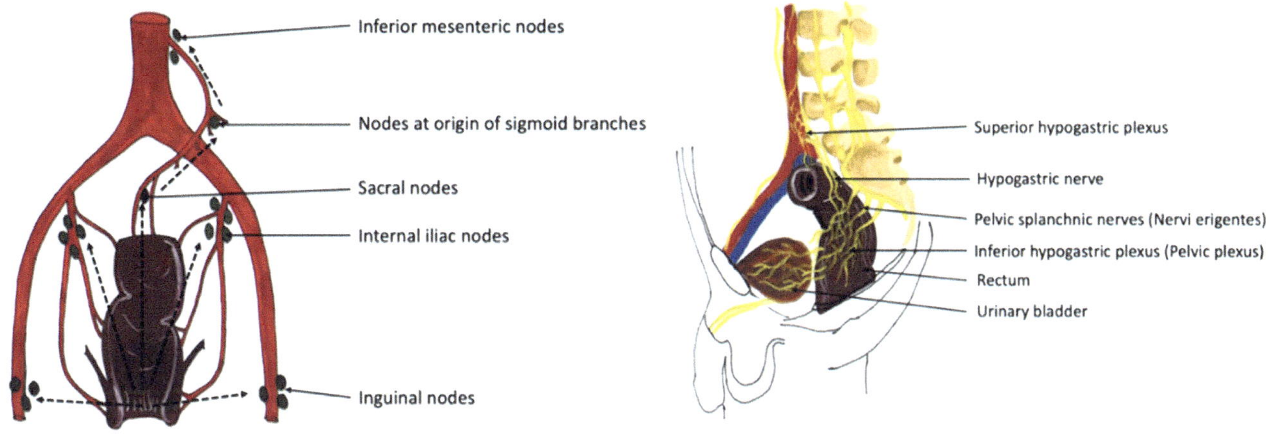

Fig. 15.3 Lymphatic drainage and nerve supply of the rectum

parasympathetic pelvic plexus results in impotence and an atonic bladder (Fig. 15.3).

Fascial Planes

The lower rectum is separated anteriorly from the prostate or vagina by a fascial layer called Denonvilliers' fascia. Posteriorly, the lower rectum is separated from the coccyx and the lower two sacral vertebrae by a fascial layer called Waldeyer's fascia.

15.2 Etiology and Risk Factors

15.2.1 Polyps

The risk of invasive carcinoma in a polyp depends on its size and histology. Villous histology is linked to a higher chance of developing invasive carcinoma. A polyp smaller than 1 cm has less than a 5% chance, while a polyp larger than 2 cm has over a 50% chance of containing invasive carcinoma. Polyps associated with hereditary disorders such as familial adenomatous polyposis (FAP) and hereditary nonpolyposis colorectal cancer syndrome (HNPCC) are especially prone to cancer development.

15.2.2 Inflammatory Bowel Disease

The incidence of colorectal cancer is 2–5% within 10 years of ulcerative colitis diagnosis. However, the risk increases by 1% each year. As a result, the cumulative risk reaches 25% at 25 years, 35% at 30 years, 45% at 35 years, and 65% at 40 years. Patients with only left-sided colitis have a lower risk of developing invasive carcinoma compared to those with pancolitis.

15.2.3 Dietary Factors and Lifestyle

High dietary fat intake, red and processed meat consumption, smoking, alcohol, obesity, and lack of physical activity have been linked to a higher risk of colorectal carcinoma.

15.3 Clinical Presentation (Table 15.1)

Table 15.1 Clinical presentation of carcinoma rectum

Bleeding per rectum
Altered bowel habits
Tenesmus
Spurious diarrhea
Sense of incomplete evacuation
Nonspecific symptoms such as: Abdominal pain and distension (in obstructing lesions) Loss of weight and appetite Intractable lower back pain

15.4 Diagnosis

Diagnosis relies on a comprehensive medical history, physical exam, and multiple diagnostic tests.

15.4.1 Abdominal Examination

The abdominal exam may appear normal in the early stages of the disease. Abdominal swelling can occur with obstructive lesions. A metastasis to the liver might sometimes be felt as a mass in the liver. Ascites can also cause abdominal swelling when the disease spreads to the peritoneum.

15.4.2 Digital Rectal Examination

The Digital Rectal Examination (DRE) is the most critical clinical examination for rectal cancer. Lesions in the mid and lower rectum can be felt per rectum. It is important to determine the lesion's distal extent in relation to the anal verge, as this greatly influences treatment planning and the ability to preserve the sphincter. Additionally, assessing sphincter tone, checking for active bleeding, evaluating circumferential involvement, and noting any fixation of the lesion to the sacrum posteriorly or to anterior organs such as the prostate or bladder are essential. In female patients, a per-vaginal exam is necessary to assess involvement of the posterior vaginal wall.

15.4.3 Tumor Markers

Serum carcinoembryonic antigen (CEA) is an important tumor marker used for prognosis and monitoring treatment response. Elevated CEA levels indicate advanced disease and poorer survival outcomes. However, 10–15% of patients may be nonsecretors and do not show increased CEA levels.

15.4.4 Colonoscopy

A colonoscopy is routinely performed in patients with suspected colorectal cancer to directly observe the tumor, determine its location, assess the extent of circumferential involvement, check for luminal obstruction, and confirm histology. It is also crucial to rule out synchronous premalignant and malignant lesions in the colon. The incidence of synchronous colorectal tumors ranges from approximately 2 to 6%, while synchronous adenomatous polyps occur in about 30%. The presence of multiple colonic polyps requires further investigation and may influence the management approach. If a complete colonoscopy cannot be performed before surgery due to obstructing lesions, it is recommended to complete the procedure 6 months after surgery (Fig. 15.4).

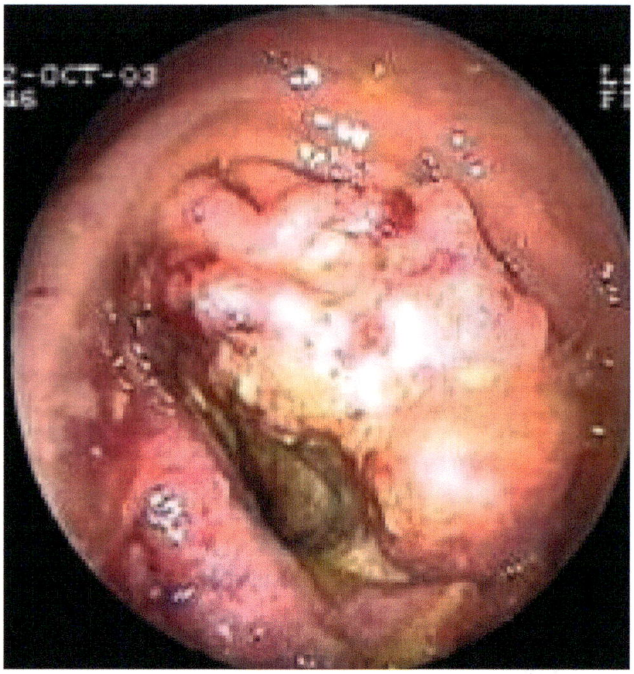

Fig. 15.4 A circumferential obstructive growth in the mid-rectum

15.4.5 Biopsy

Preoperative biopsy confirmation is essential when tumor resection may lead to a permanent stoma (colostomy/ileostomy). The same applies when initiating chemo-radiotherapy. Biopsy can be performed during proctoscopy, rigid sigmoidoscopy, or colonoscopy.

15.4.6 Imaging

Magnetic Resonance Imaging (MRI)

MRI of the abdomen and pelvis is the preferred investigation for staging rectal cancer. Pelvic MRI for rectal cancer is performed with 1. 1.5-3 T, noncontrast imaging, using a slice thickness of 3 mm (range 1–4 mm) with T 2-weighted images captured in sagittal, axial, and coronal planes. On MRI, the rectum is defined as the bowel part located below the pelvic inlet (an imaginary line drawn from the sacral promontory to the top of the pubic symphysis). The rectum is divided into three distinct layers in cross- sectional axial view: the innermost, thin, dark, hypointense mucosa; the middle hyperintense submucosa; and the outer darkly hypointense muscularis propria. The rectum is arbitrarily divided into three segments based on the distance from the anal verge—

upper, middle, and lower (0–5 cm, >5–10 cm, and > 10–15 cm, respectively). The upper rectum lies above the anterior peritoneal reflection; the mid to lower rectum is below it. The lower rectum is surrounded by mesorectal fat, enclosed by a fascial layer called the mesorectal fascia (MRF). The circumferential resection margin (CRM) is measured on MRI as the shortest distance from the tumor to the MRF. The MERCURY trial demonstrated that high-resolution MRI can accurately assess the CRM preoperatively. A CRM >1 mm is considered negative; when the tumor is within 1 mm of the MRF, or for lower third rectal cancers, within 1 mm of the levator ani muscle; and for anal rectal tumors, invasion into or beyond the intersphincteric space indicates involvement. MRI pelvis evaluates the lesion' s location relative to the anal verge, T- Stage, involvement of the anterior peritoneal reflection and adjacent organs like the prostate, seminal vesicles in males, and posterior vaginal wall in females. It also assesses mesorectal lymph nodes, perirectal tumor deposits, involvement of the mesorectal fascia, CRM, extra-mural vascular invasion (EMVI), involvement of the anal sphincter complex, intersphincteric space, levator ani muscle, and the presence of lateral pelvic nodes. MRI pelvis supports treatment planning (such as the need for neoadjuvant therapy), response assessment, and surgical planning (Fig. 15.5).

15.4.7 Contrast-Enhanced Computed Tomography (CECT)

CECT of the thorax, abdomen, and pelvis is performed with the administration of oral and intravenous contrast. It is important to assess for evidence of metastatic disease in the liver, retroperitoneal lymph nodes, any peritoneal metastatic deposits, ascites, lung metastasis, or metastasis to other distant organs (Fig. 15.6).

15.4.8 Endoscopic Ultrasound (EUS)

EUS is used selectively in early rectal cancer to differentiate between T1 and T2 tumors. On EUS, the rectal wall is visualized in five distinct layers: mucosa, muscularis mucosa, submucosa, muscularis propria, and perirectal fat. Rectal tumors are generally hypoechoic. However, EUS is highly operator-dependent, requiring experience and skill. It has difficulty distinguishing desmoplastic reactions and post-biopsy changes from local tumor invasion and is less accurate in determining nodal involvement.

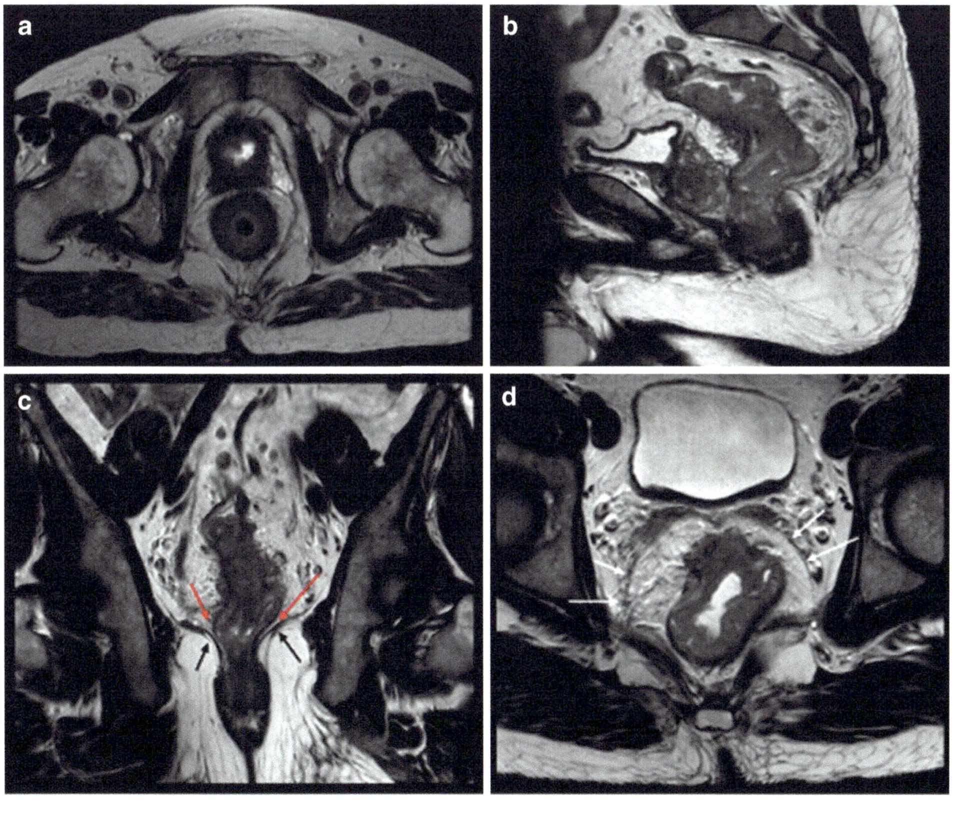

Fig. 15.5 MRI Pelvis-T2W—(**a**) Axial view showing distinct layers of normal rectum—innermost hypointense mucosa, middle hyperintense submucosa, outermost hypointense layer muscular propria; (**b**) sagittal view showing mid-low rectal tumor with mesorectal nodes' involvement and free presacral fascia; (**c**) coronal view showing relation of tumor with levator ani muscle (black arrow) and inter-sphincteric space (red arrow); (**d**) axial view showing circumferential tumor extending into mesorectum with free mesorectal fascia (white arrow)

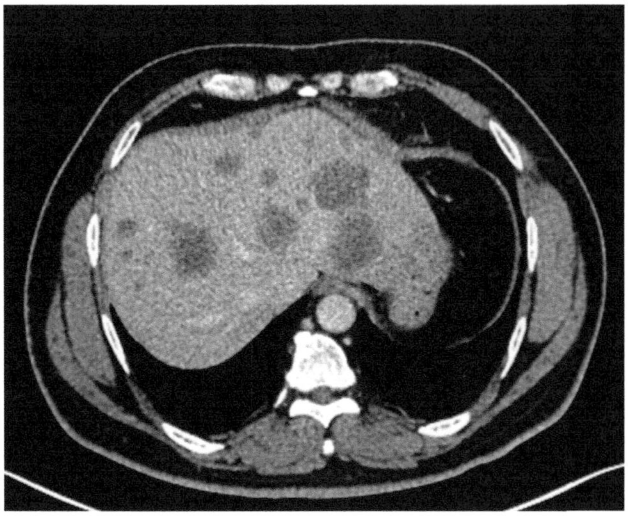

Fig. 15.6 CECT abdomen. Multiple hypodense liver lesions suggestive of liver metastasis

15.4.9 Positron Emission Tomography-Computed Tomography (PET-CT)

PET-CT is not routinely part of the preoperative workup. It is used when CT or MRI findings are unclear, when the patient has a contraindication to intravenous contrast, when CEA levels are rising during surveillance, or for restaging patients with recurrence or suspected recurrence.

15.4.10 Staging

Overall outcomes and prognosis of rectal cancer depend on the stage of the disease. The most widely used staging system is the American Joint Committee on Cancer (eighth ed., AJCC/UICC) staging system.

15.5 Management

Although colorectal cancer is often grouped and treated as a single entity, the management of rectal cancer has seen a paradigm shift in recent years with the integration of MRI in evaluation, the use of multimodal therapy (radiotherapy, chemotherapy, and surgery), organ preservation strategies, and the frequent use of minimally invasive approaches for treatment. Overall, the management of rectal cancer largely depends on the tumor's location from the anal verge. Other factors to consider before selecting a treatment method include the TNM stage at presentation.

The nonmetastatic rectosigmoid junction and select upper third rectal lesions can be generally treated on the principles of colonic cancers with upfront surgery followed by adjuvant chemotherapy if needed. The middle and lower third rectal cancer management, however, depends on the TNM stage of the disease. An algorithm for brief management of rectal cancer is presented below (Fig. 15.7).

TNM: AJCC staging eighth edition.

15.5.1 Endoscopic Management

Early rectal cancers in the middle and lower third, with the following characteristics, are suitable for endoscopic resection.

- T1, SM1 lesions (Kikuchi classification of depth of invasion into submucosa).
- Size <3 cm.
- Involving less than one-third of the circumference of the lumen.
- Low-grade/well to moderately differentiated (G1, G2).
- Within 10 cm of the anal verge.
- No evidence of lymphatic or vascular invasion on biopsy.
- Preferably superficial, mobile, polypoidal lesion.

Common endoscopic techniques include endoscopic mucosal resection (EMR) and endoscopic submucosal dissection (ESD). EMR involves using a snare through the endoscope's operative channel. Pedunculated lesions are grasped with the snare and cut below the mucosal surface. For pedunculated lesions, a solution is injected into the submucosal space to separate the mucosa from the underlying muscularis propria. The solutions used for submucosal injection are normal saline or hypertonic saline, with or without adrenaline. ESD uses a modified ESD knife. The lesion is first marked with electrocautery circumferentially at 5 mm along its margin. A submucosal cushion is created by injection, and then a circumferential incision is made with the ESD knife. Dissection is performed in the submucosal layer beneath the lesion, which is excised in its entirety.

Transanal Endoscopic Microsurgery (TEM) offers excellent access to upper and mid-rectal lesions. It uses a specially designed endoscopic device—a large proctoscope measuring 4 cm in diameter—that allows for the passage of dissecting instruments and performs various functions, including CO2 insufflation, water irrigation, suction, and intrarectal pressure monitoring. TEM enables full-thickness excision of rectal lesions up to the mesorectum.

Transanal Minimally Invasive Surgery (TAMIS) is an innovative technique for transanal excision using the SILS Port and GelPOINT Path. A pneumo-rectum is created with a CO2 insufflator, and standard laparoscopic instruments are employed for tumor excision.

Sometimes, standard surgical intervention is needed after endoscopic resection due to adverse histopathological features such as poorly differentiated adenocarcinoma, signet ring cell carcinoma, mucinous carcinoma, lymphovascular invasion, intermediate to high-grade tumor budding, T2 disease, and local recurrence following local excision.

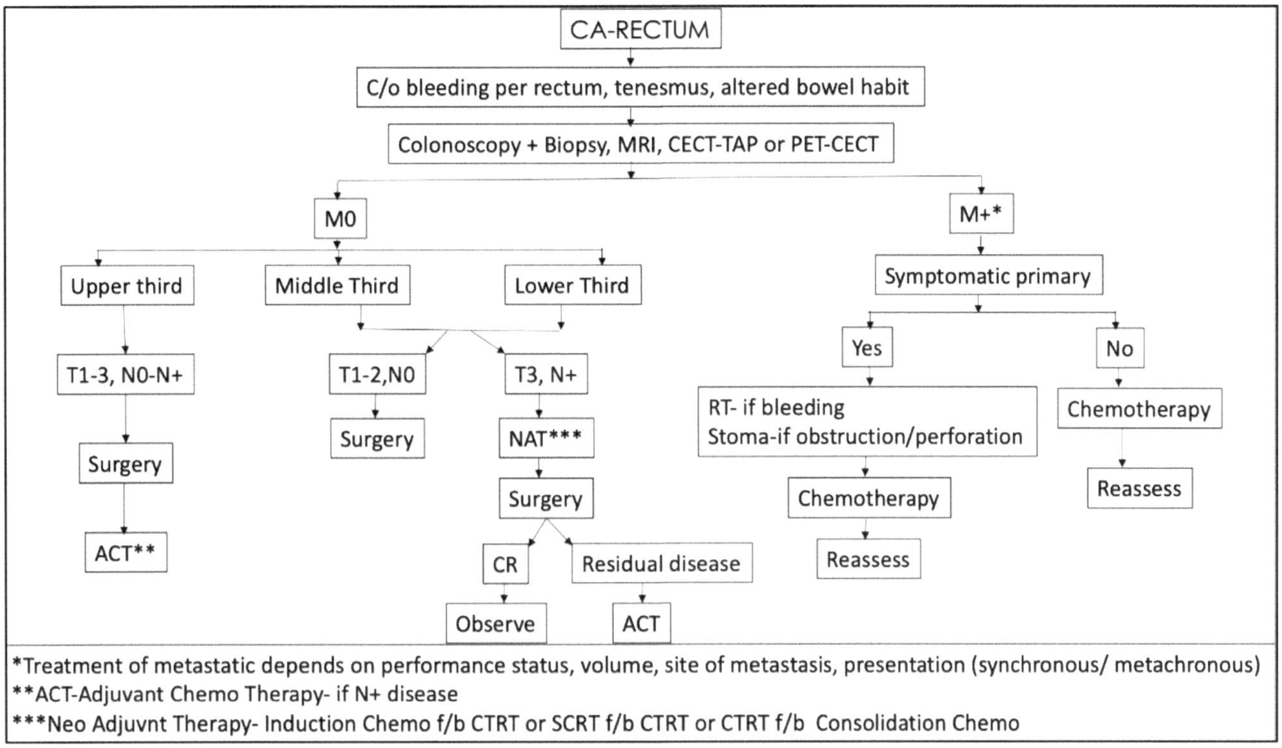

Fig. 15.7 Algorithm for management of rectal cancer

15.5.2 Role of Radiation

Before the era of Total Mesorectal Excision (TME), locoregional recurrence was a major cause of treatment failure. This led to the addition of other treatment options, like radiation, to lower local recurrence rates. Two landmark studies—the Swedish Rectal Cancer Trial and the Dutch Colorectal Cancer Trial—demonstrated that adding preoperative RT to surgery significantly decreased local recurrence.

Pre- vs Postoperative Chemoradiotherapy (CRT)
The German Colorectal Study Group provided strong evidence for the superiority of preoperative chemoradiation. The trial demonstrated significant reduction in local recurrence, less toxicity, and better sphincter-preservation rates in patients receiving preoperative chemoradiation.

Short Course Radiation Therapy (SCRT) v/s Long Course Radiation Therapy (LCRT)
SCRT and LCRT are both used in the management of rectal cancer. The standard LCRT regimen includes 45–50.4 Gy delivered in 1.8-2 Gy daily fractions over 5 to 5.5 weeks, combined with radiosensitizing chemotherapy (5-FU or capecitabine), followed by surgery after 6–8 weeks. SCRT involves 25 Gy with 5 Gy daily fractions over 5 days, followed by either immediate surgery within 1 week or delayed surgery after 6–8 weeks. The Stockholm III Trial compared LCRT with delayed surgery, SCRT with immediate surgery, and SCRT with delayed surgery. The study found no benefit in local recurrence, distant metastasis, or overall survival. However, fewer postoperative complications were observed in patients undergoing delayed surgery. Therefore, both LCRT and SCRT with a delay to surgery remain viable options.

15.5.3 Surgery (Table 15.2)

Table 15.2 Principles of surgery for rectal cancer

Total Mesorectal Excision (TME) is the standard of care for rectal cancer.
Surgery is planned 6–8 weeks after completion of neoadjuvant chemo-radiotherapy (NACTRT). If the patient has received SCRT, surgery can be scheduled immediately within 8–10 days or after 6–8 weeks of completion of SCRT.
Adequate excision of lymph nodes should be performed. For adequate nodal sampling, AJCC recommends obtaining and examining at least 12 lymph nodes. In patients who have received neoadjuvant treatment, the number of lymph nodes may be reduced.
The longitudinal as well as circumferential resection margins should be free. The adequate proximal margin should be 5 cm. The distal margin for upper rectal cancer is 5 cm; however, for mid- and low-rectal cancer, complete TME with a 1 cm distal margin is considered adequate.
Confirm the distal resection margin as free of tumor with the help of a frozen section examination, if available, before performing the anastomosis.

15.5.4 Total Mesorectal Excision

In 1986, Prof. Richard J. Heald reported very low rates of locoregional recurrence after adopting a resection technique called Total Mesorectal Excision (TME). This method is now regarded as the gold standard for treating rectal cancer. TME involves en bloc removal of the mesorectum, including the associated vascular and lymphatic structures, fatty tissue, and mesorectal fascia, through sharp dissection in an avascular plane between the fascia propria of the rectum and the presacral membrane. This avascular plane is also known as the 'Holy plane' of Heald.

15.5.5 Anterior Resection (AR), Low Anterior Resection (LAR), and Ultra Low Anterior Resection (ULAR)

The term anterior resection describes the removal of recto-sigmoid and upper rectal tumors, with the anastomosis positioned above the peritoneal reflection. Low anterior resection involves removing part of the rectum, with the anastomosis located below the anterior peritoneal reflection. TME is partial in both AR and LAR. Ultra-low anterior resection refers to the complete removal of the rectum, with the colon directly anastomosed to the anal canal about 2 cm above the dentate line.

15.5.6 Intersphincteric Resection

Intersphincteric resection is a sphincter-sparing procedure performed for low rectal cancer located less than 3 cm from the anal verge. It involves removing the rectum with at least a 1 cm distal margin along with the internal sphincter. The intersphincteric space and external sphincter are preserved. Good preoperative sphincter function is essential for the success of this procedure.

15.5.7 Abdomino-Perineal Resection (APR)

APR is indicated for low rectal cancers, less than 3 cm from the anal verge, with involvement of the external anal sphincter. It entails removing the entire rectum and anal canal through abdominal and perineal approaches, closing the perineum, and creating a permanent colostomy. There are two types of APR, depending on whether the levator ani muscles are removed based on their involvement: conventional APR (levator ani is not removed) and extra-levator APR (levator ani is removed) (Fig. 15.8).

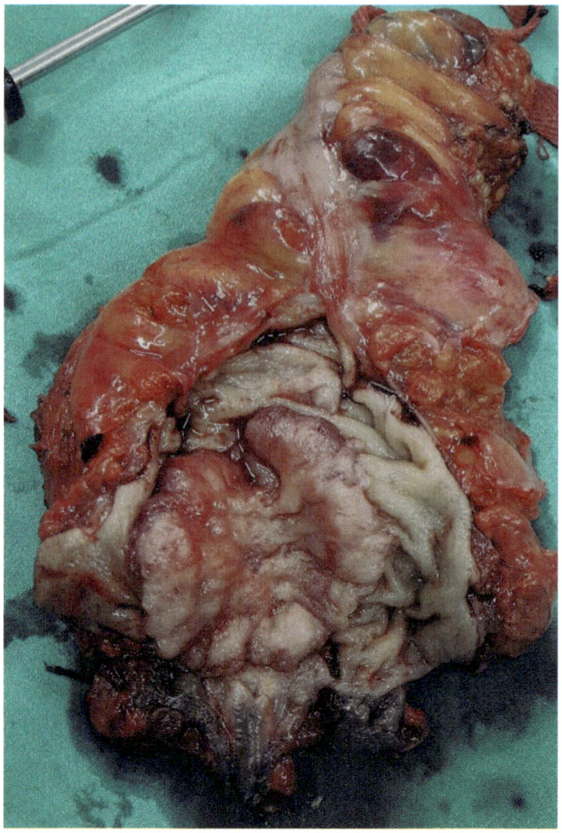

Fig. 15.8 Resected (APR) specimen of the rectum showing an ulcero-proliferative tumor just proximal to the anal verge

15.5.8 Lateral Pelvic Lymph Node Dissection (LPLND)

The lower rectum has lymphatic drainage along the iliac artery nodes on the lateral pelvic wall, which lie outside the meso-rectal template used for standard TME. The external iliac, internal iliac, common iliac, and obturator nodes are collectively called lateral pelvic lymph nodes. The most frequently involved are the internal iliac and obturator nodes, which are considered locoregional nodes. The external iliac, inguinal, and paraaortic lymph nodes are classified as nonregional or distant metastases. The involvement of lateral pelvic nodes occurs in 15–20% of T3-T4 low rectal cancers. LPLND is a technically difficult procedure associated with complications such as sexual and urinary dysfunction. Therefore, the optimal management of LPLN remains controversial. The Japan Clinical Oncology Group (JCOG) 1202 trial demonstrated improved 7-year recurrence-free survival rates in patients who underwent TME plus LPLND for Stage III low rectal cancer without clinically enlarged LPLN. Abnormal LPLN seen on initial MRI is treated with neoadjuvant therapy followed by TME and selective LPLND for patients with persistent LPLN larger than 5 mm on post-NACTRT imaging.

15.5.9 Extended Resections

Rectal cancer that invades nearby organs may require extended resections to achieve complete oncological clearance (R0 resection). Therefore, when rectal cancer involves the prostate or urinary bladder in males, total pelvic exenteration might be needed. In females, if the uterus or posterior vaginal wall is affected, an en bloc hysterectomy may be performed along with rectal resection (posterior exenteration).

15.5.10 Minimally Invasive Approach

The minimally invasive approach (laparoscopic/robotic) for rectal cancer is currently popular because it provides better access and less morbidity. The COLOR II trial has been the first to compare laparoscopic with open surgery, confirming that laparoscopic surgery is not inferior, with improved short-term outcomes such as reduced blood loss, faster return of bowel function, and shorter hospital stays. It also showed that long-term oncologic results are similar, with comparable rates of locoregional recurrence, 3-year disease-free survival (DFS), and overall survival (OS). The COREAN trial reported similar 3-year DFS results. However, the ACOSOG Z 6051 and AlaCaRT trials have failed to prove that laparoscopic surgery is not worse than open surgery for rectal cancer. Both trials found lower success rates in resection and negative circumferential resection margins (CRM) with laparoscopic approaches. Nonetheless, 2-year OS and DFS did not differ significantly between laparoscopic and open surgery in these studies. Over the past two decades, there has been an increase in the use of robotic platforms to treat rectal cancer. Robots offer advantages such as better magnification, seven degrees of freedom with articulated instruments, and 3D vision. Early evidence comparing robotic to laparoscopic surgery indicates that robotic surgery is a safe and feasible alternative. It is associated with shorter hospital stays, lower conversion rates, reduced CRM involvement, and fewer overall complications compared to laparoscopy. However, the ROLARR trial concluded that robotic surgery does not significantly decrease the likelihood of converting to open surgery and thus does not offer a clear advantage over laparoscopic surgery. Another RCT, the COLRAR trial, also found no significant improvement in TME quality with robotic surgery compared to laparoscopy. The most recent RCT, the REAL trial, reported improved oncological quality of resection with robotic surgery. The long-term results of this trial are still pending.

15.5.11 Adjuvant Therapy

Adjuvant chemotherapy is the standard care for all patients with stage III and high-risk stage II rectal cancer after NACTRT and surgery. The preferred regimens are FOLFOX or CAPOX. It is recommended that chemotherapy should begin as soon as possible after surgery, once the patient is medically fit to receive treatment.

15.5.12 Total Neoadjuvant Therapy (TNT)

TNT involves administering both radiation and full systemic chemotherapy before surgery. The goal of TNT is that delivering full-dose chemotherapy targets micrometastatic disease early, provides quick symptom relief, offers better tolerance with less toxicity, and may even allow for avoidance of surgery if a clinical complete response (cCR) is achieved. The specific radiation protocols, choice of chemotherapy, and the sequence of treatment may vary. The advantage of TNT is the significantly higher pathologic Complete Response (pCR) rate, 25%, compared to 12% in patients receiving conventional NACTRT. However, TNT is not yet considered the standard of care.

15.5.13 Nonoperative Management (NOM)

Patients who achieve cCR after TNT can be carefully considered for nonoperative management. Habr-Gama first described this method, also known as the "watch and wait" approach. Patients who achieve cCR and opt for NOM are expected to undergo strict monitoring, including digital rectal exams, flexible sigmoidoscopy, and MRI at regular intervals according to a set protocol. The risk of local regrowth with this method is about 30%, with salvage TME remaining a feasible option.

15.5.14 Follow-Up (Table 15.3)

Table 15.3 Follow-up protocol for tumor/s after resection

Surgical procedure	Follow-up protocol
Transanal excision	Proctoscopy and EUS/ MRI every 3–6 months for the first 2 years, every 6 months thereafter for 5 years
	Colonoscopy yearly if advanced adenoma (villous adenoma, polyp >1 cm or high-grade dysplasia) or else repeat at 3 years and then every 5 years
Resected stage I disease	Colonoscopy at 1 year after surgery
	Colonoscopy yearly if advanced adenoma (villous adenoma, polyp >1 cm or high-grade dysplasia) or else repeat at 3 years and then every 5 years
Resected stage II/ III disease with curative intent + adjuvant chemotherapy	History and physical examination every 3 months for 2 years, every 6 months in the third year, and then annually in the fourth and fifth years
	CEA, CA 19.9—Every 3 months for 2 years, every 6 months for the third year, and then annually for the fourth and fifth year
	CECT abdomen, pelvis, and thorax annually for 5 years
	Colonoscopy—1 year after surgery. If a presurgery colonoscopy was not complete due to an obstructing lesion, then it should be done at 6 months postsurgery. If an advanced adenoma (villous adenoma, polyp >1 cm or high-grade dysplasia) is found, then repeat in 1 year. If no advanced adenoma is present, repeat in 3 years and then every 5 years

15.5.15 Management of Metastatic Disease

Approximately 20–34% of patients with CRC present with metastatic disease to the liver, and about 50–60% of patients diagnosed with CRC will develop metastasis. Managing this group of patients is particularly challenging. The sequencing of chemotherapy and surgical procedures is crucial and tailored based on the patient's presentation. Key factors influencing the overall approach in metastatic rectal cancer include whether the presentation is synchronous or metachronous, whether the primary tumor is symptomatic or asymptomatic, and the number and location of metastases. In cases of symptomatic primary tumors, initial treatment focuses on symptom relief, such as radiation therapy for bleeding tumors or diversion stoma for obstruction or perforation, followed by chemotherapy. Patients with asymptomatic metastatic rectal cancer are directly started on conversion chemotherapy. Regular reassessment is performed to evaluate the feasibility of surgery. With advances in systemic and targeted therapies, surgical options, and liver-directed therapies, patients with favorable tumor biology and metastatic disease can potentially be offered curative treatment.

15.5.16 Management of Locally Recurrent Disease

Managing locally recurrent rectal cancer involves several challenges and depends on various factors. For resectable recurrence, treatment choices are influenced by previous treatments, the extent of the local recurrence, and the presence of distant metastasis. Patients who have not received previous radiation therapy should be considered for combined modality therapy, including NACTRT followed by surgery and adjuvant chemotherapy. Complete radical resection should only be attempted if clear microscopically negative margins can be achieved. Extensive surgical procedures, such as APR, pelvic exenteration, or sacrectomy, might be necessary. For patients who have previously undergone radiation, reirradiation may be an option in carefully selected cases.

Key Points

- Colorectal cancer is the third most common cancer worldwide.
- Common presentation symptoms are bleeding per rectum, altered bowel habits, and loss of weight and appetite.
- Digital rectal examination is vital for assessment of the tumor, its location with respect to the anal verge, mobility, and anal sphincter function.
- The work-up of the patient with rectal cancer involves tumor markers (CEA, CA-19.9), colonoscopy, MRI-pelvis for local staging, and CECT and PET-CT for metastatic staging.
- The management of rectal cancer is a multimodality approach with radiation, surgery, and chemotherapy.
- The treatment of rectal cancer is tailored according to the location of the tumor, T stage, nodal status, and metastatic status.
- T1 lesions <3 cm, with favorable histology, can be treated by local excision.
- Total mesorectal excision is the procedure of choice for resectable cancer.

Selected Reading

1. NCCN- National Cancer Comprehensive Network. Clinical Practice Guidelines in Oncology (NCCN Guidelines)-Rectal Cancer. Version 4.2024.
2. AJCC- American Joint Committee on Cancer. Colon and rectum. AJCC cancer staging manual. 8th ed. Chicago: Springer; 2017. p. 251–74.
3. Sung H, Ferlay J, Siegel RL, et al. Global cancer statistics 2020: GLOBOCAN estimates of incidence and mortality worldwide for 36 cancers in 185 countries. CA Cancer J Clin. 2021;71:209–49. https://doi.org/10.3322/caac.21660. Epub 2021 Feb 4
4. Troester AM, Gaertner WB. Contemporary management of rectal cancer. Surg Open Sci. 2024;18:17–22. https://doi.org/10.1016/j.sopen.2024.01.009.
5. Eng C, Yoshino T, Ruíz-García E, et al. Colorectal cancer. Lancet. 2024;404:294–310.
6. Cotan HT, Emilescu RA, Iaciu CI, et al. Prognostic and predictive determinants of colorectal cancer: a comprehensive review. Cancers. 2024;16:3928. https://doi.org/10.3390/cancers16233928.

Carcinoma Anal Canal

16

Rajesh S. Shinde, Deep Mashru, Saneya Pandrowala, and Shailesh V. Shrikhande

Abstract

Diagnosis of anal carcinoma is primarily clinical, with radiology and histology serving for confirmation. Squamous cell carcinoma is the most common type of histology. The treatment of anal canal cancer has modestly shifted from surgery alone to a multimodal approach involving chemoradiotherapy. Surgery in the form of APR is reserved for nonresponders; patients are showing progression of tumor or recurrence after chemotherapy or those with uncommon histology like adenocarcinoma or melanoma.

Keywords

Anal cancer · APR

The anal canal is the most distal part of the gastrointestinal (GI) tract and plays the principal function of fecal continence and defecation. Malignancies in this area are rare, with benign conditions being more frequently encountered by surgeons in everyday practice. The treatment of anal canal cancer has progressed greatly over the past 25 years. Multimodal therapy, including chemotherapy and radiotherapy, has nearly eliminated the need for surgery. Managing anal canal cancer is one of the few cancer treatments that exemplify the use of organ preservation through multimodal approaches.

16.1 Anatomy

The anal canal extends from the top of the anorectal ring, where the internal sphincter, deep external sphincter, and puborectalis muscle converge and can be felt, to the anal verge, which marks the junction between the anal canal and the keratinized, hair-bearing skin of the perineum. The dentate line is an uneven line formed by anal valves, which are the openings of anal sinuses. A zone 1–2 cm above this dentate line is called the anal transition zone (ATZ). The anal canal is split into three regions by the ATZ: below the ATZ has squamous epithelium; above the ATZ has columnar epithelium; and at the ATZ, there is cuboidal epithelium. Because of these different tissue types, various malignancies can develop in the anal canal, including squamous cell carcinoma (SCC), adenocarcinoma, lymphoma, melanoma, and others. The blood supply, venous drainage, nerve supply, and lymphatic drainage differ above and below the dentate line. The anal margin is a clearly defined area extending about 5 cm from the anal verge. Perianal cancers are tumors that originate within the skin at or beyond the squamous mucocutaneous junction. These can be fully visualized with gentle traction on the buttocks and are located within 5 cm of the anus (Fig. 16.1 and Table 16.1).

R. S. Shinde (✉) · D. Mashru · S. Pandrowala · S. V. Shrikhande
Tata Memorial Hospital, Mumbai, India

M. Ibrarullah (ed.), *Recent Concepts in Gastrointestinal (GI) Surgery*, https://doi.org/10.1007/978-981-92-1118-0_16

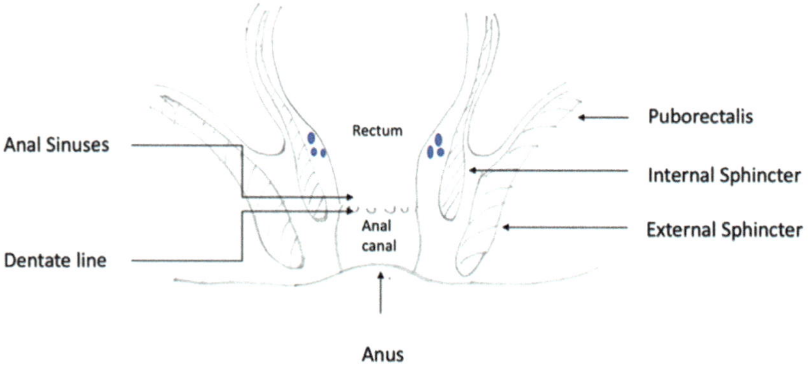

Fig. 16.1 Anatomy of the anal canal

Table 16.1 Blood supply, nerve innervation, and lymphatic drainage of anal canal

	Above the dentate line	Below the dentate line
Arterial supply	Major supply comes from the superior rectal artery, a branch of the inferior mesenteric artery. Anastomosing branches of the middle rectal artery	Major supply comes from the inferior rectal artery, which is a branch of the internal pudendal artery. Anastomosing branches of the middle rectal artery
Venous drainage	Major drainage is to the superior rectal vein, which is a tributary of the inferior mesenteric vein (portal venous system).	Major drainage is to the inferior rectal vein, which is a tributary to the internal pudendal vein (systemic venous system)
Nerve supply	Visceral innervation is through the inferior hypogastric plexus	Somatic innervation is through inferior rectal nerves, which are branches of the pudendal nerve.
Lymphatic drainage	Primary echelon nodes are the perirectal nodes, which then drain into the internal iliac group of lymph nodes.	Primary echelon nodes are the superficial inguinal group of lymph nodes

16.2 Incidence and Epidemiology

Anal canal cancer is a rare tumor. According to GLOBOCAN 2020, there were only 50,000 cases worldwide. It accounts for just 2% of all GI cancers, with an incidence of 1–2 per 100,000 people annually. The occurrence is increasing in high-income countries, likely due to rises in high-risk sexual behaviors, HIV infections, immunosuppression, and the growing prevalence of HPV infections. Females are affected more than males, with a male-to-female ratio of 5:1. The median age at diagnosis is around 60 years.

Table 16.2 Risk factors for anal canal cancer

Risk factors	Relative risk
Human Papilloma Virus (HPV)	Association in >90% cases
Human immunodeficiency virus (HIV)	RR = 2
Receptive anal intercourse	RR = 30
Smoking	RR = 2–5
Chronic immunosuppression	RR = 6

16.3 Risk Factors (Table 16.2)

Chronic inflammation caused by hemorrhoids, fissures, or inflammatory bowel disease, once thought to be a key cause, has been disproved by multiple large cohort studies.

16.3.1 Human Papilloma Virus (HPV)

HPV is the most common sexually transmitted infection worldwide and a leading cause of anal canal cancer. It is strongly associated with cancers of the cervix, vulva, oral cavity, oropharynx, and anal canal. Over 90% of anal canal cancer cases are linked to HPV, and HPV DNA can be detected in these cases. The most common HPV strains found in anal canal cancer are HPV 16, 18, 31, 33, and 45, with HPV 16 being the most frequently identified.

16.3.2 Human Immunodeficiency Virus (HIV)

HIV-positive individuals face twice the risk of anal canal cancer, particularly among men who have sex with men (MSM). Despite the use of highly active antiretroviral therapy (HAART), the incidence of anal canal cancer has risen. In individuals positive for HPV, the presence of HIV infection increases the risk of precursor lesions and anal canal cancer. The precise mechanism through which HIV contributes to anal canal cancer remains unclear.

16.3.3 Sexual Activity and Sexually Transmitted Diseases (STDs)

Receptive anal intercourse is a significant risk factor, with a relative risk (RR) exceeding 30. Having multiple sexual partners, a history of genital warts, and previous sexually transmitted infections like chlamydia trachomatis or gonorrhea are risk factors for anal cancer in both men and women. A history of cervical dysplasia or cervical cancer also raises the risk for anal cancer, possibly due to HPV infection. The highest incidence is seen in MSM with HIV and HPV coinfection.

16.3.4 Smoking

Smoking raises the risk of anal canal cancer (relative risk 2–5) and functions as a cocarcinogen.

16.3.5 Chronic Immunosuppression

Immunosuppression in patients with solid organ transplants and autoimmune diseases (on steroids) is associated with a higher risk of anal canal cancer. This may be due to an increased likelihood of HPV infection and persistence caused by the body's reduced ability to clear HPV.

16.4 Clinical Presentation

The most common age group at presentation is 60–65 years. About 50% of patients present with bleeding per rectum, often attributed to hemorrhoids or fissure in ano, which can lead to delayed diagnosis. Other symptoms may include pain, tenesmus, a mass per rectum, or a mass in the inguinal region. According to the SEER database, 50% of patients present with localized disease, while the rest have advanced disease.

16.5 Evaluation

Digital rectal examination with proctoscopy is the simplest and most effective bedside tool for diagnosing anal canal cancer. It involves a detailed assessment of the tumor's size, cranio-caudal extent, circumferential involvement, rectal involvement, and sphincter tone. A thorough gynecological examination is also recommended for female patients to rule out cervical cancer. Examination of the inguinal lymph nodes is essential to evaluate for nodal metastasis. Proctoscopic biopsy is necessary to confirm the diagnosis. Any enlarged or suspicious nodes should undergo fine needle aspiration cytology to confirm metastatic involvement. Routine blood tests and seromarkers are also recommended.

To complete the staging evaluation, magnetic resonance imaging (MRI) of the pelvis is the preferred method for assessing locoregional disease. Tumors show high signal intensity compared to skeletal muscle on T2-weighted images and low to intermediate signal intensity on T1-weighted images. Lymph node metastases usually have similar signal intensity to the primary tumor. The size of the tumor, its circumferential extent, invasion of nearby organs (vagina, urethra, prostate, and bladder), extension into the ischioanal or ischiorectal fossa, and the presence of fistulas are documented. Contrast-enhanced computed tomography (CECT) of the thorax and abdomen is performed to rule out metastatic disease. Positron emission tomography (PET) scan can differentiate between post-treatment fibrosis and active disease.

16.6 Staging

AJCC staging-eighth edition (TNM) is widely used to stage the tumor and decide the treatment modality. The perianal cancers are also staged and treated as anal canal cancer.

16.7 Management

Principles of Management

The multimodality treatment approach, including definitive chemoradiation, is now the standard of care for managing anal canal cancer. Surgery is reserved only for persistent disease after radiation therapy and early anal margin cancers. In metastatic cases, palliative chemotherapy is usually the recommended treatment.

Multimodality Management

Norman Nigro, a colorectal surgeon at Wayne State University, outlined a treatment protocol in 1974 that included administering 5-Fluorouracil (5-FU), Mitomycin-C (MMC), and radiation therapy (30 Gy in 15 sessions), followed by surgery. He noted that two-thirds of patients achieved a pathological complete response (pCR), and the third patient refused surgery and remained disease-free.

The United Kingdom Coordinating Committee for Cancer Research (UKCCCR) conducted the Anal Cancer Trial (ACT

I) study, in which 585 patients were randomly assigned to receive definitive RT versus RT combined with 5FU and MMC. In the initial report, after a follow-up of 42 months, the 3-year local failure rate was significantly lower in the chemoradiotherapy group, although this was associated with increased treatment-related toxicities. Anal cancer-related mortality was significantly lower in the combined modality treatment group, but the 3-year overall survival (OS) was similar. In a long-term follow-up of 10 years, local recurrence rates were significantly higher in the radiation-only group. Colostomy-free rates were significantly better in the combined modality group.

The European Organization for Research and Treatment of Cancer (EORTC) conducted a randomized controlled trial (RCT) with 110 anal canal cancer patients, comparing RT to combined modality treatment. At the 6-week response evaluation, a clinical complete response was observed in 80% of patients in the combined modality treatment group. After 5 years of follow-up, there was a significant improvement in locoregional control rates and colostomy-free rates in the combined modality treatment group.

These two trials have confirmed chemoradiation as the standard treatment for localized cases. Although there was no improvement in survival, locoregional control rates were higher with chemoradiation.

Similar results were observed in studies conducted by Leichman et al. and Michaelson et al. from Memorial Sloan Kettering Cancer Center (MSKCC). These studies identified groups with pCR rates and groups with residual tumors requiring surgical intervention, without a prospective randomized trial directly comparing surgery versus chemoradiation. As a result, they paved the way for accepting chemoradiation as the standard of care. Subsequently, multiple studies were conducted, leading to the decision on the most appropriate treatment protocol, which includes 5FU / Capecitabine + MMC with radiation of 45-50Gy and an additional boost of 9-16Gy for >T3 tumors or N+ disease.

Response Assessment

Response to treatment is assessed 6–8 weeks after chemoradiation. If there is a partial response or stable disease, patients continue follow-up until 6 months after finishing treatment. If there is any progression after treatment or during this period, a biopsy should be considered. Biopsy should be avoided in patients with a complete response following chemoradiation, as it can cause persistent nonhealing ulceration due to poor vascularity and may lead to necrosis. Biopsy is only recommended if there is strong clinical suspicion of recurrence, such as proliferative growth or ulceration. MRI of the pelvis is used to evaluate the local extent of disease and the possibility of surgical salvage. For suspected distant metastases, a CECT of the thorax and abdomen or a PET-CT scan is advised.

16.8 Follow-Up

Follow-up is primarily clinical. Patients are monitored every 3 months for up to 2 years, every 6 months for up to 5 years, and annually afterward. During each visit, a clinical exam—including digital rectal examination and palpation of both inguinal nodal regions—should be conducted. Fibrosis and stenosis of the anal canal resulting from radiation may hinder a complete clinical exam. MRI imaging can be considered to detect local recurrences. Most recurrences are locoregional and happen within 2 years. Long-term follow-up of the ACT-1 trial showed that after 5 years, fewer than 2% of patients experienced a locoregional relapse. Distant metastases without locoregional relapse occurred in only 7%. Therefore, during follow-up, attention should be given to early detection of recurrences and complications from chemoradiation.

16.9 Role of Surgery

Surgical management is primarily used for salvage situations (Table 16.3).

Surgery performed for anal canal malignancies is Abdomino-Perineal Resection (APR). Surgery must achieve negative margins for oncological success. Tumor invasion into adjacent organs requires en bloc resection. Invasion of local structures, such as the vagina or prostate, should be approached with the intent of resecting with negative margins. This may involve a multi-visceral resection. If inguinal nodes are positive, a groin dissection should be performed along with the APR.

Table 16.3 Indications for surgery

Anal margin cancer: in the early stage.
Control of primary in locally advanced cases: poor response or progressive local disease during/following chemoradiotherapy.
Locally recurrent tumor: local relapse (locoregional) following chemoradiation.
Failure of locally advanced cases: persistent local disease or residual lymph nodes after 6 months of completion of chemoradiation.
Persistent pain, fistula, or incontinence following chemoradiation.
Surgery is also indicated for uncommon histology such as localized non-metastatic melanoma, neuroendocrine tumors, and post-neoadjuvant chemoradiation settings in case of adenocarcinoma.
A temporary defunctioning colostomy can be done in cases of intestinal obstruction due to a large mass or due to fistulisation with the vagina.

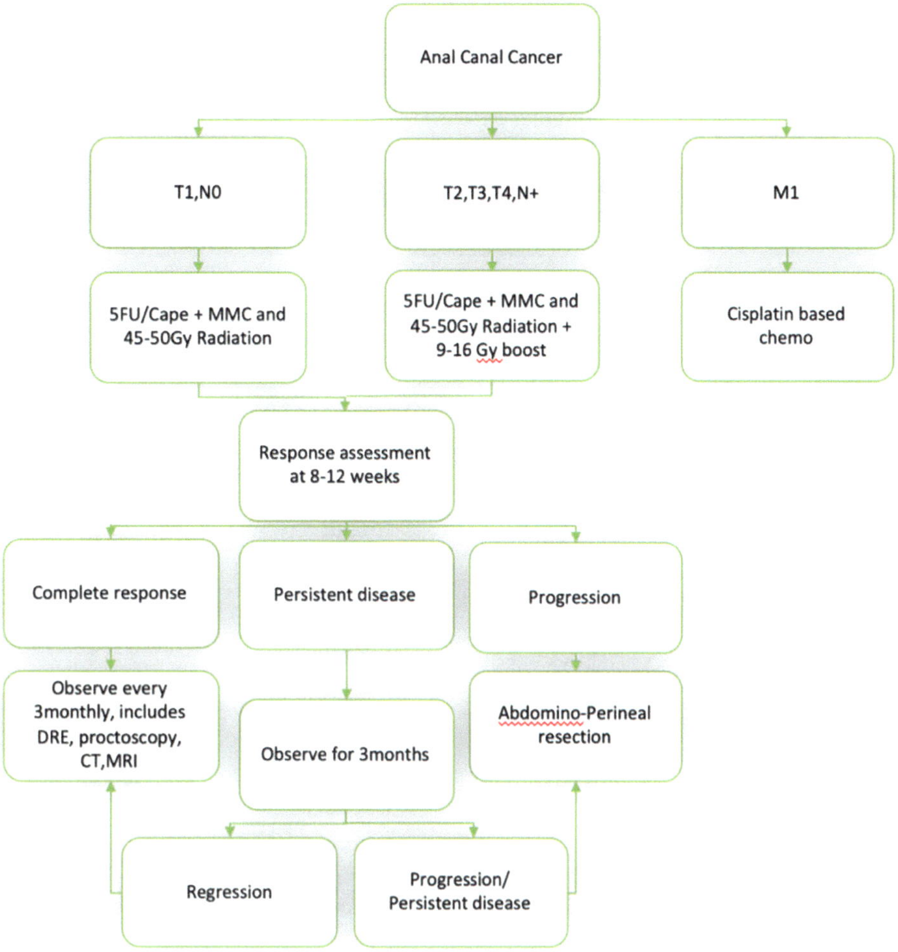

Fig. 16.2 Flowchart on management of anal canal cancer

16.10 Metastatic Disease

There are no formal studies on managing metastatic disease. However, in clinical practice, Cisplatin and 5-FU-based chemotherapy are used in this setting (Fig. 16.2).

Key Points

- There is a strong correlation between anal canal cancer and HPV infection.
- Diagnosis is primarily clinical, with radiology and histology serving for confirmation.
- Squamous cell carcinoma is the most common type of histology.
- The treatment of anal canal cancer has modestly shifted from surgery alone to a multimodal approach involving chemo-radiotherapy.
- Surgery in the form of APR is reserved for non-responders; patients showing progression of tumor or recurrence after chemotherapy or those with uncommon histology like adenocarcinoma or melanoma.

Selected Reading

1. Deo SV, Sharma J, Kumar S. GLOBOCAN 2020 report on global cancer burden: challenges and opportunities for surgical oncologists. Ann Surg Oncol. 2022;29:6497–500.
2. Clarke M, Wentzensen N. Strategies for screening and early detection of anal cancers: a narrative and systematic review and meta-analysis of cytology, HPV testing, and other biomarkers. Cancer Cytopathol. 2018;126:447–60.
3. Hillman RJ, Cuming T, Darragh T. 2016 IANS international guidelines for practice standards in the detection of anal cancer precursors. J Low Genit Tract Dis. 2016;20:283–91.
4. Kachnic L, Winter K, Myerson R, et al. Long-term outcomes of NRG Oncology- RTOG0529: A phase II evaluation of dose-painted intensity modulated radiation therapy in combination with 5-fluorouracil and mitomycin-C for the reduction of acute morbidity in anal cancer. Int J Radiat Oncol Biol Phys. 2022;112(1):146–57.
5. Correa JH, Castro LS, Kesley R, et al. Salvage abdominoperineal resection for anal cancer following chemoradiation: A proposed scoring system for predicting postoperative survival. J Surg Oncol. 2013;107:486–92.

Part IV

Liver

Surgical Anatomy of the Liver

17

Nalini Kanta Ghosh, Kausar Makki, and Vivek Vij

Abstract

The liver is divided into two lobes by Cantlie's line, which runs from the IVC to the GB fossa. The right lobe is further subdivided into anterior and posterior sectors (segments), comprising segments (V and VIII) and (VI and VII), respectively. The left lobe is subdivided into lateral (segments II and III) and medial (segment IV) sectors. The right anterior pedicle is vertical, whereas the posterior pedicle is horizontally oriented. The right, left, and middle hepatic veins drain into the IVC and lie in the intersectoral planes. The portal vein and bile duct have variable dispositions at the hepatic hilum. The hepatic artery has a variable origin, but the liver receives a robust arterial supply through a well-developed collateral circulation.

Keywords

Liver anatomy · Segmental anatomy of liver

17.1 Topographic Anatomy of the Liver

The liver is located in the right upper quadrant of the abdomen, beneath the right hemidiaphragm. Its surface anatomy can be identified clinically by percussion liver dullness over the right upper abdomen and lower thoracic areas. It is protected from trauma by the rib cage and held in position by false ligaments. The liver has two surfaces (parietal and visceral) and three borders (posterosuperior, posteroinferior, and inferior). Superiorly, it is related to the diaphragm, right lung, pleural cavity, pericardium, and heart. Posteriorly, it is related to the diaphragm, lower ribs, inferior vena cava, aorta, and esophagus. Anteriorly, it contacts the diaphragm, costal margin, sternum, and the anterior abdominal wall musculature. Two notches are palpable on an enlarged liver: the gallbladder fossa and the umbilical fissure. Inferiorly, it relates to the hepatic flexure of the colon, the proximal part of the transverse colon, hepatorenal pouch, right kidney, right adrenal gland, gallbladder, first and second parts of the duodenum, and stomach.

17.2 Peritoneal Reflections of the Liver

The liver is held in place by three main ligamentous attachments: the falciform ligament, the round ligament, and the coronary ligament. Anteriorly and posteriorly, the peritoneal coverings of the liver are reflected onto the diaphragm, forming the respective coronary ligaments. The space between these coronary ligaments is known as the bare area of the liver, which is among the sites for portosystemic shunts in patients with portal hypertension. The coronary ligaments fuse on each side to create the right and left triangular ligaments. The anterior coronary ligament folds onto itself in the midline, forming the falciform ligament. Between the two folds of this ligament, the embryological remnant of the left umbilical vein remains, called the round ligament of the liver (or ligamentum teres). The falciform ligament divides the liver into two halves in terms of morphology, which differs from the anatomical division into hemilivers. Anatomically, it separates Couinaud segments II and III from segment IV. Ventrally, the round ligament is located in the fissure for the ligamentum venosum (fossa for ductus venosus or Rex recess), which separates segments III and IV. At the porta hepatis, the peritoneal layers extend onto the lesser curvature of the stomach to form the gastrohepatic ligament. The right margin of this ligament contains three key liver structures: the hepatic artery (on the left), the bile duct (on the right), and the portal vein (posteriorly), which appears as the "Mickey Mouse" sign on ultrasonography (Figs. 17.1 and 17.2).

N. K. Ghosh (✉) · K. Makki · V. Vij
Fortis Hospital, Noida, India

M. Ibrarullah (ed.), *Recent Concepts in Gastrointestinal (GI) Surgery*, https://doi.org/10.1007/978-981-92-1118-0_17

Table 17.1 Applied anatomy

The right pleural cavity is related to the right lobe of the liver; hence, drainage of a right lobe abscess can contaminate the right pleural cavity.
Liver abscess in the right lobe can rupture into the right pleural cavity.
Left lobe abscess can rupture into the pericardial cavity.
Proximity to the stomach and duodenum makes the liver accessible for evaluation with endoscopic ultrasound.
The right adrenal gland is closely related to the right lobe of the liver and is often a site of bleeding during liver mobilization for right lobe resections.
After a right hepatectomy, the fixation of the left lobe is performed along the falciform ligament to prevent torsion and outflow obstruction.
Recanalization of the umbilical vein occurs in portal hypertension, which is a potential source of bleeding during open or laparoscopic surgeries.
The Rex recess is accessed during meso-Rex bypass or Rex shunt (for extra-hepatic portal vein obstruction).
The Rex recess is also the site for segment III bypass in cases of unresectable hilar obstructions.
Sometimes, the gastrohepatic ligament contains a replaced or accessory left hepatic artery originating from the left gastric artery, which must be preserved during hepatic or gastric surgeries.

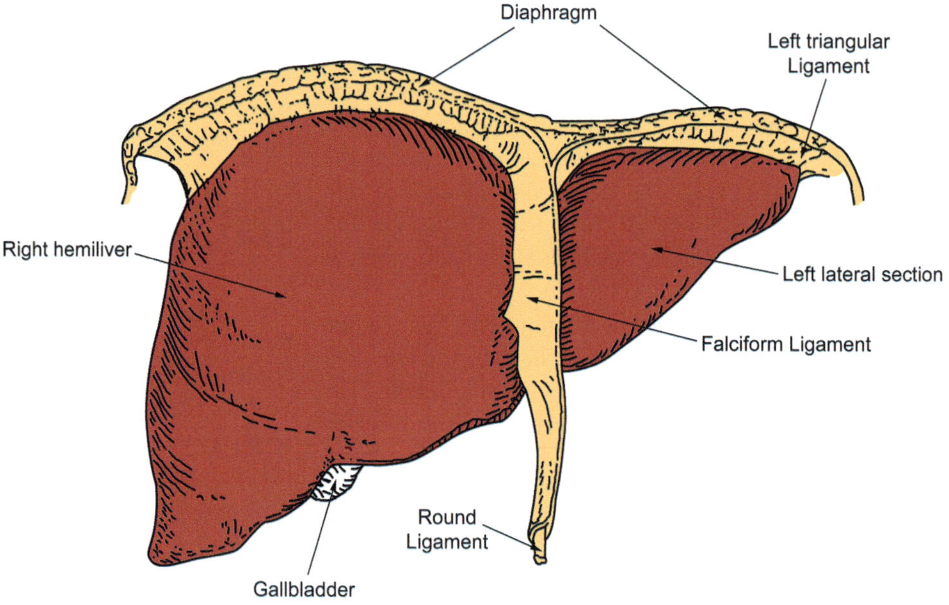

Fig. 17.1 Anterosuperior surface of the liver

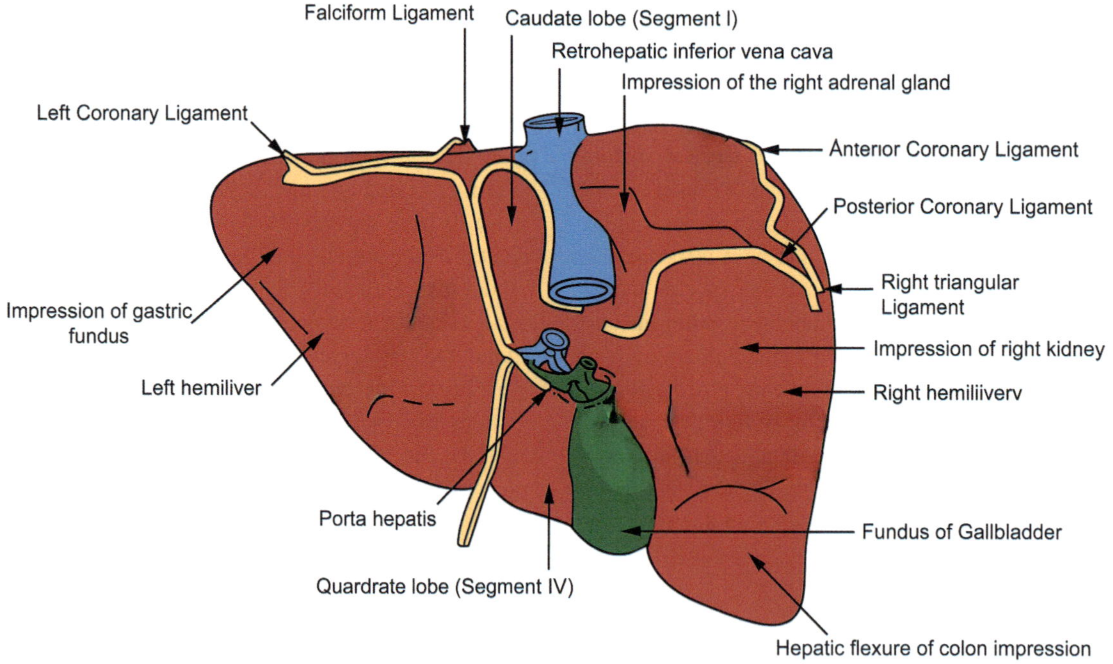

Fig. 17.2 Posteroinferior surface of the liver

17.3 Intrahepatic Anatomy

Historically, Galen proposed separate hepatic arterial and portal venous systems that end in small branches and continue as hepatic veins to drain into the inferior vena cava. James Cantlie described an imaginary line from the gallbladder (GB) fossa to the suprahepatic inferior vena cava (IVC) that divides the liver into two functional halves. This line aligns with the middle hepatic vein internally. Couinaud is credited with the modern classification of intrahepatic anatomy based on the portal venous system. The liver contains eight segments, divided into four sectors by three hepatic veins—the right hepatic vein (RHV), middle hepatic vein (MHV), and left hepatic vein (LHV)—within the hepatic scissurae. The main portal scissure, known as Cantlie's line, contains the MHV and separates the liver into two lobes with independent hepatic artery, portal vein, and biliary drainage. These lobes (right and left) are further subdivided into four segments (by Goldsmith and Woodburne) or sectors (by Couinaud). The right lobe is divided into the right anterior sector and the right posterior sector by the right portal scissure, which contains the RHV. The right posterior sector (to the right of the RHV) includes segment VI inferiorly and segment VII superiorly. The right anterior sector (between the RHV and MHV) includes segment V inferiorly and segment VIII superiorly. In contrast, the anatomy of the left lobe differs from that of the right. The left portal scissure divides the left lobe; however, the left medial and lateral sectors are separated by the left portal vein rather than the left hepatic vein. The hepatic nomenclature by Couinaud has been updated by the IHPBA (Brisbane 2000), where sectors are called sections. The left portal triad extends a long extrahepatic course (3–4 cm) at the base of segment IV. Subsequently, the left portal pedicle runs in the umbilical fissure, giving rise to branches for segments II, III, and IV (Fig. 17.3).

The caudate lobe (Segment I) is unique in its anatomy. It is located anterior to the IVC and posteroinferior to the three hepatic veins. The caudate lobe is divided into the caudate process, the paracaval portion, and the Spiegel lobe (Kumon's segmentation). The Spiegel lobe is located posterior to the gastrohepatic ligament and extends to the left of the IVC and the Arantius ligament. The Arantius ligament runs from the left branch of the portal vein and lies anterior to the caudate lobe, reaching up to the IVC just posterior to the junction of the MHV and LHV. The paracaval portion sits in front of the IVC and to the right of the Spiegel lobe. The caudate process is a small part positioned between the IVC posteriorly and the portal vein anteriorly. The caudate lobe can have a variable number of portal pedicles; however, the left pedicle is more consistently present. Portal vein branches for the caudate lobe originate independently from the right branch, left branch, or the main portal vein. The paracaval and Spiegel lobes can have 2–3 biliary drainages to the right and left ducts, respectively. The venous drainage of the caudate lobe includes short hepatic veins, the superior right hepatic vein, the caudate process hepatic vein, the accessory hepatic vein of the caudate lobe, and the proper hepatic vein of the caudate phrenic vein.

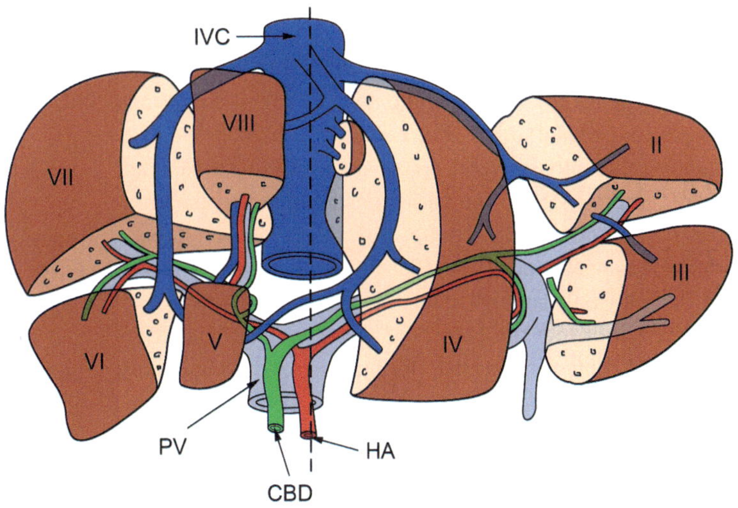

Fig. 17.3 Segmental anatomy of the liver

Table 17.2 Applied anatomy

Cantlie's line corresponds to the demarcation line on clamping the hemiportal inflow structures during hepatectomy.
In Budd-Chiari syndrome, because of hepatic venous outflow tract obstruction, alternate drainage occurs through the caudate lobe that has independent drainage to the IVC, which leads to caudate hypertrophy.
Small caudate bile ducts can lead to problematic bile leaks after hemi-hepatectomies.
The knowledge of hepatic segmentation helps to perform systematic segmental resection with less bleeding and postoperative bile leak.

17.4 Blood Supply of the Liver

The liver receives blood from two sources: the hepatic artery and the portal vein. The hepatic artery provides 25% of the blood flow and 50% of the oxygen, while the portal vein supplies 75% of the blood and the remaining 50% of the oxygen. Additionally, the hepatic arteries are the only source supplying blood to the intrahepatic bile ducts.

17.4.1 Hepatic Artery

Embryologically, there are three hepatic arteries: the left hepatic artery (LHA) originates from the left gastric artery (LGA), the right hepatic artery (RHA) originates from the superior mesenteric artery (SMA), and the middle hepatic artery originates from the celiac axis. The RHA and LHA disappear, and the middle hepatic artery from the celiac axis remains as the hepatic artery proper (Table 17.3).

Usually, the common hepatic artery lies at the superior border of the pancreatic head, posterior to a lymph node (lymph node of importance), and to the left of the common bile duct. It then divides into the hepatic artery proper and the gastroduodenal artery. The hepatic artery proper subsequently splits into the right hepatic artery (RHA) and the left hepatic artery (LHA). The RHA runs posterior to the common hepatic duct in 85% to 95% of cases. The left hepatic artery supplies segments II, III, and IV; however, in some cases, it may only supply the left lateral section. Intrahepatic, the arteries follow the course of the bile duct. The RHA divides into anterior and posterior branches, while in the left lobe, these are divided into lateral and medial branches. There is intrahepatic communication between the RHA and LHA. Therefore, accidental ligation of isolated arteries may be inconsequential in normal patients.

Table 17.3 Mitchel's classification of hepatic arterial anatomy

I	Normal anatomy
II	Replaced LHA from LGA
III	Replaced RHA from SMA
IV	Replaced LHA from LGA and replaced RHA from SMA
V	Accessory LHA from LGA
VI	Accessory RHA from SMA
VII	Accessory LHA from LGA and accessory RHA from SMA
VIII	Replaced RHA and accessory LHA or RHA, and replaced LHA
IX	CHA from SMA
X	CHA from LGA

CHA common hepatic artery, *LHA* left hepatic artery, *RHA* right hepatic artery, *SMA* superior mesenteric artery

17.5 The Portal Vein

The splenic vein and the superior mesenteric vein (SMV) merge behind the neck of the pancreas to form the portal vein (PV). It is approximately 8 cm long, with a diameter ranging from 7 to 13 mm in healthy individuals. The PV receives tributaries from the posterior superior pancreaticoduodenal vein, inferior mesenteric vein (in 50% of cases), left gastric vein, cystic vein, and small veins in the hepatoduodenal ligament. It runs within the hepatoduodenal ligament at the free edge of the lesser omentum, positioned posterior to the hepatic artery and bile duct. The main portal vein then divides into right and left branches, supplying the two lobes; however, the intrahepatic branches are not mirror images. The right portal vein divides into anterior and posterior branches, which supply their respective sectors of the right lobe. These branches further divide into superior and inferior branches, supplying individual segments of the lobe (Fig. 17.4).

The left portal vein is longer, with a horizontal part running at the base of segment IV and a vertical part running in the umbilical fissure. The vertical part divides into branches supplying segments II, III, and IV. The caudate lobe (segment I) is unique because it is supplied by both the right and left branches. The epicholedochal venous plexus of Saint and the paracholedochal plexus of Patren drain into the 3 o'clock and 9 o'clock marginal veins, which eventually drain into the gastric vein, the posterior superior pancreaticoduodenal vein, and the gastrocolic trunk. In portal vein thrombosis, these vessels dilate to form the portal cavernoma and lead to portal bilopathy in patients with chronic liver disease and noncirrhotic portal hypertension.

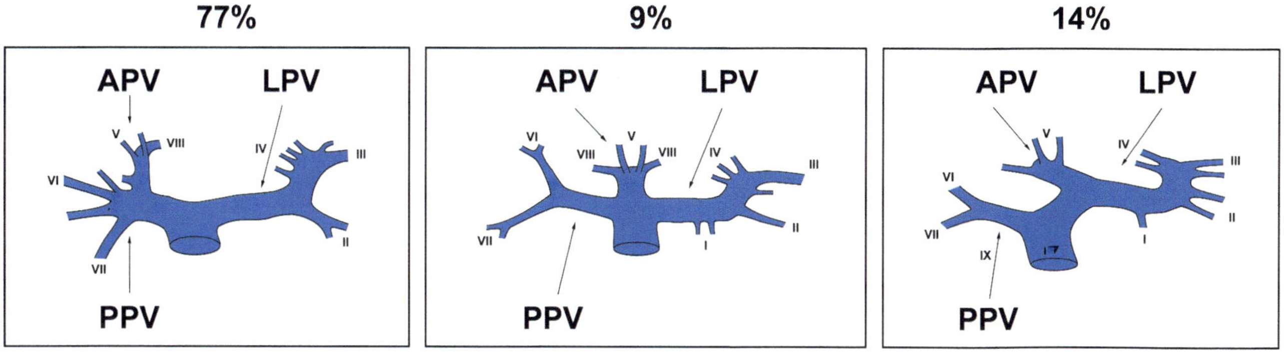

Fig. 17.4 Portal vein divisions and distribution. *APV* Anterior division, *PPV* Posterior division, *LPV* Left portal vein

17.6 Hepatic Vein

Unlike the portal triad (bile duct, hepatic artery, portal vein), which supplies individual liver segments, the hepatic veins run in the intersegmental plane, draining the corresponding segments. There are three main hepatic veins: the right, middle, and left hepatic veins (RHV, MHV, LHV). Typically, the RHV drains independently, while the MHV and LHV join before emptying into the IVC. However, variations in the drainage patterns of hepatic veins can occur. The RHV runs along the right portal fissure, which separates the right lobe into anterior and posterior sectors (segments). In about 70% of individuals, the RHV drains the right lobe as a dominant vein; in others, multiple branches may be present. Variation can also occur in the form of right inferior hepatic veins. Usually, 1–2 phrenic veins join the right and left hepatic veins. The MHV drains the anterior sector of the right lobe and the medial sector of the left lobe. The LHV drains the left lobe, dividing it into medial and lateral sectors. The MHV aligns with Cantlie's line and marks the boundary for right or left hepatic lobe resection. Variations can occur in the tributaries of the MHV. The LHV separates segments II and III and can be identified by following the Arantius ligament, an embryological remnant of the ductus venosus connecting the umbilical vein to the IVC. The caudate lobe is drained by multiple veins that empty into the IVC (Figs. 17.5 and 17.6).

Table 17.4 Applied anatomy

The portal triad in the free edge of the lesser omentum is amenable to clamping during hepatic surgeries to prevent or control bleeding (Pringle maneuver).
During pancreatic head resection or hepatic surgeries, replaced or accessory right hepatic arteries should be identified in imaging and during the procedure.
During gastric surgeries, accessory or replaced left hepatic arteries should be located in the gastrohepatic ligament.
Reduction of portal flow leads to an increase in hepatic arterial flow, known as the hepatic artery buffer response; however, the reverse does not occur.
Portal vein ligation causes atrophy of the ipsilateral side and compensatory hypertrophy of the contralateral side, which is used to augment the future liver remnant during hepatic resections.
Bile ducts are supplied solely by hepatic arteries; therefore, biliary complications can follow arterial insufficiency in cases of liver transplantation and bilio-enteric anastomosis for biliary strictures.
Intrahepatic tumors and hepatic metastases are typically supplied by the hepatic arteries, forming the basis for transarterial catheter embolization (TACE).
The Arantius ligament is a key anatomical structure to identify the left hepatic vein intraoperatively.
Phrenic veins draining the RHV must be ligated during right lobe resection and can be a source of bleeding.
The phrenic veins aid in identifying the RHV.
Hepatic vein embolization, along with portal vein embolization, enhances future liver remnant augmentation.

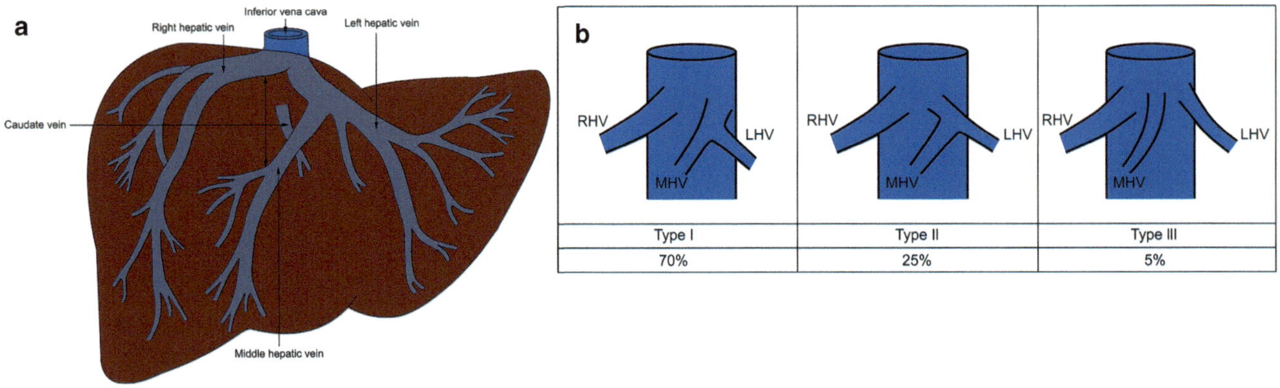

Fig. 17.5 (**a**, **b**) Hepatic venous drainage of the liver. RHV, MHV, LHV: Right, middle, and left hepatic veins, respectively. 1: LHV joins MHV to form a common trunk, II. MHV joins LHV to form a common trunk, III. RHV, MHV, and LHV draining separately

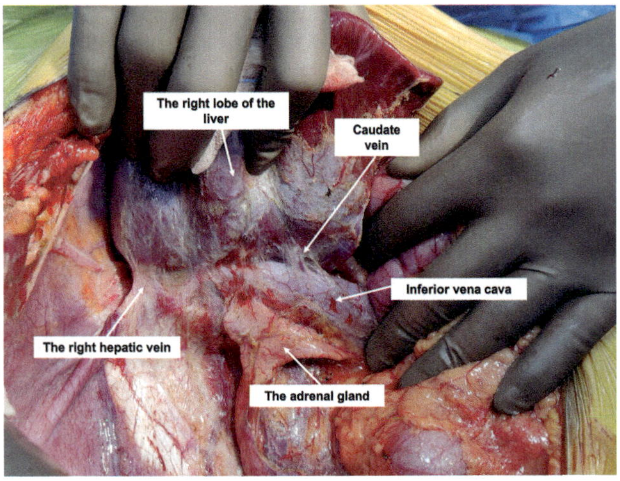

Fig. 17.6 Posterior dissection of the liver exposing the IVC and the RHV

17.7 Lymphatic Drainage of the Liver

There are two major lymphatic drainage areas of the liver, i.e., the phrenic nodes and the lymph nodes in the porta hepatis. They act as essential routes for lymphatic metastasis.

17.8 Nervous System of the Liver

The neural innervation of the liver is complex and not fully understood. Parasympathetic innervation comes from the vagus nerve. As it passes from the thorax to the abdomen around the esophagus, the vagus nerve divides into anterior and posterior branches. The hepatic branch of the anterior vagus nerve innervates the liver and runs in the gastrohepatic ligament. The sympathetic nervous system supplying the liver originates from the celiac plexus and travels through the thoracic splanchnic nerves.

17.9 Biliary Anatomy of the Liver

The bile duct is part of the portal triad and follows the portal system both outside and inside the liver. The right and left hepatic ducts drain the right and left lobes, respectively. Segment I (caudate lobe) is unique because it drains through multiple ducts to both the left and right hepatic ducts at the hilum.

The right hepatic duct (RHD) and the left hepatic duct (LHD) join to form the primary biliary confluence, which runs anterior to the right and main portal vein. This classical anatomy is seen in only 60% of people. In the remaining cases, a variable union of the sectoral ducts is observed at the hilum. Huang's classification has been proposed to categorize these variations at the biliary confluence. The right hepatic duct drains the right lobe (segments V-VIII). The ducts of segments VI and VII are called the right posterior sectoral duct (RPSD), while those of segments V and VIII are called the right anterior sectoral duct (RASD). The course of RASD is vertical and to the left of the anterior branch of the portal vein, while RPSD has a horizontal course. Usually, RPSD is epiportal and posterior to the anterior portal vein branch (the Hjortsjö crook), or less commonly (20%), it can be hypoportal and anterior to the anterior branch of the portal vein. The Hjortsjö crook may result from tethering by the caudate ducts. The RASD and RPSD join to form the right hepatic duct, which is short—about 1 cm long—and more vertical than the left hepatic duct; however, variations in this pattern can occur.

The left hepatic duct (LHD) drains segments II, III, and IV of the left hemiliver. The secondary confluence on the left side is formed by the ducts from segment III and segment II, along with a few branches from segment IV. The segment III duct runs along the left horn of the Rex recess and joins the segment II duct, providing a potential bypass area for segment III in the event of a hilar block. The LHD is longer,

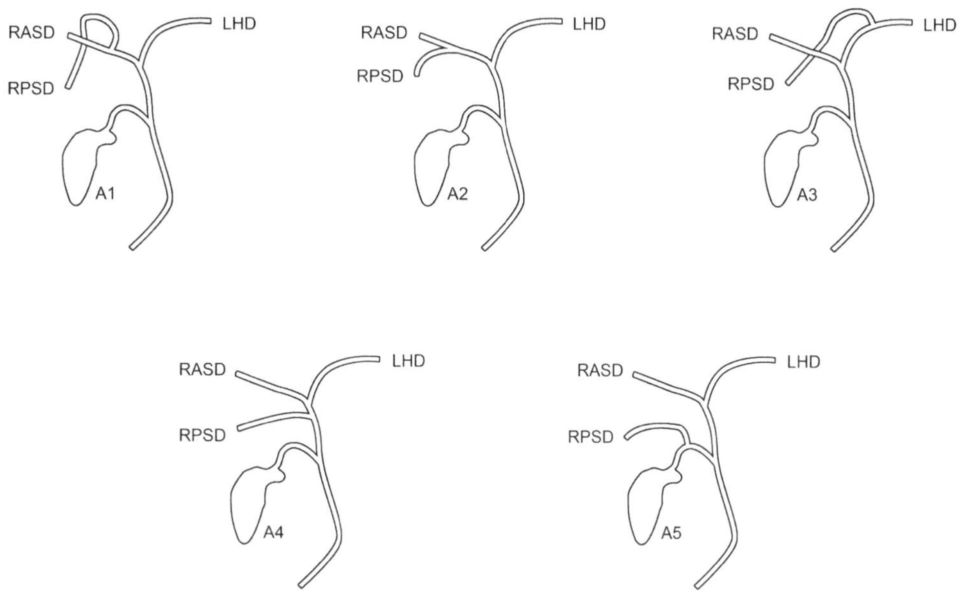

Fig. 17.7 Huang's Classification of Biliary Confluence. *RASD* Right anterior, *RPSD* Right posterior sectoral duct, *LHD* Left hepatic duct

measuring 2–5 cm, and follows a horizontal course at the base of segment IV. It initially runs superiorly and posterior to the left portal vein, but near the primary confluence with the RHD, it becomes anterior to the portal vein (Fig. 17.7).

The hilar plate is the condensation of fibroareolar tissue between Glisson's capsule and the portal structures. It is bounded above by segment IV, on the right by the cystic plate with Rouviere's sulcus and the gallbladder, and on the left by the umbilical plate. Dissection and lowering of the hilar plate are key steps in hilar dissection to isolate portal pedicles during liver resection or hepatico-jejunostomy. The right posterior pedicle runs along Rouviere's sulcus, and the right anterior pedicle runs posterior to the hilar plate on the right side. The right pedicles can be looped without dividing the hilar plate structure.

The caudate lobe can have 1 to 6 (average 3) biliary ducts to both the RHD and LHD in 80% of cases, to the RHD only in 5% of cases, and in 15% of cases, it drains into the LHD. These ducts run posterior to the portal branches and join the main duct at the back. The drainage pattern of caudate ducts into the right and left hepatic ducts has been classified based on their crossover pattern observed on intraoperative cholangiograms during liver transplant surgery: type I—left caudate ducts drain into the right duct, type II—right caudate ducts drain into the left hepatic duct, type III—bilateral crossover, and type IV—no crossover. This classification helps in managing the caudate ducts during hemi-hepatectomies.

Table 17.5 Applied anatomy

Identification of the Hjortsjö crook facilitates safe hepatic resection and liver transplantation.
Segment III bypass in cases of hilar block and rex shunt in portal hypertension can be performed in the rex recess.
Lowering the hilar plate is an essential step in safely identifying the bile duct during surgery for benign biliary stricture.
The hilar plate contains small caudate bile ducts or arterial branches and can be a source of bleeding or bile leak postoperatively.
Atrophy of one lobe and contralateral hypertrophy of the other cause rotation of the hilum around the axis toward the atrophied side, altering the relative relationships among the portal triad structures.
Due to the absence of vascular interposition at the anterior part of the hilar plate, it is also possible to separate the hilar plate from the hepatic parenchyma of segment IV.
The proximity of the caudate lobe to the biliary confluence necessitates caudate lobe resection in cases of hilar cholangiocarcinoma.
Rouviere's sulcus is the site used to identify the posterior sector pedicle, aiding the pedicular approach for posterior sectorectomy.

Key Points

- The liver is divided into two lobes by Cantlie's line, which runs from the IVC to the GB fossa.
- The right lobe is further subdivided into anterior and posterior sectors (segments), comprising segments (V and VIII) and (VI and VII), respectively.
- The left lobe is subdivided into lateral (segments II and III) and medial (segment IV) sectors.
- The caudate lobe (segment I) is considered an independent unit.
- The right anterior pedicle is vertical, whereas the posterior pedicle is horizontally oriented.
- The right, left, and middle hepatic veins drain into the IVC and lie in the intersectoral planes.
- The portal vein and bile duct have variable dispositions at the hepatic hilum.
- The hepatic artery has a variable origin, but the liver receives a robust arterial supply through a well-developed collateral circulation.

Selected Reading

1. Couinaud C. Anatomic principles of left and right regulated hepatectomy: technics. J Chir (Paris). 1954;70(12):933–66.
2. Lowe MC, D'Angelica MI. Anatomy of hepatic resectional surgery. Surg Clin North Am. 2016;96(2):183–95. https://doi.org/10.1016/j.suc.2015.11.003.
3. Surgical anatomy of the liver. OLYMPUS CONTINUUM https://www.olympusprofed.com › 2019/10 (online).

Hepatocellular Carcinoma

18

Mohammad Ibrarullah

Abstract

Cirrhosis of the liver, Hepatitis B and C infection, NASH, and NAFLD are the common predisposing factors associated with HCC. An increasing AFP and levels above 400 ng/mL are considered diagnostic of HCC when supported by clinical and imaging findings. Contrast-enhanced CT scan and MRI are reliable imaging modalities for the diagnosis of HCC. The Barcelona Clinic Liver Cancer (BCLC) system is currently the most commonly used staging system that guides management protocols. Early and very early tumors are best treated with hepatic resection. Liver transplantation is effective in HCC patients who meet the Milan criteria.

Keywords

Liver tumor · Hepatoma

Hepatocellular carcinoma (HCC) makes up over 90% of primary liver tumors. Worldwide, HCC is the fifth most common cancer and the second leading cause of cancer death after lung cancer. Its highest incidence is in Asia and Africa, likely due to the high prevalence of Hepatitis B and C-related liver disease in these areas. Early detection, achievable only through dedicated surveillance and screening programs and tumor resection, has significantly improved survival outcomes in an otherwise grim outlook.

18.1 Etiology and Predisposing Factors

Diseases that predispose to cirrhosis can de novo develop HCC (Table 18.1).

M. Ibrarullah (✉)
Department of Surgical Gastroenterology, Apollo Hospitals, Bhubaneswar, Odisha, India

Table 18.1 Etiology and predisposing factors

Common	Rare
Cirrhosis of the liver	Primary biliary cirrhosis
Alcohol abuse	Anabolic steroids
Hepatitis B virus infection	Oral contraceptives
Hepatitis C virus infection	Alpha1-antitrypsin deficiency
Nonalcoholic steatohepatitis (NASH)	Primary sclerosing cholangitis
Nonalcoholic fatty liver disease (NAFLD)	Thorotrast contrast
Diabetes mellitus	Porphyria cutaneous tarda
Obesity	
Hemochromatosis	
Aflatoxin	

18.2 Clinical Presentation

HCC is more common in males and typically presents in the sixth and seventh decades of life. In cirrhotic patients, the clinical picture is dominated by the features of chronic liver disease (CLD), such as jaundice, pruritus, hepatic encephalopathy, and ascites. The development of HCC may mark further decompensation of CLD. Anorexia, weight loss, and nodular liver may be present.

In non-cirrhotic patients, HCC may be an incidental detection as a space-occupying lesion (SOL) in the liver on routine imaging. Pain, anorexia, weight loss, and fever are other modes of presentation.

HCC may present with paraneoplastic syndromes such as hypoglycemia, hypercalcemia, polycythemia, diarrhea, or various cutaneous manifestations.

18.3 Diagnosis

The diagnostic workup primarily aims to confirm the diagnosis and identify the cause of HCC. The cause is determined mainly through laboratory tests, while the diagnosis is established via imaging and biopsy (Tables 18.2 and 18.3).

M. Ibrarullah (ed.), *Recent Concepts in Gastrointestinal (GI) Surgery*, https://doi.org/10.1007/978-981-92-1118-0_18

Table 18.2 Differential diagnosis of HCC

Dysplastic nodules in cirrhosis
Hepatic adenoma
Hemangioma
Metastatic secondaries
Mass-forming variant of cholangiocarcinoma
Hepatocholangiocarcinoma
Primary hepatic lymphoma
Organized liver abscess

Table 18.3 Hematological and biochemical tests to confirm etiology

Liver function test
Ascitic fluid analysis
Hepatitis B surface antigen
Anti-HCV antibodies
Serum copper level
Iron saturation
Alpha-antitrypsin level

18.3.1 Serum Alpha-Fetoprotein (AFP)

Serum AFP is elevated in about two-thirds of HCC cases, making it a valuable diagnostic tool. Early non-cirrhotic HCC may present with normal AFP levels. Conversely, AFP levels can be elevated in chronic active hepatitis, during recovery after toxic injury, or seroconversion following hepatitis B infection, transiently after liver resection, pregnancy, and in some germ and non-germ line tumors. The sensitivity and specificity of AFP in detecting HCC are 66% and 80%, respectively. An increasing AFP and levels above 400 ng/mL are considered diagnostic of HCC when supported by clinical and imaging findings. Due to its high specificity, it is used alongside ultrasonography for surveillance in at-risk individuals.

18.3.2 Ultrasonography (US)

When used as a screening tool in cirrhotic patients, US has 60% sensitivity and 97% specificity for HCC (Table 18.4).

Table 18.4 Ultrasound appearance of HCC

Routine (grey scale) ultrasound	Contrast-enhanced ultrasound (CEUS)
Small HCC often appears as a hypoechoic or isoechoic nodule. Larger HCCs may appear heterogeneous due to fibrosis, fat, or necrosis. Halo sign: A fibrous capsule may appear as a peripheral hypoechoic halo surrounding the tumor Mosaic pattern: A mix of hyperechoic and hypoechoic areas within the tumor. Nodule-in-nodule appearance: A smaller, brighter nodule within a larger lesion may be a feature in early HCC.	Arterial phase: The tumor often shows intense peripheral enhancement due to neo-vascularization. Portal venous phase: There may be "washout" as the tumor becomes less bright relative to the surrounding liver tissue. Tumor thrombus: Blood clots within the tumor's blood vessels may be visible.

18.3.3 Contrast-Enhanced Computed Tomography (CECT) (Table 18.5)

Table 18.5 CECT appearance of HCC

Phase	Findings
Non-contrast	Hypodense lesion compared to the surrounding liver. It may become isodense, making it detectable through abnormal contours or a mass effect on nearby vessels.
Arterial phase	Hyperenhancing with respect to the surrounding tissue due to increased vascularity
Portal venous phase	Tumor washout: The lesion becomes isodense or hypodense compared to the surrounding liver.
Delayed phase	The tumor remains hypodense. A capsule may sometimes be apparent.
Additional findings	Mosaic pattern: Variable enhancement of the tumor. Surface nodularity: Irregular margins on the surface of the liver mass. Pseudo capsule: An enhancing rim surrounding the mass. Peritumoral corona enhancement: A halo-like structure surrounding the tumor. Internal vessels: Presence of abnormal vessels within the tumor. Calcification may be present in some lesions.

18.3.4 Magnetic Resonance Imaging (MRI)

On an MRI, the tumor (HCC) typically appears as a hyperintense nodule on T2-weighted images. The tumor can be hypointense, isointense, or hyperintense on T1-weighted images. Well-differentiated tumors are usually hyperintense on T1 images and isointense on T2 images, while moderately or poorly differentiated tumors are hyperintense on T2 images and isointense on T1 images. The diagnosis is often confirmed by a dynamic contrast-enhanced MRI, which shows the lesion enhancing intensely during the arterial phase and then rapidly "washing out" its contrast in the portal-venous and delayed phases.

18.3.5 Tumor Biopsy

Preoperative biopsy confirmation is controversial and carries the risk of tumor seeding. Tumors smaller than 1 cm are usually monitored because false-negative rates are very high. Tumors between 1 and 2 cm require biopsy confirmation;

however, negative results then require close follow-up. Tumors larger than 2 cm, with cirrhosis, characteristic imaging features, and elevated AFP levels, may be managed without biopsy. Nonetheless, some surgeons still prefer a biopsy before proceeding with liver transplantation.

18.4 Staging of Hepatocellular Carcinoma

Several staging systems have been proposed, taking into consideration the clinical, pathologic, radiologic, or treatment response factors. Some more frequently used staging systems are (Tables 18.6 and 18.7)

- TNM staging, AJCC eighth edition
- BCLC: Barcelona Clinic Liver Cancer system
- CLIP: Cancer of the Liver Italian Program
- Japan Integrated Staging System

The BCLC staging system provides treatment guidelines for HCC, whereas the CLIP system is mainly used for prognostication.

18.5 Surgical Treatment

Treatment of HCC has seen significant advances in recent years. Several factors guide the choice of treatment, such as.

Location, number, and size of the tumor
Presence of metastatic disease
Presence cirrhosis
Portal vein patency
Comorbidity
Performance status
Presence or absence of metastatic disease

Table 18.6 Upgraded BCLC staging system 2022

Stage	HCC characteristics
0: Very early stage	Single ≤2 cm Preserved liver function Performance status 0
A: Early stage	Single ≤5 cm or ≤ 3 lesions each ≤3 cm Preserved liver function Performance status 0
B: Intermediate stage	Multi nodular Preserved liver function Performance status 0
C: Advanced stage	Portal invasion and/or extrahepatic spread Preserved liver function Performance status 1–2
D: Terminal stage	Any tumor burden End-stage liver function Performance status 3–4

Table 18.7 CLIP scoring system

Features	Score: 0	1	2
Child-Pugh status	A	B	C
Tumor morphology	Uninodular and extension <50%	Multinodular and extension <50%	Massive and extension >50%
Alpha fetoprotein	< 400	> 400	–
Portal vein thrombosis	Absent	Present	

Table 18.8 Poor prognostic indicators after resection

Clinical	Histology
Hepatitis C infection	Presence of cirrhosis
Preoperative AST > twice the normal level	Micro or macro vascular invasion
Preoperative AFP > 10,000 ng/ml	Poorly differentiated tumor
High intraoperative transfusion requirement	Presence of satellite nodules
	Positive resection margin
	Microvascular PV thrombosis

AST Aspartate aminotransaminase, *AFP* Alpha-fetoprotein, *PV* Portal vein

18.5.1 Liver Resection

BCCL stages 0 and 1, indicating very early and early HCC, are ideal candidates for liver resection. In the absence of cirrhosis, tumors up to 5 cm can be considered for surgery. The presence of clinically evident portal hypertension predicts poor outcomes after major liver resection (Table 18.8). Resection of more than two segments is contraindicated in patients with Child class B or C cirrhosis. Those with preserved liver function (Child A) have a 5-year survival rate exceeding 70% and a recurrence-free survival rate exceeding 30%. (Figs. 18.1 and 18.2)

18.5.2 Liver Transplantation

Orthotopic liver transplantation (OLT) was introduced as a treatment option for HCC to reduce the risk of local recurrence and to address issues related to a cirrhotic liver. In the early years, however, the recurrence and survival rates after transplantation were much lower and discouraging, leading to a more cautious approach. In later years, using much more stringent criteria and offering OLT to a select group of cirrhotic patients resulted in dramatic improvements in outcomes (Table 18.9).

A 5-year survival rate exceeding 80% and a recurrence rate below 15% have reaffirmed OLT's role as the most effective treatment option for HCC patients.

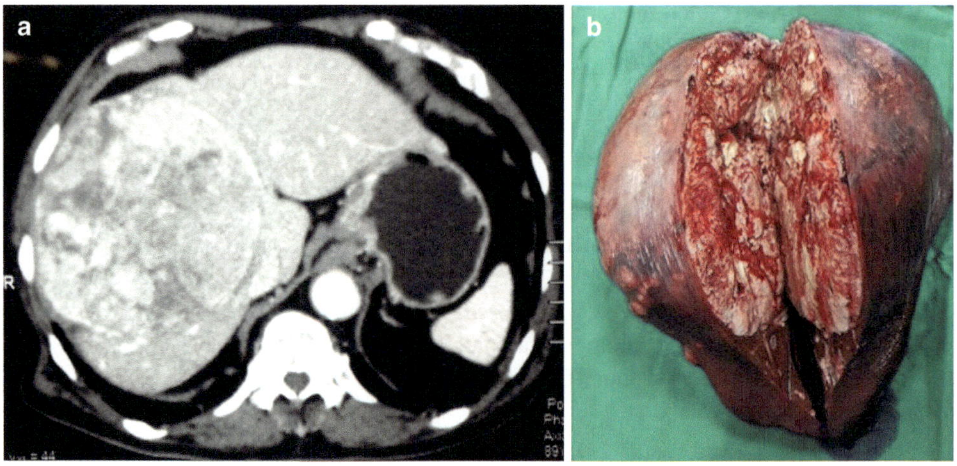

Fig. 18.1 (**a**) CECT image showing a large HCC occupying the right lobe of the liver and (**b**) right hepatectomy specimen containing the tumor

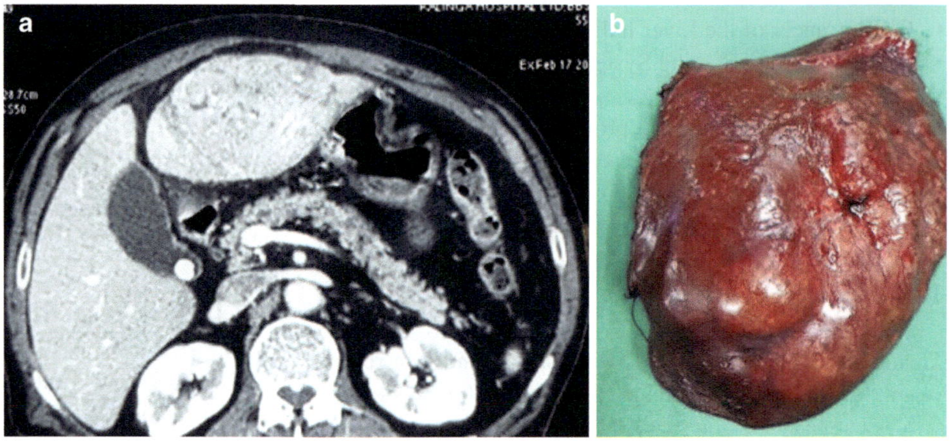

Fig. 18.2 (**a**) CECT image of a left lobe HCC and (**b**) left hepatectomy specimen containing the tumor

Table 18.9 Milan criteria of liver transplantation for HCC

Single nodule ≤5 cm in diameter
Not more than three nodules, with none larger than 3 cm in diameter
No macrovascular invasion
No extrahepatic spread.

18.6 Non-surgical Treatment

Non-surgical treatments are essentially aimed at palliation, improving resectability of large tumors, or with curative intent in individuals who are not fit for major hepatic resections or OLT.

18.6.1 Ablative Therapy

Ablative therapy is advised for individuals with BCCL stages 0 and 1 tumors, which are not suitable candidates for liver resection. The various forms of ablative treatment are.

- Percutaneous ethanol injection (PEI)
- Radiofrequency ablation (RFA)
- Cryotherapy
- Microwave ablation
- Laser ablation
- Focal external beam radiation

PEI is the earliest form of ablative treatment, where ethanol is injected into the tumor under ultrasound guidance across multiple sessions. This technique has been reported to achieve overall 3-year survival rates exceeding 70%, with about 50% in patients with Child A and B cirrhosis. RFA is also performed by inserting a needle into the tumor under image guidance or during laparoscopy. Major blood vessels near the tumor can act as dampeners for the electrical waves, reducing its tumor destruction capability. RFA appears to be more effective than PEI, with a 2-year survival rate of nearly 90%.

18.6.2 Transarterial Chemoembolization (TACE)

HCC mainly relies on arterial supply, unlike the rest of the liver, which depends on portal venous supply. TACE involves selective cannulation of the feeding artery to deliver chemotherapeutic agents such as doxorubicin, cisplatin, or mitomycin C to the tumor. The artery is then occluded to minimize systemic toxicity of the drugs. Results of TACE are inconsistent. However, adding Sorafenib to TACE has led to significantly improved survival in HCC. The procedure is usually well tolerated, with minimal side effects such as abdominal pain, fever, and elevated alanine aminotransferase (ALT). Decompensated cirrhosis is a contraindication for TACE because ischemia caused by arterial occlusion can trigger liver failure and death.

18.6.3 Stereotactic Body Radiation Therapy (SBRT)

SBRT is an advanced form of external beam radiotherapy in which a very high dose of radiation is delivered precisely to the tumors, sparing the surrounding healthy liver. In a select group of patients (tumor size <3 cm), local control of HCC is achieved in over 80%, with overall survival of 40% and progression-free survival of 33%.

18.6.4 Systemic Therapy

Systemic chemotherapy, targeted therapy, and immunotherapy are offered as palliative treatments for HCC that is not suitable for surgical or ablative procedures (Table 18.10). Chemotherapy is generally better tolerated by young individuals with hepatitis B or C infection compared to older patients with alcoholic liver disease and other co-morbidities.

Table 18.10 Drugs used for systemic therapy

Sorafenib	Atezolizumab
Regorafenib	Tremelimumab
Pembrolizumab	Durvalumab
Cabozantinib	Bevacizumab
Ramucirumab	Islelizumab
Nivolumab	Lenvatinib
Dostarlimab	Ipilimumab
Selpercatinib	

Key Points

- Hepatocellular carcinoma (HCC) makes up over 90% of primary liver tumors.
- Cirrhosis of the liver, Hepatitis B and C infection, NASH, and NAFLD are the common predisposing factors associated with HCC.
- In cirrhotic patients, the clinical picture is dominated by features of chronic liver disease. In contrast, in non-cirrhotic patients, HCC may be an incidental finding, often detected as a space-occupying lesion (SOL) on routine liver imaging. Pain, anorexia, weight loss, and fever are other modes of presentation.
- An increasing AFP and levels above 400 ng/mL are considered diagnostic of HCC when supported by clinical and imaging findings.
- Contrast-enhanced CT scan and MRI are reliable imaging modalities for the diagnosis of HCC.
- The Barcelona Clinic Liver Cancer (BCLC) system is currently the most commonly used staging system that guides management protocols.
- Early and very early tumors are best treated with hepatic resection.
- Liver transplantation is effective in HCC patients who meet the Milan criteria.
- Radiofrequency ablation (RFA) of HCC is reserved for very early or early tumors as a definitive treatment in patients who are not suitable for hepatic resection or as a bridge therapy before liver transplantation.
- Transarterial chemoembolization and systemic therapy are offered to patients with intermediate and advanced tumors, respectively.

Selected Reading

1. Marrero JA, Kulik LM, Sirlin CB, Zhu AX, Finn RS, Abecassis MM, et al. Diagnosis, staging, and management of hepatocellular carcinoma: 2018 practice guidance by the American Association for the Study of Liver Diseases. Hepatology. 2018;68(2):723–50.
2. Lucatelli P, Guiu B. 2022 update of BCLC treatment algorithm of HCC: what's new for interventional radiologists? Cardiovasc Intervent Radiol. 2022;45(3):275–6.
3. Vitale A, Romano P, Cillo U, et al. Liver resection vs nonsurgical treatments for patients with early multinodular hepatocellular carcinoma. JAMA Surg. 2024;159(8):881–9.
4. Horwitz JK, Agopian VG. Indication of liver transplant for HCC: current status and future directions. Curr Hepatol Rep. 2024;23:185–92.

Cystic and Metastatic Tumors of the Liver

19

Shikhar Tripathi, Hirak Pahari, and Samiran Nundy

Abstract

Neoplastic cysts are classified as benign and malignant mucinous neoplasms and intraductal papillary neoplasms. Simple cysts may cause symptoms due to their large size and require decompression if symptomatic. Neoplastic cysts are treated with resection because of their malignant potential. Metastatic tumors of the liver are classified into metastasis from colorectal cancer (CRLM), neuroendocrine tumors (NETs), and non-colorectal non-neuroendocrine tumors (NCNNETs). Contrast-enhanced CT scan is the diagnostic imaging of choice. CRLM, when resectable, offers good long-term survival.

Keywords

Cystic liver tumors · Liver metastasis

The liver tumors, cystic and metastatic, demonstrate diverse clinical manifestations, ranging from incidental findings during regular imaging to symptomatic cases with pain, jaundice, or liver dysfunction. The complex nature of these tumors goes beyond their clinical presentation; they create significant diagnostic challenges, as differentiating benign cystic lesions from malignant ones and distinguishing primary liver malignancies from secondary metastatic deposits often requires advanced imaging and histopathological evaluation.

19.1 Cystic Liver Tumors (Table 19.1)

Simple hepatic cysts are the most common benign cystic lesions of the liver, occurring in about 5% of the general population. They are typically congenital in origin, arising from malformations of bile ducts during liver development. Simple cysts are lined by a single layer of cuboidal or columnar epithelium, contain clear, straw-colored fluid, and have thin walls without internal septations or solid components. Biliary communication is uncommon, seen in around 25%. These cysts are often asymptomatic and found incidentally during imaging for other reasons. When symptoms occur, they are mainly due to mass and pressure effect. The cyst may cause dull pain, jaundice, or gastrointestinal symptoms like abdominal fullness and vomiting. Known complications include hemorrhage, infection, and spontaneous or traumatic rupture. Overall, simple cysts are benign with no risk of malignancy (Fig. 19.1).

Table 19.1 Classification of cystic lesions of the liver

Classification	Subtype	WHO 2010 classification	Etiology	Characteristics
Benign hepatic cysts	Simple cysts	No change	Congenital/developmental	Thin-walled, clear fluid-filled, lined by cuboidal epithelium
Parasitic cysts	Hydatid cysts	No change	Echinococcus infection	Multi-layered structure, contains daughter cysts.
Neoplastic cysts	Biliary cystadenoma	Mucinous Cystic Neoplasm (MCN)	Benign neoplasm with ovarian-like stroma	Multilocular, septate, with potential for malignant transformation
	Biliary cystadenocarcinoma	MCN with invasive carcinoma	Malignant neoplasm with ovarian-like stroma	Thick-walled, invasive, irregular margins
	Intraductal Papillary Neoplasm (IPN)	Intraductal growth with or without invasive carcinoma	Neoplastic growth within the bile ducts	Intraductal papillary projections, bile duct communication

S. Tripathi (✉) · H. Pahari · S. Nundy
Sir Ganga Ram Hospital, New Delhi, India

M. Ibrarullah (ed.), *Recent Concepts in Gastrointestinal (GI) Surgery*, https://doi.org/10.1007/978-981-92-1118-0_19

Neoplastic cysts are broadly classified as mucinous cystic neoplasm (MCN), with or without invasive carcinoma, and intraductal papillary neoplasm (IPN) (Fig. 19.2). These tumors develop from abnormal epithelial proliferation within the bile ducts, leading to the formation of multilocular cystic masses filled with mucinous fluid. The pathogenesis involves genetic mutations, such as changes in KRAS, TP53, and β-catenin, which contribute to the neoplastic transformation and progression of these cysts. As MCNs grow, they develop internal septations, mural nodules, and irregular walls, indicating a higher risk of malignant transformation. In cases where MCNs progress to invasive carcinoma, additional genetic mutations drive epithelial-mesenchymal transition (EMT), promoting invasiveness, local infiltration, and potential metastasis of MCN. Unlike benign MCN, malignant forms often present with more aggressive clinical features, such as abdominal pain, jaundice, weight loss, and sometimes systemic symptoms like anorexia and fatigue. Early diagnosis and prompt surgical treatment are essential, as complete resection offers the best chance for prolonged survival.

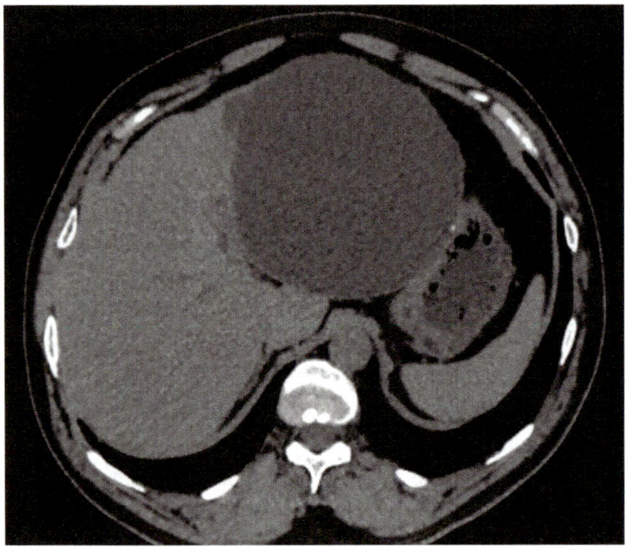

Fig. 19.1 Simple hepatic cyst on CT scan

IPN refers to a tumor that exhibits intraductal growth, similar to intraductal papillary mucinous neoplasm (IPMN) of the pancreas. It is characterized by papillary proliferation of the epithelial lining, excessive mucin production, and dilatation of the affected bile ducts. Genetic mutations in GNAS, KRAS, and RNF43 have been linked to the development of IPNs, with progression to invasive carcinoma occurring through a series of genetic changes that promote tumor cell proliferation and mucin production. Its similarity with that of the pancreas, both in behavior and progression, suggests a shared pathway of pathogenesis involving mucin-secreting epithelial cells. Common presenting symptoms include intermittent or progressive cholestatic jaundice, cholangitis, anorexia, and weight loss.

19.2 Diagnosis

The diagnosis of cystic liver tumors involves a combination of laboratory tests, imaging techniques, and histopathological examination. A systematic approach is essential for differentiating between benign and malignant lesions, guiding appropriate management, and improving patient outcomes. The following diagnostic strategies are commonly used:

Laboratory tests facilitate the initial evaluation of cystic liver tumors. Liver Function Tests (LFTs), including bilirubin, alkaline phosphatase (ALP), alanine aminotransferase (ALT), and aspartate aminotransferase (AST), provide insights into liver function and can help detect biliary obstruction. Although LFT abnormalities are nonspecific, elevated bilirubin and ALP levels may indicate bile duct

Fig. 19.2 (**a**) CT scan of a MCN (Biliary cystadenoma) in the right liver and (**b**) operative image of the same

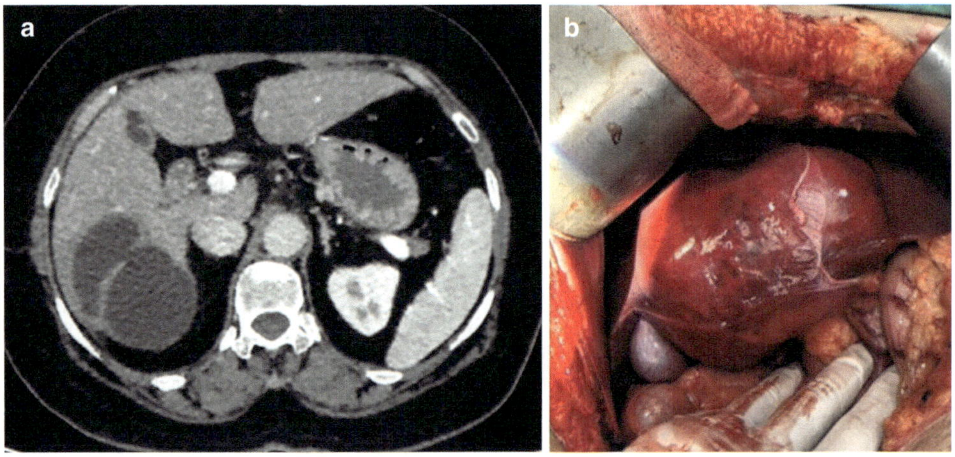

compression caused by large or peri-biliary cystic lesions. Additionally, tumor markers such as carcinoembryonic antigen (CEA) and CA 19-9 are used to evaluate neoplastic cysts, especially MCN and IPN. Elevated levels of these markers suggest malignant potential but are not definitive for diagnosis. In endemic areas, hydatid serology is a crucial diagnostic tool to rule out hydatid cysts. Serological tests, such as enzyme-linked immunosorbent assays (ELISA) for Echinococcus antibodies, support imaging findings and confirm parasitic etiology.

Ultrasound is commonly used as the first imaging technique because it is widely accessible, affordable, and effective at distinguishing simple cysts from more complex lesions. On ultrasound, simple hepatic cysts appear as anechoic, well-defined structures with thin walls. Conversely, complex cysts such as MCN and IPN may display internal septations, mural nodules, and varying levels of echogenicity. Ultrasound also helps detect daughter cysts or calcifications in cases of hydatid disease, making it valuable for initial screening in endemic areas. However, ultrasound has limitations, including difficulty evaluating deep-seated lesions or differentiating small cystic parts within solid tumors.

Contrast-enhanced CT scans offer precise visualization of cyst features, including wall thickness, septations, and enhancement patterns. They can differentiate benign cystic lesions from malignant ones by identifying characteristics such as irregular walls, solid components, and mural nodularity.

MRI, especially when combined with gadolinium-based contrast, offers superior soft tissue characterization and is especially useful for evaluating the internal structure of MCNs and IPNs. It can also distinguish MCNs, which are typically non-communicating, from IPNs, which exhibit intraductal growth patterns. In cases of hydatid cysts, CT or MRI can identify specific features like the water-lily sign (floating membranes) or calcified cyst walls, confirming the diagnosis and assisting in surgical planning.

Histopathological evaluation remains the gold standard for a definitive diagnosis, especially when imaging results are ambiguous or suggest malignancy. Fine-needle aspiration (FNA) or core biopsy can be performed under ultrasound or CT guidance to collect samples of cystic fluid or tissue. FNA helps analyze the cyst fluid for cytological features and biochemical markers, such as CEA and CA 19-9, which are often elevated in neoplastic cysts. However, FNA may be limited in differentiating benign from malignant cysts, particularly in mucinous neoplasms, due to sampling error or insufficient cellular material. In such cases, core biopsy, which provides a more substantial tissue sample, is preferred. Core biopsy is especially useful for identifying ovarian-like stroma in MCNs or confirming invasive carcinoma. In the context of IPNs, histopathological analysis can detect papillary proliferation and assess for invasive components.

19.3 Management

The management of cystic liver tumors is based on the type, size, and risk of malignancy or complications (Table 19.2).

Table 19.2 Management and prognosis of cystic liver tumors

Tumor type	Management	Comments	Prognosis
Simple hepatic cysts	Observation/aspiration/ sclerotherapy/laparoscopic deroofing	Intervention only for symptomatic or large cysts (prone to rupture)	Good, low recurrence
Mucinous cystic neoplasms (MCN)	Complete excision	Excision because of malignant potential	Low incidence of recurrence
MCN with invasive carcinoma	Wide excision, adjuvant therapy if indicated	Aims for negative margins; high risk of recurrence, close monitoring needed	Variable; depends on completeness of resection and stage of the disease.
Intraductal papillary neoplasm (IPN)	Complete resection; biliary drainage if needed	Prevents recurrence and progression; regular surveillance required	A non-invasive tumor has a good prognosis

19.4 Metastatic Liver Tumors

Metastatic liver tumors are much more common than primary liver cancers. Due to its unique anatomical position and dual blood supply—receiving blood from both the portal vein (75%) and the hepatic artery (25%)—the liver is highly susceptible to metastasis. This extensive vascular network allows circulating tumor cells from distant organs to lodge in the liver, making it one of the most common sites for metastasis. Metastases from gastrointestinal (GI) cancers, especially colorectal cancer, are among the most frequent in the liver. It is estimated that up to 50% of patients with colorectal cancer will develop liver metastases at some point. Liver metastasis is also common in cancers of the breast, lung, pancreas, stomach, and other solid tumors, highlighting the liver's role as a central hub in the systemic spread of cancer cells.

The nature of liver metastases varies greatly depending on the primary tumor. GI cancers often show multiple nodular liver lesions, while breast and lung cancer metastases may present as single or multiple nodules, sometimes with spread to other sites.

Early detection and intervention are vital in managing liver metastases, as prompt treatment can greatly boost survival chances. For example, surgically removing isolated liver metastases from colorectal cancer can lead to 5-year survival rates of 35–60%, compared to poorer outcomes with untreated or advanced metastases. However, the treatment plan depends on factors such as the number, size, and location of liver metastases, the presence of disease outside the liver, and the patient's overall health (Table 19.3).

Table 19.3 Classification of metastatic liver tumors

Category	Primary tumor origin	Key characteristics
Metastasis from Colorectal Cancer (CRLM)	Colorectal cancer	Common, often bilobar, multiple nodular lesions, rim enhancement on imaging. It spreads to the liver via the portal vein.
Metastasis from Neuroendocrine Tumors (NETs)	GI NETs, extra-GI NETs	Large, hypervascular lesions, indolent growth pattern, often asymptomatic initially, can be hormone-secreting
Metastasis from Non-colorectal Non-neuroendocrine Tumors (NCNNETs)	Breast, kidneys, lungs, pancreas, and others	Varies based on primary site. Can be hyper hypervascular. Indicates advanced-stage disease

19.4.1 Metastasis from Colorectal Cancer

Colorectal liver metastasis (CRLM) is the most common type of liver metastasis because of the direct venous drainage from the colon to the liver through the portal vein. Up to 50% of patients with colorectal cancer develop liver metastases during their disease course. CRLM usually appears as multiple nodular lesions of varying sizes, often found across both hepatic lobes.

19.4.2 Metastasis from Neuroendocrine Tumors (NETs)

Neuroendocrine liver metastasis is different from CRLM because of the slow growth pattern and often well-differentiated nature of neuroendocrine tumors (NETs). Liver metastases can develop from GI or extra-GI NETs. NET liver metastases frequently appear as large, enhancing lesions on arterial-phase CT scans, which shows their abundant blood supply. These metastases may remain symptom-free for long periods, making them suitable for potential curative resection or debulking surgery. The sub-classification system categorizes based on the number and spread (or pattern) of liver metastases seen on radiologic imaging: a single metastasis (type I) of any size or location, an isolated metastatic mass with smaller lesions (type II), and widespread metastatic spread involving both liver lobes (type III) (Figs. 19.3 and 19.4).

19.4.3 Metastasis from Non-colorectal Non-neuroendocrine Tumors (NCNNETs)

This broad category includes metastases from a wide variety of primary cancers, such as breast, lung, pancreas, kidneys, and other solid organs, each exhibiting distinct behavior and prognosis. NCNNET liver metastases often represent advanced-stage disease and may present as single or multiple nodular lesions, depending on the primary tumor.

19.4.4 Pathogenesis

The pathogenesis of metastatic liver tumors involves a complex interplay of hematogenous spread, microenvironmental adaptation, and genetic alterations. These mechanisms

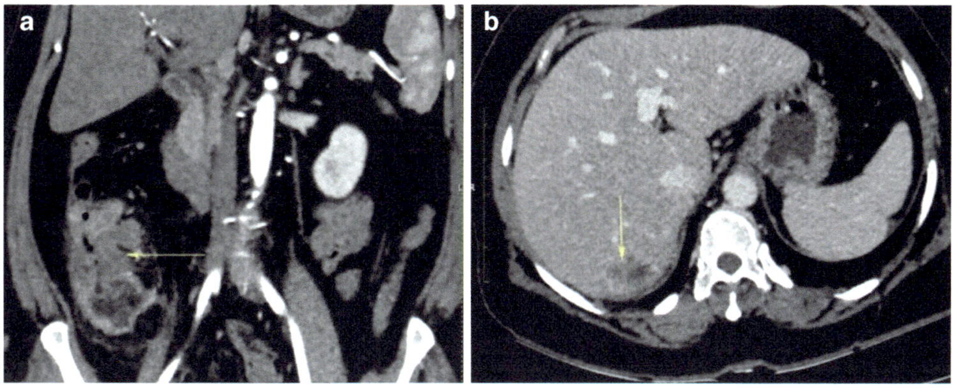

Fig. 19.3 (**a**): Carcinoma of the cecum (arrow) with (**b**) metastatic liver nodule (arrow)

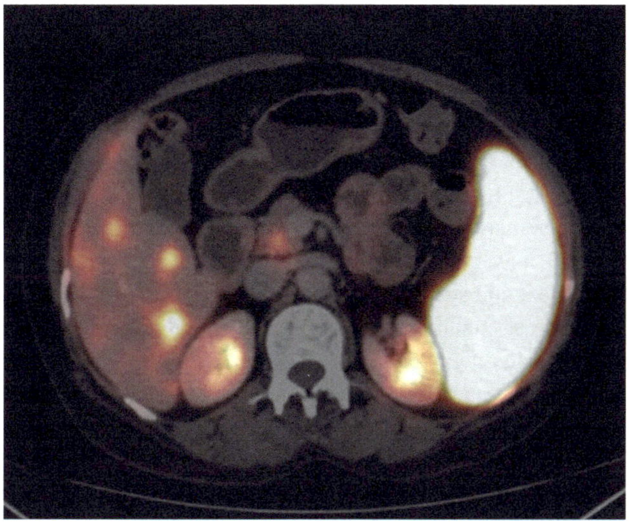

Fig. 19.4 PET scan showing liver metastasis secondary to p-NET

enable tumor cells originating from primary sites elsewhere in the body to survive, establish, and proliferate within the liver. Hematogenous spread is the primary pathway through which liver metastasis occurs, particularly for GI tumors. The portal venous system plays a crucial role in this process. Tumor cells from primary cancers of the colon, rectum, pancreas, stomach, and small intestine are carried to the liver via the portal vein, making it the first major organ to encounter circulating cancer cells from the gastrointestinal tract. Additionally, some non-GI tumors, such as breast or lung cancers, can reach the liver via the hepatic artery. Once in the liver, the tumor cells extravasate through the fenestrated sinusoidal capillaries, facilitating their entry into the liver parenchyma. Microenvironment adaptation is critical for the survival and growth of metastatic cells within the liver. The hepatic microenvironment, composed of various cell types like Kupffer cells (liver macrophages), hepatic stellate cells, and liver sinusoidal endothelial cells (LSECs), plays an essential role in tumor progression.

- Kupffer cells are among the first immune cells to interact with circulating tumor cells (CTCs). Depending on their activation state, they can either promote or inhibit tumor growth. In some cases, Kupffer cells release pro-inflammatory cytokines that enhance tumor cell adhesion and growth.
- Hepatic stellate cells are activated by tumor-derived factors, leading to the production of extracellular matrix components that create a pro-metastatic environment. These stellate cells also secrete growth factors such as TGF-β, VEGF, and HGF, which promote tumor cell proliferation and angiogenesis.
- Liver sinusoidal endothelial cells (LSECs) facilitate the attachment and migration of tumor cells, helping them establish within the liver tissue. The slow blood flow in hepatic sinusoids also supports the retention and survival of metastatic cells.
- Genetic mutations are crucial in the metastatic process, helping tumor cells gain the traits needed to survive in the liver. Several genetic changes have been found in metastatic liver tumors, reflecting mutations from their primary locations along with additional mutations that support metastasis.
- KRAS mutations are especially common in metastatic colorectal cancer, present in up to 40–50% of cases. These mutations promote cell proliferation, survival, and invasiveness, contributing to liver colonization. KRAS mutations are linked to a more aggressive disease, lower response to EGFR inhibitors, and worse outcomes.
- TP53 mutations, found in a wide range of primary tumors, promote tumor cell survival by disrupting cell cycle regulation. This allows cells to evade apoptosis and develop resistance to therapy. TP53 mutations are frequently observed in liver metastases originating from gastrointestinal, breast, and lung cancers.
- Additional mutations, such as those in the BRAF, PIK3CA, and SMAD4 genes, also play a role in liver metastasis by

supporting processes like epithelial-mesenchymal transition (EMT), immune evasion, and angiogenesis. For example, BRAF mutations, especially in colorectal cancer, are associated with more aggressive liver metastases, early liver involvement, and a poor prognosis.

19.4.5 Clinical Presentation

The clinical presentation of metastatic liver tumors varies widely, ranging from asymptomatic incidental findings to severe systemic manifestations, depending on the tumor burden, location within the liver, and extent of extrahepatic disease. Many patients remain asymptomatic in the early stages, while symptomatic cases often present with signs related to liver enlargement, biliary obstruction, or systemic effects of widespread disease. Due to the liver's large size and ability to function even when partially affected, many metastatic lesions are found incidentally during imaging done for staging or assessing the primary cancer. Therefore, patients may not show any liver-specific symptoms until there is a significant tumor burden or secondary complications develop. Symptoms may include:

- Firm or nodular enlargement of the liver, which may be palpable on physical examination. Hepatomegaly is often accompanied by right upper quadrant pain or discomfort, which may be referred to the right shoulder due to diaphragmatic irritation.
- Jaundice can develop if liver metastases compress or invade the intrahepatic bile ducts, leading to biliary obstruction.
- Weight loss: Unintentional weight loss is common in patients with metastatic liver disease, often due to a combination of reduced appetite, increased metabolic demand, and tumor-associated cachexia.
- Fatigue: Patients frequently report generalized fatigue, which can be severe and debilitating. It is often associated with anemia, liver dysfunction, and the overall impact of systemic cancer.
- Anorexia: Loss of appetite is another frequent symptom, further contributing to weight loss and overall debility.
- Paraneoplastic syndromes: Certain primary tumors, especially neuroendocrine tumors (NETs), can produce hormonal substances that cause paraneoplastic syndromes.
- In NET liver metastasis, symptoms can include flushing, diarrhea, wheezing, or even carcinoid heart disease, reflecting the systemic effects of secreted hormones like serotonin or vasoactive intestinal peptides.
- Other paraneoplastic manifestations, such as hypoglycemia, hypercalcemia, or coagulopathy, can be seen depending on the primary tumor type and its secretory profile.

19.4.6 Diagnosis

The diagnosis of metastatic liver tumors requires a comprehensive approach, integrating laboratory tests, imaging modalities, and histopathological confirmation. This multistep diagnostic strategy is essential for accurately characterizing liver metastases, assessing resectability, detecting extrahepatic disease, and guiding treatment planning.

- Liver function tests help assess hepatic function and detect possible biliary obstruction. Elevated ALP and bilirubin levels are common when metastases compress or infiltrate the bile ducts.
- Carcinoembryonic Antigen (CEA): Elevated levels of CEA are often seen in CRLM and can be used to monitor treatment response and detect recurrence.
- CA 19-9: Elevated levels suggest a pancreatic origin of the liver metastasis, although they can also be seen in other GI tumors (e.g., biliary or gastric cancers).
- Other markers such as AFP (alpha-fetoprotein) and CA 15-3 may also be evaluated, depending on the clinical context and suspected primary site.
- Contrast-enhanced CT is often the initial imaging choice for evaluating liver lesions, offering detailed visualization of tumor characteristics, vascular involvement, and potential biliary obstruction. It can distinguish between hypervascular (NET) and hypovascular (CRM) metastases, aiding in determining the primary source.
- MRI, particularly with gadolinium-based contrast, offers superior soft-tissue contrast and is useful for further characterizing metastases. It can detect smaller lesions, assess vascularity, and evaluate bile duct involvement. MRI is particularly valuable in differentiating between benign liver lesions and metastases, as well as in cases where the primary cancer is neuroendocrine, due to its sensitivity in detecting hypervascular lesions.
- Positron Emission Tomography-Computed Tomography (PET-CT) is an important tool for identifying extrahepatic disease, particularly when there is a need to stage advanced cancers comprehensively. PET-CT is useful for detecting occult metastasis that may not be visible on CT or MRI, such as small nodal or peritoneal metastases, which can alter treatment plans.
- Biopsy is the gold standard for confirming the diagnosis of metastatic liver tumors, especially when the primary tumor origin is uncertain or before considering chemoradiotherapy. Percutaneous fine-needle aspiration (FNA) or core biopsy under ultrasound or CT guidance allows for histopathological examination, confirming the primary tumor type and assessing receptor status or other molecular markers relevant for treatment planning.

19.4.7 Management

The management of metastatic liver tumors varies based on the primary tumor origin, extent of liver involvement, and presence of extrahepatic disease. Treatment aims to achieve tumor control, improve overall survival, and maintain quality of life. The primary approaches include surgical resection, liver-directed therapies, and systemic therapy, each tailored according to the type of liver metastasis.

19.4.8 Metastasis from Colorectal Cancer (CRLM)

Surgical Resection Surgical resection remains the gold standard for isolated and resectable colorectal liver metastases. Complete removal with negative margins provides the best chance for extended survival, with 5-year survival rates ranging from 35% to 60%. Surgical methods include one-stage hepatectomy for localized disease or two-stage hepatectomy for bilobar metastases. In select cases, portal vein embolization (PVE) may be utilized to increase the future liver remnant, enabling safer resection. Preoperative chemotherapy is often administered to downstage initially unresectable lesions or to improve resectability by decreasing tumor size. This usually involves a 2–3 month regimen followed by re-evaluation for operability. In cases of extensive disease where traditional resection is not feasible, Associating Liver Partition and Portal vein Ligation for Staged hepatectomy (ALPPS) may be considered to stimulate hypertrophy of the future liver remnant rapidly.

Liver-Directed Therapies For unresectable CRLM, liver-directed therapies like Radiofrequency Ablation (RFA), Transarterial Chemoembolization (TACE), and Selective Internal Radiation Therapy (SIRT) are vital. RFA is mainly used for small lesions (<3 cm), often as an adjunct to resection or when resection is not possible. TACE and SIRT can target larger or multiple lesions, especially in patients with good liver function and limited extrahepatic disease. These treatments provide local tumor control, symptom relief, and can sometimes downstage tumors to make them resectable.

Systemic Therapy Chemotherapy remains the primary treatment for both resectable and unresectable CRLM, utilizing regimens like FOLFOX (5-FU, leucovorin, oxaliplatin) or FOLFIRI (5-FU, leucovorin, irinotecan). Targeted agents such as anti-VEGF (e.g., bevacizumab) and EGFR inhibitors (e.g., cetuximab, panitumumab) are added based on molecular profiling, including KRAS, NRAS, and BRAF mutation status. Immunotherapy is considered for patients with microsatellite instability-high (MSI-H) tumors, using checkpoint inhibitors like pembrolizumab.

19.4.9 Metastasis from Neuroendocrine Tumors (NETs)

Surgical Resection In cases of isolated liver metastases from NETs, surgical resection is often feasible and can be curative. In cases of extensive disease, surgery can significantly reduce tumor burden. The choice of surgery depends on the pattern of liver involvement. Simple pattern (Type 1): Unilobar, low-grade (G1/G2) tumors are treated with resection. Complex pattern (Type 2): Bilobar, extensive, low-grade disease may require a two-step hepatectomy or ALPPS (Associating Liver Partition and Portal Vein Ligation for Staged Hepatectomy), sometimes combined with ablation for optimal debulking. Diffuse Pattern (Type 3): Resection is rarely possible; instead, systemic therapies are the mainstay of treatment.

Liver-Directed Therapies Liver-directed therapies, such as TACE, TA, or SIRT, are often used for NET liver metastases, especially in patients who are not suitable candidates for surgery. These treatments help control symptoms related to hormone secretion (e.g., flushing, diarrhea) and manage tumor growth, often used in conjunction with systemic treatments.

Systemic Therapy Systemic treatments for neuroendocrine liver metastases include somatostatin analogs (SSA) for symptom relief and growth suppression in low-grade NETs. For progressive or high-grade disease, options include targeted therapies (e.g., Everolimus, Sunitinib) and Peptide Receptor Radionuclide Therapy (PRRT), which delivers radiolabeled isotopes directly to the tumor. Chemotherapy (e.g., Streptozocin-based regimens) is reserved for high-grade tumors (G3) or refractory cases.

19.4.10 Metastasis from Non-colorectal Non-neuroendocrine Tumors (NCNNETs)

Surgical Resection Surgical resection for NCNNET liver metastases is less common because they are usually diagnosed at an advanced stage. It is considered only when liver involvement is limited and the primary cancer (such as breast, renal, or ovarian) is well-controlled. Selected patients with renal cell carcinoma, melanoma, or breast cancer might benefit from resection of liver metastases, especially when combined with effective systemic therapy.

Liver-Directed Therapies RFA, TACE, or SIRT may be employed for local control, especially in patients with limited liver lesions and no significant extrahepatic disease. Liver-directed therapies are frequently used to attain tumor control, alleviate symptoms, and, in some cases, convert unresectable disease to resectable status. *Systemic Therapy:* The primary treatment for NCNNET liver metastases is systemic therapy, tailored to the primary tumor's molecular profile and treatment guidelines. Standard regimens include chemotherapy, targeted agents (e.g., HER2-targeted therapy for breast cancer, VEGF inhibitors for renal cell carcinoma), and immunotherapy (e.g., PD-1/PD-L1 inhibitors for melanoma or lung cancer). Systemic therapy aims to manage both liver and extrahepatic disease, with liver-directed therapies sometimes added in specific cases.

19.4.11 Role of Liver Transplant

Liver transplantation has emerged as a potential treatment option for highly selected patients with CRLM and NET with liver metastasis. While traditionally reserved for primary liver diseases, advances in patient selection criteria, perioperative care, and immunosuppressive protocols have allowed liver transplantation to be considered for specific metastatic liver diseases, particularly when other treatment options are not feasible or effective. Criteria for liver transplant in CRLM include:

- Limited extrahepatic disease: Only patients with controlled, minimal extrahepatic disease (e.g., isolated lung metastasis) are considered, as widespread systemic disease decreases survival outcomes.
- No progression on systemic therapy: Patients should maintain stable disease after neoadjuvant chemotherapy, indicating disease control and response to treatment.
- Long disease-free interval (DFI): Patients who remain disease-free for a longer period after initial treatment of the primary tumor and liver metastases (usually over 2 years) are more likely to benefit from transplantation.
- Low metastatic burden: Candidates should have a limited number of liver metastases, ideally confined to the liver, with an extent of liver involvement that rules out surgical resection.

Recent studies have shown 5-year survival rates of 50–60% in highly selected CRLM patients undergoing liver transplantation, comparable to outcomes in other indications for transplantation. However, recurrence remains a significant concern, necessitating a strict selection process and close postoperative monitoring.

Liver transplantation is a more established option for patients with NET and liver metastasis, especially those with low-grade, well-differentiated tumors that are often slow-growing but cause significant symptoms due to hormone secretion or liver dysfunction. NETs exhibit a more indolent course compared to CRLM, making liver transplantation a more feasible consideration when other treatments fail. Selection criteria for liver transplant in NET-liver metastasis include:

- Well-differentiated (G1/G2) tumors: Transplantation is usually considered only for Grade 1 or 2 NETs, as high-grade tumors (G3) tend to have a poorer prognosis and higher recurrence rates.
- Stable disease on systemic therapy: Similar to CRLM, patients should show disease stability with systemic therapy, which indicates a more favorable tumor biology.
- No extrahepatic disease: Patients should have no detectable extrahepatic disease, confirmed through comprehensive imaging (e.g., PET-CT) and/or staging laparotomy.
- Liver-dominant disease: Transplantation is most effective for patients with liver-dominant NETs, where the liver metastases are the main source of morbidity, especially in cases with debilitating hormone-related symptoms that are not managed by other therapies (e.g., somatostatin analogs, liver-directed treatments).
- Age and performance status: Candidates should generally be under 60 years old with good performance status to tolerate the surgery and immunosuppressive therapy.
- Well-differentiated (G1/G2) tumors: Transplant is generally considered only for Grade 1 or 2 NETs, as high-grade tumors (G3) have a poorer prognosis with higher recurrence rates.
- Stable disease on systemic therapy: Similar to CRLM, patients should demonstrate disease stability with systemic therapy, indicating a more favorable tumor biology.
- No extrahepatic disease: Patients should have no detectable extrahepatic disease, confirmed through comprehensive imaging (e.g., PET-CT) and/or staging laparotomy.
- Liver-dominant disease: Transplantation is most beneficial for patients with liver-dominant NETs, where the liver metastases are the primary source of morbidity, particularly in cases with debilitating hormone-related symptoms that are not controlled with other therapies (e.g., somatostatin analogs, liver-directed therapies).

Long-term survival rates after liver transplantation for NETs are encouraging, with 5-year survival rates exceeding 70% in selected patients, making it a potentially curative option for liver-dominant NETs. Despite this, the risk of recurrence remains, requiring ongoing surveillance and systemic therapy after the transplant.

Key Points

- Simple hepatic cysts are the most common benign cystic lesions of the liver, congenital in origin, arising from malformations of the bile ducts.
- Neoplastic cysts are classified as benign and malignant mucinous neoplasms and intraductal papillary neoplasms.
- Simple cysts may cause symptoms due to their large size and require decompression if symptomatic.
- Neoplastic cysts are treated with resection because of their malignant potential.
- Metastatic tumors of the liver are classified into metastasis from colorectal cancer (CRLM), neuroendocrine tumors (NETs), and non-colorectal non-neuroendocrine tumors (NCNNETs).
- Contrast-enhanced CT scan is the diagnostic imaging of choice.
- CRLM, when resectable, offers good long-term survival.
- Metastatic NETs are classified into three variants from a treatment point of view. Simple pattern (Type 1): Unilobar, low-grade (G1/G2) tumors are treated with resection. Complex pattern (Type 2): Bilobar, extensive, low-grade disease may require a two-step hepatectomy or ALPPS (Associating Liver Partition and Portal Vein Ligation for Staged Hepatectomy), sometimes combined with ablation for optimal debulking. Diffuse Pattern (Type 3): Resection is rarely possible; instead, systemic therapies are the mainstay of treatment.
- Liver-directed therapies, such as TACE, TA, and SIRT, or systemic therapy, are often used for liver metastases in patients who are not suitable candidates for surgery.
- Liver transplantation has emerged as a potential treatment option for highly selected patients with CRLM and NET with liver metastasis.

Selected Reading

1. Rawla P, Sunkara T, Muralidharan P, Jeffrey RP. An updated review of cystic hepatic lesions. Clin Exp Hepatol. 2019;5(1):22–9. https://doi.org/10.5114/ceh.2019.83153.
2. Pitchaimuthu M, Duxbury M. Cystic lesions of the liver—a review. Curr Probl Surg. 2017;54:514–42. https://doi.org/10.1067/j.cpsurg.2017.09.001.
3. European Association for the Study of the Liver. EASL Clinical Practice Guidelines on the management of cystic liver diseases. J Hepatol. 2022;77:1083–108.
4. Cicerone O, Basilico G, Tassi C, et al. Mucinous cystic neoplasms of the liver: literature review and case series. World J Clin Oncol. 2025;16(8):108557. https://doi.org/10.5306/wjco.v16.i8.108557.
5. Clift AK, Hagness M, Lehmann K, et al. Transplantation for metastatic liver disease. J Hepatol. 2023;78:1137–46.
6. Sharma A, Meena RN, Khanna R, et al. Liver metastasis: current concepts in management and future perspectives. Int J Oncol Res. 2023;6:053. https://doi.org/10.23937/2643-4563/1710053.

Portal Hypertension

20

Sharad C. Kantharia, Sharvari G. Pujari,
and Chetan V. Kantharia

Abstract

Portal hypertension is defined as a pressure gradient of >6 between the portal venous system and the inferior vena cava or hepatic vein. Cirrhosis, NCPF, and EHPVO are the three most common causes of portal hypertension. Variceal bleeding is an essential complication of portal hypertension. Endoscopic treatment is often successful in controlling acute bleeding. TIPS has currently replaced shunt surgery for control of variceal bleeding in cirrhotic patients and serves as a bridge for liver transplant. PSRS is the preferred treatment for EHPVO, particularly for those presenting with symptomatic hypersplenism and bleeding

Keywords

Portal hypertension · Liver cirrhosis

The term portal hypertension, first introduced by Gilbert and Villaret in 1906, refers to an increase in pressure within the portal venous system. More precisely, it is an increase in the pressure gradient between the portal venous system and the inferior vena cava or hepatic vein. Normally, this pressure gradient is 5 mm Hg or less. A pressure gradient of 6 mm Hg or more indicates portal hypertension. A pressure gradient greater than 10 mm Hg is considered clinically significant portal hypertension.

20.1 Classification (Table 20.1)

Table 20.1 Classification based on site of resistance and etiology

Prehepatic	Increased blood flow	Tropical splenomegaly, AV malformations, or fistula, PV or SV thrombosis, compression of PV by tumor
Intrahepatic	Presinusoidal	Schistosomiasis, congenital hepatic fibrosis, early primary biliary cirrhosis, sarcoidosis, chronic active hepatitis, and toxins such as vinyl chloride, arsenic, and copper
	Sinusoidal	Cirrhosis, non-cirrhotic portal fibrosis, alcoholic hepatitis, vitamin A intoxication, and cytotoxic drugs
	Postsinusoidal	Sinusoidal obstruction syndrome or veno-occlusive disease
Posthepatic	Outflow obstruction	Hepatic vein involvement: Stenosis and or obstruction (Budd-Chiari syndrome) Inferior vena cava involvement: Stenosis, thrombosis, webs, or tumor invasion Involvement at the level of the heart: Constrictive pericarditis leading to a rise in atrial pressure

AV arteriovenous, *PV* portal vein, *SV* splenic vein

S. C. Kantharia · S. G. Pujari · C. V. Kantharia (✉)
Seth GS Medical College & KEM Hospital, Mumbai, India

M. Ibrarullah (ed.), *Recent Concepts in Gastrointestinal (GI) Surgery*, https://doi.org/10.1007/978-981-92-1118-0_20

20.2 Pathophysiology

Portal pressure is determined by the product of portal blood flow and the vascular resistance opposing that flow. An increase in portal blood flow, vascular resistance, or both, therefore, results in higher portal pressure.

Increase in Vascular Resistance: In cirrhosis, an increased resistance to portal blood flow is the main cause of portal hypertension. Though resistance to portal blood flow can occur at any site within the portal venous system, the intrahepatic resistance occurs primarily due to alterations in the architecture following cirrhosis.

Increase in Splanchnic Blood Flow: The precise cause of hyper-dynamic splanchnic circulation is not clear. It is linked to overproduction of endogenous vasodilators and decreased vascular responsiveness to vasoconstrictors. Peripheral vasodilatation triggers activation of endogenous neuro-humoral systems. This results in sodium retention and expansion of plasma volume, which in turn raises the cardiac index. An increased cardiac index leads to a higher portal pressure gradient, causing portal hypertension.

20.3 Pathways of Collateral Circulation in Portal Hypertension

- The left gastric vein (LGV) anastomoses with the esophageal veins, which drain into the azygos vein (AV).
- The superior rectal vein (SRV) anastomoses with the middle and inferior rectal veins (IRV), which are tributaries of the internal iliac and the pudendal veins, respectively
- The paraumbilical vein (PUV) anastomoses with subcutaneous veins in the anterior abdominal wall.
- Tributaries of the splenic and pancreatic veins anastomose with the left renal vein in the retroperitoneum
- Short veins also connect the splenic and colic veins to the lumbar veins of the posterior abdominal wall.
- The veins of the bare area of the liver communicate with those of the diaphragm, as well as the right internal thoracic vein

- The left gastric vein (LGV) anastomoses with the esophageal veins, which drain into the azygos vein (AV).
- The superior rectal vein (SRV) anastomoses with the middle and inferior rectal veins (IRV), which are tributaries of the internal iliac and the pudendal veins, respectively
- The paraumbilical vein (PUV) anastomoses with subcutaneous veins in the anterior abdominal wall.
- Tributaries of the splenic and pancreatic veins anastomose with the left renal vein in the retroperitoneum
- Short veins also connect the splenic and colic veins to the lumbar veins of the posterior abdominal wall.
- The veins of the bare area of the liver communicate with those of the diaphragm, as well as the right internal thoracic vein

The collaterals or the varices are classified as esophageal, gastric, esophagogastric, and ectopic varices. Ectopic varices occur anywhere in the GI tract other than the esophagogastric region. Though commonly located in the duodenum, they may also be seen within the jejunum, ileum, colon, rectum, omentum, gallbladder, bile duct, uterus, vagina, diaphragm, and urinary bladder, and at enterostomy stoma and anastomotic sites.

Table 20.2 Clinical manifestations of portal hypertension

GI bleed	Hematemesis
	Melena
Liver failure	Ascites
	Hepatic encephalopathy
	Hepato-renal syndrome
	Porto-pulmonary hypertension
Hypersplenism	Splenomegaly
	Cytopenia
	Bleeding disorder
	Growth retardation

20.4 Diagnostic Investigations (Table 20.3)

Table 20.3 Basic laboratory studies

Test	Parameter	Diagnosis
Hemogram	Hemoglobin and hematocrit	Low values indicate hypersplenism or GI bleed
	Cytopenia	Hypersplenism
Liver function test	Deranged liver enzymes and raised serum bilirubin	Hepatic dysfunction
	Low serum albumin with consequent alteration in albumin: globulin ratio	Loss of the synthetic function of the liver in cirrhosis
	Deranged PT, APTT, and INR	Loss of the synthetic function of the liver in cirrhosis
Viral serology	Hepatitis B and C	Viral cause of liver cirrhosis
Renal Function Test	Blood urea nitrogen (BUN) and Creatinine levels	serves as a baseline in patients who progress to develop HRS

20.5 Ultrasonography (Table 20.4)

The first sign of portal hypertension on Doppler ultrasonography is the loss of the normal triphasic pattern of portal blood flow. Additional features evaluated on ultrasonography include the status of the left renal vein and IVC in patients being assessed for porta-systemic shunt surgery.

Table 20.4 Ultrasonography evaluation

Parameter	Findings	Diagnosis
Liver size and echotexture	Shrunken, coarse echotexture	Liver cirrhosis
Speno-portal axis	Dilated (SV > 10 mm, PV > 12 mm)	Liver cirrhosis, NCPF
	Obstructed by thrombus	EHPVO
Portal cavernoma	Collaterals replacing PV	EHPVO
Ascites	–	Liver cirrhosis

SV splenic vein, *PV* portal vein, *NCPF* non-cirrhotic portal fibrosis, *EHPVO* extrahepatic portal venous obstruction

20.6 CT Scan and Magnetic Resonance Imaging (MRI)

Contrast-enhanced CT scan and MRI are useful qualitative studies when ultrasonographic evaluations are inconclusive. Spiral CT scanning and three-dimensional (3D) angiographic reconstruction techniques help visualize the portal vasculature more accurately. MRI also provides quantitative data on portal venous and azygos blood flow. These assessments are performed before surgical intervention to evaluate the portal venous anatomy.

20.7 Hemodynamic Measurement of Portal Pressure

Direct portal pressure measurements involve cannulating the portal vein and assessing its pressure. This can be done through percutaneous transhepatic, transjugular, or endoscopic ultrasound-guided portal pressure gradient measurement. However, direct portal pressure measurements are usually not performed due to their invasive nature and the risk of complications. Instead, measurement of the hepatic venous pressure gradient (HVPG) is used, and it is considered the gold standard for this assessment.

20.8 Esophagogastroduodenoscopy

Endoscopy is an essential diagnostic and therapeutic tool in patients with portal hypertension. It helps determine the presence of gastro-esophageal varices. Endoscopic grading of varices is based on size, shape, location, and presence of high-risk stigmata. These gradings help predict bleeding risk and guide treatment decisions. Over the years, various classifications have been proposed. The classification commonly used in clinical practice for diagnosing and managing variceal bleeding is the American Association for the Study of Liver Diseases (AASLD) classification. It categorizes esophageal varices into "small" and "large." The presence of variceal red color signs (cherry red spots, red wale markings—longitudinal red streaks on varices, blue varices) and the "white nipple sign" (platelet fibrin plug overlying a varix) indicates an increased risk of rebleeding. Classification of gastric varices has also been proposed.

20.9 Diagnostic Paracentesis of Ascites

Total protein concentration and calculation of the serum ascites albumin gradient (SAAG): In patients with portal hypertension, the SAAG value is greater than 1.1 g/dL (or 11 g/L).

Spontaneous bacterial peritonitis (SBP) should be ruled out in all cirrhotic patients with ascites on hospital admission. The diagnosis of SBP is confirmed when ascitic neutrophil count is >250 cells/mm^3 in the absence of an intra-abdominal and surgically treatable source of sepsis.

20.10 Management

Management of portal hypertension is aimed at measures to reduce portal pressure and prevent bleeding. This includes pharmacotherapy, endoscopic and interventional radiology procedures, and surgery.

20.10.1 Specific Management of Acute Variceal Hemorrhage

Emergency Upper GI endoscopy: Upper GI endoscopy is performed to confirm variceal bleeding and to rule out other causes of hematemesis. Varices should be treated if they show signs of recent hemorrhage. Bleeding esophageal varices are managed with endoscopic band ligation (EVL) or sclerotherapy (EST). Bleeding gastric varices are treated with cyanoacrylate glue injection. Control of acute variceal hemorrhage is defined as cessation of bleeding with hemodynamic stability for 24 h after therapy. On the other hand, failure of endo-therapy is defined as rebleeding occurring after 48 h of index endo-therapy.

Administration of Vasoactive Agents: Vasoactive drugs include somatostatin and its analogues (such as octreotide), as well as vasopressin and its analogues (like Terlipressin) (Table 20.5). These drugs cause vasoconstriction in the splanchnic circulation, which reduces portal pressure. Octreotide is the preferred vasoactive agent for managing variceal hemorrhage because of its safety profile. Vasopressin is not recommended due to the high risk of cardiovascular adverse events. Terlipressin may also cause abdominal pain, chest pain, diarrhea, and hyponatremia. It is contraindicated in patients experiencing hypoxia, worsening respiratory symptoms, or with ongoing coronary, peripheral, or mesenteric ischemia.

Mechanical Tamponade: Balloon tamponade is reserved for patients with refractory bleeding. Commonly used tamponade devices include the Sengstaken–Blakemore tube and the Minnesota tube. The tube is inserted through the nose or mouth and guided into the stomach. The gastric balloon is inflated with 250 ml saline, and the tube is secured with countertraction on the ala nasi or attached to a helmet for stabilization. This countertraction anchors the gastric bal-

Table 20.5 Vasoactive agents and their dose scheduled for acute variceal bleeding

Drug	Standard regimen	Duration (days)
Octreotide (somatostatin analogue)	50 mg IV bolus, followed by continuous IV infusion at 50 mg/h; additional IV boluses can be given in case of ongoing bleeding	2–5
Somatostatin	250 mg IV bolus, followed by continuous IV infusion at 250–500 mg/h; additional IV boluses can be given in case of ongoing bleeding	2–5
Terlipressin (vasopressin analogue)	Initial 48 h: 2 mg IV every 4 h until bleeding is controlled. Maintenance: 1 mg IV every 4 h	2–5

loon at the GE junction, a common site of bleeding from esophageal varices. If the gastric balloon fails to control bleeding, an esophageal balloon is inflated with saline, up to 30 mm Hg pressure, which can be increased to 45 mm Hg if necessary to stop the bleeding.

Self-Expandable Metal Stents (SEMSs): In refractory esophageal variceal bleeding, self-expandable metal stents (SEMSs) are recommended as a bridge to more definitive treatment. SEMSs compress the varices after expansion in the lower esophagus, exerting a tamponade effect similar to mechanical balloon tamponade. The advantage of SEMS is that it can be deployed without radiological assistance or even an endoscope, as it has a built-in gastric balloon that guides stent placement. An additional benefit of SEMS is that it can be kept in place for 7 days, allowing oral feeding with the stent in situ. Compared to mechanical balloon tamponade, the risk of aspiration and esophageal perforation is much lower with SEMS.

Transjugular Intrahepatic Portosystemic Shunt (TIPS): TIPS, with the assistance of an interventional radiologist, can be considered if variceal bleeding is unresponsive to the treatments mentioned above.

Balloon-Occluded Retrograde Transvenous Obliteration (BRTO): In patients with gastric varices and ectopic varices, BRTO may be considered based on its feasibility (shunt type and diameter) and the availability of local expertise.

Emergency Surgery: In patients with acute variceal bleeding unresponsive to initial endoscopic, pharmacologic treatment and/or mechanical balloon tamponade, and when facilities for TIPS and SEMS are unavailable, surgery remains the only option to control hemorrhage. In an emergency setting, esophagogastric devascularization is the preferred procedure. In a select subgroup of patients who are hemodynamically stable, Child A, and have had their portal venous anatomy mapped beforehand, a shunt surgery may be performed (Table 20.6).

Table 20.6 Portal decompressive procedures

Procedure	Type of shunt	Indications	Contraindications	Complications
End-to-side Portocaval shunt	Non-selective	Acute variceal bleed	Refractory ascites, decompensated liver PV thrombosis	Encephalopathy, liver failure
Side-to-side Portocaval shunt (direct/interposed graft)	Non-selective	Acute variceal bleeding, intractable ascites	Decompensated liver PV thrombosis	Encephalopathy, liver failure
Mesocaval shunt	Non-selective	Acute variceal bleeding, intractable ascites	Mesenteric vein thrombosis	Encephalopathy, liver failure, graft thrombosis
Proximal splenorenal shunt (PSRS)	Non-selective	Acute variceal bleeding, EHPVO with symptomatic hypersplenism	Thrombus extending to SV, SV <1 cm in diameter	Shunt thrombosis, liver decompensation[a]
Distal splenorenal shunt (DSRS)[b]	Selective	Variceal bleeding	SV thrombosis, Gross ascites, massive splenomegaly with symptomatic hypersplenism	Loss of selectivity without splenopancreatic disconnection, aggravation of ascites, and shunt thrombosis
Inokuchi shunt (LGV to IVC)	Selective	Variceal bleeding, ascites	Variability of LGV	Shunt thrombosis
Small diameter (8 mm) interposition portocaval shunt	Partial (prograde flow to the liver is maintained)	Acute variceal bleeding	PV thrombosis	Shunt thrombosis
Rex shunt (SMV to left PV through vein graft)	Selective	Variceal bleeding, EHPVO	–	Shunt thrombosis
TIPS[c]	Non-selective	Variceal bleeding. Ascites (usually as a bridge to transplant)	Heart failure, pulmonary hypertension, liver failure, PV or HV thrombosis	Shunt thrombosis, occlusion
Esophago-gastric devascularization procedures	–	Acute variceal bleeding, PHT with symptomatic hypersplenism, when shunt surgery is contraindicated	Ectopic varices, PHG bleeding	Esophageal leak

PV portal vein, *SV* splenic vein, *IVC* inferior vena cava, *SMV* superior mesenteric vein, *LGV* left gastric vein, *HV* hepatic vein, *PHT* portal hypertension, *EHPVO* extrahepatic portal vein obstruction

[a]Liver decompensation is rare in EHPVO

[b]Reversal of splenomegaly and hypersplenism is rare with massive splenomegaly

[c]Interventional radiological procedure

20.10.2 Prophylactic Treatment for Varices in Portal Hypertension

Prophylactic EVL is recommended for high-risk varices. Prophylactic shunt surgery, however, is not indicated for cirrhosis or NCPF due to the risk of encephalopathy. In selected patients with EHPVO, splenectomy and PSRS may be considered in cases such as symptomatic hypersplenism, growth retardation, a grossly enlarged spleen vulnerable to trauma, or patients living in remote areas without access to emergency treatment facilities.

Key Points

- Portal hypertension is defined as a pressure gradient of >6 between the portal venous system and the inferior vena cava or hepatic vein.
- Cirrhosis, NCPF, and EHPVO are the three most common causes of portal hypertension.
- The diagnosis is confirmed through LFT, viral markers, and imaging of the liver, spleen, and splenoportal axis.
- Variceal bleeding is an essential complication of portal hypertension.
- Endoscopic treatment is often successful in controlling acute bleeding.
- TIPS has currently replaced shunt surgery for control of variceal bleeding in cirrhotic patients and serves as a bridge to liver transplant.
- PSRS is the preferred treatment for EHPVO, particularly for those presenting with symptomatic hypersplenism and bleeding

Selected Reading

1. Wolff M, Hirner A. Current state of portosystemic shunt surgery. Langenbecks Arch Surg. 2003;388:141–9. https://doi.org/10.1007/s00423-003-0367-5.
2. Sarin SK, Kumar A, Chawla YK, et al. Noncirrhotic portal fibrosis/idiopathic portal hypertension: APASL recommendations for diagnosis and treatment. Hepatol Int. 2007;1:398–413.
3. Garcia-Tsao G, Abraldes JG, Berzigotti A, Bosch J. Portal hypertensive bleeding in cirrhosis: risk stratification, diagnosis, and management: 2016 practice guidance by the American Association for the Study of Liver Diseases. Hepatology. 2017;65:310–35.
4. Lopez-Verdugo F, Sánchez-García J, Gagnon A. Surgical portosystemic shunts: history, evolution, and current applications. Digest Dis Interv. 2020;04(02):157–67. https://doi.org/10.1055/s-0040-1713371.
5. Kotani K, Kawada N. Recent advances in the pathogenesis and clinical evaluation of portal hypertension in chronic liver disease. Gut Liver. 2023; https://doi.org/10.5009/gnl230072.
6. Guixé-Muntet S, Quesada-Vázquez S, Gracia-Sancho J. Pathophysiology and therapeutic options for cirrhotic portal hypertension. Lancet. 2024;9:646–63.

Liver Transplantation

21

S Sreejith, Subash Gupta, and Peush Sahni

Abstract

Liver transplantation is frequently performed for decompensated liver disease and acute liver failure. DDLT is the most common form in the Western world, while LDLT is the most common in the Eastern world, including India. The right lobe of the liver typically constitutes 60–70% of the total volume, while the left lobe accounts for 30–40%. In LDLT, a healthy donor can donate up to 70% of their liver, which will regenerate to 85% of its original volume in 11–14 days and reach full size in 3 months. To prevent rejection post-transplant, a triple immunosuppressive regimen is used, which includes tacrolimus, mycophenolate mofetil, and prednisolone.

Keywords

Liver transplantation · Hepatic transplantation

The first human liver transplant (LT) was performed by Thomas Starzl on March 1, 1963, at the University of Colorado. It was a deceased donor liver transplantation (DDLT); however, the patient did not survive, and the same outcome occurred with the next nine consecutive patients. Finally, on July 23, 1967, the first successful DDLT was performed at the University of Colorado. While DDLT is considered the ideal form of LT, it is limited by the availability of organs. This scarcity of liver grafts from deceased donors led to the successful introduction of living donor liver transplants (LDLT) in the late 1990s, which was a significant breakthrough in addressing the donor liver shortage. The availability of improved immunosuppressive agents such as Tacrolimus, Cyclosporine, and Mycophenolate Mofetil, along with refinements in surgical techniques and multidisciplinary care in both peri-operative and post-operative settings, has contributed to an increase in LT procedures worldwide, with an operative mortality rate of less than 5% and a 1-year survival rate exceeding 90% at most centres globally.

Table 21.1 Types of liver transplantation

Deceased Donor Liver Transplant (DDLT)	The most common and ideal type of liver transplant globally A healthy liver is surgically removed from a brain dead donor and transplanted into the recipient, replacing his diseased liver
Living Donor Liver Transplant (LDLT)	Part of the liver from a living donor is transplanted, and it is the most common type in India The donated segment is usually the right lobe for an adult or the left lateral segment for a paediatric recipient
Split Liver Transplant	The whole liver from a deceased donor is split into two sections and transplanted into two different recipients Usually, the smaller left lobe goes to a child and the bigger right lobe to an adult
Domino Liver Transplant	Liver from a patient with metabolic diseases is used as a donor organ for another patient. The donor, in this case, receives a healthy liver from another source. The native liver from the initial recipient has a genetic defect. Still, it is structurally normal and healthy enough to be transplanted into someone else with end-stage liver disease without any genetic defect
Auxiliary Liver Transplantation	A part of healthy liver is transplanted, retaining the recipient's own liver, with a possibility of recovery in the future

21.1 Transplantation of Human Organs and Tissues Act

In India, the Transplantation of Human Organs Act (THOA) was enacted into law by the Parliament in 1994. The Act established a system for the procurement, storage, and transplantation of organs for designated patients who are registered for transplantation. It also created a mechanism to

S. Sreejith (✉) · S. Gupta
Max Super Speciality Hospital, Saket, New Delhi, India

P. Sahni
Centre for Liver and Biliary Sciences, Max Super Speciality Hospital, Saket, New Delhi, India

M. Ibrarullah (ed.), *Recent Concepts in Gastrointestinal (GI) Surgery*, https://doi.org/10.1007/978-981-92-1118-0_21

facilitate living donor transplantation between related family members and altruistic donors. Additionally, the Act provided a legal framework for the declaration and certification of brain death and set minimum criteria for hospitals where organ donation and transplantation can take place. This Act was amended in 2011 and is now known as the Transplantation of Human Organs and Tissues Act (THOTA).

21.2 Indications for Liver Transplant

The indications for LT can be broadly classified as: decompensated chronic liver disease (CLD), acute liver failure (ALF), hepatic malignancies, congenital or metabolic liver diseases, and re-transplantations. Recently, acute-on-chronic liver failure (ACLF) has been commonly used to describe a clinical syndrome of chronic liver disease accompanied by multi-organ failure and increased short-term mortality (Table 21.2).

Table 21.2 Indications for liver transplantation

Decompensated chronic liver disease (CLD) (a) Cholestatic liver disease (b) Parenchymal liver disease	Alcoholic liver disease Metabolically-dysfunction-associated steatotic liver disease (MASLD) Chronic viral hepatitis due to hepatitis B or C Autoimmune causes (Autoimmune hepatitis, primary sclerosing cholangitis, primary biliary cirrhosis) Vascular causes: Budd–Chiari syndrome Drug induced
Acute liver failure (ALF)	Drug/Toxin (ATT drugs, Paracetamol, Zinc phosphide-Ratol poisoning) Hepatitis A/E Acute Wilson's disease Autoimmune hepatitis
Hepatic malignancies	Hepatocellular carcinoma (HCC) Hepatoblastoma A small subset of cholangiocarcinoma Epithelioid haemangio-endothelioma Liver-only metastasis without extra-hepatic disease in neuroendocrine and colorectal tumours
Congenital or metabolic liver diseases	Wilson's disease Cholestatic liver disease, like biliary atresia and primary familial intra-hepatic cholestasis (PFIC) Congenital hepatic fibrosis Maple syrup urine disease Urea cycle defects Amino acid defects Glycogen storage diseases Alagille syndrome Polycystic liver disease Primary hyperoxaluria
Retransplantation	Chronic rejection Hepatic artery thrombosis (HAT) Primary non-function

21.3 Contraindications for Liver Transplant

With the advent of advanced intensive care, the contraindications for LT have narrowed. However, bacterial or fungal septicaemias are generally considered a contraindication. Any potential recipient who has multiple-organ failure (usually more than three) is also regarded as unsuitable for LT.

21.4 Recipient Assessment

A comprehensive history and physical exam of all potential liver recipients is crucial, especially regarding alcohol abstinence, blood transfusions, and viral hepatitis treatment history. Blood grouping is the first step, followed by biochemistry tests to assess liver function, renal function with electrolytes, coagulation parameters, viral markers, and blood gas analysis. A cross-sectional imaging study, preferably a multiphase contrast-enhanced CT or MRI of the liver, is essential for planning a liver transplant. This imaging helps define liver morphology, vasculature, portal vein thrombus, space-occupying lesions (SOL), and the presence and location of porto-systemic shunts. In cases of hepatocellular carcinoma (HCC), extrahepatic disease should be excluded with either an HRCT of the chest or a PET-CT scan, based on institutional protocols. Patients with diabetes should be evaluated for diabetic nephropathy, diabetic retinopathy, and carotid Doppler with brain imaging. Those over 60 years old need brain imaging to assess cerebral vasculature and carotid Doppler, as neck manipulation during intubation and intravenous access might dislodge plaques, potentially leading to a stroke. Cardiac assessment includes 2-D echocardiography or dobutamine stress echocardiography (DSE), as appropriate. All patients should undergo a psychological evaluation, and women are required to have a gynaecological exam, which serves as a mandatory prerequisite.

21.5 Deceased Donor Liver Transplantation

Deceased donor transplants involve the donation of organs or tissues after the determination of brain death (DBD). Currently, this is the most common form of deceased donation worldwide. However, donations after circulatory determination of death (DCDD) are another form in the Western world but are less common in India. DDLT is the most common and ideal form of LT, as there is no live donor surgery involved; however, the scarcity of organs has resulted in the concept of LDLT. Brain death usually results from head trauma or cerebrovascular accidents, leading to irreversible brain damage and loss of cranial nerve activity. An apnoea test is performed to confirm the absence of respiratory effort despite hypercarbia. The test is repeated twice, with at least a 6-h interval, to confirm brain death. Organs donated after cardiac arrest experience a period of hypoperfusion known as warm ischaemia time. This period is characterized by low flow followed by circulatory arrest. Hypoperfusion is thought to be most damaging when systolic blood pressure falls below 50 mmHg or when SpO2 drops below 70% for more than 2 min.

21.6 Living Donor Assessment

Liver donation is strictly voluntary with informed consent, and donors are never coerced. Ideal liver donors are aged between 18 and 60 years, have normal blood biochemistry, no active substance abuse, and a healthy liver. Blood group compatibility is preferred, with AB blood group serving as a universal recipient and O blood group as a universal donor. Rhesus typing is not relevant. ABO-incompatible LDLT has also become more common with the use of Rituximab for desensitization when ABO-compatible donation is unavailable. Donors with fatty livers should be excluded. Traditionally, this is assessed by comparing liver attenuation to that of the spleen in CT scans, known as the Liver Attenuation Index (LAI). If the liver attenuation exceeds that of the spleen, the liver is considered non-fatty. Recently, MRI is increasingly used to evaluate fatty changes in the liver by calculating the proton fat fraction. When the liver quality is deemed adequate, intravenous contrast is administered, and a triple-phase CT angiogram is performed to evaluate the hepatic artery, portal vein, and hepatic veins during different phases of contrast circulation. Additionally, the scan helps determine total liver volume, the volume of each lobe, and the remnant liver volume with the help of CT volumetry. The anticipated volume of the graft (either right or left lobe) is used to determine the graft-to-recipient weight ratio (GRWR). The GRWR is the ratio of graft weight to the recipient's body weight. For example, if the graft weighs 700 g and the recipient's body weight is 85 kg, then the GRWR would be 0.82. In ideal situations, the GRWR should be at least 0.8. The remnant liver volume is also calculated and must be at least 30% to prevent post-hepatectomy liver failure. Magnetic resonance cholangiopancreatography (MRCP) is used to delineate biliary anatomy and can be combined with magnetic resonance spectroscopy to quantify the fat fraction within the liver. Cardiorespiratory evaluation, including 2D echocardiography and, if necessary, a dobutamine stress test, is mandatory for major surgery. Liver biopsy may sometimes be indicated in donors to rule out steatohepatitis with fibrosis, which makes them unsuitable for donation, but the advent of MR elastography has limited this invasive procedure. Human Leukocyte Antigen (HLA) tissue typing and cross-matching are not essential in liver transplant because the liver is an immune-privileged organ. However, if there is a potential one-way mismatch with the donor, HLA tissue typing should be conducted, and such donors are rejected due to the near-fatal risk of Graft-versus-Host Disease (GVHD) post-transplant. Under the Human Transplant Act, donor and recipient relationships must be definitively proven, and the Hospital Authorization Committee may request DNA tissue typing to confirm the relationship. All donors must undergo psychiatric evaluation by law.

21.7 Recipient Surgery

The recipient surgery starts with thorough preparation for anaesthesia because there are significant haemodynamic fluctuations during the surgery. Rapid infusers, central lines, arterial lines, transoesophageal echocardiography, and sometimes cell saver and venovenous bypass may be necessary to prevent massive blood transfusions.

Access to the Abdomen: A bilateral subcostal incision with a midline extension or an inverted "T" incision is used to gain access. Large venous collaterals are often encountered and must be ligated.

Liver Mobilization: The falciform and round ligaments (Ligamentum teres hepatis) are divided. The round ligament often contains a recanalized paraumbilical vein and should be secured with ligatures. The division of the falciform ligament is carried cranially until it divides into the right and left coronary ligaments, which are also divided to expose the bare area of the liver. Once the bare area of the liver is exposed, the junction of the right, middle, and left hepatic veins with the inferior vena cava (IVC) becomes visible. Fixed abdominal wall retractor systems (Omnitract or Thompson) are placed to provide good exposure of the operative field. The left half of the gastro-hepatic ligament (lesser omentum) is divided to reveal the caudate lobe of the liver. A replaced or accessory left hepatic artery is present in the lesser omentum in nearly 12%–20% of patients. It should be safeguarded, as it may serve as a valuable inflow in case of dissection of the recipient hepatic artery.

Dissection of the Retrohepatic IVC: This step is vital for liver mobilization, and bleeding often occurs when entering the retroperitoneum. The assistant rotates the right lobe of the liver to expose the retrohepatic cava and right adrenal gland. The right adrenal gland is often adherent to segment VII of the liver and must be dissected off for proper exposure of the IVC. Division of the right adrenal vein is performed during adrenal dissection and aids in mobilizing the IVC. It is prudent to sling the lower cava as soon as possible after mobilizing the right lobe or even at the start if feasible. Multiple inferior hepatic veins and short hepatic veins of varying sizes are encountered while separating the liver from the IVC. These are meticulously divided between ligatures or titanium clips. Large venous branches are best transfixed to prevent slippage and possible torrential bleeding from the IVC. Division of the hepatocaval ligament between clamps is necessary, as it almost always contains a draining hepatic vein that can cause significant blood loss and air embolism. Once the extrahepatic portion of the right hepatic vein (RHV) is exposed, water dissection may be used to open the space between the right and middle hepatic veins, followed by looping of the right hepatic vein with a vascular sling.

Portal Dissection: Mobilization of portal structures begins with a cholecystectomy in the usual manner. Attention then turns to careful dissection of the left hepatic artery (LHA), which is often used for inflow reconstruction to the graft's right hepatic artery. Frequently, a middle hepatic artery (MHA) is present on the left side of the biliary tissue, entering the umbilical fissure, which supplies the segment IV. The left portal vein branch becomes visible after dissecting and dividing the left hepatic artery between ligatures. An incision is then made on the peritoneum over the main portal vein, separated from the biliodigestive sheath to allow looping of the portal vein by directing the right angle to the exposed left portal vein and reversing the right angle to divide the retroportal tissue. After looping the portal vein, an effort should be made to identify and ligate the branches of the right hepatic artery. Upward traction on the bile duct with an eyelid retractor will expose the bifurcation of the portal vein. Once the inflow vasculature is controlled, the next step is lowering the hilar plate to visualize the division of the right and left bile ducts separately. In LDLT, it is preferable to divide the right and left hepatic ducts separately, as donor grafts may have two or more ducts. The three arteries (LHA, RHA, and MHA) to the liver are divided between ligatures, and the portal vein is divided as it branches into right and left veins, which marks the start of the "anhepatic phase," during which haemostasis may require antifibrinolytic agents like tranexamic acid due to common clot lysis.

Completion of Liver Explantation: Once the liver is anhepatic, only the draining veins of the caudate lobe and the three hepatic veins remain attached. The caudate lobe is dissected from the IVC by incising the peritoneum along its left border and individually dividing the caudate veins draining into the IVC. The next step involves dividing the RHV after applying a Satinsky clamp at the RHV–IVC junction. The final step is dividing the common stump of the middle hepatic vein (MHV) and left hepatic vein (LHV) after applying another Satinsky clamp. The cirrhotic liver is then removed from the abdominal cavity. The hepatic vein stumps are secured with a 4-0 polypropylene running suture. The anhepatic phase should ideally be as short as possible. A temporary end-to-side porto-caval shunt using 5-0 polypropylene running suture may be done till the donor liver is available for implantation. Methylprednisolone in a dose of 10 mg/kg is administered during the anhepatic phase to reduce the incidence of ischaemia-reperfusion injury and early acute allograft rejection after implantation of the graft liver.

Haemostasis and Preparation of the Liver Bed: The anhepatic phase can be used to achieve haemostasis on the raw surfaces and prepare the inflow and outflow vessels for subsequent revascularization of the liver graft. Portal hypertension often causes significant blood loss from the raw surfaces created during explantation. The retroperitoneal, retrohepatic and paracaval areas are common sites of bleeding, which can be easily identified and managed during the anhepatic phase. Time should be taken to locate and secure each bleeding vessel through suturing, ligating, clipping, or using an energy device (Fig. 21.1).

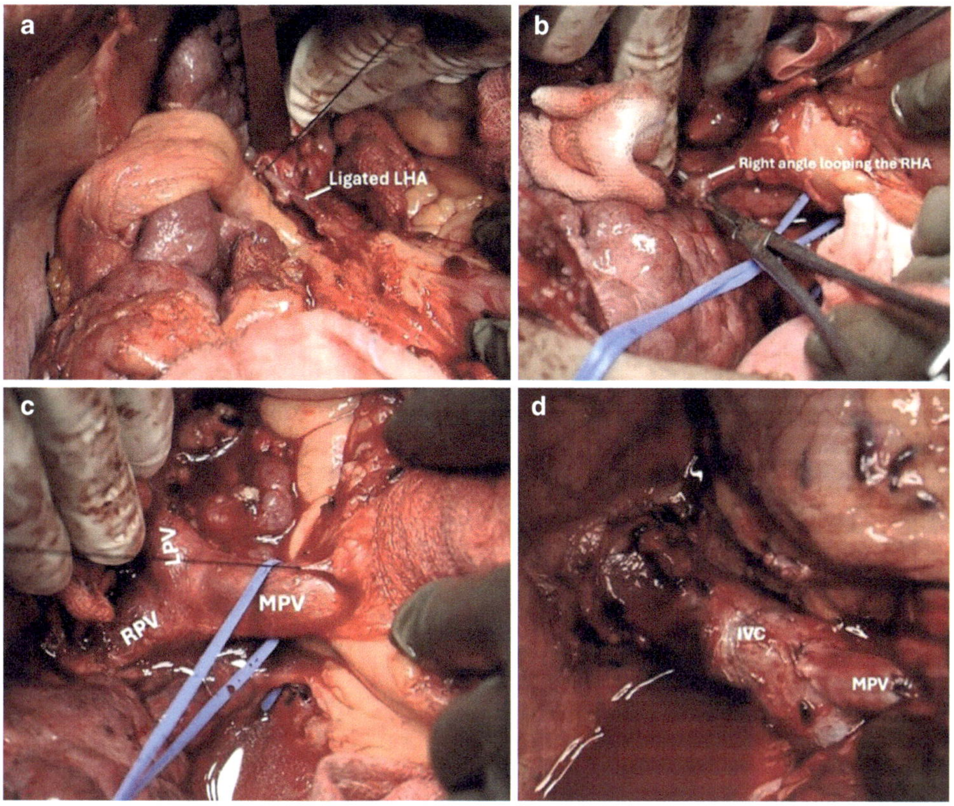

Fig. 21.1 Illustration of the hilar dissection: (**a**) The porta dissection showing ligated left hepatic artery (LHA); (**b**) the right hepatic artery (RHA) being looped; (**c**) the main portal vein (MPV) looped which bifurcates into right portal vein (RPV) and left portal vein (LPV); (**d**) completed temporary end-to-side porto-caval shunt

21.8 Deceased Donor Graft

In DDLT, the entire liver is removed from the donor along with the retrocaval IVC, common hepatic artery, often including the celiac trunk, portal vein, and bile duct. The procedure begins with an incision from the suprasternal notch to the pubic symphysis, requiring extensive access to the thorax and abdominal cavity, often necessitating a cruciate incision on the abdomen. The organs needing procurement are evaluated for functionality and quality. The liver is mobilized, and a Cattell–Braasch manoeuvre is performed to expose the IVC and aorta. To perfuse the organs with organ preservation solution, the aorta is cannulated, followed by the inferior mesenteric vein (IMV) or superior mesenteric vein (SMV) for portal perfusion. The supra-coeliac aorta is also looped for the aortic cross-clamp before organ removal. Once the recipient team is informed and prepared, the abdomen is cooled with crushed ice, a process known as pre-cooling. Subsequently, the aorta is cross-clamped, and cold preservation solution is perfused through the aortic cannula and the IMV/SMV cannula, followed by opening the right atrium or suprahepatic vena cava to drain the perfusate. After the effluent runs clear, the organ is systematically retrieved.

21.9 Donor Hepatectomy

21.9.1 Living Donor Hepatectomy

In live donor hepatectomy, either the right lobe or the left lobe of the liver can be retrieved, depending on the recipient's condition, weight, anatomy, and volume of the donor liver. The left lobe donor hepatectomy is safe since the right lobe constitutes 50%–70% of the liver, ensuring a good remnant liver. However, the right lobe is generally preferred for adult recipients due to its larger volume. the principles and major steps of donor hepatectomy are (Fig. 21.2 and Tables 21.3, 21.4 and 21.5)

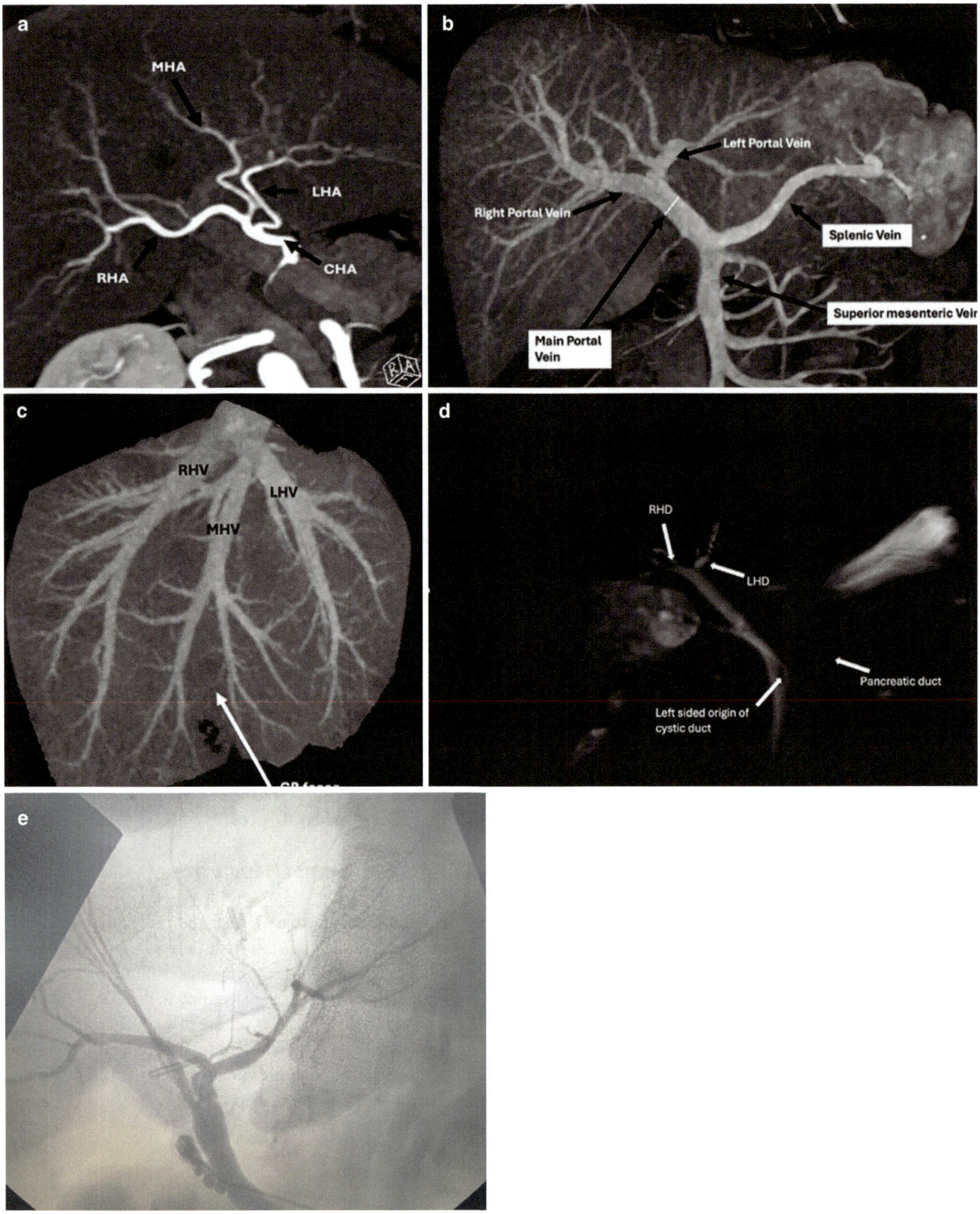

Fig. 21.2 Reconstructed donor vascular and biliary anatomy to plan donor hepatectomy in LDLT; (**a**) standard hepatic arterial anatomy; (**b**) Type A portal venous anatomy; (**c**) venous reconstructed image with arrow showing GB fossa (line drawn from right of MHV to the middle of GB fossa is the Cantlie's line or the transection line in donor hepatectomy); (**d**) MRCP image. (**e**) Intra-operative Cholangiogram showing a Type IIIA biliary anatomy with metallic clip used as marker to define the anterior right hepatic duct

Table 21.3 The possible grafts from a living donor

Right lobe graft (standard, modified or extended-comprising the MHV)
Right posterior segment graft
Left lobe graft (with or without caudate lobe)
Left lateral segment graft
Mono-segment grafts
(The left lateral segment and mono-segment grafts are usually taken for children)

Table 21.4 Essential steps in right lobe donor hepatectomy

Dissection of the suprahepatic IVC with delineation of RHV-MHV groove
Mobilization of the right lobe
Dissecting the right lobe from the IVC by dividing the inferior hepatic vein (IHV) and the short hepatic veins
Division of the hepatocaval ligament
Delineation of the RHV and looping with a vascular sling
Cholecystectomy with cannulation for intra-operative cholangiogram with a metallic marker to decide the site of duct division as shown in picture (Picture 21.2e)
Delineation of right portal vein (RPV) and RHA
Lowering of hilar plate and check-cholangiogram with metallic markers to identify the right hepatic duct (RHD)
Temporary occlusion of the RPV and RHA to mark the transection plane or Cantlie's line.
Transection of the liver parenchyma with preservation of the middle hepatic vein (MHV) on the remnant side and serial division of the segment V and segment VIII veins
Completion of parenchymal transection
Division of the RHD
Division of the RHA and RPV
Division of the RHV and retrieval of the graft for static cold storage-wherein flushing the graft with heparinized cold organ perfusion solution
Careful closure of the stumps of RHV, RPV, RHA, and the RHD
It is preferable to perform a check cholangiogram to rule out any leak or narrowing of the CBD
Careful haemostasis on all the stumps as well as on the cut surface of the liver
Fixation of the remnant left lobe to the anterior wall to prevent rotation of the lobe or kinking of the vascular inflow/outflow

Table 21.5 Essential steps in left lobe donor hepatectomy

Dissection of the suprahepatic IVC with delineation of RHV-MHV groove
Mobilization of the left lobe
Dissecting the left lobe and caudate off the IVC by dividing the caudate veins
Delineation of MHV-LHV and subsequent looping with a vascular sling whenever feasible
Cholecystectomy with cannulation for intra-operative cholangiogram
Delineation of left portal vein (LPV), LHA and MHA when present
Lowering of the hilar plate and a check-cholangiogram with metallic markers to identify the left hepatic duct (LHD)
Temporary occlusion of the LPV and LHA (with MHA) to mark the transection plane or Cantlie's line
Transection of the liver parenchyma with sequential division of segment V and segment VIII veins
Completion of parenchymal transection
Division of the LHD
Division of the LHA and LPV
Division of the MHV-LHV and retrieval of the graft for cold storage as done for right lobe graft
Careful closure of the stumps of LHV-MHV, LPV, LHA, and LHD
Check haemostasis and cholangiogram as in right hepatectomy

21.10 Postoperative Care

The donor is monitored with serial arterial blood gases, haemogram, renal function tests, PT-INR, and liver function tests. A Doppler study is usually performed on the first postoperative day to assess flow patterns in the vascular inflow and outflow.

21.11 Static Cold Storage of the Graft

The aortic cross-clamp time in DDLT and in LDLT, once the graft liver is out of the donor body, it is immediately perfused with cold solution, which marks the beginning of "cold ischaemia time." The retrieved liver graft is flushed with cold (0–4 °C) organ preservation solution. This solution can be

Table 21.6 Warm and cold ischaemia in a liver graft

First warm ischaemia: It is the time taken from ligation of the hepatic artery through the retrieval of the graft in live donor hepatectomy till cold storage
Cold ischaemia time: It is the time taken from the perfusion of cold organ perfusion solution till the liver is out of ice just before implantation
Second warm ischaemia time: It is the time starting when the graft is taken out of ice till reperfusion of the portal blood in graft liver in the recipient
The first warm ischaemia in a DDLT: It is the time taken for liver removal after it has been perfused and cooled

either the University of Wisconsin (UW) solution or the Histidine–Tryptophan–Ketoglutarate (HTK) solution, depending on the institutional protocol. The purpose is to flush the liver graft with cold organ perfusion solution to remove blood and clots from the graft and to supply nutrients to the hepatocytes during cold preservation. The organ perfusion solution contains electrolytes and other chemical substances to provide nutrients and prevent cellular oedema (Table 21.6).

21.12 Benchwork

Benchwork or back table preparation of the liver allograft mainly involves preparing the graft liver for implantation into the recipient. In DDLT, this includes removing all diaphragmatic muscles and tendinous attachments from the liver, suture ligating the phrenic vein openings on the suprahepatic IVC, and clearing the portal vein, hepatic artery, and bile duct tissues from the surrounding connective tissue and fat. In LDLT, bench work involves assessing the graft liver's portal vein stump, RHV stump, and reconstructing the so-called neo-MHV from the segment V and VIII veins using either an autologous vein graft or a synthetic graft such as PTFE to facilitate implantation in a modified right lobe graft. A left lobe or left lateral lobe graft usually does not require bench work unless venoplasty is needed.

21.13 Implantation

The allograft must be flushed with at least 1 L of cold normal saline before implantation to remove air and prevent potassium-rich preservative fluid from entering the recipient's circulation, especially when UW solution is used as the organ preservation solution (Table 21.7).

Table 21.7 Steps in implantation

Preparation of the inflow and outflow
Outflow-hepatic vein reconstruction
Inflow-portal vein reconstruction
Inflow-hepatic artery reconstruction
Bile duct anastomosis

21.13.1 Preparation of the Inflow and Outflow

Aim for quick and efficient implantation because warm ischaemia time should be minimized. A wide outflow is crucial for good function, and once the graft has been reperfused, the remaining steps can be done more slowly. Next reconstruct the hepatic artery, followed by the bile duct anastomosis. Any major porto-systemic shunts seen on pre-operative imaging should be looped, and portal flow should be evaluated after clamping the shunts, with subsequent ligation of the shunts.

21.13.2 Reconstruction of the Outflow in DDLT

The implantation process begins with reconstruction of the vascular outflow. Three techniques are used for this purpose in DDLT: classical technique, piggyback technique, and longitudinal cavo-cavostomy.

Classical or Caval Replacement Technique: This was described by Sir Thomas Starzl, where the recipient's retrohepatic IVC is replaced with the donor's retrohepatic IVC, involving two end-to-end anastomoses connecting the donor's suprahepatic and infrahepatic IVC to the recipient IVC. It requires cross-clamping the recipient IVC, which can cause hemodynamic instability and negatively affect renal function. As a result, this technique is rarely used today. The main indications include a stenosed or unhealthy recipient IVC, such as in patients undergoing re-do liver transplants, those with Budd–Chiari syndrome, or when the IVC is involved by a large hepatocellular carcinoma.

Piggyback Technique: This technique was initially described by Sir Roy Calne and popularized by Tzakis. In the classical "piggyback" technique, an end-to-side anastomosis is created between the common funnel made by joining the stumps of the recipient RHV, MHV, and LHV and the superior end of the donor suprahepatic IVC using a 4-0 polypropylene running suture. The main advantage of this technique is that cross-clamping of the IVC is avoided, leading to

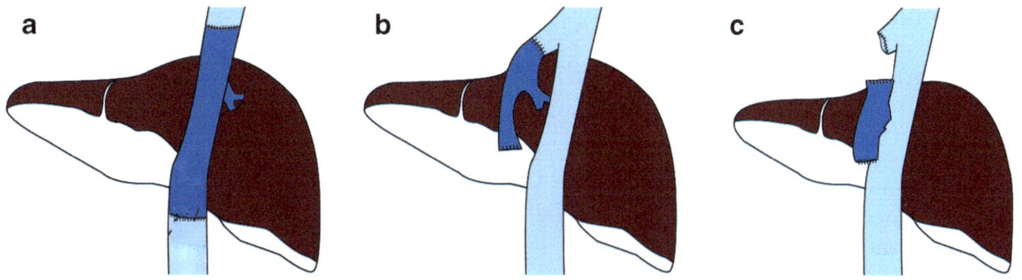

Fig. 21.3 Reconstruction of the outflow tract. (**a**) The classical caval replacement technique, (**b**) the piggyback technique, and (**c**) the cavo-cavostomy

better haemodynamic stability in the recipient. Also, the flushing of the liver graft may be avoided as the inferior part of the liver graft IVC can be opened to flush out blood after reperfusion.

Cavo-cavostomy: In this technique, a long (10–12 cm) side-to-side anastomosis is made between the recipient IVC and graft retrohepatic IVC using running 4-0 polypropylene sutures (Fig. 21.3).

21.13.3 Reconstruction of the Outflow in LDLT

Implantation in LDLT can be performed either by cross-clamping the cava, and if this approach is planned, haemodynamic assessment should be conducted after caval clamping. Alternatively, it is possible to implant with partial clamping, and anastomosis time can be minimized by consolidating all outflows into one during benchwork. Regardless of the method selected, large inferior hepatic veins must be included in the outflow anastomosis. In a left lobe graft, the outflow typically involves the common stump of the MHV-LHV, which is anastomosed to the recipient's common opening of the RHV-MHV-LHV, often requiring cross-clamping.

21.13.4 Reconstruction of Graft Inflow in DDLT and LDLT

The portal vein anastomosis is performed before the hepatic artery and is done in an end-to-end fashion using a continuous 6-0 polypropylene suture. Care should be taken to avoid redundancy or twisting of the portal vein, and a "growth factor" should be left to allow for expansion of the anastomosis after reperfusion. Few centres perform portal vein anastomosis with continuous sutures on the posterior wall and interrupted sutures on the anterior wall; however, this approach may be time-consuming. The technique for portal vein anastomosis is determined mainly by institutional protocols or the surgeon's preference.

21.13.5 Reperfusion

After completing the portal vein anastomosis, release the vascular clamps on the recipient's IVC/RHV/MHV first, followed by the clamp on the portal vein to allow blood to reperfuse the liver allograft. This reperfusion marks the end of the warm ischaemia time. Once adequate reperfusion occurs, the liver surface turns uniformly pink from a pale brown colour. Any significant bleeding from the anastomotic sites or the IVC should be controlled with sutures or clips after re-perfusion.

21.13.6 Hepatic Artery Anastomosis

Successful hepatic artery reconstruction is crucial for graft function, and various methods have been described. In DDLT, a Carrel's patch of donor coeliac artery or common hepatic artery is anastomosed end-to-end to the recipient's common hepatic artery or to a branch patch of the bifurcation of the gastroduodenal artery and the proper hepatic artery using 6-0 or 7-0 polypropylene interrupted or continuous sutures. In LDLT, the graft hepatic artery is anastomosed with the recipient's RHA, LHA, or CHA, depending on the caliber and length of the graft artery.

21.13.7 Intraoperative Doppler

The intraoperative Doppler study is usually performed after completing the vascular anastomoses to assess the patency of the arterial and venous connections, as well as the blood flow pattern and volume across these anastomoses. The hepatic artery flow velocity should be greater than 25 mL/min, and the resistive index should be between 0.5 and 0.9. The portal

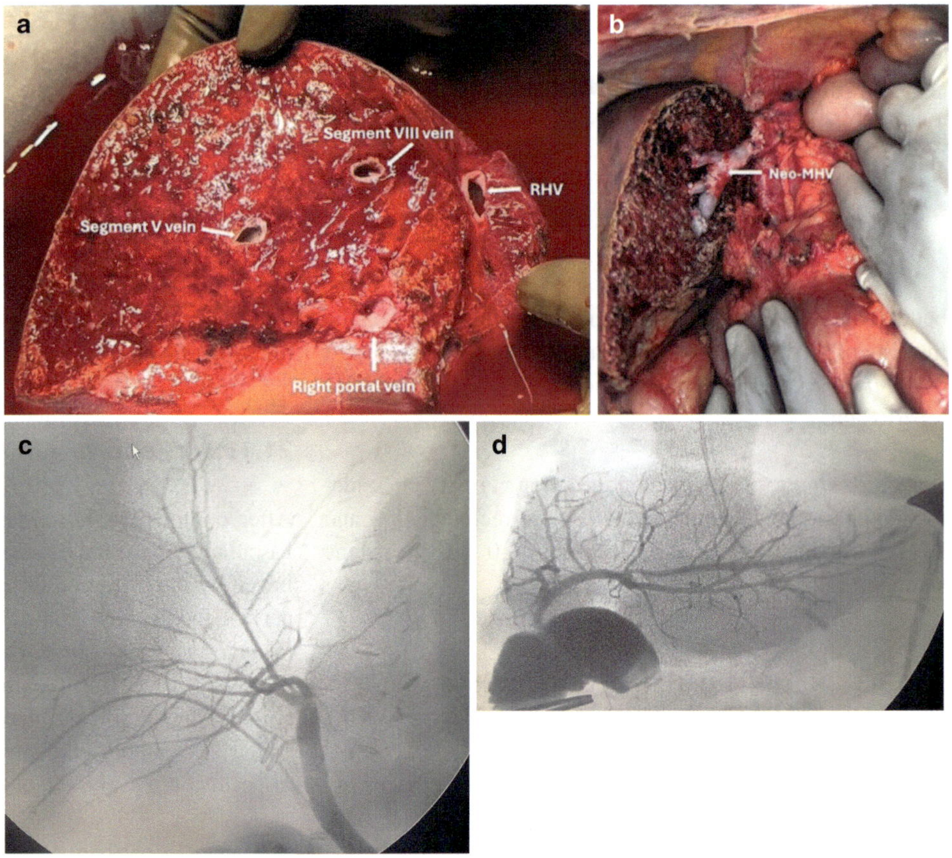

Fig. 21.4 (**a**) A typical right lobe donor graft showing single segment V, VIII, RHV, and RPV; (**b**) The final appearance of the graft liver after implantation, showing neo-MHV (reconstructed using autologous vein graft from the explant portal vein of the recipient by anastomosing segments V and VIII veins) in LDLT ; (c) Recipient Cholangiogram after completion of duct to duct anastomosis in adult showing right anterior and posterior ducts; (d) Pediatric recipient's cholangiogram after completion of Roux-en Y hepatico-jejunostomy following a left lateral lobe implantation

vein anastomosis is examined for proper alignment, luminal patency, and the flow volume is measured. The portal flow volume should range from 150 to 400 mL per 100 g of liver tissue. Low portal flow may require flow modulation, such as ligation of any significant lienorenal shunt or other large collateral vessels. The flow through the hepatic veins should be hepatofugal and display a triphasic pattern.

21.13.8 Restoration of Biliary Continuity

The bile duct in DDLT and the hepatic duct in LDLT are anastomosed in a duct-to-duct fashion between the donor and recipient bile ducts. An end-to-end anastomosis between donor and recipient bile ducts is preferred because it is more physiological. The anastomosis can be performed either with a continuous running suture or with interrupted sutures using absorbable material usually a 6-0 polydioxanone. Care must be taken to avoid redundancy of either side of the bile duct, as it can lead to bilio-stasis, obstruction, or stone formation. A Roux-en-Y hepaticojejunostomy is preferred in children or in patients with bile duct diseases such as PSC or after prior surgery. It is advisable to perform a completion cholangiogram after completing the biliary anastomosis to confirm the patency and to check for any leaks or narrowing. The cholangiogram can be done through either the cystic duct stump or the end of the Roux limb in cases of hepaticojejunostomy (Fig. 21.4).

21.13.9 Haemostasis and Drain Placement

Post-implantation, meticulous haemostasis should be performed with particular attention to the retroperitoneum, paracaval area, and porta hepatis. A 24–28 Fr abdominal drain is placed in Morrison's pouch and brought out through the right flank. Some centres use two drains through the right and left flanks.

21.13.10 Closure

The abdominal wall incision is closed in either one or two layers, with the muscle and sheath sutured using number 1 polypropylene or nylon. The subcutaneous tissue and skin are typically closed with absorbable sutures or surgical clips. The surgical site is covered with a sterile dressing. If the abdominal closure appears tight, a prosthetic mesh may be used to prevent the serious complication of compartment syndrome, though this should generally be avoided.

Table 21.8 Complications in donor hepatectomy in LDLT

Bleeding
Bile leak
Post-hepatectomy liver dysfunction or failure
Torsion of the remnant liver following right lobe hepatectomy
Bile duct stricture
Portal vein thrombosis

Table 21.9 Complications in the recipient

Bleeding
Bile leak
Hepatic vein stricture
Portal vein thrombosis
Hepatic artery thrombosis
Recurrent Ascites
Early allograft dysfunction/Primary non-function mostly in DDLT
Rejection
Infection: intrabdominal/blood borne (bacterial/fungal/viral)
Bile duct stricture
Chronic rejection
Graft vs host disease (GVHD)

21.14 Immunosuppression

The liver is an immune-privileged organ with lower rejection rates than other solid organs. The goal of immunosuppression after a liver transplant is to prevent the host immune system from rejecting the allograft while maintaining immune control over infections and neoplasias. Current immunosuppressive regimens use various combinations of calcineurin inhibitors (CNIs), corticosteroids, molecular target of rapamycin (mTOR) inhibitors, antimetabolites, and biological agents. These combination protocols allow the use of drugs at lower doses without increasing the risk of allograft rejection and simultaneously reduce the toxicity of individual agents. Immunosuppressive medications are gradually adjusted over time based on graft function. CNIs include tacrolimus and cyclosporine, with tacrolimus being preferred because of fewer rejection episodes. The initial dose of tacrolimus is 0.1–0.15 mg/kg/day divided into two doses. The dose of cyclosporine is 10–15 mg/kg/day, divided into doses. Mycophenolate mofetil is administered at 500–1000 mg twice daily. Corticosteroids start at 5–10 mg/kg and are tapered over time. The dose of CNI is adjusted according to the trough levels and titrated as needed.

Induction of tolerance is desirable after liver transplant but is uncommon. Many case reports have documented natural haematopoietic chimerism, and numerous studies have aimed to achieve "operational tolerance" or haematopoietic chimerism—where graft function and histology remain stable and normal without immunosuppression, while immune competence is maintained. Natural tolerance has been observed in both adult and paediatric recipients, with up to 15% of paediatric cases allowing for the withdrawal of immunosuppression. The immune-privileged features of the liver are related to active intra- and extra-hepatic processes, including lymphocyte and dendritic cell migration to lymph nodes and the thymus; the release of soluble major histocompatibility complex (MHC) molecules; clonal deletion or exhaustion of allo-reactive T-cells; suppression by CD4+ T-cells; immune anergy resulting from deficient co-stimulation; and the transfer of passenger donor immune cells to the recipient, establishing a form of microchimerism.

21.15 Short-Term and Long-Term Outcomes After Liver Transplant

The short-term outcome after a transplant mainly depends on the patient's pre-operative condition, including the MELD score (a lower score indicates a better prognosis), involvement of other organs such as the kidneys or lungs, absence of infection, quality donor liver graft without steatosis, and a GRWR >0.8. Intraoperative factors like minimal blood loss with fewer transfusions also play a role, along with maintaining optimal immunosuppression without bacterial, fungal, or viral sepsis. Currently, the 30-day mortality rate at high-volume centres is less than 5%, and the 1-year mortality rate is under 10%. Long-term outcomes are influenced by adherence to medical therapy, disease recurrence (e.g., HCC, autoimmune hepatitis), chronic rejection, kidney dysfunction secondary to CNI use, cardiac or cerebrovascular events, and the development of malignancies.

Presently, the survival rates after liver transplantation are approximately 85–95% at 1 year, 70–80% at 5 years, and 60–70% at 10 years.

Key Points

- Liver transplantation is frequently performed for decompensated liver disease and acute liver failure.
- DDLT is the most common form in the Western world, while LDLT is the most common in the Eastern world, including India.
- In DDLT, a healthy liver is obtained from a brain-dead patient; in LDLT, a healthy donor donates a part of the liver.
- Cold ischaemia time refers to the period from perfusion of the cold (0–4 °C) organ preservation solution until the graft liver is removed from ice just before implantation. 8–10 h of cold ischaemia is tolerable for a healthy, non-steatotic graft liver.
- The right lobe of the liver typically constitutes 60–70% of the total volume, while the left lobe accounts for 30–40%.

(continued)

- In LDLT, a healthy donor can donate up to 70% of their liver, which will regenerate to 85% of its original volume in 11–14 days and reach full size in 3 months.
- During right lobe donor hepatectomy, preserving 30% of the remnant liver with the middle hepatic vein (MHV) is essential to prevent post-hepatectomy liver failure.
- The sequence of implantation involves the hepatic veins, portal vein, hepatic artery, and finally the bile duct.
- Bile duct anastomosis remains one of the most challenging aspects of liver transplantation.
- To prevent rejection post-transplant, a triple immunosuppressive regimen is used, which includes tacrolimus, mycophenolate mofetil, and prednisolone.

Selected Reading

1. Starzl TE, Iwatsuki S. Van thiel DH Evolution of liver transplantation. Hepatology. 1982;2(5):14–36. https://doi.org/10.1002/hep.1840020516.
2. Tiwari P, Nundy S. The status of liver transplantation in India. Natl Med J India. 2025;38:30–4.
3. Gadour E. Lesson learnt from 60 years of liver transplantation: advancements, challenges, and future directions. World J Transplant [Internet]. 2025;15(1) [cited 2025 Jun 20]. Available from: https://www.wjgnet.com/2220-3230/full/v15/i1/93253.htm
4. Chen CL, Fan ST, Lee SG, Makuuchi M, Tanaka K. Living-donor liver transplantation: 12 years of experience in Asia. Transplantation. 2003;75(Supplement):S6–11.
5. Rastogi R, Gupta S, Garg B, Vohra S, Wadhawan M, Rastogi H. Preoperative liver fat quantification in. Indian J Radiol Imaging. 2016;26(1)
6. Sreejith S, Ghimire R, Bappaditya H, Acharya MR, Inbaraj B, Nidoni R, et al. Comparison of outcomes of recipient in living donor liver transplantation with donor age less than 55 years and more than 55 years: a propensity score matched study. J Liver Transplant. 2022;7:100087.
7. Eikmans M, Van Halteren AG, Van Besien K, Van Rood JJ, Drabbels JJ, Claas FH. Naturally acquired microchimerism: Implications for transplantation outcome and novel methodologies for detection. Chimerism. 2014;5(2):24–39.
8. Pillai AA, Levitsky J. Overview of immunosuppression in liver transplantation. World J Gastroenterol. 2009;15(34):4225.

Part V

Biliary Tract

Surgical Anatomy of the Extrahepatic Biliary System

22

Mohammad Ibrarullah

Abstract

Variations related to GB include agenesis, floating, and left-sided GB. The right hepatic duct (RHD) is less angulated than the left hepatic duct (LHD). The LHD has a longer extrahepatic course (2–3 cm) and is located at the base of segment IV. Variation in the hilar confluence is noted in nearly 40% due to segmental ducts, more commonly that of the RHD, joining at different levels. Cholecystectomy involves the identification of specific landmarks to guide safe dissection, exposure of the hepatocystic triangle (HCT) to delineate the cystic duct and artery, and mobilization of the GB from the cystic plate. Rouviere's sulcus (RS) represents the plane of the extrahepatic portal pedicle. Cystic artery is the most variable structure in the HCT. To achieve CVS, the HCT is cleared of all fibrofatty tissue, leaving behind only two structures: the cystic duct and the cystic artery. The distal 1/3 of the GB is dissected off the cystic plate (CP).

Keywords

Biliary anatomy · Gallbladder · Bile duct

22.1 Gallbladder

The gallbladder (GB) is a pear-shaped, sea-green in appearance, approximately 7–10 cm in length, 3–4 cm in width, and less than 3 mm thick, with a normal volume of 30–50 ml. It is situated on the inferior surface of the right lobe of the liver, between segments IV and V. The GB fossa is located on the inferior aspect of the Cantle's line, which marks the boundary between the right and left hepatic segments. The GB is divided arbitrarily into the fundus, body, and neck. The tapered part of the neck is called the infundibulum, which joins the common hepatic duct (CHD) via the cystic duct (CD). An outpouching of the infundibulum caused by a lodged stone is known as Hartman's pouch. Developmental anomalies, such as multiple GBs (double or triple) with single or multiple cystic ducts, have been anecdotally reported. Variations in shape, including Phrygian cap, bilobed, trilobed, or septate GB, are typically acquired conditions resulting from recurrent inflammation or adenomyosis. The GB receives blood supply from the cystic artery (CA), which arises from the right hepatic artery (RHA). Cystic veins drain directly into the portal veins. The cystic lymph node, located between the GB neck and the CA, acts as the sentinel node for lymphatic drainage of the GB. Parasympathetic innervation originates from the hepatic branch of the vagus nerve, while sympathetic supply comes from the celiac plexus. The position and vascular supply of the GB can vary, which may have important implications during cholecystectomy.

The abnormal position of the GB (ectopic GB) indicates its arrest at various stages of development, from the pars cystica of the hepatic diverticulum to its final location on the undersurface of the right liver. Reported abnormalities include agenesis, floating GB, intrahepatic GB, or its location in the hepatoduodenal ligament, mesocolon, abdominal wall/falciform ligament, and retroduodenal area. Congenital atrophy of the right lobe of the liver can result in a subdiaphragmatic or retrohepatic GB (Figs. 22.1 and 22.2).

22.1.1 Gallbladder Agenesis

The prevalence of GB agenesis ranges from 0.007% to 0.13%. In the absence of the GB, the common bile duct (CBD) assumes its function. Bile flow stasis may lead to stone formation. Non-visualization of the GB on ultrasound (US) is often interpreted as a contracted or diseased GB, and agenesis is only discovered during surgery and confirmed through peroperative cholangiogram. Imaging techniques such as MRCP or EUS can diagnose agenesis preoperatively. Congenital anomalies in other organ systems have been

M. Ibrarullah (✉)
Department of Surgical Gastroenterology, Apollo Hospitals, Bhubaneswar, Odisha, India

M. Ibrarullah (ed.), *Recent Concepts in Gastrointestinal (GI) Surgery*, https://doi.org/10.1007/978-981-92-1118-0_22

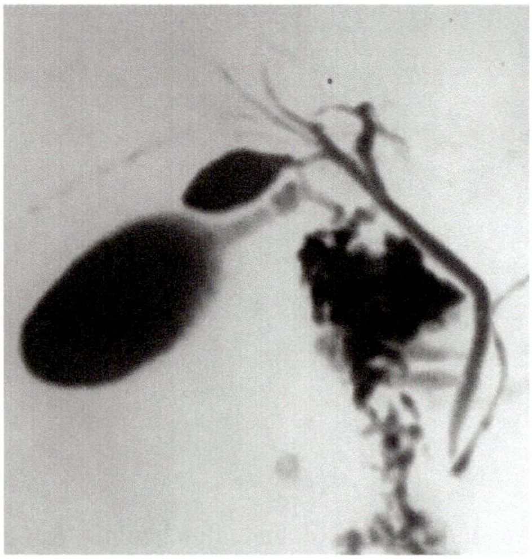

Fig. 22.1 Double GB, incidentally detected on MRCP. (Photo courtesy—Sadaf Ali)

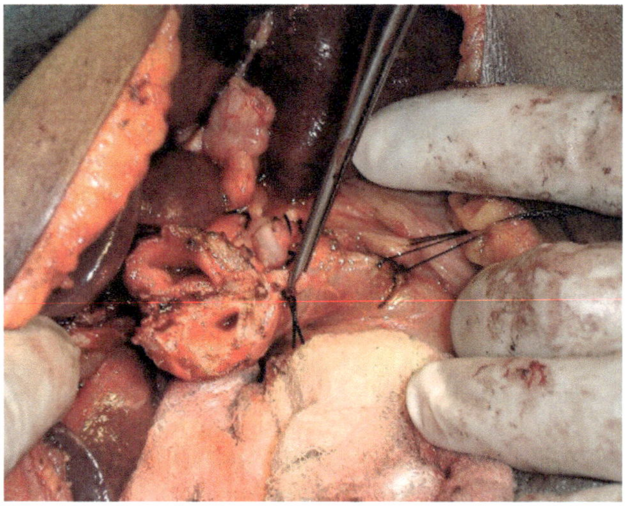

Fig. 22.2 Septate GB. A thick septum divides the GB into two. Displayed after transecting the GB at the body

reported in up to 30% of cases, making complete patient evaluation crucial in suspected cases of GB agenesis.

22.1.2 Floating Gallbladder

A floating GB is the most common variant of ectopic GB, characterized by poor development of the mesentery between the GB and liver. Four variants are recognized: I—absence of mesenteric attachment with the liver except at the cystic duct and artery, II—the mesentery is present but the GB is long, redundant, and tortuous, III—the GB fundus is freely mobile, and IV—poor GB mesenteric attachment due to liver atrophy or cirrhosis and fat loss secondary to aging or weight loss.

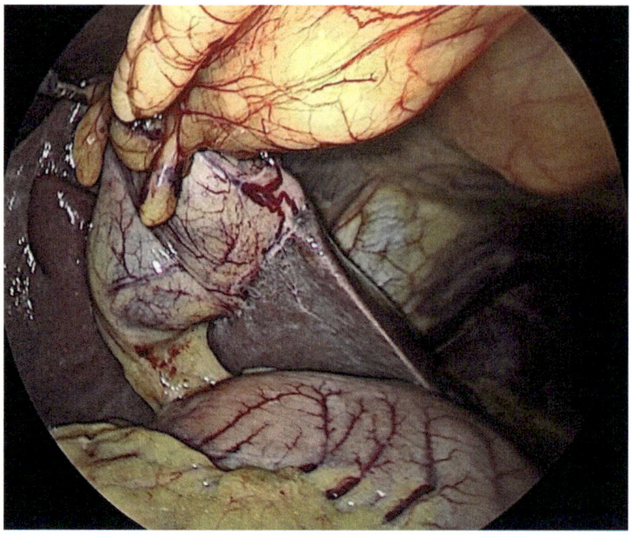

Fig. 22.3 Left-sided GB, appearance during laparoscopic cholecystectomy. (Note the GB fundus is clearly to the left of the falciform ligament)

These abnormal attachments predispose the GB to torsion, strangulation, herniation, and increased stone formation.

22.1.3 Left-Sided Gallbladder

A left-sided GB, with an estimated prevalence of 0.04–1.1%, is located on the left side of the falciform ligament. It results from its positional arrest during development or congenital atrophy of the right lobe or segment 4 of the liver. Three variants have been identified: I—associated with situs inversus, with GB lying in the left upper quadrant of the liver; II—true left-sided, also called sinistroposition, where the cystic duct joins the hepatic duct from the left side and the celiac artery crosses the bile duct from right to left to supply the GB; and III—false left-sided GB, also called medioposition, where the GB is normally located but the falciform ligament shifts to the right due to atrophy of the left lobe and persistence of the right umbilical vein. There may be associated anomalies of the bilio-vascular structures and atrophy of segment IV, along with developmental defects in other organ systems (Fig. 22.3).

Ectopic GB is more prone to develop complications such as cholelithiasis and cholecystitis due to poor emptying, abnormal blood supply, and inappropriate location. Failure to anticipate and localize it may lead to delays in diagnosis, further complicating the issue. Laparoscopic cholecystectomy in such patients is technically challenging and has a higher risk of bile duct injury, ranging from 4.4 to 7.3%, compared to 0.3–0.5% in routine cholecystectomy.

22.2 Extrahepatic Bile Duct

The right hepatic duct (RHD) is less than 1 cm long and less angulated than the left hepatic duct (LHD). The LHD has a longer extrahepatic course (2–3 cm) and is located at the base of segment IV. The hilar plate is a condensation of fibrous tissue between the portal structures and Glisson's capsule at the hilum. Mobilizing the hilar plate (lowering of the hilar plate) exposes the hepatic hilum and the extrahepatic segment of the LHD, providing additional length of the duct for an optimal hepatico-jejunostomy. The larger extrahepatic segment and the angulation with the common hepatic duct (CHD) make the LHD more vulnerable to stasis and stone formation compared to the RHD. The common bile duct (CBD) continues from the CHD beyond the cystic duct insertion. It measures about 6.0–8.0 cm in length and is divided into supraduodenal, retroduodenal, retropancreatic, and intraduodenal segments. The supraduodenal segment is located in the free border of the hepatoduodenal ligament, anterior to the portal vein (PV) and to the right of the hepatic artery (HA). The normal CBD diameter is approximately 6–8 mm. Physiological dilation up to 1 cm can occur after cholecystectomy or with aging. The retroduodenal segment passes behind the first part of the duodenum, lies to the right of the gastroduodenal artery (GDA), and in front of the PV. In over 80% of cases, the CBD descends through the pancreatic tissue, while in the remaining cases, it lies in a groove behind the pancreatic head.

Variations in Hilar Confluence: Hilar confluence is formed by RHD and LHD in the majority. However, variation is noted in nearly 40% of cases due to segmental ducts, more commonly found in the RHD, joining at different levels. A detailed description of the variations with respective incidences is presented below (Fig. 22.4).

Arterial Supply: The proximal bile duct is supplied by the hepatic arteries—right, left, and middle—as well as the cystic artery. The distal bile duct receives arterial blood from the posterior superior pancreaticoduodenal artery (SPDA), supraduodenal artery, gastroduodenal artery (GDA), and retroportal artery (RPA). The RPA arises either from the celiac trunk (42%) or the superior mesenteric artery (58%) and supplies the mid and distal parts of the bile duct. This artery ascends on the posterior surface of the portal vein and pancreas head to join the PSPDA or ascends on the posterior surface of the supraduodenal bile duct to join the RHA. The mid-CBD is mainly supplied by two axial vessels, the 3 o'clock and 9 o'clock arteries, which arise from the SPDA or GDA and connect with the right hepatic artery (RHA) and cystic artery, respectively. These arteries form the epicholedochal plexus, connecting with the intramural and subepithelial plexuses of the bile duct. Both ends of the bile duct have a richer blood supply compared to the mid-CBD. The junction between the cystic duct CD and the CBD is considered a watershed area of vascularity between the proximal and mid-bile duct. The limited vascularity of the mid-segment makes it more vulnerable to ischemic damage following injury during cholecystectomy. In cases of accidental CBD transection, end-to-end repair has a high failure rate due to disruption of the axial vessels. Similarly, a high hepatico-jejunostomy using the well-vascularized proximal segment results in a lower incidence of stricture compared to an anastomosis lower down (Fig. 22.5).

Venous Drainage: The venous drainage of the bile duct follows the arterial pattern. The epicholedochal venous plexus, a fine reticular plexus on the surface of the bile duct, joins two distinct marginal veins at the 3 o'clock and 9 o'clock positions. In some cases, an additional 6 o'clock marginal vein can be seen on the posterior surface of the bile duct.

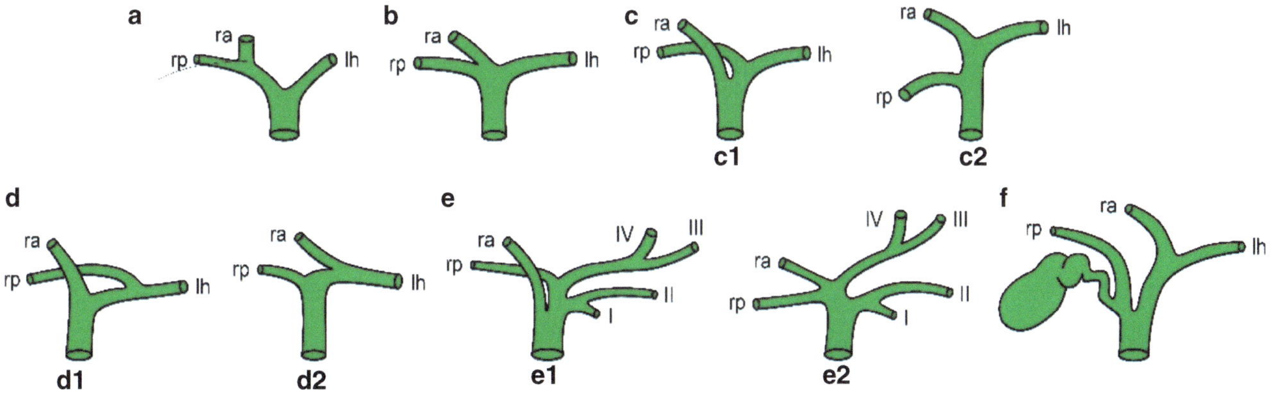

Fig. 22.4 Variations in hilar anatomy. (**a**) Normal biliary confluence formed by RHD and LHD (57%). (**b**) Triple confluence formed by right anterior (ra), posterior (rp) segmental ducts, and LHD (12%). (**c**) Right anterior or posterior segmental duct joining CHD (20%). (**d**) Right posterior or anterior segmental duct joining LHD (6%). (**e**) Absent hepatic duct confluence (3%). (**f**) Right posterior duct joining the cystic duct (2%). *ra* right anterior segmental duct, *rp* right posterior segmental duct, *lh* LHD

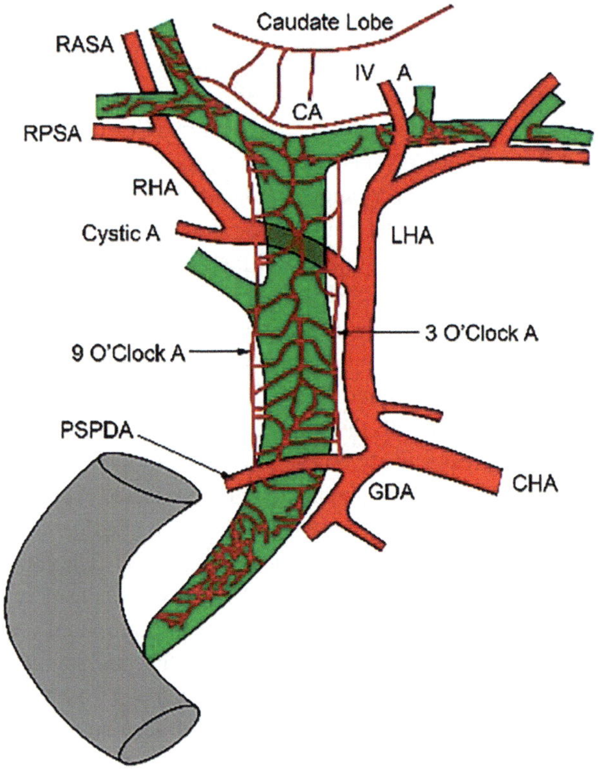

Fig. 22.5 Arterial supply of the extrahepatic biliary system

Inferiorly, the marginal veins and the venous plexus communicate with gastric veins, the posterior superior pancreaticoduodenal vein (PSPDV), and the gastrocolic trunk (GCT). Superiorly, the marginal veins enter the hepatic substance or join the hilar venous plexus, which eventually drains into the portal vein. The hilar venous plexus communicates with the cystic veins or veins of the caudate lobe. Portal cavernoma results from the massive enlargement of the parabiliary venous system due to thrombosis of the portal vein.

Lymphatic Drainage: Lymphatics from the GB drain first to the cystic node located in the hepatocystic triangle close to the cystic artery. It subsequently drains to the lymph nodes in the hepatoduodenal ligament, and then to the coeliac lymph nodes along the common hepatic artery. Superior pancreaticoduodenal nodes, para-aortic nodes, and superior mesenteric lymph nodes are the distant nodes. Lymph from the part of the gallbladder adjacent to the liver passes into the intrahepatic lymph vessels.

22.3 Surgical Anatomy Related to Cholecystectomy

Cholecystectomy involves the identification of specific landmarks to guide safe dissection, exposure of the hepatocystic triangle (HCT) to delineate the cystic duct and artery, and mobilization of the GB from the cystic plate.

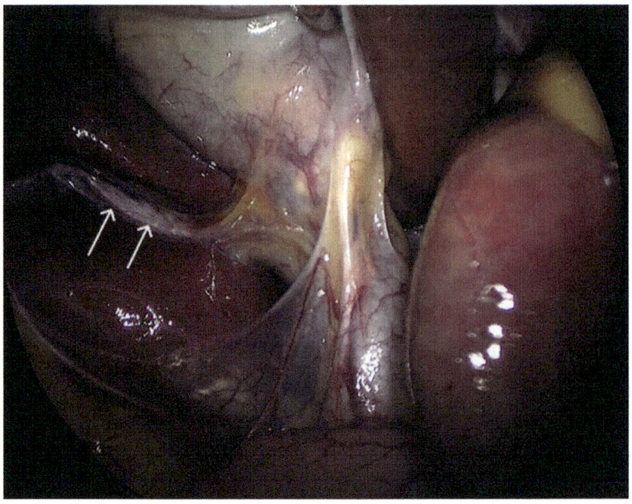

Fig. 22.6 Rouviere's sulcus (arrows) seen after lifting the Hartman's pouch. In 70% of patients, the RS contains the right portal pedicle

22.3.1 Rouviere's Sulcus

Rouviere's sulcus (RS) is the first anatomical landmark identified during cholecystectomy. The sulcus lies below the GB fossa and can be seen after lifting Hartman's pouch upward and medially. It represents the plane of the extrahepatic portal pedicle. To avoid injury to the CBD, the dissection of the GB should stay ventral to the plane connecting the sulcus and the base of segment 4 (Fig. 22.6 and Table 22.1).

22.3.2 Hepatocystic Triangle

The hepatocystic triangle (HCT) is bounded by the common hepatic duct (CHD), gallbladder (GB), and the undersurface of the liver. Careful dissection of this triangle is the most important step in cholecystectomy to achieve the critical view of safety (CVS). In clinical practice, HCT is often mistakenly called Calot's triangle, although the latter is actually part of the HCT, bounded by the common hepatic duct, cystic artery, and cystic duct (Fig. 22.7).

22.3.3 Cystic Artery

CA is the most variable structure in the HCT. In approximately 80% of cases, it arises from the RHA and crosses the CBD to supply the GB. In the remaining cases, it can originate from any named branch of the celiac trunk, such as the common hepatic artery, left or middle hepatic artery, gastroduodenal artery, or directly from the main trunk itself. It runs close to the cystic lymph node, which serves as an important landmark for its (artery's) isolation during cholecystectomy. At the GB neck, it divides into superficial and deep branches. The superficial branch runs along the

Table 22.1 Ibrarullah and Sikora's classification of Rouviere's sulcus

Type	Description	Incidence (%)
0	Absent or rudimentary sulcus	23
1	Deep sulcus	53
	Medial end of the sulcus is open	40
	Medial end of the sulcus is fused	11
	Sulcus is fused in the middle	02
2	Slit—small and shallow (<1 cm) sulcus away from the hepatic hilum	05
3	Scar—completely fused sulcus, appearing as a white linear scar	03
4	Double sulcus	0.2
NI	Sulcus is not identifiable (NI) because of subhepatic adhesions	15

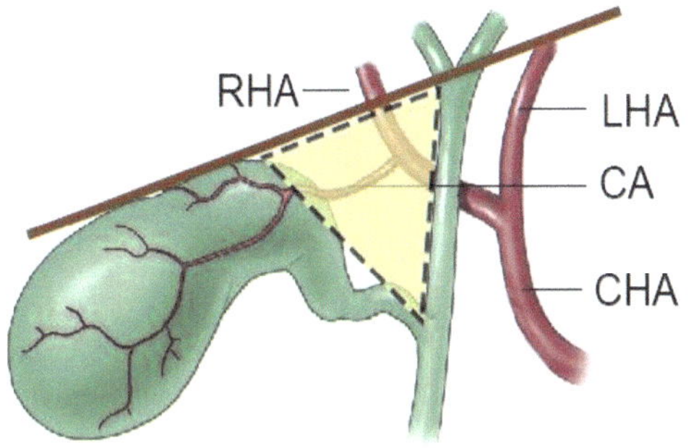

Fig. 22.7 The hepatocystic triangle

anterior surface of the GB toward the neck and infundibulum, while the deep branch travels in the GB bed toward the fundus, ends there, or dips into the liver parenchyma. Depending on its course around the GB, a classification has been proposed. The various types and their respective incidences are as follows (Fig. 22.8 and Table 22.2).

22.3.4 Cystic Duct

The CD typically measures 2–4 cm in length and 2–3 mm in width. It joins the extrahepatic bile duct at various levels and in different configurations. The most common variation is angular insertion of the CD in 75%, followed by a parallel CD in 20%, and a spiral CD in 5% of cases. Occasionally, it may join the RHD or right sectoral duct in 0.6–2.3% of cases. The CD is rarely absent, but when it is, this is often due to inflammatory shortening or erosion from a stone, as seen in Mirizzi syndrome. For a safe cholecystectomy, it is essential to identify its junction with the GB rather than the point where it joins the CBD (Fig. 22.9).

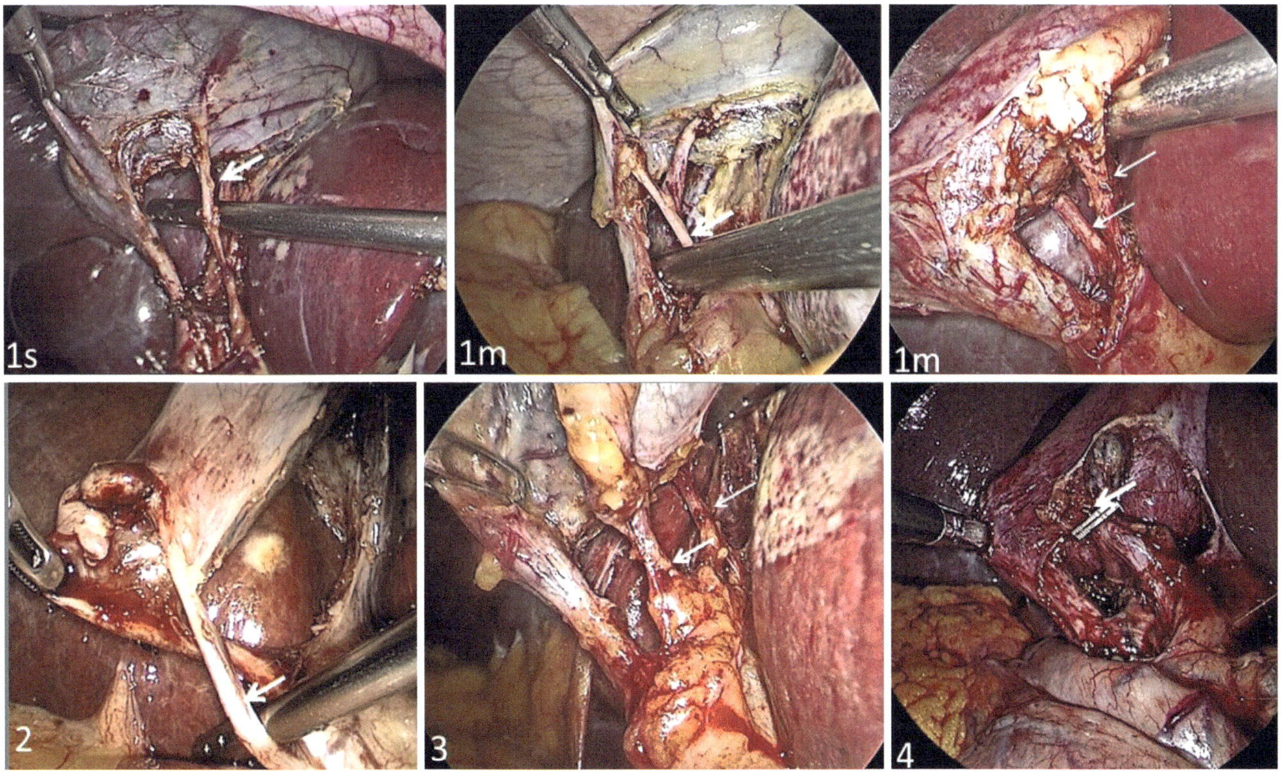

Fig. 22.8 Cystic artery (arrows) classification

Table 22.2 Cystic artery classification

Type	Description	Incidence (%)
1	S—single CA superomedial to CD in the HCT M—multiple arterial branches in the HCT due to early division of the CA	77 5
2	Inferior CA, i.e., artery arising inferolaterally, usually from GDA or CHA, runs behind or crosses the CD to enter the HCT to supply the GB	8
3	Double CA—Both the arteries appear to arise at different planes and, unlike the early division of CA	02
4	Small CA arising from the aberrant RHA in the HCT (caterpillar hump)	2.4
NI	CA not identifiable due to inflammation/fibrosis/multiple small branches	06

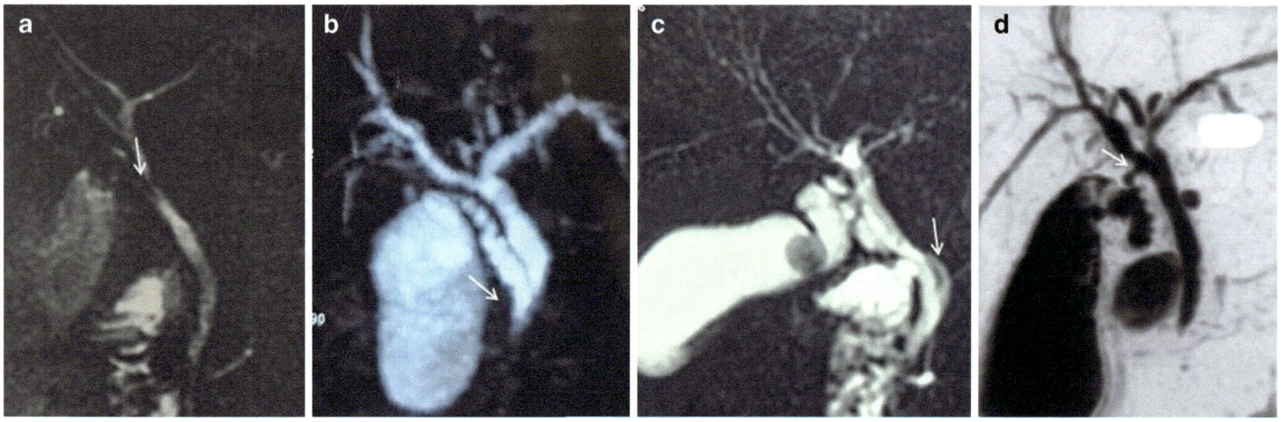

Fig. 22.9 MR cholangiogram showing variations in cystic duct (arrow) insertion. (**a**) angular insertion, (**b**) parallel and low insertion, (**c**) spiral insertion, and (**d**) cystic duct joining RHD

22.3.5 Subvesicle Duct

Subvesicle duct, located close to the GB bed, is present in 3%–10% of cases. The average diameter of the duct is usually less than 2 mm. Four types of ducts have been identified.

Type 1: A segmental: Right posterior segmental duct that runs close to the GB bed to join the main duct.

Type 2: An accessory duct: Arising from the right anterior or posterior segmental duct, drains into the main duct.

Type 3: Cholecystohepatic duct: The duct drains into the GB.

Type 4: A series of minute ducts that end blindly in the connective tissue of the GB bed. This is the only variant originally described by Luschka in his study. Therefore, it is wrong to use the terminology "duct of Luschka" for all variants of the subvesicle ducts.

22.3.6 Anatomy of the Critical View of Safety (CVS) (Fig. 22.10)

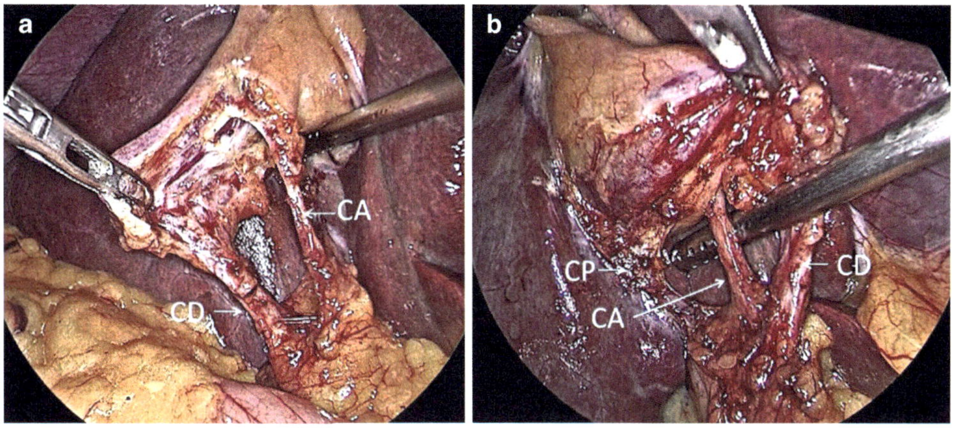

Fig. 22.10 CVS (**a**) anterior view and (**b**) posterior view. Hepatocystic triangle cleared of all fibrofatty tissue, leaving behind only two structures: the cystic duct (CD) and the cystic artery (CA). The distal 1/3 of the GB is dissected off the cystic plate (CP)

Key Points

- Variations related to GB include agenesis, floating, and left-sided GB.
- The right hepatic duct (RHD) is less angulated than the left hepatic duct (LHD). The LHD has a longer extrahepatic course (2–3 cm) and is located at the base of segment IV. The hilar plate is a condensation of fibrous tissue between the portal structures and Glisson's capsule at the hilum. Mobilizing the hilar plate (lowering of the hilar plate) exposes the hepatic hilum and the extrahepatic segment of the LHD, providing additional length of the duct for an optimal hepatico-jejunostomy.
- The larger extrahepatic segment and the angulation with the common hepatic duct (CHD) make the LHD more vulnerable to stasis and stone formation compared to the RHD
- Variation in the hilar confluence is noted in nearly 40% due to segmental ducts, more commonly that of the RHD, joining at different levels.
- The proximal bile duct is supplied by the hepatic arteries—right, left, and middle—as well as the cystic artery. The distal bile duct receives arterial blood from the posterior superior pancreaticoduodenal artery (SPDA), supraduodenal artery, gastroduodenal artery (GDA), and retroportal artery (RPA).
- The mid-CBD is mainly supplied by two axial vessels, the 3 o'clock and 9 o'clock arteries, which arise from the SPDA or GDA and connect with the right hepatic artery (RHA) and cystic artery, respectively.
- Cholecystectomy involves the identification of specific landmarks to guide safe dissection, exposure of the hepatocystic triangle (HCT) to delineate the cystic duct and artery, and mobilization of the GB from the cystic plate.
- Rouviere's sulcus (RS) represents the plane of the extrahepatic portal pedicle. To avoid injury to the CBD, the dissection of the GB should stay ventral to the plane connecting the sulcus and the base of segment 4.
- Careful dissection of the HCT is the most essential step in cholecystectomy to achieve the critical view of safety (CVS).
- Cystic artery is the most variable structure in the HCT.
- Cystic duct insertion into the CBD is variable; angular insertion is seen in 75%.
- To achieve CVS, the HCT is cleared of all fibrofatty tissue, leaving behind only two structures: the cystic duct and the cystic artery. The distal 1/3 of the GB is dissected off the cystic plate (CP).

Selected Reading

1. Adkins RB, Chapman WC, Reddy VS. Embryology, anatomy, and surgical applications of the extrahepatic biliary system. Surg Clin North Am. 2000;80:363–79.
2. Ibrarullah M, Mohanty L, Mishra A, Panda A, Sikora S. Anatomical appraisal of safe cholecystectomy: a prospective study. ANZ J Surg. 2023;93:1329–34.

Cholelithiasis

23

Mohammad Ibrarullah

Abstract

More than two-thirds of GS cases are asymptomatic when first detected. During follow-up, approximately 10–25% develop symptoms over the next 5–15 years. About 10–20% of all patients with GS are likely to develop acute cholecystitis, accounting for 1–2% of all symptomatic cases. Diagnosis of acute cholecystitis is based on clinical evaluation, laboratory tests, and imaging. The US is the primary imaging test for diagnosis. More advanced imaging, such as a CT scan or an MRI, is necessary to identify complications.

Keywords

Gallstone · Cholelithiasis · Cholecystitis

Cholelithiasis, or gallstones (GS), is the most common abdominal problem worldwide that requires surgery for treatment. The prevalence of GS varies widely based on age, sex, ethnicity, and geographical location. It is rare in the first two decades of life, but the incidence steadily increases with age. GS is 1.5–2 times more common in females than in males. Among different ethnic groups, Hispanics and Native Americans have very high prevalence rates, ranging from 20 to 40% and from 50 to 70%, respectively. The reported incidence in Asian countries is 3–10%, compared to 10–20% in Western countries.

23.1 Pathogenesis

The types of stones encountered in the biliary tract are cholesterol, black pigment, brown pigment, and mixed stones. Cholesterol stones account for more than two-thirds of all stones in Europe and America, whereas pigment stones are more common in Asian countries. The cholesterol and black pigment stones arise exclusively in the gallbladder (GB), while brown pigment stones develop in the bile duct, resulting from biliary infection (Table 23.1).

Supersaturation of bile with cholesterol, combined with accelerated nucleation facilitated by GB hypomotility, are the initial events in the formation of cholesterol crystals. These crystals, along with mucin in the GB, form biliary sludge that eventually leads to stone formation. Supersaturation of bile with calcium hydrogen bilirubinate is crucial for pigment stone formation. Its nucleation and polymerization in the GB, along with the deposition of inorganic salts like calcium carbonate and phosphate, result in black pigment stones. Brown pigment stones typically do not develop in the GB. Their pathogenesis has been discussed elsewhere (Fig. 23.1).

M. Ibrarullah (✉)
Department of Surgical Gastroenterology, Apollo Hospitals, Bhubaneswar, Odisha, India

M. Ibrarullah (ed.), *Recent Concepts in Gastrointestinal (GI) Surgery*, https://doi.org/10.1007/978-981-92-1118-0_23

Table 23.1 Conditions predisposing to gallstones

Genetic
Forty (years of age), female, fatty, fair, and fertile (5 "F"s)
Diabetes mellitus
Excessive calorie and fat consumption
Prolonged fasting and dieting
Bariatric surgery
Hyperlipidemia
Chronic liver disease
Inflammatory bowel disease
Short bowel syndrome
Pregnancy
Hemolytic anemia
Medications: Oral contraceptive pills, estrogen and progesterone supplements
GB hypomotility/stasis

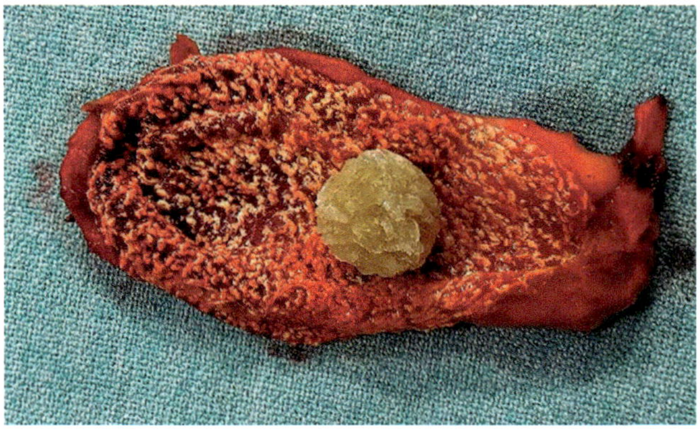

Fig. 23.1 Solitary cholesterol stone. The GB mucosa is showing extensive cholesterosis

23.2 Clinical Presentation

Gallstone presents in one of the following ways.

- Silent gallstone
- Biliary pain
- Acute cholecystitis and its complications
  - Empyema gallbladder
  - Gangrenous cholecystitis
    Gallbladder perforation
- Chronic cholecystitis and its complications
  - Cholecysto-enteric fistula and gallstone ileus
  - Mirizzi syndrome
    Xanthogranulomatous cholecystitis
- Choledocholithiasis ± cholangitis
- Acute pancreatitis
- Gallbladder cancer

23.3 Silent Gallstone

An estimated 50–75% of GS are silent at the time of detection. On follow-up, nearly 10–25% become symptomatic over the next 5–15 years, with an average of about 2% per year. When symptoms develop, chronic cholecystitis is the most common presentation, and GB cancer is the least frequent, at 8.8% and 0.4%, respectively. The predictors of symptomatic GS include female gender, young age, obesity, multiple stones, large stones, GB polyps, and chronic hemolytic anemia.

Most often, GS are found incidentally during ultrasound exams done for other conditions or routine health screenings. In women, GS are usually discovered incidentally on antenatal scans during pregnancy evaluations. Detecting GS requires a thorough assessment of the patient, including factors that may signal the need for cholecystectomy (Table 23.2).

Contrary to earlier practice, current guidelines do not recommend diabetes mellitus as an indication for prophylactic cholecystectomy. The risk of surgery in a well-controlled diabetic is the same as in a nondiabetic individual.

Table 23.2 Indications for cholecystectomy in silent gallstones

Porcelain GB
Associated GB polyps >1 cm in diam
Solitary large stone
Associated choledocholithiasis
Abdominal surgery for concomitant pathology
Patient scheduled for organ transplant and/or immunosuppression therapy
Geographical endemicity of gallbladder cancer
Long term parenteral nutrition
Chronic hemolytic conditions like sickle cell anemia

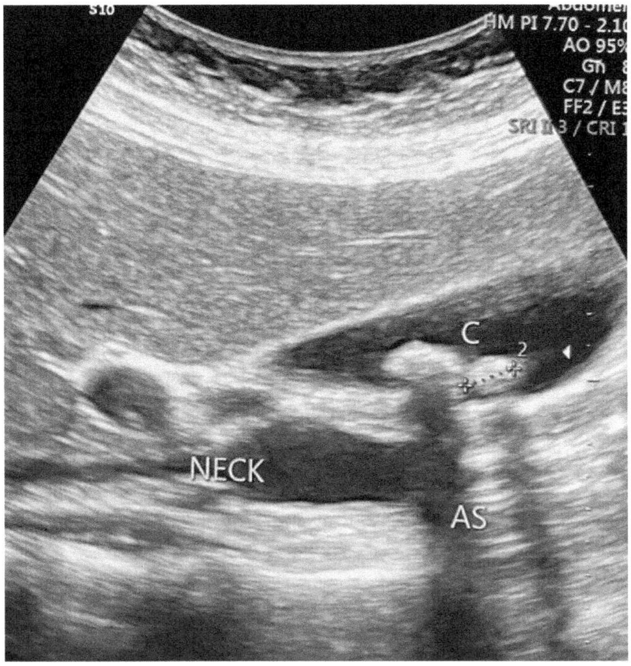

Fig. 23.2 Cholelithiasis with posterior acoustic shadowing on US examination

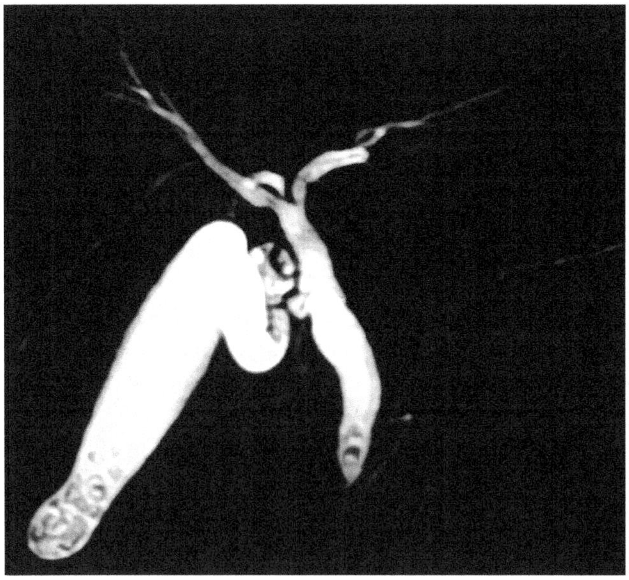

Fig. 23.3 Magnetic resonance cholangio-pancreatogram (MRCP) showing cholelithiasis and choledocholithiasis

23.4 Biliary Pain

Pain is the most common presenting symptom of GS. Biliary pain occurs due to smooth muscle contraction following a transient obstruction of the cystic duct by stone(s). The biliary pain usually lasts from a few minutes to several hours. Pain lasting more than 6 h suggests persistent obstruction and the development of acute cholecystitis. The pain may occur after a heavy fatty meal, but this is not specific. It is typically felt in the epigastrium or right upper quadrant of the abdomen, radiating to the interscapular region or right shoulder. Less frequently, the pain may be felt in the retrosternal area, left hypochondrium, or the central or lower abdomen.

Diagnosis is confirmed through ultrasound examination, which has an accuracy of over 95%. More advanced imaging techniques, such as CT scan, MRI, or endoscopic ultrasound (EUS), may be necessary to confirm or rule out any associated complications of GS. Blood tests are nonspecific if no complication is present. The pain usually subsides on its own but may require oral or parenteral analgesic and antispasmodic medications (Figs. 23.2 and 23.3).

23.5 Acute Cholecystitis

An estimated 10–20% of all patients with GS are likely to develop acute cholecystitis. It represents 1–2% of all cases of symptomatic GS.

23.5.1 Pathogenesis

Persistent obstruction of the cystic duct by GB stone leads to distention, stretching, and ischemia of the GB wall, initiating an inflammatory response. Bile in the obstructed GB gets infected by the transmigration of gut bacteria. The incidence of infection in unobstructed GB bile is less than 10%, but it increases to 70–80% in cases of acute cholecystitis. Continued inflammation can result in gangrene, perforation of the GB and biliary peritonitis.

23.5.2 Clinical Presentation

- Persistent biliary pain (as described above). Pain may be absent or quite vague in diabetics, immunocompromised, or elderly patients.

- Nausea, vomiting
- Fever, tachycardia, high-grade fever with chills indicate empyema GB
- Mild icterus may result from temporary liver dysfunction or compression of the bile duct by the distended GB. Moderate to severe icterus could indicate associated choledocholithiasis or GB gangrene, or perforation.
- Guarding, rigidity, and tenderness of the right upper quadrant (Murphy's sign)
- Generalized guarding, rigidity of the abdomen, and signs of peritonitis and systemic sepsis appear when inflammation continues unabated and GB gangrene or perforation develops.

23.6 Acute Acalculous Cholecystitis

Acalculous cholecystitis accounts for 5–10% of all cases of acute cholecystitis. It is seen in the following clinical settings:

- Patients in the intensive care unit
- Trauma
- Burn
- Multiorgan failure
- Sepsis
- Immunodeficiency

The pathogenesis of acalculous cholecystitis is not well understood. It is likely caused by a combination of factors such as GB stasis, infection, ischemia, increased cortisol and decreased cholecystokinin levels, and gut-derived toxins, which trigger inflammation. Usually painless at the start, acalculous cholecystitis presents with worsening abdominal signs and ongoing sepsis in a critically ill patient. The gallbladder is more vulnerable to complications, possibly due to these underlying factors or the delay in diagnosis. A high level of suspicion and routine abdominal screening are essential to identify the disease.

23.7 Gallbladder Perforation (Modified Niemier's Classification)

The incidence of GB perforation is 2–10% of all cases of acute cholecystitis (Table 23.3).

Table 23.3 Gallbladder perforation: Classification

Type	Presentation	Clinical features
1	Acute perforation	Biliary peritonitis and sepsis
2	Subacute perforation. Pericholecystic abscess	Pain, fever, ongoing sepsis
3	Chronic perforation. Cholecystobiliary or cholecystoenteric fistula	Features of Mirizzi syndrome. Cholecystoenteric fistula may present as recurrent fever, gallstone ileus, or aerobilia
4	Acute on chronic perforation. GB perforation in a case of preexisting cholecysto-biliary/enteric fistula	Biliary peritonitis and sepsis

23.7.1 Investigations

- Hematological: Polymorphonuclear leucocytosis is often present. However, leucopenia at this stage may indicate severe sepsis.
- Inflammatory markers: Raised CRP
- Biochemical: All liver enzymes—such as serum transaminase, transpeptidase, alkaline phosphatase, and gamma-glutamyl transpeptidase—may show mild to moderate elevation. However, in about 10% of patients, these enzymes can be elevated up to ten times, indicating sepsis-induced hepatic dysfunction. The levels usually return to normal quickly once sepsis is under control. Mild elevation of serum bilirubin is observed in 10–20% of patients. A bilirubin level higher than 4 mg/dL requires ruling out a concomitant common bile duct stone or GB perforation.
- Ultrasonography (US): US has a sensitivity of 80% and a specificity of 88% for diagnosing acute calculous cholecystitis. The typical findings are,
  - Distended and thick-walled GB. The wall thickness is usually >4 mm
  - Stone impacted in Hartman's pouch or cystic duct
  - GB wall edema
  - Pericholecystic fluid. A thin rim of fluid around GB suggests acute inflammation. A fluid pocket and/or breach in the GB wall suggest gangrene/perforation.
  - A linear echogenic structure appearing as an intraluminal flap is suggestive of gangrenous cholecystitis
  - Probe tenderness in the right hypochondrium (Murphy's sign)
- Contrast-enhanced computed tomography (CECT): CECT is indicated to assess the severity of cholecystitis and also to diagnose complications. The various findings are,
  - Hypo or hyperattenuating GS. It is important to note that GS may not be delineated clearly on a CT scan.
  - Pericholecystic inflammatory fat stranding.
  - Edematous hyperattenuation of the adjacent liver bed known as "transient hepatic attenuation difference."
  - Presence of intraluminal or intramural gas suggesting emphysematous cholecystitis.
  - Gangrenous cholecystitis is diagnosed by the presence of intraluminal membranes, gas within the GB wall or lumen, irregular or discontinuous mural enhancement,

or a breach in the GB wall. Alternating mural hypo- and hyperattenuating foci are said to be specific signs of necrosis on CT.

- Magnetic resonance imaging (MRI): MRI scan is indicated to confirm acute cholecystitis, identify complications, and choledocholithiasis in patients with altered liver function test and jaundice. The diagnostic criteria are
  - GB enlargement (long axis >8 cm, short axis >4 cm)
  - GB wall thickness >4 mm
  - Fluid accumulation around the GB
  - Linear shadows in the fatty tissue around the GB
  - Asymmetry and focal intramural hyperintensity on fat-suppressed T2-weighted image signifying ulceration, hemorrhage, or microabscess due to the GB wall gangrene

Though MRI provides the same information as a CT scan with respect to GB, stones are delineated better on MRI as compared to CT scan. Hence, this can be used as an alternative in patients in whom a CT scan is contraindicated. MRI is the investigation of choice to rule out choledocholithiasis in a patient with elevated liver enzymes and serum bilirubin.

- Cholescintigraphy (Tc99m HIDA scan) is a much-hyped investigation in the diagnosis of acute cholecystitis. The diagnosis relies on the non-visualization of the GB and the visualization of the rest of the biliary tract, along with the excretion of the radioisotope into the duodenum. Cystic duct obstruction, which causes non-visualization of the GB, can also occur in longstanding cholelithiasis and chronic cholecystitis, thereby limiting its usefulness in these patients when an acute attack occurs. Additionally, the test has limitations in assessing the severity of acute cholecystitis. However, it remains useful for diagnosing acalculous cholecystitis. Both non-visualization of the GB when the cystic duct is obstructed and bile leaks from a perforated GB with a patent cystic duct can be reliably confirmed by isotope scan.

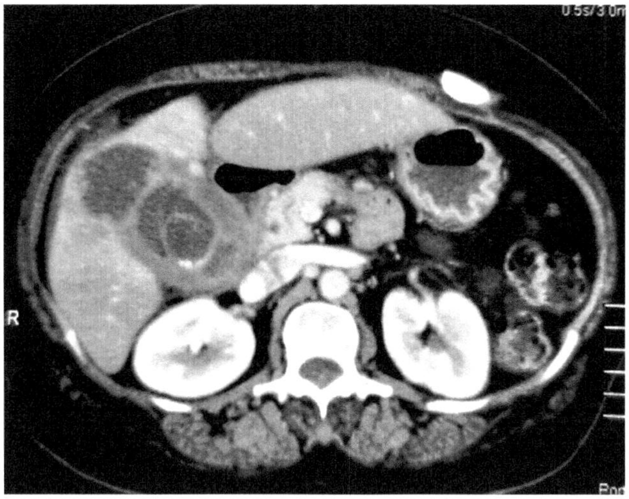

Fig. 23.4 CT scan image of acute gangrenous cholecystitis. Note the thick GB wall, intraluminal membrane, and the localized perforation at the fundus

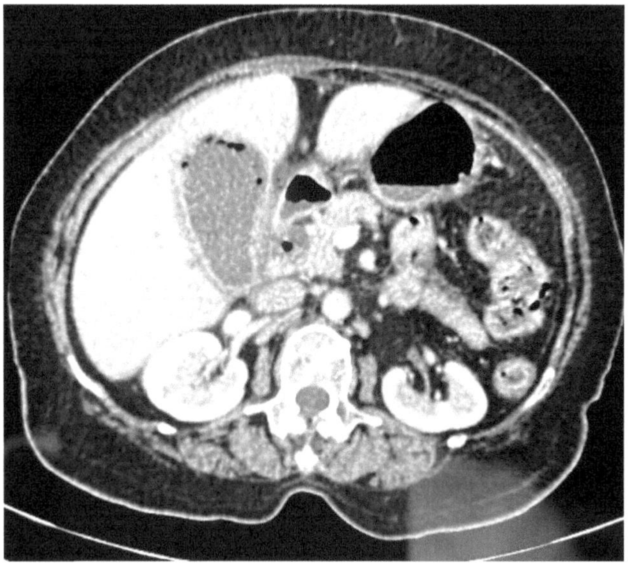

Fig. 23.5 Emphysematous cholecystitis. (Note the air bubbles inside GB)

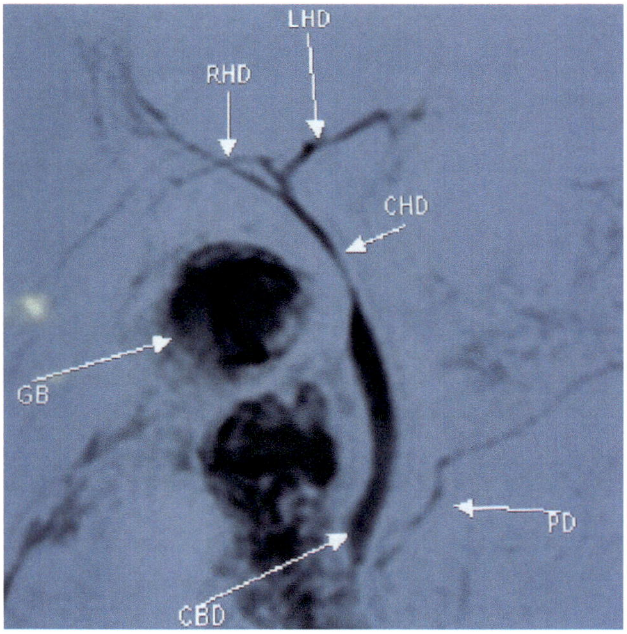

Fig. 23.6 MRCP showing smooth eccentric compression of the common hepatic duct by the distended GB in acute cholecystitis

23.7.2 Management

Moderate to severe acute cholecystitis requires the patient to be hospitalized. Oral intake is restricted; intravenous fluid, analgesics, and broad-spectrum antibiotics are started. After initial resuscitation, blood tests and imaging are performed to confirm the diagnosis and assess severity. Presence of any organ system dysfunction and co-morbidity is ascertained for risk stratification for cholecystectomy (Tables 23.4 and 23.5).

23.7.3 Cholecystectomy in Acute Cholecystitis

The current concept and recommendations are as follows.

- Early cholecystectomy is considered as safe as delayed elective cholecystectomy and offers the advantage of earlier recovery from the disease and lower hospitalization costs.
- Early cholecystectomy is advised within 10 days of symptom onset.

Table 23.4 Diagnosis of acute cholecystitis

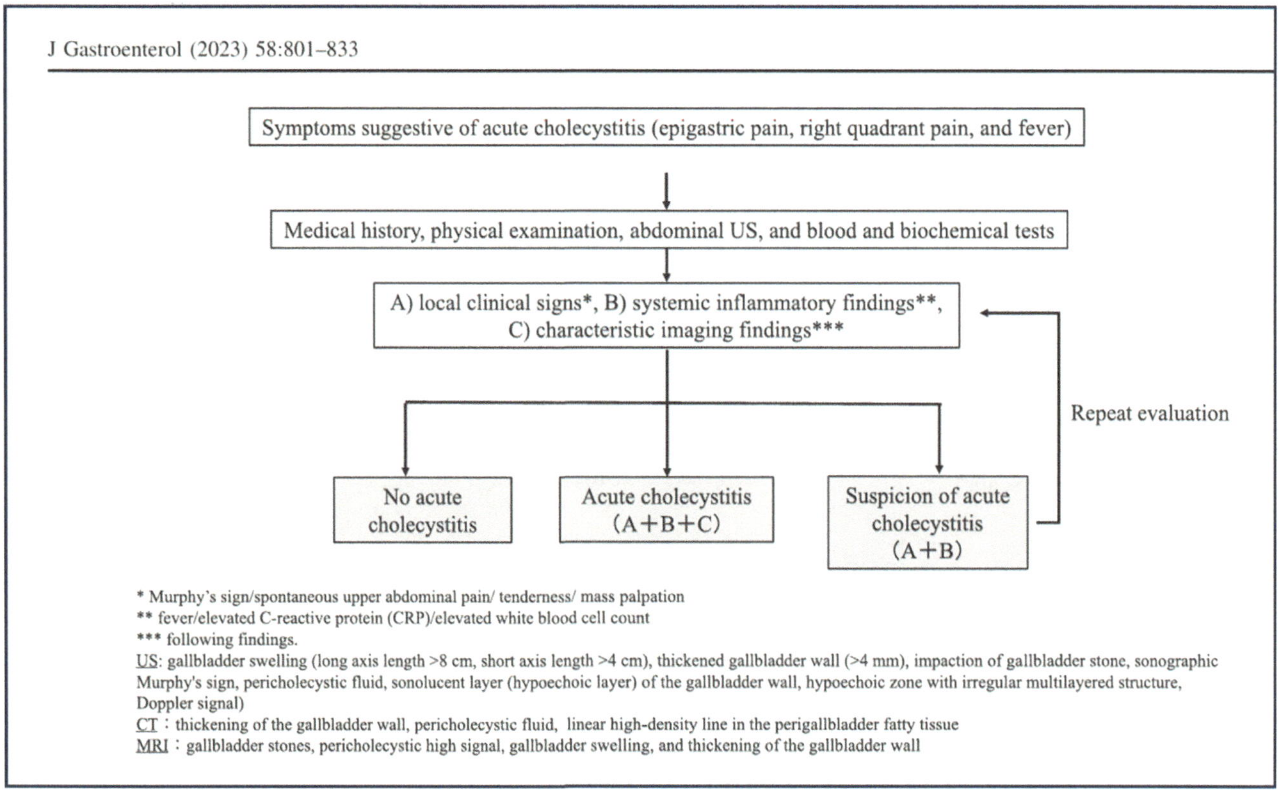

Reproduced from Ref. [2] (open access)

Table 23.5 Severity assessment criteria of acute cholecystitis (Tokyo Guidelines- TG 18)

Grade	Features
I (mild)	Mild inflammatory changes in the GB No organ dysfunction
II (moderate)	Elevated WBC count (>18,000/mm^3) Palpable tender mass in the right upper abdominal quadrant Duration of complaints >72 h Marked local inflammation (gangrenous cholecystitis, pericholecystic abscess, hepatic abscess, biliary peritonitis, emphysematous cholecystitis)
III (severe)	Cardiovascular dysfunction: hypotension requiring vasopressor support Neurological dysfunction: decreased level of consciousness Respiratory dysfunction: PaO_2/FiO_2 ratio <300. Renal dysfunction: oliguria, creatinine >2.0 mg/dl Hepatic dysfunction: PT-INR >1.56 Hematological dysfunction: platelet count <100,000/mm

- When early cholecystectomy is not feasible, surgery should be scheduled electively after a waiting period of 4–6 weeks to allow inflammation to subside.
- Cholecystectomy during this period is considered unsafe and should only be attempted in cases of unresolving cholecystitis, complications like gangrene or perforation, or recurrence of an attack.
- Laparoscopic cholecystectomy, despite initial reservations, is the preferred procedure and has better outcomes compared to open cholecystectomy for acute cholecystitis.
- Mild and moderately severe cases with minimal systemic comorbidities are candidates for laparoscopic cholecystectomy.
- Individuals with a severe form of the disease should be resuscitated in the intensive care unit. Early cholecystectomy should only be attempted if the patient responds adequately to resuscitative measures. Non-surgical GB drainage is performed for ongoing sepsis despite adequate conservative measures.
- *Laparoscopic cholecystectomy for acute cholecystitis should only be performed by an experienced surgeon and in centers properly equipped to manage complications and care for seriously ill patients.*

23.7.4 Gallbladder Drainage Procedures

Gallbladder drainage is indicated in high-surgical-risk patients with ongoing sepsis. The available techniques are

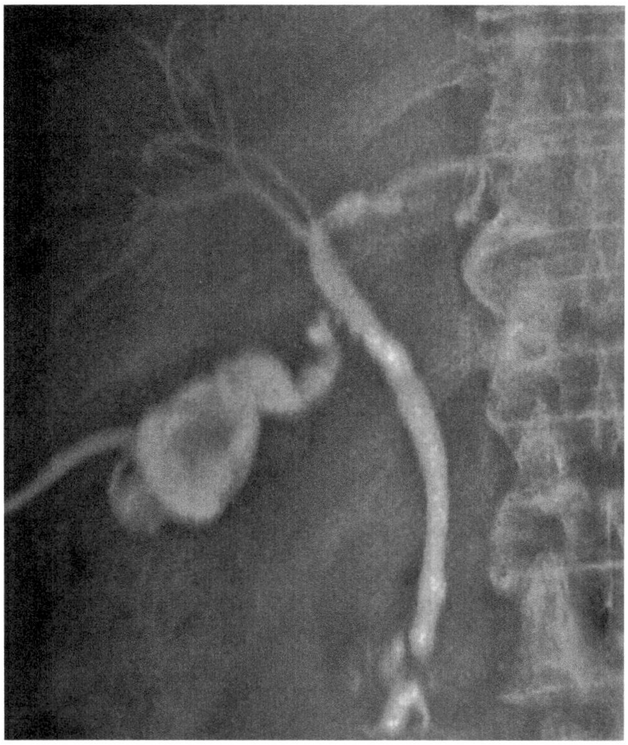

Fig. 23.7 Tube cholangiogram in a patient with PTGBD for acute acalculous cholecystitis

- Percutaneous transhepatic GB drainage (PTGBD)
- Endoscopic transpapillary GB drainage (ETGBD)
- EUS-guided GB drainage (EUS-GBD)

PTGBD (percutaneous cholecystostomy), performed under image guidance, is the technically easiest and most effective procedure. It is successful in over 90% of patients, and the percutaneously placed catheter helps drain the inflamed GB as well as any localized perforation (type-2 GB perforation). However, the procedure is contraindicated in cases of ascites or coagulation disorders. Golden yellow bile through the drainage catheter indicates that the cystic duct has reopened. A tube cholangiogram confirms this and can also detect stones in the GB or bile duct. In cases of acalculous cholecystitis, the drainage catheter can be removed after 4–6 weeks. For patients with blocked cystic ducts or gallstones, drainage should continue until they are fit for elective cholecystectomy (Fig. 23.7).

ETGBD is an alternative to PTGBD and also helps drain the obstructed bile duct to relieve cholangitis. It requires a skilled endoscopist to perform, and accessing an obstructed cystic duct for gallbladder drainage may not always be possible. In EUS-GBD, the GB is drained internally by placing a lumen-apposing stent. This procedure has not yet gained widespread acceptance due to limited experience and its technical difficulty. Successful GB drainage controls sepsis and alleviates the patient's symptoms.

Key Points

- Cholelithiasis is a global problem
- Cholesterol is the dominant component of gallstones.
- Supersaturation of bile with cholesterol or bile pigment is the initiating event in the formation of gallstones. Cholesterol and black pigment stones develop in the gallbladder, while brown pigment stones form in the bile duct due to infection.
- More than two-thirds of GS cases are asymptomatic when first detected. During follow-up, approximately 10–25% develop symptoms over the next 5–15 years.
- Not all cases of asymptomatic GS require cholecystectomy; there are specific indications for it.
- 10–20% of all patients with GS are likely to develop acute cholecystitis, accounting for 1–2% of all symptomatic cases.
- Diagnosis of acute cholecystitis is based on clinical evaluation, laboratory tests, and imaging.
- The US is the primary imaging test for diagnosis. More advanced imaging, such as a CT scan or an MRI, is necessary to identify complications.
- Early cholecystectomy within 10 days of disease onset is recommended for mild and moderately severe disease.
- Severe disease should be managed conservatively in the intensive care unit; GB drainage is necessary for ongoing sepsis.
- Percutaneous GB drainage is feasible and effective in most cases.
- Laparoscopic cholecystectomy is regarded as better than open cholecystectomy in cases of acute cholecystitis.
- Avoid surgery in the second week unless it is necessary due to unresolved cholecystitis or complications.
- Patients responding to conservative treatment should undergo an elective cholecystectomy 4–6 weeks later.

Selected Reading

1. Morris-Stiff G, Sarvepalli S, Hu B, et al. The natural history of asymptomatic gallstones: a longitudinal study and prediction model. Clin Gastroenterol Hepatol. 2023;21:319–27.
2. Fujita N, Yasuda I, Endo I, et al. Evidence-based clinical practice guidelines for cholelithiasis 2021. J Gastroenterol. 2023;58:801–33.
3. Yokoe M, Hata J, Takada T. Tokyo guidelines 2018: diagnostic criteria and severity grading of acute cholecystitis (with videos). J Hepatobiliary Pancreat Sci. 2018;25:41–54.
4. Kohji Okamoto K, Suzuki K, Takada T, et al. Tokyo guidelines 2018: flowchart for the management of acute cholecystitis. J Hepatobiliary Pancreat Sci. 2018;25:55–72.

Chronic Cholecystitis and Its Complications

24

Mohammad Ibrarullah

Abstract

Cholecysto-duodenal fistula is the most common type of cholecystoenteric fistula (CEF). Mirizzi syndrome is defined as bile duct obstruction by impaction or erosion of stone/s in Hartman's pouch or cystic duct. Xanthogranulomatous cholecystitis is a complication of longstanding cholelithiasis that closely mimics gallbladder cancer—clinically, radiologically, and during surgery.

Keywords

Cholecystitis · Mirizzi syndrome · Xanthogranulomatous cholecystitis

Chronic cholecystitis, characterized by fibrosis of the gallbladder (GB) wall and infiltration by chronic inflammatory cells, develops from the continued presence of stones within the GB. The GB becomes thick-walled and contracted. Uncomplicated chronic cholecystitis may be asymptomatic (silent GB) or present with recurrent biliary pain. Persistent stones, their migration through the cystic duct, or pressure necrosis can lead to various complications such as choledocholithiasis, cholecysto-enteric fistula, Mirizzi syndrome, xanthogranulomatous cholecystitis, or carcinoma.

24.1 Cholecysto-Enteric Fistula and Gallstone Ileus

Recurrent inflammation causes adhesion between the GB and the digestive tract. Erosion caused by a stone and inflammatory rupture of the GB lead to the formation of a cholecysto-enteric fistula (CEF). In over 90% of cases, the fistula involves the stomach or duodenum, with less frequent involvement of the small and large intestines. Gallstone ileus, which is an intestinal obstruction caused by a gallstone (GS), has been reported in 0.3–0.5% of patients with symptomatic disease. The obstructing stone typically enters the intestine through the CEF. The terminal ileum is the most common site of obstruction (60%), followed by the proximal ileum (24%) and the jejunum (9%). Duodenal obstruction due to GS, known as Bouveret's syndrome, is rare and accounts for 1–3% of all gallstone ileus cases. The typical symptoms include signs of intestinal or duodenal obstruction in patients with a history of cholelithiasis.

On a plain X-ray, a radio-opaque stone, changes in its position on serial X-rays, pneumobilia, and intestinal obstruction (Rigler's triad and tetrad) when present (in less than 50%) are considered diagnostic. Additional findings of chronic cholecystitis on ultrasound (US) increase diagnostic sensitivity to 74%. Contrast-enhanced CT scan has a specificity and sensitivity of over 90% in diagnosing GS ileus. However, the findings of cholecystoduodenal fistula on endoscopy, chronic cholecystitis with or without GS on US, and features of intestinal obstruction on X-ray can form an important triad (Ibrarullah's triad) in diagnosing GS ileus.

Endoscopic fragmentation and extraction or dislodgment of the impacted stone often suffice to relieve duodenal obstruction. Rarely, a duodenotomy may be necessary to remove the offending stone. In cases of intestinal obstruction, enterotomy and stone removal can be performed on a very sick patient, postponing cholecystectomy for another day, particularly if the GB is already emptied of stones (which is often the case). However, an attempt should be made to perform a complete surgery in a patient who is fit. The cholecysto-enteric fistula should be disconnected, and cholecystectomy performed along with enterotomy and stone extraction (Fig. 24.1).

M. Ibrarullah (✉)
Department of Surgical Gastroenterology, Apollo Hospitals, Bhubaneswar, Odisha, India

M. Ibrarullah (ed.), *Recent Concepts in Gastrointestinal (GI) Surgery*, https://doi.org/10.1007/978-981-92-1118-0_24

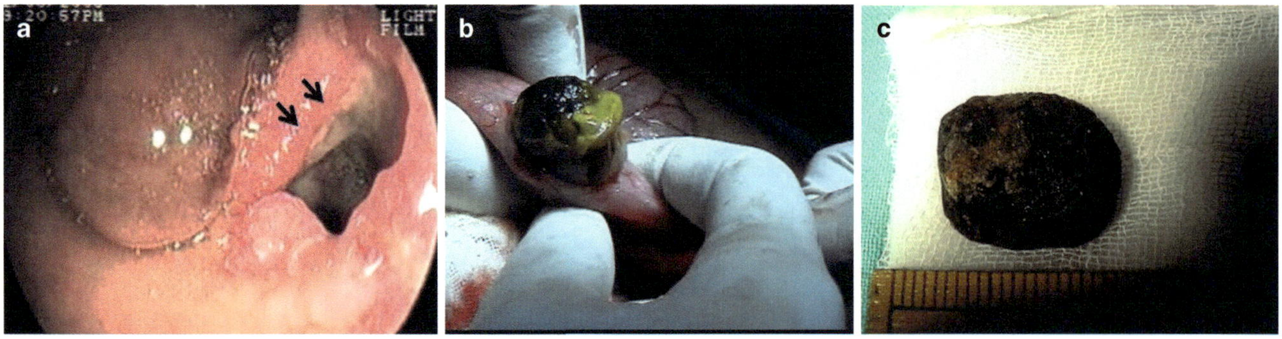

Fig. 24.1 (**a**) Endoscopic appearance of the duodenal bulb showing cholecysto-duodenal fistula (arrows) that allowed passage of a big stone, causing intestinal obstruction. (**b**) Retrieval of the offending stone by enterotomy. (**c**) The retrieved stone

24.2 Mirizzi Syndrome

Mirizzi syndrome, as described by PL Mirizzi in 1948, referred to biliary obstruction caused by stone(s) in the cystic duct, leading to inflammation and spasm of the common hepatic duct sphincter; the entity was therefore called "functional hepatic syndrome." However, subsequent studies refuted the existence of any such sphincter, and the obstruction was shown to be purely mechanical. Currently, it is defined as bile duct obstruction due to impaction or erosion of stone(s) in Hartman's pouch or the cystic duct.

Pathogenesis and Classification: The incidence of MS ranges from 0.3% to 6% among all cases of cholelithiasis and from 0.05% to 4% in all patients undergoing cholecystectomy. Cystic duct occlusion caused by stones and inflammation leads to GB distension and causes Hartman's pouch to come into contact with the common hepatic duct or common bile duct (hereafter called the common duct). Continued presence of stones and inflammation results in pressure necrosis and fistula formation. McSherry classified MS into two types: Type I—bile duct obstruction by external compression, and Type II—cholecystobiliary fistula (CBF). Cendes further subclassified the CBF based on the extent of circumferential erosion of the common duct (CD) and proposed a new classification. The different types according to this classification and their relative incidence are shown in the table. Each type is considered to represent a more advanced stage than the previous one (Table 24.1).

However, since the extent of bile duct erosion, which forms the basis of this classification, is not amenable to detection on preoperative imaging, the original classification as proposed by McSherry is still popular with surgeons and also the radiologists who play an essential role in the preoperative diagnosis of these patients.

24.2.1 Clinical Feature

Mirizzi syndrome occurs more frequently in females, likely due to the higher prevalence of GS in this group. The average age at presentation ranges from 21 to 90 years, highlighting that the syndrome is a complication of long-standing cholelithiasis. Pain is the most common presenting symptom, reported in 54–100% of patients, followed by jaundice in 24–100%, and cholangitis in 6–35%. Charcot's biliary triad is present in 44–71% of cases. Painless jaundice may often mimic malignant biliary obstruction. About one-third of patients have also been reported to have acute cholecystitis. Less common presentations include acute pancreatitis, gallbladder perforation, gallstone ileus, and weight loss. Hepatomegaly is common, and a hard GB lump mimicking carcinoma may be palpable in 22% of patients. Rarely, patients may be asymptomatic despite complete erosion of the common duct. The frequent association of xanthogranulomatous cholecystitis and GB cancer in MS may reflect longstanding cholelithiasis.

24.2.2 Diagnosis

Liver function tests show a cholestatic pattern similar to choledocholithiasis. Serum bilirubin levels range from normal to as high as 30 mg/dl, with an average of 7–10 mg/dl. Serum alkaline phosphatase may increase approximately three to tenfold. However, imaging studies remain the primary method for preoperative diagnosis. Ultrasound (US) is a good screening test with a sensitivity of 23–46%. Although the most common diagnosis suggested is choledocholithiasis, specific findings of MS on US include a small, contracted GB containing stones, an echogenic nodule or calculus in the CD, mild to moderate dilatation of the proximal biliary radicals, and a normal-sized or untraced bile duct distal to the nodule or stone. The demonstration of a longitudinal septum-like structure in the CD, resulting from the dilated cystic duct running parallel to the bile duct, may also suggest MS in suspected cases. Intraductal ultrasound (IDUS) has been reported to be highly sensitive (97%) and specific (100%). When performed, computed tomography (CT) can confirm US findings. Additionally, an irregular cavity near the neck of the GB containing a protruding stone is quite characteristic of MS. The duodenum and colon may appear in close proximity to the GB, indicating a bilioenteric fistula, which

Table 24.1 Types, incidence, and management of Mirizzi syndrome

Type	Pathology	Incidence	Management
1	Obstruction of the CD by stone/s impacted in the Hartman's pouch or the cystic duct	11%	Partial cholecystectomy
II	CBF with erosion of less than 1/3 of the circumference of the CD	41%	Repair of the fistula or choledochoplasty over T-tube
III	Erosion of up to 2/3 of the circumference of the CD	44%.	Choledochoplasty, T-tube drainage
IV	Complete or near destruction of the CD wall by the offending stone	4%	Bilio-enteric anastomosis
V	CBF with cholecystoenteric fistula (a) without gallstone ileus and (b) with gallstone ileus	Up to 29%[a]	Partial cholecystectomy ± choledochoplasty/bilioenteric anastomosis + repair of the enterotomy

[a]Includes all variants of Mirizzi syndrome with bilioenteric fistula

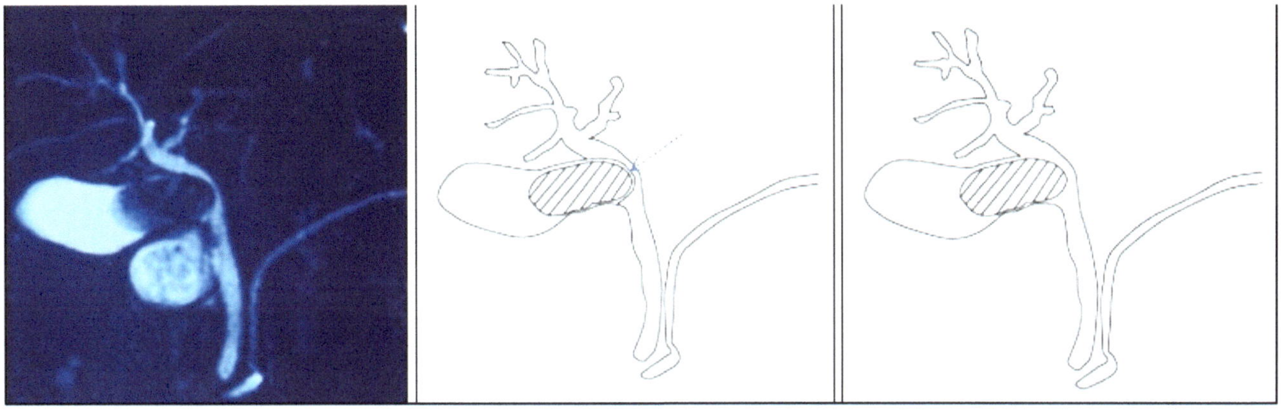

Fig. 24.2 (**a**) Magnetic resonance cholangiopancreatogram (MRCP) showing the typical appearance of Mirizzi syndrome. A large protruding GB stone, causing an eccentric filling defect in the mid-bile duct. (**b**) Mirizzi syndrome type I: Representative sketch to depict external compression of the bile duct by the stone in the Hartman's pouch. Note the intact GB wall (arrow) in relation to the bile duct. (**c**) Mirizzi syndrome type II: Erosion of the stone into the bile duct, causing cholecystobiliary fistula. Note the missing common wall between Hartman's pouch and the bile duct

is common in these patients. Cholangiography remains the most reliable method for preoperative diagnosis. Typical findings include (i) a contracted GB, (ii) a smooth, eccentric, or excavating defect on the lateral wall of the common duct or a "peg"-shaped deformity of the mid-common bile duct containing a large stone, (iii) dilated intrahepatic biliary radicals, and (iv) dilatation of the CD proximal to the obstruction with a normal distal duct. Similar cholangiographic features may also result from GB or cystic duct cancer. However, the contour of the filling defect may be irregular in malignancy, contrasting with the smooth outline of a stone. Magnetic resonance cholangio-pancreatogram (MRCP) is preferred over endoscopic retrograde cholangiogram (ERC) because it is non-invasive. Additionally, T2-weighted images can differentiate a neoplastic mass from an inflammatory one, which may not be possible with US or CT scan. Combining MRCP and CT scan in diagnosis offers a specificity, sensitivity, and accuracy over 90%. ERC and stenting are less often used for diagnosis but more commonly for preoperative biliary drainage and for identifying and protecting the bile duct during cholecystectomy (Figs. 24.2, 24.3, 24.4 and 24.5).

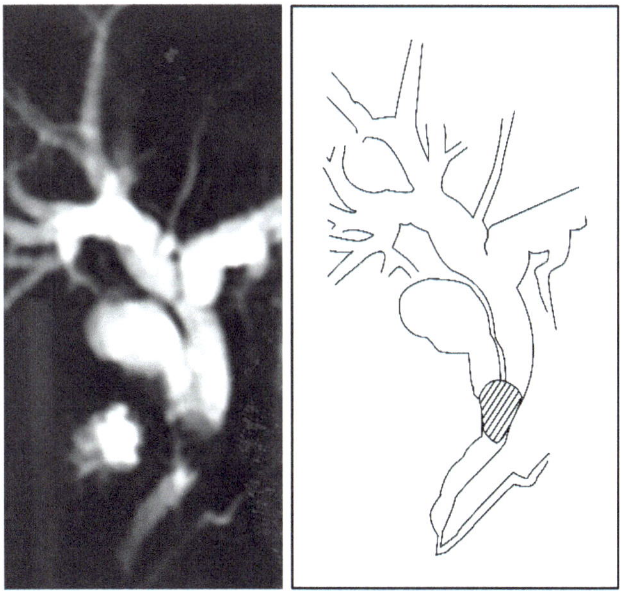

Fig. 24.3 (**a**) MRCP showing obstruction by a cystic duct stone eroding into the bile duct. (**b**) Representative sketch of the same

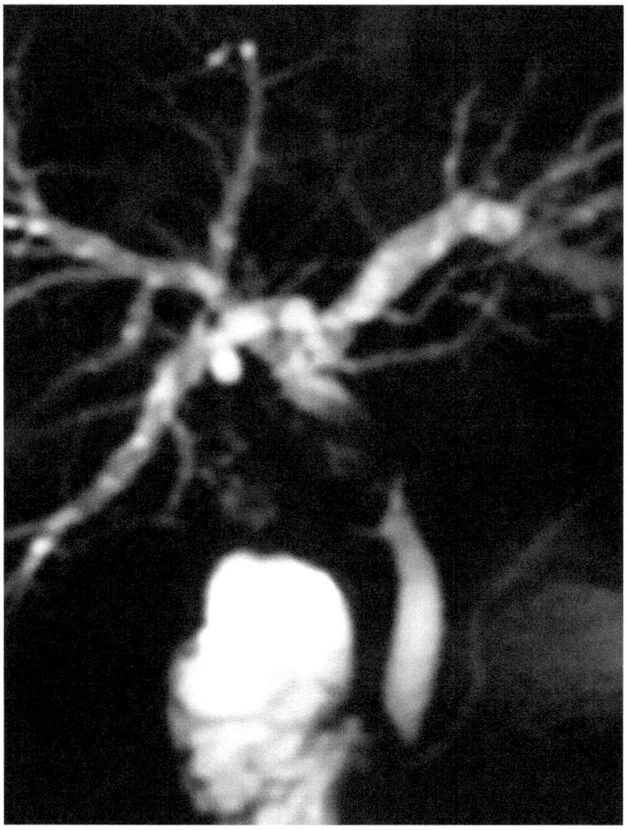

Fig. 24.4 Mirizzi syndrome: Typical appearance on cholangiogram. Contracted GB, a large stone in GB causing eccentric filling defect in the mid-bile duct, dilated proximal bile duct and intrahepatic ducts, and Collapsed distal bile duct with a peg-shaped filling defect

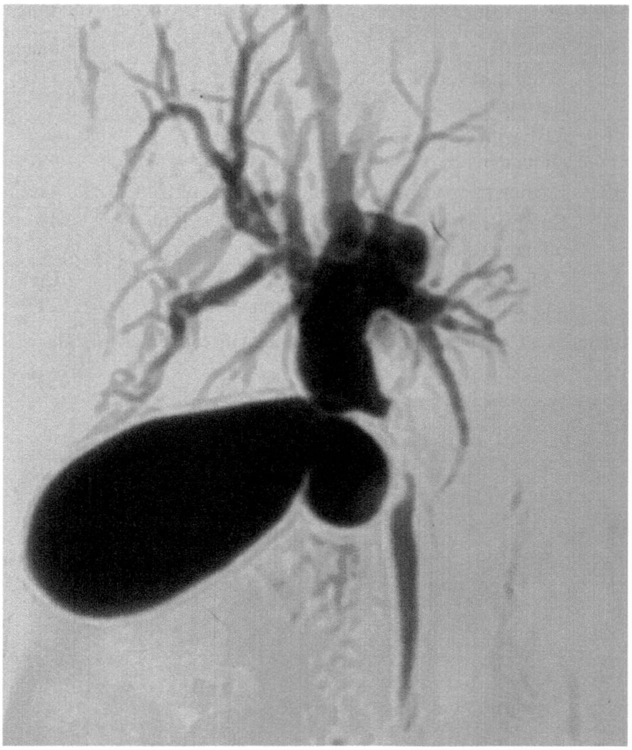

Fig. 24.5 Carcinoma of the GB neck region mimicking Mirizzi syndrome on MRCP. Smooth eccentric filling defect in the mid common duct by the tumor is unusual

24.2.3 Management

Frozen Calot's triangle, presence of a bilioenteric fistula, and coexistence of carcinoma in a significant number of patients require extra caution during cholecystectomy. Inadequate or improper surgery risks bile duct injury or long-term stricture formation.

Operative Strategy: MS was initially considered an absolute contradiction for laparoscopic cholecystectomy. However, with experience, laparoscopy can be attempted with the readiness to convert if dissection and identification of structures become difficult. A very high conversion rate, nearly half of the patients, has been reported with this approach. An antegrade approach is the standard recommendation for suspected or confirmed cases of MS. The fundus of the GB is opened, and the stone(s) are extracted. In rare instances, when the Hartman's pouch or cystic duct lies behind the CBD, retrieving the offending stone may be challenging. A transcholedochal approach has been suggested in such cases. A gush of bile when the stone is removed indicates the presence of CBF. Assessing the extent of bile duct erosion at this point guides the subsequent management. In the absence of bile duct erosion, i.e., type I variety, partial cholecystectomy alone is sufficient. After removing the stone, the Hartman's pouch or the parallel cystic duct is left intact. The inflammatory adhesion between these structures and the bile duct prevents dissection in this area and may cause injury if insisted upon. In most cases of CBF, the defect in the CD can be managed by leaving a cuff of the GB around the fistula, which is then approximated—a procedure known as choledochoplasty (Fig. 24.6). The CD in such cases should be drained with a T-tube placed either through the fistula itself or through a fresh choledochotomy, preferably. An increased incidence of bile leak has been reported when the tube is brought out through the fistula rather than through a choledochotomy. When bile duct erosion is extensive, performing a bilioenteric anastomosis is the most appropriate option to prevent late stricture formation. Possible procedures include hepatico-jejunostomy (end-to-side or side-to-side), choledocho-duodenostomy, or cholecysto-

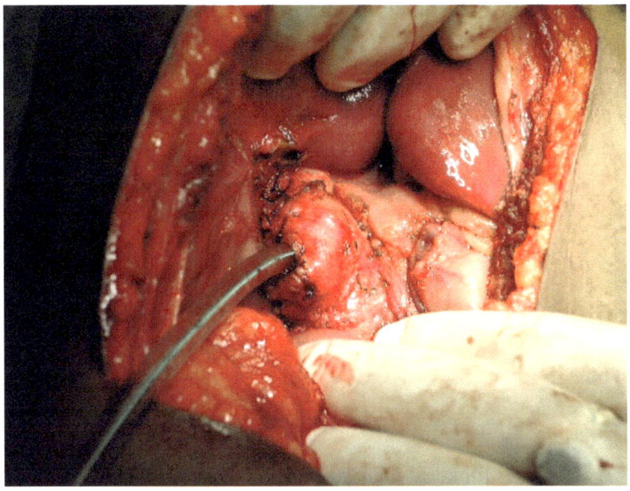

Fig. 24.6 Choledochoplasty for Mirizzi syndrome type II: Repair of the cholecystobiliary fistula with a GB cuff around the T-tube placed in the bile duct

choledocho-duodenostomy. Treatment options based on the extent of bile duct erosion are outlined in the table. Concomitant choledocholithiasis has been reported in 35–62% of patients with MS, requiring preoperative endoscopic clearance or intraoperative exploration of the common duct. Cholangioscopy-guided lithotripsy has also been used to fragment and clear obstructing stones. A frozen section biopsy may be performed if malignancy is suspected.

24.3 Xanthogranulomatous Cholecystitis

Xanthogranulomatous cholecystitis (XGC) is considered a complication of long-standing cholelithiasis, recurrent acute, and chronic cholecystitis (CC). The condition is significant because of its clinical, radiological, and morphological similarities to, as well as its association with, gallbladder cancer (GBC). The incidence of XGC varies geographically, ranging from 1% to 2% of all cholecystectomy specimens in reports from Europe and America, to as much as 10% in reports from India.

24.3.1 Pathogenesis

Mucosal ulceration and/or rupture of the Rokitansky-Aschoff sinuses, caused by cholelithiasis, cystic duct obstruction, and acute or chronic cholecystitis, results in the extravasation of bile into the interstitial tissue. This triggers an intense inflammatory response, leading to the accumulation of fibroblasts and granuloma formation, which includes foamy histiocytes (lipid-laden macrophages or xanthoma cells), lymphocytes, plasma cells, polymorphonuclear leukocytes, and giant cells. Extensive fibrosis, with focal xanthogranulomas, is characteristic of the disease. These xanthogranulomas appear as yellow submucosal nodules or confluent bands in the GB wall. Inflammation extending beyond the GB wall to adjacent organs can cause fistula formation. The xanthomatous process can also involve the common bile duct (CBD), leading to stricture formation. Concurrent gallbladder carcinoma (GBC) is found in 1–5% of all XGC cases, though some reports from India indicate a high incidence of up to 20%. Similarly, 10–20% of GBC specimens can show coexisting XGC.

24.3.2 Clinical Features

XGC occurs with equal frequency in both males and females, unlike cholelithiasis, which is three to four times more common in females than in males. The mean age of presentation is in the fifth and sixth decades of life. Pain is present in more than 80% of patients. Nausea, vomiting, anorexia, and weight loss are less common symptoms. A positive Murphy's sign is noted in approximately 50%, jaundice in 20%, and a right upper quadrant mass in 10% of patients.

24.3.3 Diagnosis

Laboratory investigations are non-specific. A preoperative diagnosis is often made on imaging studies.

24.3.4 Ultrasonography

US findings in XGC include diffuse thickening of the GB wall with hypoechoic nodules or bands. Intramural hypoechoic nodules strongly suggest XGC but are not specific, as this appearance is also seen in conditions like intramural abscesses, cholesterosis, and adenomyomatosis. Cholelithiasis is present in the majority. Additional findings in XGC include a GB mass, subhepatic fluid collection, obliteration of the GB and liver interface, and, rarely, aerobilia when a bilioenteric fistula (such as with the duodenum or colon) is present.

24.3.5 Contrast-Enhanced Computed Tomography (CECT)

CECT findings: (Figs. 24.7 and 24.8)

- Cholelithiasis
- Diffuse and symmetrical thickening of the GB wall, measuring between 5 and 15 mm, in over 85% of cases. Focal or asymmetric thickening is less common and may suggest malignancy.
- Intramural hypodense nodules or bands representing xanthogranuloma.

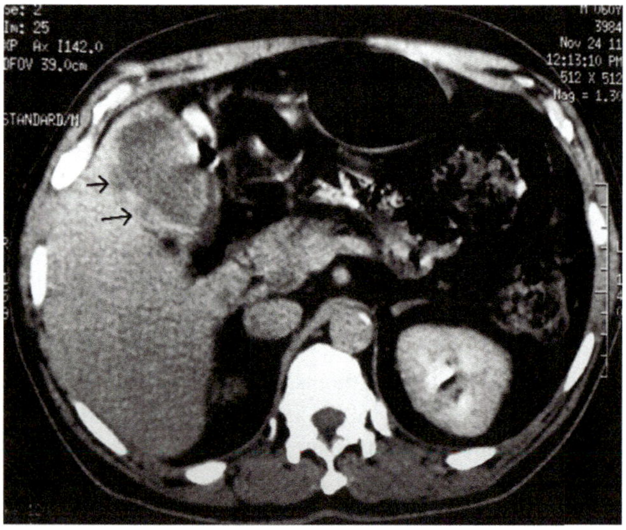

Fig. 24.7 CT scan showing intramural hypodense nodules (arrows)

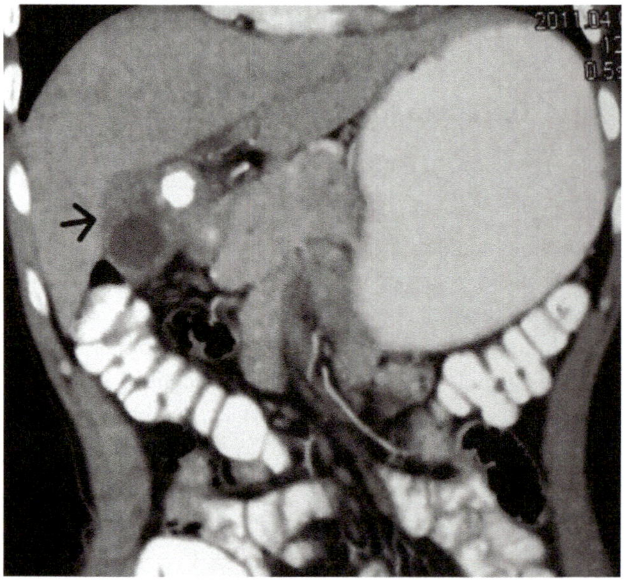

Fig. 24.8 XGC resulting in grossly thickened and contracted GB (arrow)

- Luminal surface enhancement (LSE), which refers to the enhancement of the GB epithelium and is more prominent in the portal venous phase, is observed in nearly 75–85% of patients. This indicates a continuous mucosal lining, further supporting XGC as a submucosal disease. Focal mucosal breach is reported in about 20–25% of XGC cases, compared to over 80% in GBC.

24.3.6 Magnetic Resonance Imaging (MRI)

The MRI features of XGC are

- Gallstones
- GB wall thickening (same as in CT). Hypointense nodules on T1-weighted images corresponding to xanthogranulomas.

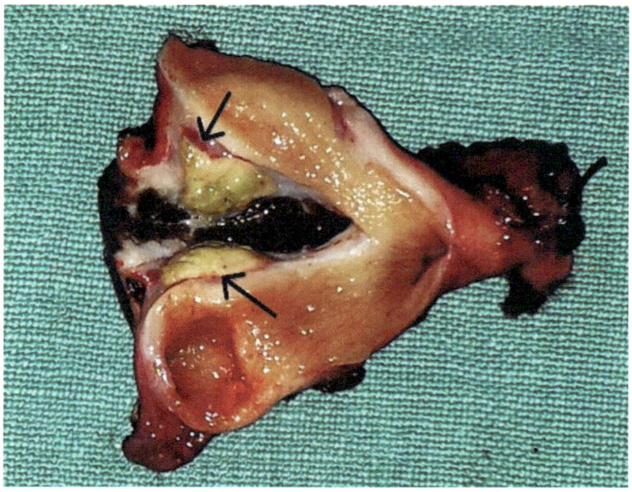

Fig. 24.9 GB specimen. Incised mucosa showing a yellowish intramural xanthogranuloma nodule (arrow)

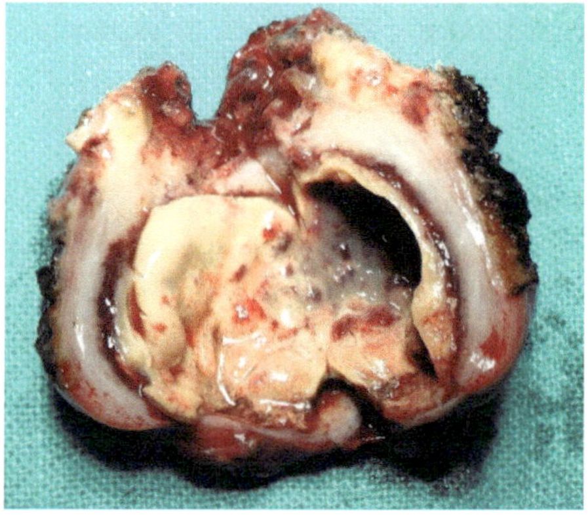

Fig. 24.10 Grossly contracted, fibrotic thickening of the GB wall in XGC. (Note the intact but sclerotic mucosa)

Table 24.2 Similarities and differences between XGC & GBC

Features	XGC	GBC
Longstanding cholelithiasis	+	+
Anorexia, weight loss	Less common	More common
GB wall thickening	Diffuse, symmetrical, uniform	Focal, asymmetrical, non uniform
Intramural nodules on imaging	+	–
Luminal surface enhancement (LSE) and mucosal continuity	+	–
Mucosal breach	Less common	Common
Mass replacing GB, intra-luminal polypoidal mass	–	+
Infiltration into the adjacent liver, bowel, and parietes	May be present	May be present
Intrahepatic biliary radical dilatation (IHBRD)	–	+
FDG-PET	May be false-positive due to inflammation	Positive
Locoregional lymphadenopathy	Variable Shows homogenous enhancement	Common More often non-homogeneous

- Hyperintense signals within the GB wall on T2-weighted images indicate inflammation, edema, and fibrosis.
- Inflammation extending to the GB bed in the adjacent liver.
- Lymphadenopathy.
- Diffusion-weighted images (DWI) may help differentiate wall-thickening in XGC from GBC. Diffusion restriction is more frequently associated with GBC, and the mean apparent diffusion coefficient (ADC) value of XGC is higher than that in GBC.

24.3.7 Treatment

A diagnostic confusion with GBC may result in undertreatment or overtreatment in about 10% of cases of XGC. Table 24.2 summarizes the clinical, radiological, and morphological overlaps between the two entities. Preoperative targeted FNAB, particularly using endoscopic ultrasound (EUS), has nearly 90% specificity and sensitivity in diagnosing GBC. Cholecystectomy is recommended for all cases of XGC. Laparoscopic approach is technically difficult, and the need for conversion to open cholecystectomy in about 16–80% has been reported. Presence of dense pericholecystic adhesions, obliterated anatomy, cholecystoenteric fistula, and the association—real or fortuitous—with GBC make open cholecystectomy a more desirable option in XGC. Frozen section biopsy is often required to exclude malignancy. Disconnection and repair of the cholecystoenteric fistula and subtotal cholecystectomy can be performed when complete surgery appears technically hazardous. The entire treatment plan for XGC has been summarized in Table 24.3.

Table 24.3 Management plan for XGC

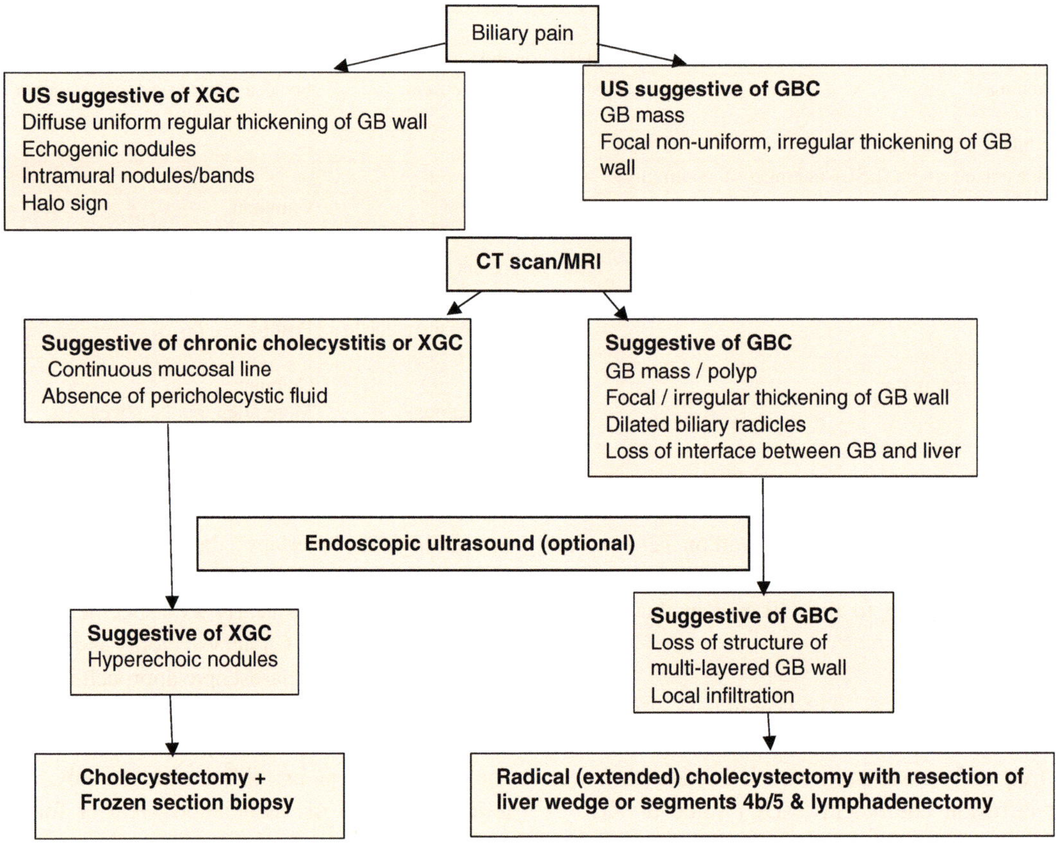

Key Points

- Cholecysto-duodenal fistula is the most common type of cholecystoenteric fistula (CEF)
- Passage of a large gallstone (GS) through the CEF and its subsequent impaction may cause intestinal obstruction.
- The terminal ileum is the most common site of obstruction, while the duodenum is the rarest.
- Though the diagnosis can be reliably made with a CT scan, findings of a cholecystoduodenal fistula on endoscopy, chronic cholecystitis with or without GS on ultrasound, and features of intestinal obstruction on X-ray can form an important triad in diagnosing GS ileus.
- Duodenal obstruction can be relieved by endoscopy. Enterotomy and removal of the offending stone are required for intestinal obstruction. Cholecystectomy and dismantling of the CEF should ideally be performed in the same sitting.
- Mirizzi syndrome is defined as bile duct obstruction by impaction or erosion of stone/s in Hartman's pouch or cystic duct.
- Clinical presentation and liver function tests mimic choledocholithiasis. A cholangiogram is the primary diagnostic tool that shows eccentric or peg-shaped filling defects in the mid-CBD, with proximal dilation and collapsed duct distally.
- Partial cholecystectomy, choledochoplasty, and/or bilioenteric anastomosis are performed depending on the extent of erosion of the common duct.
- A high occurrence of choledocholithiasis and malignancy may necessitate further treatment.
- Xanthogranulomatous cholecystitis is a complication of longstanding cholelithiasis that closely mimics GBC—clinically, radiologically, and during surgery.
- Bile leakage into the GB wall causes severe inflammation, fibrosis, and xanthogranuloma formation.
- On imaging, diffuse symmetrical thickening, and continuous mucosal lining differentiate it from XGC.
- Concomitant malignancy occurs in up to 10% of XGC specimens.
- Intraoperative frozen section should be performed to rule out suspicion of GBC.
- Conversion occurs in 16–80% of cases, making laparoscopic cholecystectomy a challenging procedure in XGC. Open cholecystectomy is preferred, especially when the possibility of GBC cannot be ruled out.

Selected Reading

1. Ibrarullah M, Mishra T, Das AP. Mirizzi syndrome. Indian J Surg. 2008;70:281–7.
2. Koo JGA, Tham HY, Toh EQ, et al. Mirizzi syndrome—the past, present, and future. Medicina. 2024;60:12. https://doi.org/10.3390/medicina60010012.
3. Hale MD, Roberts KJ, Hodson J, Scott N, Sheridan M, Toogood GJ. Xanthogranulomatous cholecystitis: a European and global perspective. HPB. 2013;16:448–58.
4. Singh VP, Rajesh S, Bihari C, et al. Xanthogranulomatous cholecystitis: what every radiologist should know. World J Radiol. 2016;8(2):183–91.

Surgery for Choledocholithiasis

25

Ragini Kilambi and Naren Mandalapu

Abstract

CBD stones are present in 10–15% patients with gallstones. They may present with biliary colic, jaundice, cholangitis, and pancreatitis or may be asymptomatic. Where expertise is available, a single-stage laparoscopic approach is the treatment of choice in good-risk patients. ERCP and CBD clearance, followed by laparoscopic cholecystectomy in two stages, or performing ERCP and CBD clearance during the same session after laparoscopic cholecystectomy, are alternative approaches.

Keywords

Choledocholithiasis · CBD stone

Choledocholithiasis or common bile duct (CBD) stone is reported in about 3–20% of patients undergoing cholecystectomy for gallstones (GS). The presentation can range from being entirely asymptomatic to experiencing mild biliary colic or more severe complications such as jaundice, cholangitis, or pancreatitis. While spontaneous passage of stones has been reported in up to a third of cases without any treatment, most patients will require some form of intervention, either endoscopic or surgical. This is particularly true for those who present with symptoms or biochemical abnormalities. If left untreated, bile duct stones can be life-threatening, leading to complications like cholangitis or pancreatitis (Table 25.1).

Table 25.1 Classification of choledocholithiasis

Types	Characteristics
Primary	Brown pigment in appearance, soft and multiple Uncommon, <5% of all choledocholithiasis Resulting from bile stasis and infection, the alteration in bile solubility and pH leads to the formation of stones in the bile duct
Secondary	More commonly, approximately 95% of all choledocholithiasis Arise in the gallbladder, migrate to the bile duct through the cystic duct, or by erosion (Mirizzi syndrome)

25.1 Clinical Presentation

Biliary Colic: This is the most common presentation of CBD stones. The pain results from the distension of the bile duct caused by partial or complete blockage by the stone. This pain is usually felt in the right upper quadrant and the epigastric region, often accompanied by nausea and vomiting. The pain tends to be more severe and lasts longer than typical biliary colic, lasting over 6 h, and is not influenced by posture. Pain may be relieved if the stones move spontaneously backward into the proximal duct or, in cases of small stones, into the duodenum. The pain can recur when the stone shifts back and forth within the duct, and a history of similar episodes is often present. Rome IV criteria can be used to diagnose biliary pain, which includes pain in the epigastrium or right hypochondrium lasting at least half an hour, occurring at variable intervals. The pain should be

R. Kilambi (✉) · N. Mandalapu
Institute of Liver and Biliary Sciences, New Delhi, India

M. Ibrarullah (ed.), *Recent Concepts in Gastrointestinal (GI) Surgery*, https://doi.org/10.1007/978-981-92-1118-0_25

severe enough to disrupt activities and is unrelated to posture, bowel movements, or acid-suppressive medications. However, distinguishing this pain from that caused by gallbladder (GB) stones can be challenging. Complications such as jaundice, cholangitis, and pancreatitis frequently follow bile duct obstruction, affecting up to 25% of patients.

Obstructive Jaundice: Jaundice may sometimes be the first symptom to appear in some patients, and a detailed history can reveal previous episodes of biliary colic, providing clues to the diagnosis. Larger stones tend to become impacted, while smaller ones may move back and forth, causing a waxing and waning pattern of jaundice. This is often accompanied by dark-colored urine and clay-colored stools, and there may also be associated pruritus.

Cholangitis: This is a more serious and potentially life-threatening complication of CBD stones. Patients with stones have associated bactibilia in 36–51% of cases. Acute cholangitis presents with characteristic symptoms such as jaundice, fever, and right upper quadrant pain (Charcot's triad). In more severe cases, it may progress to shock and altered mental status (Reynold's pentad). However, it is essential to remember that most patients do not exhibit classic symptoms and signs, so clinicians should maintain a high index of suspicion. The 2018 Tokyo guidelines have established criteria for diagnosing cholangitis accurately, including two of the three Charcot criteria, laboratory evidence of systemic inflammation, abnormal LFTs, imaging suggestive of biliary dilation, and evidence of any underlying cause.

Acute Pancreatitis: Smaller stones can either become lodged at the sphincter of Oddi or cause edema as they pass, leading to blockage of the common channel and resulting in acute biliary pancreatitis. Patients typically present with epigastric pain that radiates to the back, often accompanied by nausea and vomiting. The pain can range from mild to severe and may be relieved by stooping forward.

25.2 Physical Examination

On examination, patients may appear jaundiced. Abdominal exam might show tenderness in the right upper quadrant and epigastric area. The gallbladder (GB) is usually not palpable, and Murphy's sign is typically absent. A palpable GB or positive Murphy's sign suggests a mucocele or acute cholecystitis. Patients with pancreatitis may have epigastric tenderness and guarding. Those with cholangitis may exhibit tachycardia, fever, hypotension, and appear toxic.

25.2.1 Diagnosis

The diagnostic evaluation for suspected choledocholithiasis starts with a thorough history, and the first-line investigations comprise basic biochemical tests, including hemogram, liver function tests (LFT), and abdominal ultrasonography (USG). This preliminary assessment may prevent the need for additional comprehensive testing in patients who are deemed to be at low risk of having CBD stones (normal LFT, and an unobstructed bile duct on ultrasound with a CBD diameter of less than 9 mm).

Liver Function Tests: A completely normal LFT is considered sufficient to rule out CBD stones. Elevated levels of total and direct bilirubin, gamma-glutamyl transferase (GGT), and serum alkaline phosphatase (SAP) are better predictors of CBD stones, with high sensitivity and specificity, compared to elevated transaminases, aspartate transaminase (AST), and alanine transaminase (ALT). Yang et al. found that GGT, with a 97.9% negative predictive value, was the most powerful biochemical predictor of the absence of CBD stones. AST and ALT levels increase during the first 48 to 72 h after biliary obstruction, followed by a steadier rise in SAP and bilirubin levels, which correlates with the duration and severity of the obstruction. Elevated bilirubin, SAP, and GGT have a positive predictive value of only 25–50%. Bilirubin levels above 1.7 mg/dL show about 60% specificity for CBD stones in patients with GS scheduled for cholecystectomy, increasing to 87.5% when bilirubin exceeds 4 mg/dL. However, fewer than a third of patients with choledocholithiasis will have such high bilirubin levels, highlighting the need for further evaluation with imaging.

Ultrasonography: USG is usually the first-line investigation for patients presenting with abdominal pain or abnormal liver function tests. However, it is highly operator-dependent, which limits its sensitivity. Despite this, it is inexpensive, widely available, and does not involve ionizing radiation, making it an important screening tool for CBD stones. Direct visualization of stones is often not possible due to their location in the distal CBD, where bowel gas can obscure the view. Nonetheless, it can detect CBD dilation with high sensitivity, serving as a marker for biliary obstruction. When combined with the presence of GS, the likelihood of CBD stones increases as the cause of dilation. Another indirect sign is multiple small gallstones, which suggest they may have migrated into the CBD. However, a negative ultrasound does not rule out CBD stones, especially when liver function tests are abnormal. A study involving 195 patients with suspected CBD stones showed that ultrasound had a specificity of 79%, but a negative predictive value of only 38%.

Computed Tomography (CT): CT is not the preferred imaging method for patients with suspected choledocholithiasis. However, it can be used to rule out other conditions when the likelihood of a CBD stone is low or to identify specific complications like pancreatitis. CBD stones may also be incidentally found on CT scans performed for other reasons. The low sensitivity is due to most biliary stones not being radiopaque. Contrast-enhanced CT has a sensitivity for choledocholithiasis ranging from 65 to 88%. Its sensitivity and accuracy can be improved with biliary-excreted contrast agents. Still, these are not commonly used because of their potential toxicity, allergic reactions, and the fact that obstructive cholestasis reduces their excretion into the biliary system. Additionally, CT scans cannot detect biliary stones smaller than 3 mm because of limited resolution and 5 mm slice acquisition. Finally, the risks associated with ionizing radiation and low diagnostic accuracy often limit its use in diagnosing CBD stones.

Magnetic Resonance Cholangiopancreatography (MRCP): In cases with high suspicion of CBD stones and a normal USG, the next step often involves imaging with MRCP. It reveals a stone as a filling defect in heavily T2-weighted images. MRCP is considered the gold standard for noninvasive imaging of the biliary tree (Fig. 25.1). It is now widely accessible, noninvasive, does not require contrast or anesthesia, and maps the entire biliary system, acting as a guide for future procedures. Its sensitivity ranges from 81% to 100% and its specificity from 92% to 100%. The primary limitation is that any detected stone typically necessitates another intervention for removal. Additionally, its sensitivity decreases for stones smaller than 5 mm, where ERCP and endoscopic ultrasound (EUS) offer better performance. Other factors to consider include limited availability in smaller centers, cost, and technical challenges in patients with metallic implants, claustrophobia, or severe obesity. Nevertheless, it has overtaken ERCP as the diagnostic gold standard for CBD stones due to its noninvasive approach and comparable accuracy. A randomized trial demonstrated that performing a pre-ERCP MRCP prevented the need for ERCP in 50% of patients, sparing them from unnecessary procedures and associated complications.

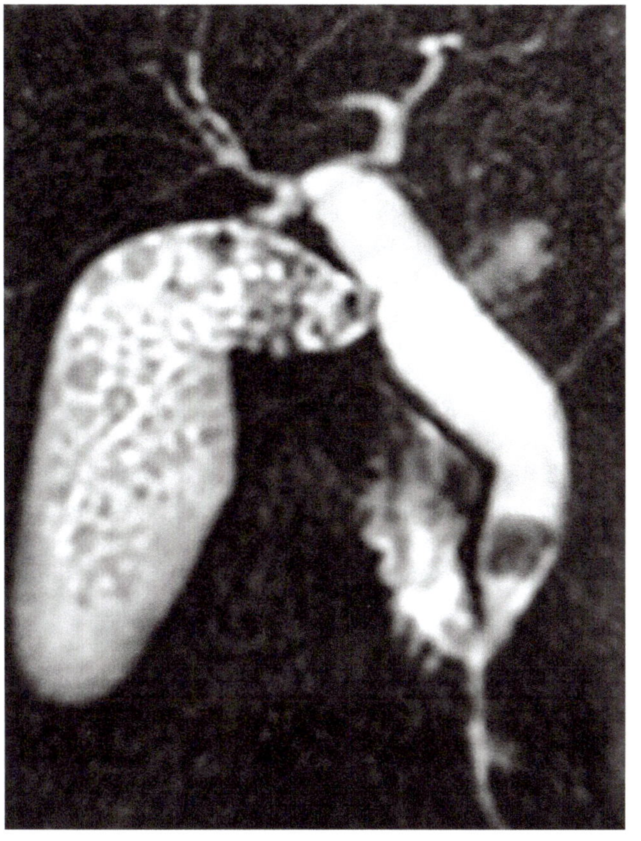

Fig. 25.1 MRCP showing multiple gallstones, dilated CBD, and a stone at its lower end

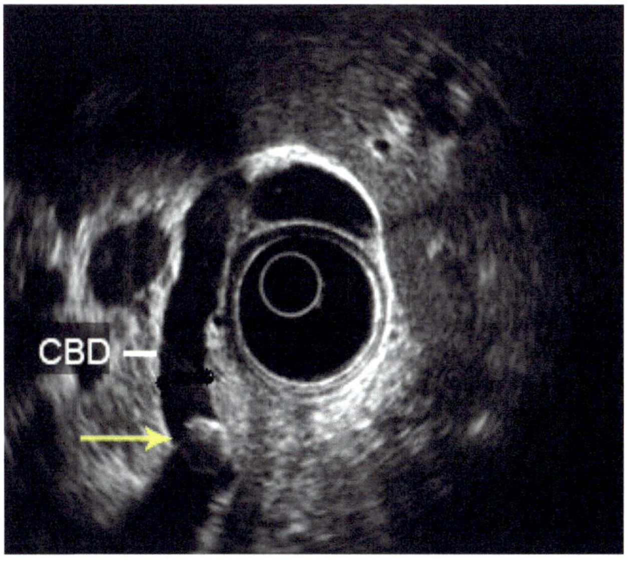

Fig. 25.2 EUS image: dilated CBD with a stone at the lower end

Endoscopic Ultrasonography (EUS): Endoscopic ultrasound detects CBD stones (Fig. 25.2) with a sensitivity ranging from 75% to 100% and a specificity of 85% to 100%. Its sensitivity is comparable to diagnostic ERCP, despite being less invasive and associated with minimal complications.

Compared to MRCP, a Cochrane review concluded that EUS has equivalent sensitivity and specificity. However, EUS is more sensitive for detecting small stones <5 mm. Its main advantage over MRCP is that ERCP can be performed during the same session for stone removal. Like MRCP, using EUS before ERCP reduces the number of nontherapeutic procedures. When EUS is performed, nearly two-thirds of patients avoid ERCP, which also lowers complication rates. However, EUS remains a user-dependent procedure with limited availability, high cost, and a small but definite risk of complications due to its invasive nature.

Endoscopic Retrograde Cholangiopancreatography (ERCP): Although ERCP has high sensitivity and specificity as a diagnostic tool and was once considered the gold standard for diagnosis, it is now reserved only for patients with a high likelihood of choledocholithiasis who require therapeutic intervention for stone removal or biliary drainage.

Intraoperative Cholangiogram (IOC): IOC is performed during cholecystectomy to visualize biliary anatomy and confirm or rule out bile duct stones. It has a sensitivity of 59–100% and a specificity of 93–100% for CBD stones. Currently, its use is limited due to the widespread availability of MRCP.

Laparoscopic Ultrasound (LUS): LUS helps diagnose CBD stones intraoperatively during cholecystectomy. However, it is operator-dependent and has a longer learning curve than IOC. It has a sensitivity of 80% to 100% and a specificity of 96% to 100%.

25.3 Risk Stratification

Diagnosis of CBD stone is based on clinical, biochemical, and imaging findings. Based on these, risk stratification has been proposed by several scientific societies (Table 25.2).

Table 25.2 Risk of CBD stone based on clinical, biochemical, and imaging parameters

Risk of CBD stone	ASGE	ESGE	SAGES	BSG
High	Cholangitis or CBD stone on USG or a combination of total bilirubin >4 mg/dL and CBD dilation on USG	Cholangitis or CBD stone on USG	Presence of any two of the following: CBD stone on USG Clinical evidence of acute cholangitis Total bilirubin >1.7 mg/dL Dilated CBD	CBD stone on USG or features of cholangitis or pain, duct dilation, and jaundice in a patient with a history of gallstones
Intermediate	Abnormal LFT or age >55 years or CBD dilation on ultrasound	Abnormal LFT and/or CBD dilation on	Not meeting criteria for high and low risk	Abnormal LFTs with normal biliary system or CBD dilation on USG with normal LFT
Low	Normal LFT and ultrasound (no CBD dilation on USG ult	Normal LFT and no CBD dilation on USG	No jaundice and normal bile duct on ultrasound	Normal results

ASGE American Society for Gastrointestinal Endoscopy, *ESGE* European Society of Gastrointestinal Endoscopy, *SAGES* Society of American Gastrointestinal and Endoscopic Surgeons, *BSG* British Society of Gastroenterology

25.4 Management

The natural history of CBD stones remains unclear. There is evidence to suggest that small stones, found incidentally on intraoperative cholangiogram, may pass spontaneously. However, because of potential serious and life-threatening complications, consensus favors removing the CBD stone once detected, either surgically or endoscopically.

Management of choledocholithiasis was relatively straightforward during the era of open surgery, with predefined treatment plans for all clinical situations. Open CBD exploration was the treatment of choice for all patients with CBD stones, with or without GS. In 1968, McCune et al. first reported the endoscopic cannulation of the papilla, and by 1974, it was being used therapeutically following the introduction of the sphincterotome. Though endoscopy (ERCP) was increasingly used for CBD stones, open CBD exploration remained the treatment of choice, along with open cholecystectomy. However, the scenario changed with the advent of laparoscopic cholecystectomy, which became the gold standard for managing cholelithiasis. This led to ERCP clearance of stones, with laparoscopic cholecystectomy becoming the standard of care, since skills for laparoscopic CBD exploration had yet to be mastered. However, in the present era of advanced laparoendoscopy, treatment options for CBD stones when detected with GS have been reasonably standardized to either laparoscopic or endoscopic CBD clearance.

The treatment options mainly depend on when the diagnosis is made in relation to cholecystectomy—whether it is identified preoperatively, intraoperatively, or postoperatively. If diagnosed preoperatively, there are three options for CBD clearance: (i) a two-step approach, which involves ERCP clearance of the CBD stone followed by laparoscopic cholecystectomy 24–48 h later; (ii) same-sitting open or laparoscopic cholecystectomy followed by CBD exploration; and (iii) same-sitting laparoscopic cholecystectomy followed by ERCP clearance of the CBD. If suspected during cholecystectomy, further confirmation can be obtained using IOC or LUS. If confirmed, it can be managed by CBD exploration in the same sitting or an intraoperative or postoperative ERCP clearance. However, leaving the CBD stone behind for postoperative endoscopic clearance carries the risk of cystic duct blow-out due to the obstructing stone and is therefore not recommended. In cases of retained bile duct stones after surgery, the preferred method for duct clearance is the transpapillary endoscopic technique. An algorithm for suggested management is shown in (Table 25.3).

25.5 Common Bile Duct Exploration

25.5.1 Open Approach

Essential steps for open CBD exploration include confirming the presence, number, and position of CBD stones through preoperative or intraoperative cholangiography, which is crucial before CBD exploration. After cholecystectomy, the peritoneum is removed to expose the CBD. The duodenum is

Table 25.3 Proposed management algorithm for choledocholithiasis

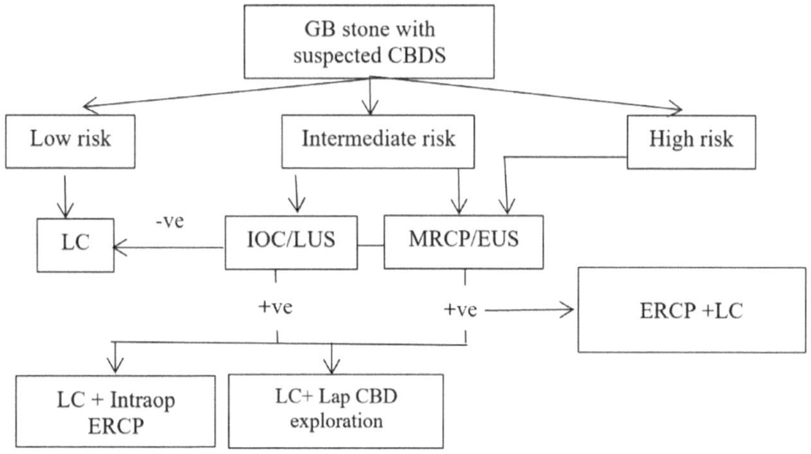

GB gallbladder, *CBDS* common bile duct stones, *LC* laparoscopic cholecystectomy, *IOC* intraoperative cholangiogram, *LUC* laparoscopic ultrasound, *MRCP* magnetic resonance cholangiopancreatogram, *EUS* endoscopic ultrasound, *ERCP* endoscopic retrograde cholangiopancreatogram, *Intraop* intraoperative, +ve CBD stone present, –ve CBD stone absent

Kocherized to palpate and manipulate stones in the distal CBD. Stay sutures are placed, and bile is aspirated to confirm the CBD. The CBD is opened with a stab knife usually longitudinally, and the incision is enlarged on either side. Using fingers in the foramen of Winslow, CBD stones are palpated and milked out. Remaining stones are extracted with Desjardin forceps and flushing. An 8-French infant feeding tube is passed across the papilla to rule out obstruction. Both the proximal and distal biliary tree are irrigated with normal saline to remove residual stones, fragments, or sludge. A choledochoscopy or completion cholangiogram is performed to confirm complete CBD clearance. An appropriately sized (12–16 F) T-tube is trimmed and guttered, then placed inside the CBD, with the long limb exiting through one end of the choledochotomy incision. The incision is closed with interrupted Vicryl 3-0 sutures. Alternatively, an indwelling transpapillary plastic stent may be placed, or the choledochotomy may also be closed primarily after confirming complete CBD clearance without any stents. A subhepatic drain is inserted, and the abdomen is closed.

25.5.2 Laparoscopic Transcholedochal Approach

Dilated CBD with a limited number of stones is suitable for laparoscopic transcholedochal exploration. All the basic steps of CBD exploration are as described above. Choledocholithotomy, however, is performed with a Dormia basket or an endoscopic balloon introduced through the side of the epigastric port. This usually suffices when the number of CBD stones is small and can be counted with a preoperative cholangiogram. Alternatively, a flexible choledochoscope introduced via the epigastric port can retrieve the CBD stones under direct vision using a transendoscopic Dormia basket. After ensuring complete clearance, primary closure of the CBD with an indwelling transpapillary CBD stent is preferred over T-tube drainage. Alternatively, the CBD may be closed primarily without any stents after ensuring complete stone clearance. The success rate for stone clearance ranges from 91% to 95%. Morbidity ranges from 5% to 10%, and mortality is under 1%. Complications include postoperative bile leak, retained stones, and stricture formation. However, long-term studies have demonstrated the safety of this approach, with the risk of stricture formation being negligible (Fig. 25.3).

25.5.3 Laparoscopic Transcystic Approach

Approach through the cystic duct is preferred for normal or minimally dilated CBD because a choledochotomy in such patients can be risky. The other requirements for a transcystic CBD exploration are:

1. Small stones <10 mm.
2. Located distal to the point where the cystic duct joins the CBD.
3. Cystic duct diameter >4 mm to allow instrumentation.
4. The cystic duct should enter laterally, angulated downward, and not be tortuous.

After cholecystectomy, the cystic duct is incised and then dilated with a balloon to facilitate instrumentation and stone removal. This method offers the advantage of being minimally invasive but is limited by the size and anatomy of the

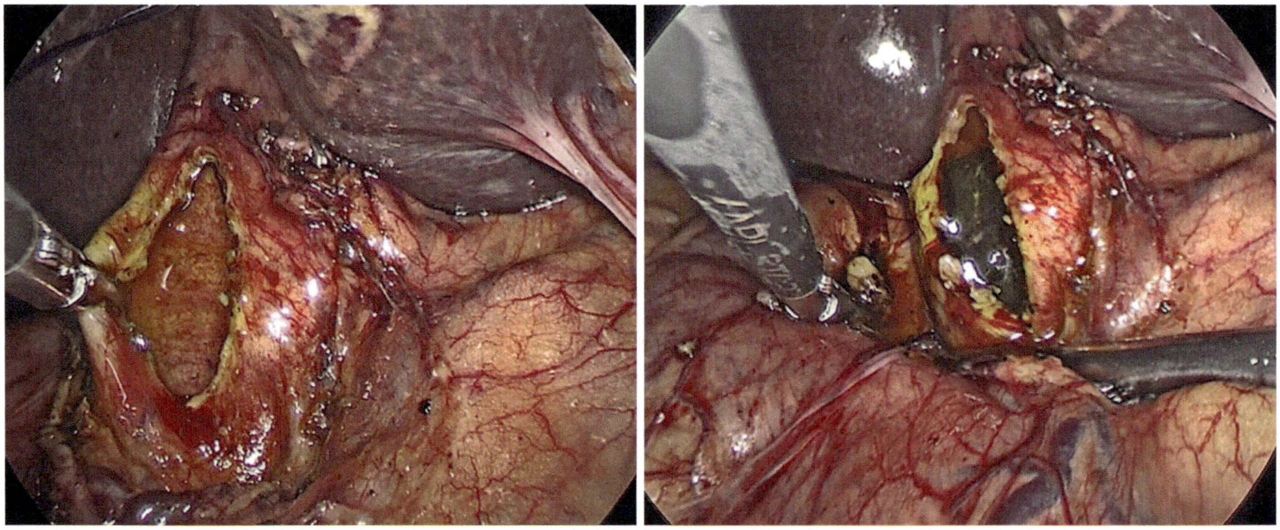

Fig. 25.3 Laparoscopic CBD exploration. (i) Wide choledochotomy; (ii) a large stone is being removed by applying pressure from below

cystic duct. Complications of transcystic exploration include bile leak, pancreatitis, or cystic duct tear. Although this technique is recommended for an undilated CBD and small stones, it is cumbersome and constrained by several limitations. Consequently, it has not gained broad acceptance, especially since endoscopic transpapillary intervention is more successful and more widely available.

25.6 ERCP Followed by Laparoscopic Cholecystectomy

ERCP followed by laparoscopic cholecystectomy is one of the most common approaches for preoperatively diagnosed CBD stones. Therapeutic ERCP is performed for stone removal. After an endoscopic sphincterotomy, stones are extracted using a balloon sweep, basket, or lithotripter. This may or may not be followed by stent placement. Stent placement protects the patient from biliary obstruction if there is incomplete clearance, retained stone fragments, or repeated slippage of stones into the bile duct before cholecystectomy. Cholecystectomy is ideally performed 24–48 h later. This interval allows any post-ERCP complications to become apparent. Laparoscopic cholecystectomy immediately after ERCP should be avoided, as bowel distention following endoscopy can obscure the operative field and make dissection almost impossible.

25.7 Rendezvous Technique/ Intraoperative ERCP

Laparoscopic cholecystectomy with intraoperative ERCP clearance of the CBD stones is a very appealing concept because it offers the benefits of two-stage approaches in a single stage, thereby reducing the hospital stay and treatment cost. As explained above, laparoscopic cholecystectomy should always precede ERCP. In the rendezvous technique, after cholecystectomy, a guidewire is passed through the cystic duct across the papilla, which facilitates subsequent retrograde cannulation by the endoscopist for endoscopic papillotomy and CBD clearance. This technique can be performed in a left lateral or supine position. After endoscopic stone extraction, the cystic duct is clipped, and the cholecystectomy is completed. Alternatively, after finishing the cholecystectomy, the patient is turned prone, and ERCP is conducted. The decision to perform ERCP during or after the cholecystectomy largely depends on the policies of the respective surgical and endoscopy teams. The only disadvantage of this procedure is logistical: the need for proper coordination between the two teams.

25.7.1 Robotic CBD Exploration with Cholecystectomy

Robotic surgery offers improved instrumentation and easier intracorporeal suturing. These benefits have contributed to robotic CBD exploration becoming a viable alternative to laparoscopic CBD exploration.

25.8 Choosing the Best Treatment Option

Various trials have shown comparable success rates for pre- and intraoperative ERCP clearance of CBD stones and laparoscopic CBD exploration. Preoperative ERCP is the most commonly used method since it involves only a cholecystectomy after ductal clearance. However, ERCP carries certain risks such as pancreatitis, cholangitis, perforation, and bleeding. Additionally, there is a realistic risk of losing follow-up after ERCP, with a potential for recurrent biliary events in the interim. Nonetheless, in situations where the patient has cholangitis, poor performance status (making them unfit for general anesthesia), minimally dilated CBD, or limited laparoscopic skills, ERCP remains the treatment of choice. Intraoperative ERCP is limited in its use due to logistical challenges. Postoperative ERCP is justified only in cases where stones are detected after cholecystectomy, making it the preferred treatment in such situations. Regarding laparoscopic CBD exploration, several meta-analyses have demonstrated that single-stage laparoscopic cholecystectomy combined with CBD exploration is superior to staged endoscopic and laparoscopic management, as it results in shorter hospital stays and lower treatment costs.

25.9 Drainage Procedures

These are not the primary management options for choledocholithiasis but are indicated only in specific situations, such as significantly dilated ducts (>2 cm), recurrent or primary CBD stones, hepatolithiasis, and in patients at risk for ongoing biliary stasis, like those with periampullary diverticula, papillary stenosis, and biliary strictures. The procedures include choledochoduodenostomy, Roux-en-Y choledochojejunostomy, and transduodenal sphincteroplasty. These can be performed either through open surgery or laparoscopically.

Choledochoduodenostomy: After exploring and clearing all stones from the CBD, the duodenum is widely Kocherized to allow a tension-free anastomosis. The CBD is incised vertically, and the duodenum along its long axis (transverse

Key Points

- CBD stones are present in 10%–15% patients with gallstones.
- They may present with biliary colic, jaundice, cholangitis, and pancreatitis or may be asymptomatic.
- Ultrasound with LFT is the first line of investigation.
- MRCP is the investigation of choice in patients with suspected CBD stones.
- Surgical and endoscopic approaches are available for management.
- The procedure of choice in an individual patient depends on the available expertise, instruments, and the patient's performance status.
- Where expertise is available, a single-stage laparoscopic approach is the treatment of choice in good-risk patients.
- ERCP and CBD clearance, followed by laparoscopic cholecystectomy in two stages, or performing ERCP and CBD clearance during the same session after laparoscopic cholecystectomy, are alternative approaches.
- The endoscopic approach is especially suitable for nondilated or minimally dilated CBD and those with residual CBD stones after cholecystectomy.
- Drainage procedures may be needed in patients with recurrent stones, primary stones, dyskinetic CBD, papillary stenosis, or hugely dilated CBD.

incision). Both structures are approximated with interrupted, delayed absorbable sutures to create a diamond-shaped anastomosis, at least 2.5 cm long, which improves drainage, reduces strictures, and helps prevent sump syndrome postoperatively.

Roux-en-Y Choledochojejunostomy or Hepaticojejunostomy: An end-to-side or side-to-side Roux-en-Y choledochojejunostomy or hepaticojejunostomy is especially indicated for patients with CBD stones who may also have distal strictures or an eroded duct due to Mirizzi syndrome.

Transduodenal Sphincteroplasty: In the pre-ERCP era, transduodenal sphincteroplasty was considered an alternative to lateral choledochoduodenostomy. However, with the widespread availability of ERCP and endoscopic sphincterotomy, the indication for transduodenal sphincterotomy is now primarily limited to a stone firmly impacted at the ampulla that cannot be retrieved through supraduodenal choledochotomy. It is contraindicated in cases of periampullary inflammation, suprasphincteric CBD stricture, duodenal diverticulum, and dilated CBD (>2 cm). After a wide Kocherization, the second part of the duodenum is opened with an oblique incision. The papilla is identified at the junction of the vertical and transverse mucosal folds. Subsequently, the papilla is incised for 4–5 mm between the 11 and 1 o'clock positions, avoiding the pancreatic duct, which lies at the 5 o'clock position. Fine absorbable sutures are placed on the outer, lateral margin to suture the CBD to the duodenum. This ensures hemostasis, provides traction for further extension of sphincterotomy, and prevents duodenal leak. The sphincterotomy is extended for 10–12 mm. Stones are then removed using forceps, flushing, balloon, or basket extraction. Check choledochoscopy is performed to confirm complete stone clearance.

Selected Reading

1. Wu X, Yang Y, Dong P, et al. Primary closure versus T-tube drainage in laparoscopic common bile duct exploration: a meta-analysis of randomized clinical trials. Langenbeck's Arch Surg. 2012;397(6):909–16. https://doi.org/10.1007/s00423-012-0962-4.
2. Bencini L, Tommasi C, Manetti R, Farsi M. Modern approach to cholecysto-choledocholithiasis. World J Gastrointest Endosc. 2014;6(2):32–40. https://doi.org/10.4253/wjge.v6.i2.32.
3. Singh AN, Kilambi R. Single-stage laparoscopic common bile duct exploration and cholecystectomy versus two-stage endoscopic stone extraction followed by laparoscopic cholecystectomy for patients with gallbladder stones with common bile duct stones: systematic review and meta-analysis of randomized trials with trial sequential analysis. Surg Endosc. 2018;32(9):3763–76.
4. Manes G, Paspatis G, Aabakken L, et al. Endoscopic management of common bile duct stones: European Society of Gastrointestinal Endoscopy (ESGE) guideline. Endoscopy. 2019;51(5):472–91. https://doi.org/10.1055/a-0862-0346.
5. Williams E, Beckingham I, El Sayed G, et al. Updated guideline on the management of common bile duct stones (CBDS). Gut. 2017;66(5):765–82. https://doi.org/10.1136/gutjnl-2016-312317.
6. Nie S, Fu S, Fang K. Comparison of one-stage treatment versus two-stage treatment for the management of patients with common bile duct stones: a meta-analysis. Front Surg. 2023;10. Frontiers Media S.A https://doi.org/10.3389/fsurg.2023.1124955.
7. Kumar Hari Rajah. Current management of choledocholithiasis-narrative review article. Asian J Med Health. 2024;22(4):32–40. https://doi.org/10.9734/ajmah/2024/v22i4999.

Complications of Cholecystectomy

26

Vishal Gupta, Ajeet P. Maurya, and Gaurav Jain

Abstract

Common postoperative complications of laparoscopic cholecystectomy include bleeding (0.79%), retained common bile duct (CBD) stones (0.5%), and bile duct injury (BDI) (0.3–0.5%). A bile leak after surgery appears as an external biliary fistula when there is a subhepatic drain. The presence of acute cholecystitis, adhesions, aberrant arterial anatomy, cirrhosis of the liver, and portal cavernoma is an important cause of bleeding during LC. Residual or recurrent stone in the gallbladder or cystic duct remnant, or CBD can cause ongoing postoperative symptoms. Its management involves revision surgery and endoscopic removal for CBD stones, respectively.

Keywords

Bile duct injury, Bile leak, Biliary stricture · Cholecystectomy complications

Laparoscopic cholecystectomy (LC) is associated with an overall morbidity of 1.6–5.3% and a mortality rate of 0.08–0.14%. Common postoperative complications include bleeding (0.79%), retained common bile duct (CBD) stones (0.5%), bile duct injury (BDI) (0.3–0.5%), respiratory (0.48%), cardiac (0.36%), intra-abdominal abscess (0.34%), bowel injury (0.15%), sepsis (0.14%), pancreatitis (0.14%), and deep venous thrombosis or pulmonary embolism (0.13%). Factors such as operative approach (including open surgery and open conversion), higher Nassar operative difficulty grade, higher American Association of Anesthesiologists (ASA) physical status, emergency surgery, and older age are important predictors of postoperative complications. Overall conversion rates range from 4.2% to 6.2%. Long-term complications of cholecystectomy include postcholecystectomy syndrome, diarrhea, and recurrent stones in the remnant gallbladder (GB) stump.

V. Gupta (✉)
Department of Surgical Gastroenterology, All India Institute of Medical Sciences, Bhopal, India

A. P. Maurya
Department of General Surgery, All India Institute of Medical Sciences, Bhopal, India

G. Jain
Arora St Lukes Medical Center, Milwaukee, WI, USA

26.1 Biliary Complications

Biliary and vascular injuries are considered the most serious complications following LC. Biliary injuries during cholecystectomy are more common after laparoscopic than open cholecystectomy, with an incidence of 0.3–0.5% compared to 0.1–0.2% after open cholecystectomy. Over time, BDI rates have decreased; however, morbidity and mortality rates have remained the same.

26.1.1 Risk Factors

Several risk factors have been identified that predispose individuals to biliary injuries during LC. In general, these risk factors are categorized as related to an altered or abnormal anatomy, pathological changes, and surgical techniques (Table 26.1).

26.1.1.1 Surgical Technical Error

Achieving CVS is unquestionably the safest method to prevent injury during LC. In this process, the hepatocystic triangle (HCT) is cleared of all fibrofatty tissue. The cystic artery and cystic duct, the two target structures, are clearly delineated, and at least the lower one-third of the GB is dissected away from the cystic plate. The cystic duct and artery are then clipped and divided. Errors often occur from not following the principles of safe cholecystectomy, such as improper GB traction, dissecting in unsafe zones and below

M. Ibrarullah (ed.), *Recent Concepts in Gastrointestinal (GI) Surgery*, https://doi.org/10.1007/978-981-92-1118-0_26

Table 26.1 Risk factors for biliary injury during laparoscopic cholecystectomy

Dangerous anatomy	Aberrant ductal anatomy—aberrant right segmental/sectoral duct Caterpillar turn/Moynihan's hump of the right hepatic artery Short cystic duct
Dangerous pathology	Mirizzi syndrome Acute cholecystitis Chronic cholecystitis with a small contracted gallbladder Cholecysto-enteric fistula Large impacted stone at the neck Prior acute pancreatitis, especially moderately severe or severe Prior attempt at cholecystectomy Liver cirrhosis Portal cavernoma
Dangerous surgical technique	Inadequate training Overconfidence Inability to appreciate aberrant anatomy Infundibular technique of LC instead of the "critical view of safety" (CVS) technique Injudicious use of energy sources Faulty surgical equipment, e.g., poor quality image system, damaged hand-instruments

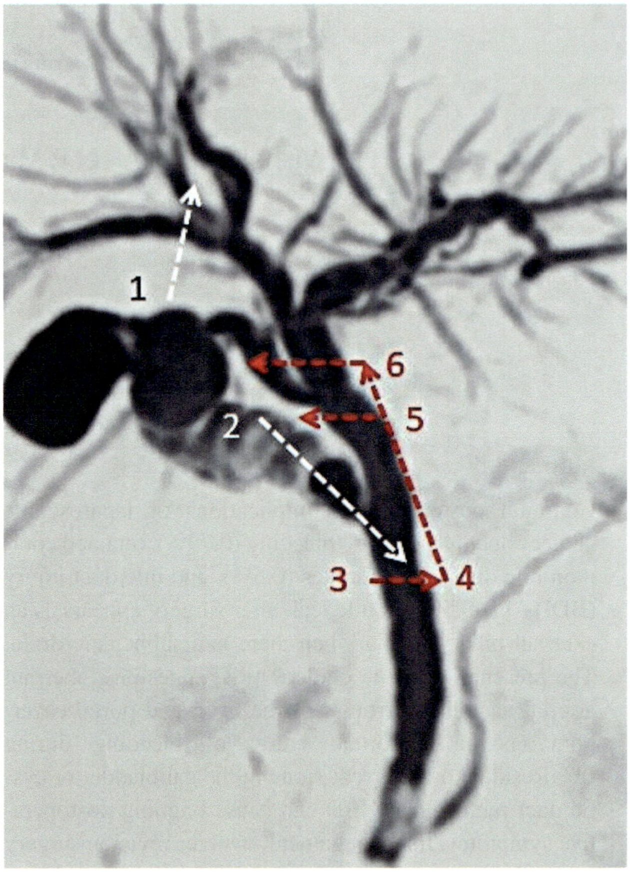

Fig. 26.1 Usual mechanism of bile duct injury. (1) Medial retraction of the neck or an obliterated HCT causes (2) cystic duct to align with the CBD (3) the CBD is mistaken for the cystic duct and transected (4) dissection continues in the wrong plane medial to the CBD (5) the CBD /CHD is transected again as dissection proceeds laterally to remove the GB (6) further proximal transection can cause sectoral duct injury (Bismuth type V)

the R4U line, dividing structures without proper or conclusive identification or without achieving CVS, not staying close to the GB during dissection, or going deep into the liver bed or hepatic hilum. Other common mistakes include not using bailout options in difficult cases, insecure clipping of the cystic duct, or placing clips on the junction of the cystic duct and CBD.

26.1.1.2 Misidentification of Anatomy/Perception Error

Most of the BDI during cholecystectomy results from misinterpretation of anatomy during dissection. The most common error is misidentifying the CBD as the cystic duct (Fig. 26.1). Predisposing factors, in addition to those already mentioned, include a short cystic duct, obliterated HCT caused by inflammation, fibrosis, or the presence of a large stone in Hartman's pouch.

26.1.2 Classification of Biliary Injury

Several classification systems for biliary injury have been proposed. However, the most commonly followed are the Bismuth classification (1982) and the Strasberg classification (1995) (Fig. 26.2, Tables 26.2 and 26.3). Bismuth classification primarily describes established biliary strictures, while the Strasberg classification includes acute injuries as well. Vascular injuries are not included in either, but are described in others, like the Stewart and Way and Hannover classification.

These classification systems help determine the complexities of these biliary injuries, guide management planning, assess outcomes, and predict prognosis. Strasberg type A and D may be managed with endoscopic therapy, while severe injuries like type E3, E4, and E5 almost always require surgical intervention. Less severe injuries like type E1 and E2 have favorable outcomes after surgical repair, whereas more severe injuries (E3/4) tend to do worse.

26.1.3 Clinical Presentation

Biliary injuries may be detected during surgery, in the immediate postoperative period, or later (delayed presentation) after many months or even years. The majority of BDIs

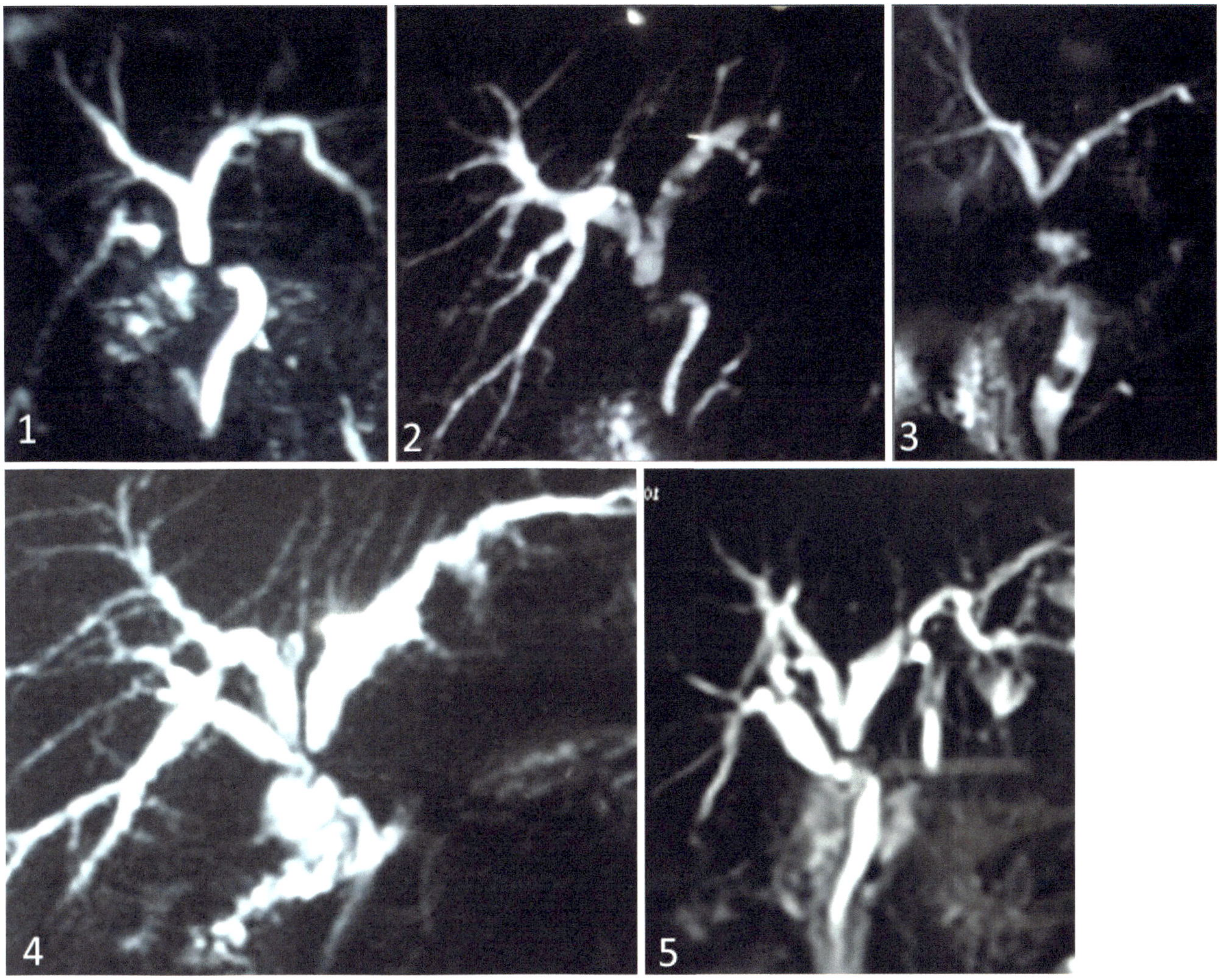

Fig. 26.2 MRCP depicting various Bismuth types (types 1–5) of post cholecystectomy biliary stricture. See Table 26.2 for details

Table 26.2 Bismuth classification of post-cholecystectomy biliary stricture

Type 1	Stricture level ≥2 cm below the confluence, i.e., common hepatic duct stump ≥2 cm
Type 2	Stricture level <2 cm below the confluence, i.e., common hepatic duct stump <2 cm
Type 3	Stricture at the primary biliary confluence; confluence patent; right and left biliary systems communicating with each other
Type 4	Stricture involving the primary biliary confluence; confluence not patent; right and left biliary systems not communicating with each other
Type 5	Stricture involving an aberrant right bile duct with/without common hepatic duct stricture

Table 26.3 Strasberg classification of post-cholecystectomy biliary injuries

Type A	Bile leak from the cystic duct stump or cholecystohepatic duct/duct of Luschka
Type B	Injury to the aberrant right bile duct with ligation and division; no bile leak
Type C	Injury to the aberrant right bile duct with only division; bile leak present
Type D	Lateral injury to the common bile duct/hepatic duct
Type E	Similar to Bismuth classification: E1–E5

present postoperatively; only about one-third are identified intraoperatively.

26.1.3.1 Intraoperative Presentation

Several intraoperative signs can indicate BDI, provided the operating surgeon is aware of and attentive to these clues (Table 26.4 and Figs. 26.3, 26.4, 26.5, 26.6). The appearance of golden yellow bile at any point during GB dissection should raise a red flag. The surgeon must pause and try to determine the source of the bile. Bile leak from the GB, resulting from instrument injury, rupture, or loose clip, is usually green unless it is very close to the cystic duct. BDI is

Table 26.4 When to suspect biliary injury during laparoscopic cholecystectomy?

Stage of the procedure	Alarming findings	Likely injury
During dissection in the HCT (to identify the cystic duct and artery) (Fig. 26.3)	Bile leak (or ICG dye leak) from the hepatic hilum during dissection or after GB removal	Injury to the CBD, CHD, or aberrant bile duct
After division of the (presumed) cystic duct	Retraction of (presumed) cystic duct stump vertically down behind the duodenum	Transected CBD/CHD
During GB mobilization after (presumed) cystic duct division	Encountering another tubular structure near the hilum	Transected CBD or presence of sectoral duct
During or after GB removal from the liver (Fig. 26.5)	Appearance of golden yellow bile in the GB bed; closer inspection reveals the source as a small tubular structure	Division of the cholecystohepatic duct
Inspection of GB after extraction (Fig 26.6)	Presence of a segment of a tubular structure attached to the GB specimen, especially with two openings with or without bile leak in the hepatic hilar area	Excision of a CBD segment
During an intraoperative cholangiogram	Nonopacification of the proximal/intrahepatic biliary system (on conventional cholangiogram) Nonvisualization of the distal biliary system (on NIRFC-ICG cholangiogram)	CBD occluded by a clip with/without excision

HCT hepatocystic triangle, *ICG* indocyanine green, *NIRFC* near infrared fluorescence cholangiography, *GB* gallbladder, *CBD* common bile duct, *CHD* common hepatic duct

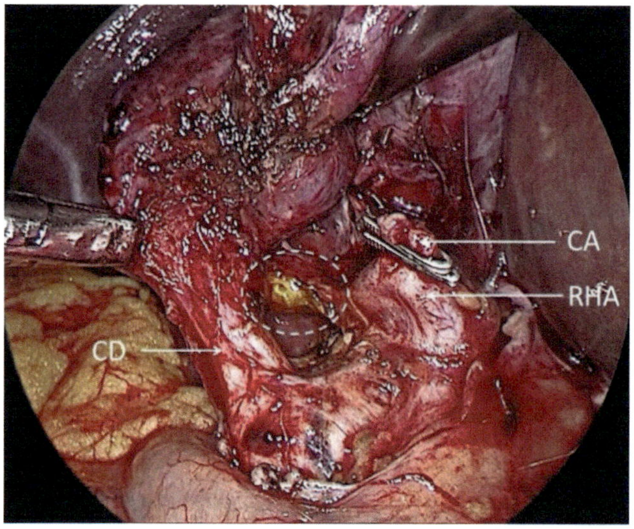

Fig. 26.3 Cautery injury to the sectoral duct (dotted circle) during dissection of the hepatocystic triangle. Note the small nick and bile staining in the duct. The sectoral duct was opening into the cystic duct. *CD* cystic duct, *CA* cystic artery, *RHA* right hepatic artery

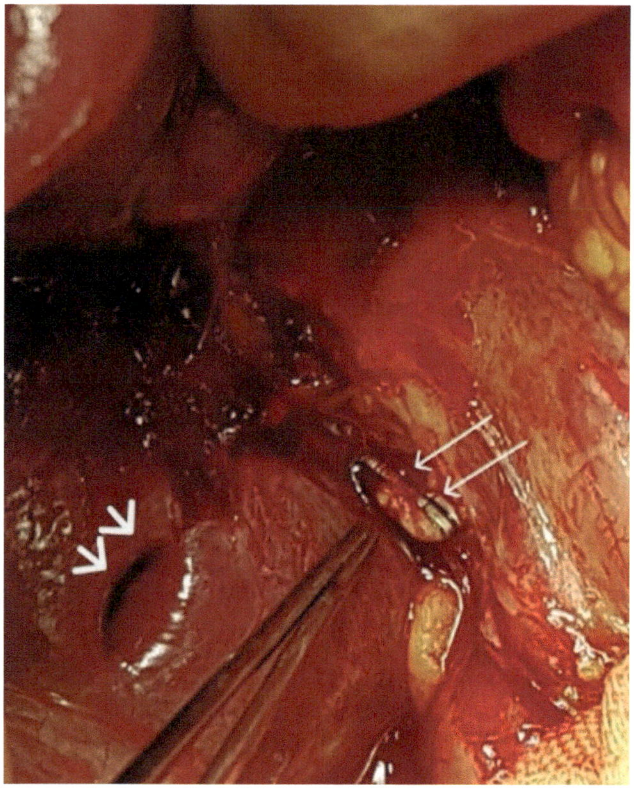

Fig. 26.4 Common bile duct mistaken for cystic duct, clipped and divided. Clipped distal cut end (arrows). Note the cut end is below the plane of Rouviere's sulcus (thick and short arrows)

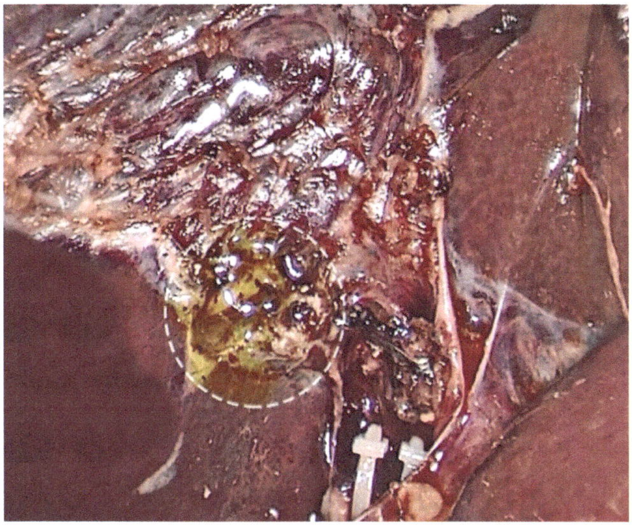

Fig. 26.5 Injury to the cholecystohepatic duct manifesting as bile staining in the gallbladder bed after its removal

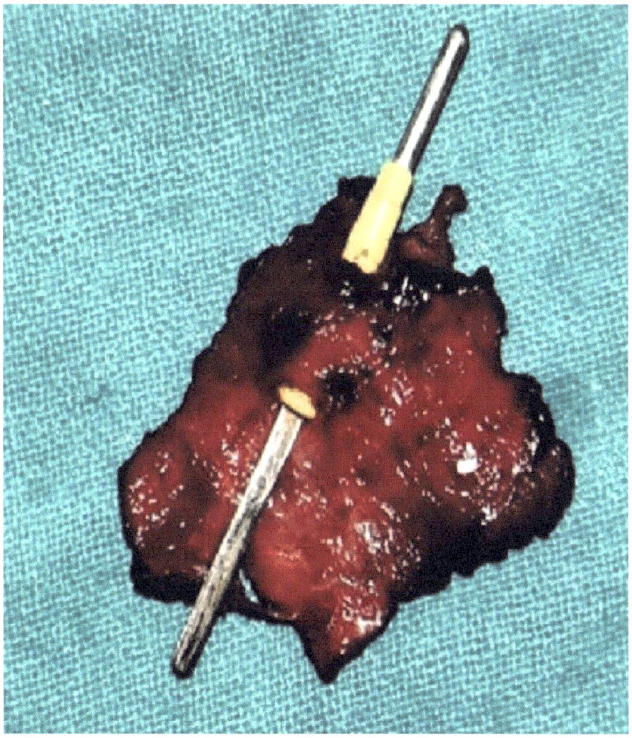

Fig. 26.6 Excised segment of the common bile duct attached to the cholecystectomy specimen

suspected if there is a bile leak from the hepatic hilar area during or after GB removal.

26.1.3.2 Presentation in the Immediate Postoperative Period

In the immediate postoperative period, biliary injury should be strongly suspected and ruled out if the patient is unwell, the abdomen is not settled, or vital signs are unstable, and the patient is not recovering as expected. Biliary injury may present with bile leak and or jaundice.

Bile leak presents in one of the following ways:

(a) External biliary fistula when a subhepatic drain is present: The patient is minimally symptomatic if it is a controlled fistula.
(b) Biliary peritonitis: Manifesting with signs of systemic sepsis, such as tachycardia, tachypnea, fever, abdominal distension with guarding, rigidity, and rebound tenderness.
(c) Bilioma: A localized collection of bile, usually in the subhepatic space or lesser sac (Figs. 26.7 and 26.8). The patient may experience mild to moderate symptoms, including tachycardia and fever.
(d) Bile ascites: Presence of several liters of bile in the peritoneal cavity with minimal signs and symptoms. Low-grade fever, mild to moderate tachycardia, and abdominal distention may be the only presenting features.

Jaundice may be mild, resulting from sepsis or peritoneal absorption of bile. Progressive jaundice indicates an occluded (clipped or ligated) main bile duct (CHD or CBD). In the latter event, the peritoneal cavity may be dry. However, as the bile duct stump sloughs out or the pressure builds up in the divided bile duct stump, the clip(s)/suture may give way, resulting in delayed bile leak and peritonitis.

26.1.3.3 Delayed Presentation

Late presentation of biliary injury includes jaundice with or without cholangitis, abdominal pain or discomfort, and/or fever, mainly caused by an established biliary stricture.

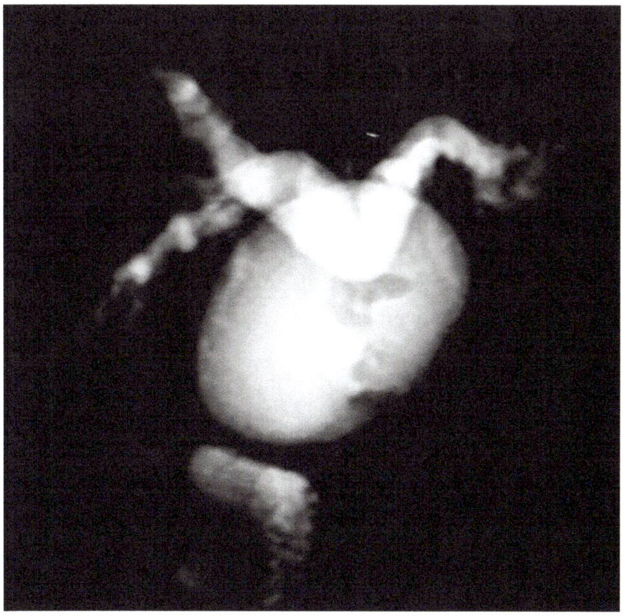

Fig. 26.7 MRCP showing subhepatic bilioma and Bismuth type 3 stricture

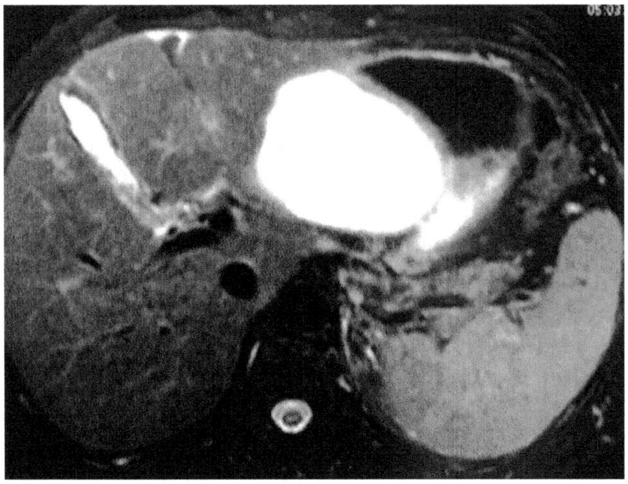

Fig. 26.8 Lesser sac bilioma; fluid collection between the stomach and the left lobe of the liver

These symptoms may be mild and intermittent and often ignored by the patient. If left undiagnosed and untreated for an extended period, the patient may develop hepatic fibrosis or secondary biliary cirrhosis (SBC), which can present with features of portal hypertension like variceal bleeding and splenomegaly, and/or hepatolithiasis.

Table 26.5 Management principles of bile duct injury detected or suspected intraoperatively

	What NOT to do	What to do
1	Panic	Time-out
2	Further dissection to know what has happened	Wash the area, try to locate the site of the bile leak, and assess the extent of the injury
3	Open conversion to know what has happened *(unless the surgeon has sufficient expertise to assess and repair the injury)*	Call a surgical colleague with expertise in biliary repair—physically or online—to discuss the situation and obtain an independent opinion, then decide on the further line of management
4	Attempt to place a feeding tube or T-tube in the injured duct (hepaticostomy)	If halfway through the dissection and the gallbladder (GB) is still attached to the liver/hilum—stop and do not do further dissection, leave the gallbladder in situ—put abdominal drains and close
5	Tying/clipping the injured end of the duct	Place multiple wide-bore drains in the subhepatic region, close to the GB/GB bed/hepatic hilum
6	End-to-end repair or hepaticojejunostomy if the surgeon lacks sufficient experience to manage biliary injuries	

26.1.4 Management

The most essential part of management is the early detection of biliary or any other visceral injury so that these complications can be managed promptly and appropriately.

26.1.4.1 Intraoperative Management

If bile duct injury is suspected during cholecystectomy, further dissection should be stopped immediately. Time-out should be exercised without panic. The area of dissection should be thoroughly inspected; the field should be cleaned with saline, and the site of the bile leak/suspected injury should be clearly exposed and assessed.

Once biliary injury is confirmed or highly suspected, the surgeon must follow certain principles of management (Table 26.5). Further management varies according to the scenario.

- If bile leak is observed from the GB bed away from the hilum, injury to the cholecystohepatic duct or segmental duct is suspected. Once the entire gallbladder is dissected from the liver, a leaking duct can be safely ligated using suture or clip if it is 3–4 mm or smaller in size. Larger ducts in this location are rare.
- Bile leak from the hepatic hilar area or GB bed near the hepatic hilum requires thorough assessment. This type of leak suggests a problem with a major duct, such as the common hepatic, right hepatic, or an aberrant sectoral duct. Proper management depends on accurately identifying the leak and having the necessary surgical expertise for biliary repair, as well as facilities for intraoperative cholangiography, appropriate instruments, sutures, retractors, and expert assistance. *It is advised not to convert to open surgery solely for the purpose of assessing the injury.*
- If appropriate expertise and facilities are available, these injuries are assessed further after open conversion with an intraoperative cholangiogram. In case of major injuries or duct transection, on-table repair may be performed provided biliary injury assessment is complete (to determine the type and extent of injury), there is no associated vascular injury, and the patient is hemodynamically stable.
- Repair methods range from simple suture repairs using fine 4-0/5-0 absorbable sutures for lateral injuries to Roux-en-Y hepaticojejunostomy for Strasberg type E injuries.
- In cases of complete transection *without* segmental loss or periductal dissection with healthy ductal ends and good vascularity, end-to-end repair may be considered over a T-tube (Fig. 26.9) or a plastic biliary stent, provided these can be placed easily and without further injuring the duct, which is usually undilated and thin-walled. However, such repairs have a high failure rate (29–64%) but can be

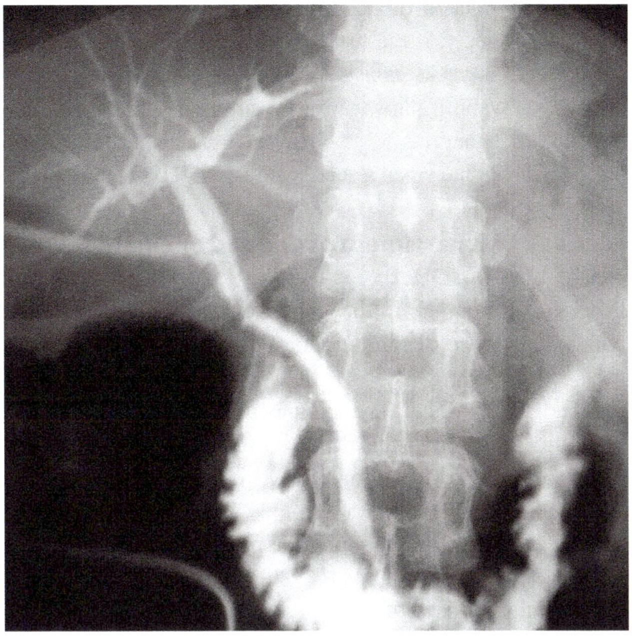

Fig. 26.9 Repair of the common bile duct over T-tube: T tube cholangiogram showing no contrast leak or stricture with free passage of contrast into the duodenum

managed endoscopically. This repair may be relatively simpler compared to Roux-en-Y reconstruction.
- If it is realized that the bile duct has been tied or clipped during the procedure, the tie or clip should be removed immediately. However, removal of a locking clip (Hem-o-lock) may be extremely difficult and may further damage the duct during the attempt. Since the CBD wall and/or its vascularity may be compromised by such clipping or tying, the affected segment may develop necrosis later, leading to delayed bile leaks or strictures. A drain should be placed, and the patient should be monitored closely with regular liver function tests and imaging.

26.1.4.2 Management in the Immediate Postoperative Period

In a stable patient with minimal abdominal signs, biliary scintigraphy (HIDA scan) can confirm or exclude any bile leak. Assessment of bilious drainage through the abdominal drain should include its nature (yellow or green, thin, turbid, or mucoid, possibly containing food particles) to rule out gut injury. Additionally, the output volume and its daily trend should be recorded.

Basic laboratory tests, such as a complete blood count, liver function tests (LFTs), C-reactive protein (CRP), renal function tests, and electrolyte levels, should be performed. Elevated leukocyte counts, CRP, and abnormal LFTs in a patient with an unsettled abdomen or unstable vitals necessitate further evaluation, including at least sonography to

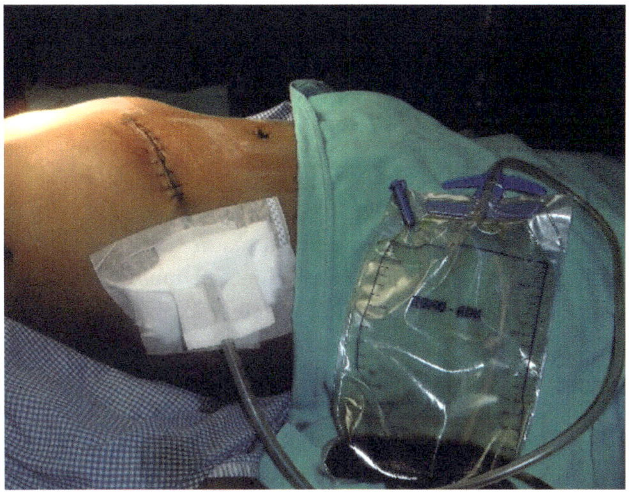

Fig. 26.10 Controlled external biliary fistula after surgical exploration for uncontrolled intrabdominal bile leak

check for intra-abdominal collections, biliary duct dilation, CBD stones, or pancreatitis. Mild collections may be observed in the GB fossa after cholecystectomy; however, significant collections require drainage.

If sonographic findings are inconclusive, a contrast-enhanced computed tomography (CECT) scan should be performed in a patient who is septic. Alternatively, Magnetic Resonance Imaging (MRI) may be resorted to if deranged renal function prohibits a CECT scan. CT imaging can reveal intra-abdominal collections, liver vascular status, and the biliary system and help rule out acute pancreatitis and intestinal injury. If the patient is not severely ill, Magnetic Resonance Cholangiopancreatography (MRCP) should be performed to determine the extent and cause of dilation and to identify the nature and type of biliary injury, ideally after draining any intra-abdominal collections (especially perihepatic) to allow an accurate assessment of biliary anatomy.

For bile leaks with significant intra-abdominal collections (bilioma), ascites, or bile peritonitis, the primary goal is to drain the collection to control sepsis and convert an uncontrolled intra-abdominal leak into a controlled external biliary fistula (EBF). Bilioma can be managed with image-guided percutaneous catheter drainage (PCD). Sometimes multiple drains are necessary to evacuate all collections.

Surgical intervention is needed for generalized collection (bile peritonitis), ascites/collections with loculations, collections that are not suitable for PCD, and persistent sepsis or uncontrolled leaks despite PCD, or in cases of suspected or confirmed bowel injury or management of associated or isolated vascular injury. The goal of surgical exploration is to drain all collections, control sepsis, and contain the leak, thereby converting an uncontrolled fistula into a controlled one (Fig. 26.10). *Repair of the injury at this stage is not rec-*

ommended because such repair is likely to fail in the presence of local inflammation with edematous, friable tissues in a patient with sepsis and hemodynamic instability.

26.1.4.3 Management of Controlled External Biliary Fistula

Endotherapy: A low-output fistula, showing a decreasing output trend, can be observed and may resolve on its own with conservative management. Smooth muscle relaxants (e.g., hyoscine butylbromide), which relax the sphincter of Oddi, may expedite the fistula closure. Persistent high output fistula (>200 ml/d for >1 week) with biliodigestive continuity intact is treated with endoscopic retrograde cholangiogram (ERC) and biliary stenting. Any missed CBD stone that might have caused cystic duct blow-out can also be removed during ERCP. A low-output fistula, exhibiting a decreasing output trend, can be observed and may resolve on its own without the need for endotherapy. Complications of ERCP (acute pancreatitis, bleeding) may outweigh its benefits in this situation. Endotherapy may be therapeutic for Type A, C, and minor D injuries, but not advisable for Type E acute injuries, especially when there is biliary discontinuity or when the divided duct is occluded by the clip or suture tie.

Surgical Repair: Lateral injuries most often heal after endotherapy. However, extensive loss of the CBD wall or complete excision of the CBD eventually leads to stricture formation, which coincides with fistula closure. If there is no cholangitis and the fistula output shows a decreasing trend, it is advisable to wait for local inflammation to subside, stricture to form, allowing the bile duct to dilate, which will facilitate a successful repair. Conversely, if the fistula output remains high and constant after 2–3 weeks, consider hepaticojejunostomy (HJ) after 4–6 weeks. Waiting allows sepsis to settle, hilar inflammation to subside, duct margins to stabilize (after ischemic retraction), and possibly dilate when a successful repair (HJ) is carried out.

26.1.4.4 Management of Clipped or Ligated Bile Duct

Progressive jaundice in the immediate postoperative period without evidence of bile leak or abdominal symptoms suggests a clipped/ligated bile duct or, though uncommon, a retained CBD stone. The diagnosis is confirmed through screening ultrasound and MRCP. Such patients are candidates for early intervention if associated vascular injury is ruled out. During exploration, if only a clip or ligature across the bile duct is found, it should be removed, and a T-tube or stent should be placed across the clipped segment for 6 weeks to 3 months. In case of a clipped and transected duct, HJ is the treatment of choice. It is important to emphasize that such treatment must be performed at a tertiary care center or by a specialist hepatobiliary surgeon.

26.1.4.5 Delayed Management

Standard management of established stricture involves biliary reconstruction via Roux-en-Y hepaticojejunostomy (Fig. 26.11). This is usually performed at least 6–8 weeks after the injury or control of sepsis. The interval may be longer in patients with associated vascular injury or ongoing bile leak. This waiting period allows local inflammation to sub-

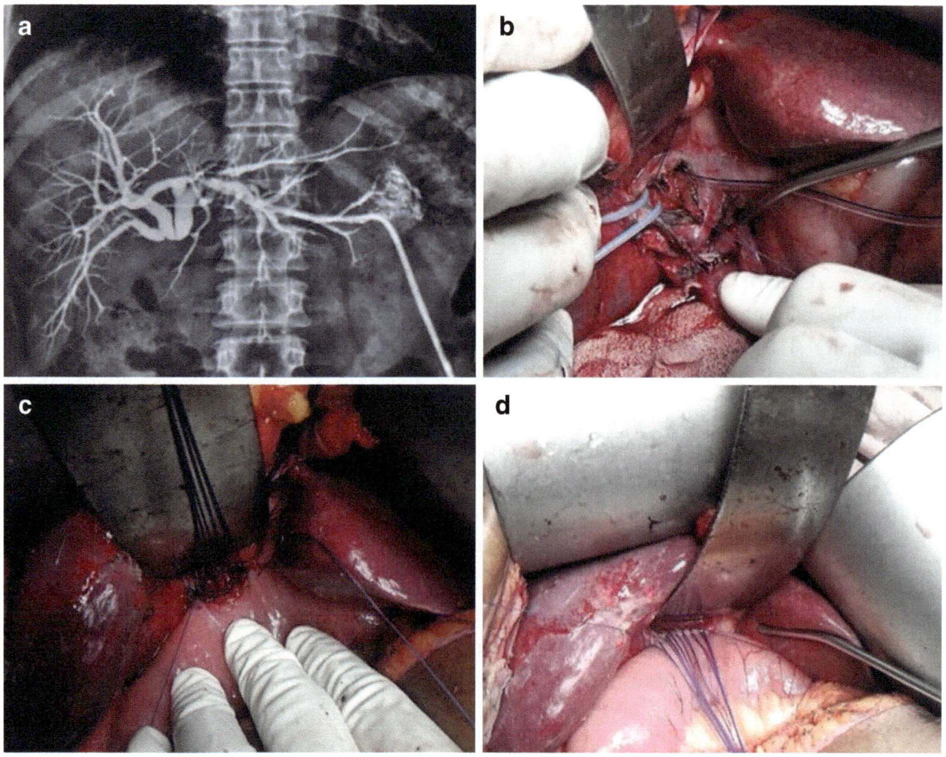

Fig. 26.11 (**a**) Strasberg E3 stricture: Preoperative percutaneous biliary catheterization with cholangiogram, (**b**) intraoperative photographs showing all three ducts—right anterior, right posterior sectoral, and left hepatic ducts—exposed and catheterized in preparation for hepaticojejunostomy, (**c**) hepaticojejunostomy: posterior layer of the anastomosis completed, and (**d**) anterior layer of the anastomosis completed

side, the extent of the biliary stricture to be clearly defined, and sufficient collaterals to develop across the hepatic hilum in cases of arterial injury. Preoperatively, complete biliary anatomy should be mapped with imaging studies such as MRCP or PTBD cholangiogram.

Achieving excellent long-term outcomes requires adherence to the basic tenets of surgical repair (Table 26.6). While a single anastomosis is necessary for Types E1, E2, and E3 injuries, two separate anastomoses may be required for E4 and E5. Since an anastomosis is a side-step, the presence of a dilated bile duct, although preferred, is not mandatory for performing the procedure. It is most commonly performed in a single layer with interrupted fine (3-0/4-0) delayed absorbable sutures; however, continuous suturing can also be used, especially in dilated ducts during minimally invasive repairs, such as laparoscopic or robotic procedures. Higher strictures (Type E3, E4, E5) may require preoperative biliary catheterization (PTBC) to delineate the anatomy of the stricture, identify the ducts during surgery, and serve as trans-anastomotic stents (Fig. 26.12). The use of a stent across the HJ stoma can be routine or optional. Optional use is recommended when the bilioenteric anastomosis is at risk, such as in cases with thin and friable ducts, undilated ducts, inability to achieve mucosa-to-mucosa anastomosis, or when the anastomosis is under tension. In such cases, stents should be retained for at least 3 months to allow the healing process to mature.

Endoscopic management may be considered in highly selected cases with low strictures (Type E1 or E2) when the patient is not a surgical candidate or is unwilling to undergo surgical treatment. However, endoscopic therapy typically requires multiple sessions and stents, often taking about a year to complete, unlike surgical repair, which is a one-time

Table 26.6 Principles of bilioenteric anastomosis for repairing biliary stricture

A side-to-side hepaticojejunostomy using the Hepp-Couinaud technique; this involves lowering the hilar plate to gain additional length of the healthy hepatic duct, specially in higher stricture
Tension-free, mucosa-to-mucosa anastomosis using a healthy duct and a 45–60 cm long Roux limb of the jejunum
Drainage of all segments of the liver through (single or multiple) bilio-enteric anastomosis
Ensure the stoma is at least 2 cm in size; this might necessitate extending the incision onto the left duct, which has an extrahepatic course at the base of segment 4
Anastomosis using fine, delayed absorbable sutures

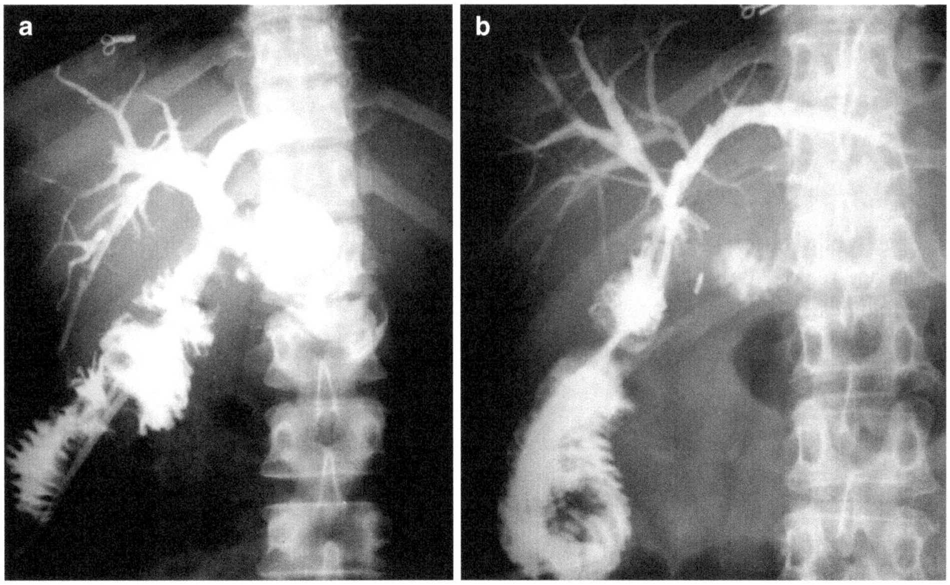

Fig. 26.12 Hepatico jejunostomy (**a**) using one transanastomotic stent, (**b**) two stents

procedure. Strong patient compliance for multiple scheduled visits is essential for the success of endoscopic management).

26.2 Bleeding and Vascular Complications

Bleeding during LC is another potentially serious complication that can result in open conversion, longer operative time, higher risk of biliary injury, and extended hospital stay. Preoperative identification, assessment, and appropriate planning can decrease the risk of bleeding during cholecystectomy (Table 26.7). Management depends on the cause and site of the bleeding (Table 26.8).

Table 26.7 Predisposing factors for bleeding during laparoscopic cholecystectomy

Inflammation and adhesions	Chronic cholecystitis, previous abdominal surgery, prior attempt at cholecystectomy, prior percutaneous cholecystostomy, and prior acute pancreatitis. Inflammation around the gallbladder (GB) makes dissection more difficult. It may also obscure normal or aberrant anatomy and increase the risk of injury to blood vessels
Acute cholecystitis	The acutely inflamed and friable GB is more prone to bleeding during dissection The surrounding tissues may also exhibit inflammatory changes, making it more challenging to identify biliary and vascular structures
Liver cirrhosis	Cirrhotic patients pose a higher risk due to the liver's increased vascularity, decreased coagulability, and presence of portal hypertension with collaterals The friable nature of the cirrhotic liver increases the likelihood of bleeding from the liver capsule or parenchyma during GB separation
Portal cavernoma	Portal cavernoma due to extrahepatic portal vein obstruction with portal hypertension increases the risk of bleeding from venous collaterals around the GB and in the HCT
Aberrant anatomy	Unidentified anatomical anomalies, like a caterpillar hump, a replaced right hepatic artery, or an accessory cystic artery, increase the risk of vascular injury during dissection
Obesity	Excess fat can sometimes obscure important anatomical landmarks and structures in the HCT, thereby increasing vulnerability to injury during dissection
Coagulopathies	Patients who have bleeding disorders or are taking blood thinners are more likely to experience bleeding during and after surgery

HCT hepatocystic triangle

Table 26.8 Bleeding during laparoscopic cholecystectomy: Causes, prevention, and management

Stage of cholecystectomy	Site and cause of bleeding	Prevention and management
Port placement	Port site, mesentery, aorta (rarely)	Use the open technique (under vision) for trocar insertion. Be extra careful in case of a previous laparotomy. Inspect all port sites and cauterize if a bleeding point is identified. Major bleeding from the mesentery or the aorta requires immediate conversion
Separation of pericholecystic adhesions	Torn omental vessels	Identify and cauterize
Fundal retraction	Liver parenchymal tear at the base of the falciform ligament	Release the lateral part of the ligament. Cauterize the bleeding point(s)
Cystic artery isolation	Avulsed cystic artery	Isolate the CA close to the cystic lymph node. Divide using a vessel sealer (e.g., Harmonic scalpel (Ethicon)) or sharply with scissors without excessive traction after applying two clips proximally. Divide before cystic duct division to prevent undue traction with GB retraction. In the event of accidental avulsion or a slipped clip, apply pressure by flipping the GB onto the liver or using a gauze piece. Release the tamponade after ten minutes, identify the bleeding point, reapply the clip, or coagulate with bipolar cautery
Posterior dissection of the GB infundibulum	Injury to the deep branch of the CA	Apply pressure for ten minutes. Clip or cauterize after identifying the bleeding point

(continued)

Table 26.8 (continued)

Stage of cholecystectomy	Site and cause of bleeding	Prevention and management
Dissection of the HCT	Accidental injury to the accessory CA	More than one arterial twig is present due to the early division of the CA, multiple CA, or RHA hump in the HCT in about one quarter of patients. Carefully dissect to isolate all arterial branches, then clip and divide them. In the event of bleeding, use tamponade followed by coagulation or clipping
Dissection of HCT	Accidental clipping of the RHA	Expect RHA if the arterial trunk appears unusually thick and pulsating. Dissect and divide the CA near the GB surface, laterally to the cystic lymph node. Remove the clip if RHA has been clipped but not divided. Most often, repair of the RHA is not required unless ischemic discoloration of the right lobe appears
Dissection of the GB from the liver bed	Deep branch of the CA Parenchymal bleeding Hepatic vein tributaries	Dissect superficial to the cystic plate. Diffuse oozing can be controlled by pressure packing, spray coagulation, followed by application of Surgicel or Gelfoam. Prolonged pressure with the mobilized GB or gauze piece often controls venous bleeding. Suture ligation may be required to control avulsed venous tributaries
Dissection in patients with liver cirrhosis	GB bed diffuse ooze	Leave behind the adherent posterior wall of the GB adherent to the liver
Dissection in patients with portal cavernoma	Torn collaterals	Use advanced energy device / vessel sealerfor dissection. Consider the "fundus first" technique and subtotal cholecystectomy, avoiding the dissection of Hartman's pouch and HCT having significant collateral veins. Considerable bleeding may require conversion to open for control

CA cystic artery, *HCT* hepatocystic triangle, *RHA* right hepatic artery, *GB* Gallbladder

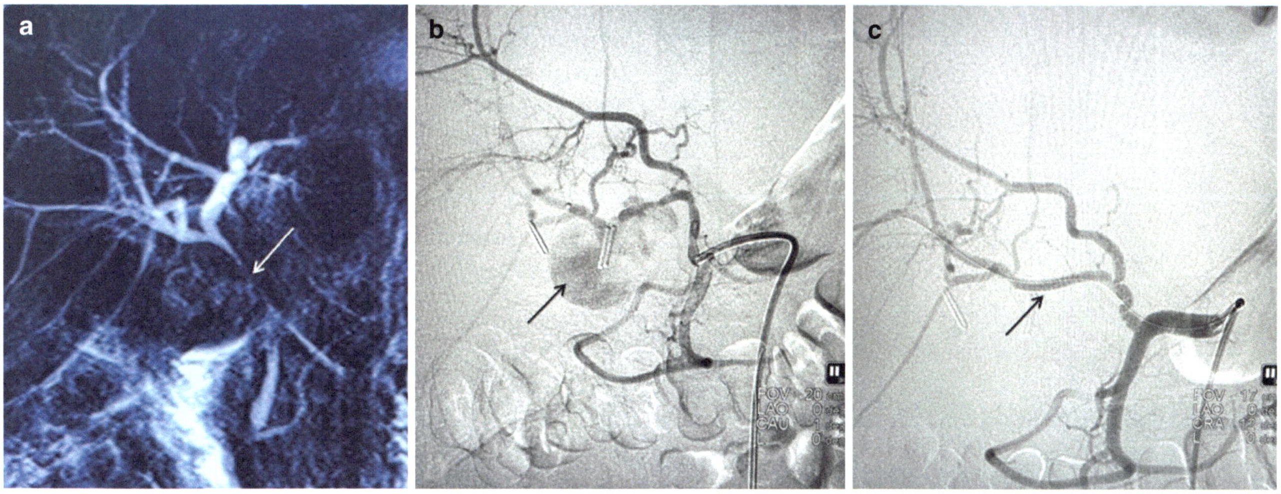

Fig. 26.13 Right hepatic artery (RHA) pseudoaneurysm following laparoscopic cholecystectomy. (**a**) MRCP showing pseudoaneurysm and hematoma compressing the CBD (arrow). (**b**) Selective angiography confirms the diagnosis (arrow). (**c**) An endovascular stent is placed across the breach in the RHA

26.2.1 Delayed Presentation of Vascular Complications

Pseudoaneurysm of the CA or RHA, resulting from cautery injury, is more commonly reported with LC than with open cholecystectomy. It typically presents late after surgery with subhepatic bleeding, hematoma, or gastrointestinal bleeding if it erodes into the duodenum. A CT angiogram confirms the diagnosis. Angio-embolization for CA or endovascular stenting for RHA involvement is the treatment of choice (Fig. 26.13).

26.3 Bowel Injury During Cholecystectomy

Bowel injury during LC is an uncommon but serious complication. Most often, it involves the small intestine (58%) and large intestine (32%), and less frequently the stomach (7%) and duodenum (0.04%). This complication mainly results from mechanical injury that occurs during Veress needle insertion, port placement, retraction, and dissection, as well as from thermal injury. Risk factors for bowel injury include prior abdominal surgery, extensive and/or dense intrabdominal adhesions, difficult cholecystectomy with significant pericholecystic adhesions, distended bowel, and suction injuries when an active suction cannula is used for retraction.

Bowel injuries are detected intraoperatively in only half of the cases. Remaining cases manifest in the immediate postoperative period or even later due to delayed perforation, as seen in cases of thermal injury. Missed cholecystoenteric fistula can also manifest postoperatively clinically and radiologically like bowel injury.

Detection of these injuries in the postoperative period requires a high index of suspicion. A deviant postoperative course with increasing abdominal distension, vomiting, tachycardia, hypotension, fever, ileus, sepsis, increasing drain output after resuming oral intake, and features of peritonitis should raise the suspicion of bowel injury. Drainage of greenish/yellowish fluid, mucoid in nature, with increasing output with oral intake, should raise the suspicion of duodenal injury, while thick yellowish foul-smelling content suggests colonic injury.

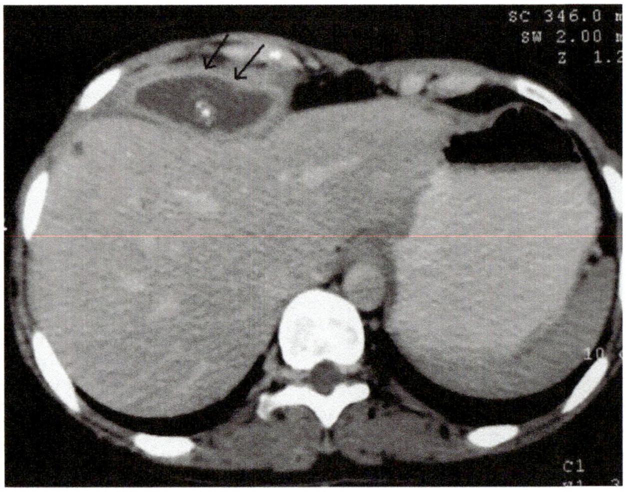

Fig. 26.14 An organized abscess with spilled gallstone in the center (arrows), located between the liver surface and parietes. The patient presented with recurrent abdominal pain and fever

When suspected, these injuries should be ruled out by prompt investigations. A CT scan with positive oral contrast is a highly sensitive and accurate modality for detecting bowel injuries. Per-rectal positive contrast is helpful in ascertaining colonic injury. A CT scan also allows assessment of an intrabdominal collection.

Management includes immediate abdominal exploration, repair of the injury, drainage of abdominal collections, and peritoneal lavage. A colonic injury may require a protective diverting ileostomy or colostomy.

26.4 Gallstone Spillage

Most often, incomplete retrieval of spilled gallstones is inconsequential, with adverse events reported in only a minority (~7%) of the cases. The complications of lost gallstones include abdominal pain, abdominal phlegmon or mass or abscess (Fig. 26.14), intestinal obstruction, intrabdominal sepsis, fever, chronic wound infection, port site sinus or fistula. Every effort should be made to prevent iatrogenic GB perforation. When it occurs, efforts should be made to retrieve all spilled stones. Morrison's pouch should be thoroughly examined by retracting the liver (by subcostal port) and the duodenum/omentum/colon (through lumbar port as spilled stones tend to get lost in deep spaces. Spilled bile and stone should be thoroughly cleared from the port site if spillage occurs during GB retrieval.

26.5 Wound Sinus and Nonhealing Port Sites

A nonhealing port site with surrounding cellulitis is an uncommon but challenging problem following LC. Brawny induration with multiple discharging sinuses in the affected area, lasting for days to weeks after the initial surgery, is the typical presentation (Fig. 26.15). The usual causes include spilled gallstones or infection by *Mycobacterium tuberculo-*

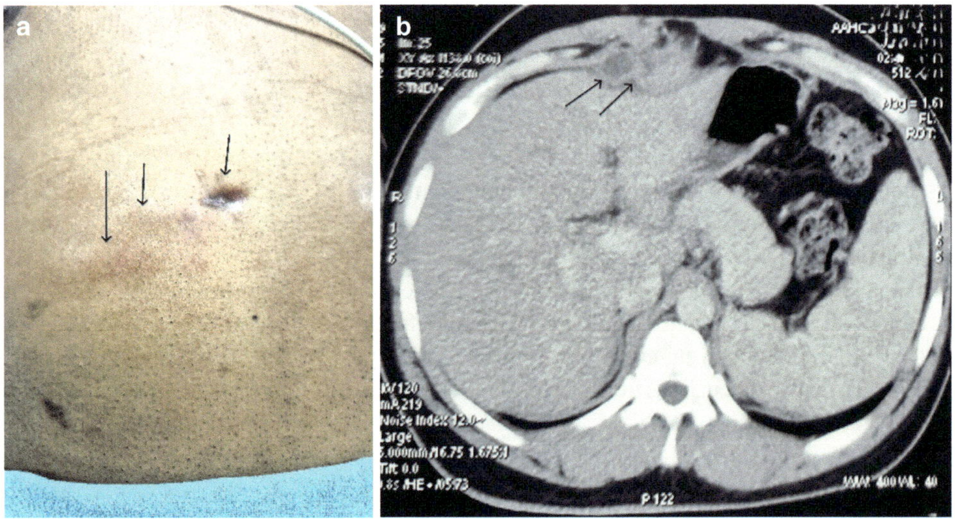

Fig. 26.15 Port site sinus following laparoscopic cholecystectomy. (**a**) A nonhealing epigastric port with purulent discharge, cellulitis, and brawny induration (arrows) around it. (**b**) CT scan showing a subcutaneous phlegmon (arrows)

sis or *Mycobacterium chelonae*. The latter is an atypical mycobacterium found in contaminated tap water. Improper sterilization of instruments is the sole cause of this infection. Diagnosis is confirmed by MRI or CT scan, with MRI being more accurate in delineating the sinus tract. Biopsy of the sinus tract and the indurated tissue confirms the presence of caseating or noncaseating granulomas, indicating a Mycobacterial infection. If spilled stones are involved, exploration of the sinus tract to remove the offending stone is necessary. Mycobacterial infections require wound debridement, excision of the indurated tissue, and a six to nine-month course of antituberculosis treatment.

26.6 Postcholecystectomy Syndrome/Symptoms

Postcholecystectomy syndrome encompasses a wide range of symptoms due to a variety of causes. After cholecystectomy, preoperative symptoms are relieved in about 60% of patients while 40% remain symptomatic in long-term follow-up, as noted in the PERFECT and SUCCESS trials. These may be persistent symptoms that existed before cholecystectomy or new-onset symptoms.

Residual or newly formed gallstones may be seen in 0.2–23% of cases. Residual stones are most commonly diagnosed as retained stones in the CBD, cystic duct, or in the remnant GB. Stone may reform in the GB remnant or within the CBD as well. These residual or recurrent stones may present with symptoms of biliary colic, jaundice, or cholangitis. High index of suspicion should be there for residual or recurrent stones in the GB remnant after subtotal cholecystectomy (especially reconstituting type). Besides sonography, MRI with MRCP is a valuable and important imaging modality for assessment and planning management. It is essential to assess the size of the GB remnant, cystic duct, and extrahepatic biliary tract anatomy for more accurate surgical planning. Management is directed at surgically removing the GB remnant, cystic duct stump, or endoscopic or surgical clearance of the CBD. Depending on the intraoperative difficulty and expertise available, the GB remnant can be excised laparoscopically. However, such cases are associated with higher open conversion and need for further bailout, as a complete stump cholecystectomy may not be feasible for the same reason that prohibited a complete cholecystectomy at index surgery. The primary aim in reoperative surgery for recurrent stump gallstones is complete cholecystectomy; if complete cholecystectomy is not feasible due to unfavorable anatomy, the aim should be to clear the GB remnant of the stones completely, excise it as much as possible, and leave the stump open, preferably after closing the cystic duct opening from inside the stump lumen (fenestrating subtotal cholecystectomy).

Most postcholecystectomy persistent symptoms are due to coexisting diseases, and symptoms are nonbiliary. Gastroesophageal reflux, peptic ulcer, irritable bowel disease, and constipation are common causes. These causes are often overlooked and not thoroughly evaluated before cholecystectomy.

New onset symptoms may be due to postcholecystectomy complications (1–3%), including bile duct injury, spilled stones, port site hernia, or physiological changes. Later changes are common, occurring in 16–58% of cases, and primarily result from the loss of GB reservoir function, leading to continuous bile flow in the duodenum and increased duodeno-gastric reflux, which may cause gastritis or dyspepsia. A reduced bile salt pool after cholecystectomy may result in diarrhea and flatulence due to fat malabsorption or decreased gut transit caused by bile acid-induced secretion and motility. Postcholecystectomy diarrhea is seen in as many as 57% cases. Prevention and treatment include a low-fat and low-animal protein diet, a high-fiber diet, antidiarrheals (loperamide), ursodeoxycholic acid, bile acid sequestrants (cholestyramine), and newer therapies such as bile acid receptor agonists (farnesoid X receptor (FXR) agonist), Glucagon-like peptide 1 receptor agonist, and targeting intestinal microbiota.

Sphincter of ODDI dysfunction and psychological distress may also result in persistent or recurrent abdominal symptoms after cholecystectomy.

The most important approach to managing the most persistent symptoms is proper case selection for cholecystectomy, achieved through an adequate preoperative workup that includes necessary investigations and assessments, such as esophagogastroduodenoscopy. Proper counseling of the patient selected for cholecystectomy is also essential, explaining realistic outcomes for symptom resolution, as conditions like functional dyspepsia and irritable bowel syndrome may be present in 20–30% and 20% of cases, respectively. Patients with predominant functional symptoms should be reassessed after some time, and expectant management should be considered for gallstones in the absence of typical symptoms. An online tool (gallbladderresearch.shinyapps.io/SUCCESS/) may assist both physicians and patients in making appropriate decisions.

Key Points

- Laparoscopic cholecystectomy (LC) has an overall morbidity rate of 1.6–5.3% and a mortality rate of 0.08–0.14%.
- Common postoperative complications include bleeding (0.79%), retained common bile duct (CBD) stones (0.5%), and bile duct injury (BDI) (0.3–0.5%).
- Misidentification of anatomy or perception errors during LC is the most common cause of BDI.
- Less than one-third of BDI cases are detected during the index surgery; the remaining cases appear in the early or late postoperative period.
- A bile leak after surgery may appear as an external biliary fistula when there is a subhepatic drain.
- Without a subhepatic drain, it may manifest as biliary peritonitis, bilioma, or bile ascites.
- Initial management of bile leak involves evaluation through CECT and/or MRCP and control of sepsis.
- Controlling sepsis involves properly draining all the collected bile and establishing a controlled external biliary fistula (EBF) as the initial step.
- After establishing a controlled EBF, lateral injury or cystic duct leak is primarily treated with ERC and bile duct stenting.
- For major BDI delayed hepaticojejunostomy (HJ) after at least 4–6 weeks of EBF is recommended to allow EBF and inflammation to resolve, the bile duct stump and stricture to mature and ducts to dilate.
- Early HJ can be considered in selected cases for a clipped or ligated duct if there is no bile leak, sepsis, or vascular injury.
- Intraoperative bleeding is a significant cause of conversion.
- Presence of acute cholecystitis, adhesions, aberrant arterial anatomy, cirrhosis of the liver, and portal cavernoma/portal hypertension are important causes of bleeding during LC.
- Careful dissection and identification of the bleeding point after compression are necessary to control the bleeding. Blind control of bleeding with cautery or clips must not be attempted in a desperate attempt to control bleeding.
- Pseudoaneurysm of the cystic artery or right hepatic artery is a rare but recognized complication of LC that usually occurs in the late postoperative period.
- When detected, angio-embolization or endovascular stenting is the preferred treatment for pseudoaneurysm.
- Bowel injury is a serious complication of LC that requires quick recognition and treatment.
- Residual or recurrent stone in the GB or cystic duct remnant, or CBD can cause ongoing/recurrent postoperative symptoms. Its management involves revision surgery and endoscopic removal for CBD stones, respectively.

Selected Reading

1. Alexander HC, Bartlett AS, Wells CI, et al. Reporting of complications after laparoscopic cholecystectomy: a systematic review. HPB (Oxford). 2018;20(9):786–94. https://doi.org/10.1016/j.hpb.2018.03.004.
2. Abdallah HS, Sedky MH, Sedky ZH. The difficult laparoscopic cholecystectomy: a narrative review. BMC Surg. 2025;25(1):156. https://doi.org/10.1186/s12893-025-02847-3.
3. Kapoor VK, editor. Post-cholecystectomy bile duct injury. Singapore: Springer; 2020.
4. Brunt LM, Deziel DJ, Telem DA, The Prevention of Bile Duct Injury Consensus Work Group, et al. Safe cholecystectomy multi-society practice guideline and state of the art consensus conference on prevention of bile duct injury during cholecystectomy. Ann Surg. 2020;272(1):3–23. https://doi.org/10.1097/SLA.0000000000003791.
5. Bansal VK, Misra M, Agarwal AK, et al. SELSI consensus statement for safe cholecystectomy – prevention and management of bile duct injury – Part A. Indian J Surg. 2021;83(Suppl 3):592–610. https://doi.org/10.1007/s12262-019-01993-2.
6. Bansal VK, Misra M, Agarwal AK, et al. SELSI consensus statement for safe cholecystectomy – prevention and management of bile duct injury – Part B. Indian J Surg. 2021;83(Suppl 3):611–24. https://doi.org/10.1007/s12262-019-01994-1.

27 Choledochal Cyst

Phani Krishna Ravula and Suresh Sepuri

Abstract

In Todani's classification, five types of choledochal cysts are identified; types I and IV make up the majority. Considered to be developmental in origin, APBJ is an important predisposing factor associated with choledochal cyst in 60–90% of cases. MRCP is the investigation of choice that not only delineates the cyst but also displays APBJ, the presence of stones, stricture, or malignancy. Resection of the extrahepatic segment of the cyst is recommended. Multiple intrahepatic cysts (types IVa and V) are difficult to manage and may ultimately require liver transplantation.

Keywords

Choledochal cyst

Choledochal cysts, also known as bile duct cysts, are characterized as focal or segmental dilatations of the biliary tree. Believed to be of developmental origin, the majority are diagnosed during childhood, with two-thirds of cases presenting before the age of 10 and approximately 25% diagnosed in adulthood. While more common in Asian populations, with an estimated incidence of 1 in 1000, choledochal cysts are also seen in Western populations, albeit less frequently, at around 1 in 13,000. A notable gender disparity exists, with females affected three to four times more often than males.

27.1 Etiopathogenesis

The exact cause of choledochal cysts remains elusive, with several theories proposed, none of which fully explain all cases. The two most widely recognized hypotheses are:

1. Babbitt's hypothesis (Reflux theory): This theory addresses the frequent association of choledochal cysts with an abnormal pancreatobiliary junction (APBJ). In these cases, a longer-than-normal common channel allows pancreatic juice to reflux into the biliary system. This reflux, which contains enzymes such as amylase, trypsinogen, and phospholipase A2, is thought to cause inflammation and subsequent dilation of the bile duct due to increased pressure. Over time, this chronic inflammation may result in dysplasia and, potentially, malignancy. Between 60% and 90% of choledochal cysts are linked to ABPJ.
2. Kusunoki's congenital hypothesis (distal bile duct weakness) proposes that a congenital deficiency in ganglion cells within the distal common bile duct (CBD) leads to inherent weakness and subsequent dilation. This mechanism is similar to the pathogenesis of Hirschsprung's disease and achalasia, both of which are characterized by a lack of ganglion cells in specific areas of the gastrointestinal tract.

It's important to note that neither of these theories can fully explain the diverse spectrum of choledochal cyst presentations, and multiple factors likely contribute to their development. Further research is required to clarify the complex etiopathogenesis of these cysts.

27.2 Classification

Choledochal cysts are categorized according to the Todani classification, which is a modification of the Alonso-Lej classification (Fig. 27.1; Table 27.1).

P. K. Ravula (✉) · S. Sepuri
Pace Hospitals, Hyderabad, India

M. Ibrarullah (ed.), *Recent Concepts in Gastrointestinal (GI) Surgery*, https://doi.org/10.1007/978-981-92-1118-0_27

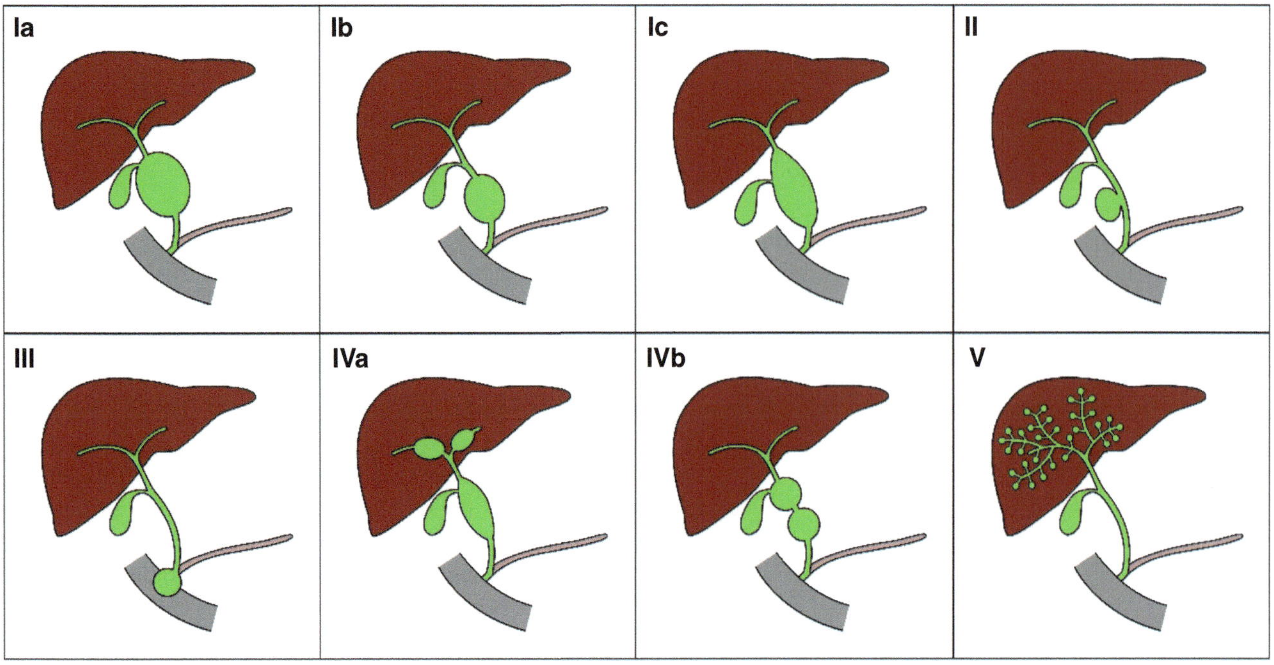

Fig. 27.1 Todani classification of choledochal cyst

Table 27.1 Modified Todani classification of choledochal cyst

Type	Appearance	Incidence
1	(a) Saccular dilation of the extrahepatic bile duct, frequently associated with APBJ (b) Focal dilation of the CBD typically occurs in the suprapancreatic region. The cystic duct arises separately. These cysts are not associated with APBJ (c) Fusiform dilation of the extrahepatic biliary system extending from the intrapancreatic CBD to CHD and sometimes extrahepatic right and left ducts (d) Cystic dilatation of the CBD, CHD, and cystic duct	50%–80%
II	A diverticular outpouching of the CBD typically arises from the right lateral wall of the CHD and mimics duplication of the gallbladder	2%–3%
III	Cystic dilation of the intraduodenal portion of the CBD (a) The bile duct opens into the duodenum through the cyst (b) The bile duct opens directly into the duodenum	2%
IV	(a) Involves both the intra- and extrahepatic biliary systems. Intrahepatic involvement is usually either both sides or the isolated left side, with a stenosis or membrane at the level of the hilum (b) Multiple cysts are present involving the extrahepatic biliary system, resembling a "string of beads"	15%–30%
V	Caroli's disease is characterized by multiple intrahepatic cystic dilatations of the biliary system with no involvement of the extrahepatic biliary tree	20%
VI	Isolated dilatation of the cystic duct	
Forme fruste	Minimal or no dilation of the biliary system, but with an associated abnormal APBJ	

APBJ abnormal pancreatobiliary junction, *CBD* common bile duct, *CHD* common hepatic duct

27.3 Abnormal Pancreatobiliary Junction

APBJ is defined as the union of the bile duct and pancreatic duct outside the duodenal wall, leading to a long common channel. A length of 5 mm (range 2–20 mm) is considered normal. The common channel in APBJ, as reported by various authors, measures between 22 mm and 28 mm (range 13–67 mm). APBJ is associated with choledochal cysts in 60%–90% of cases, most commonly of the type I and type IV variants. A higher frequency has also been noted with choledochal cysts that develop malignancy. Initially, APBJ was classified as C-P (bile duct joining pancreatic duct) or P-C (pancreatic duct joining the bile duct) variants. A third variant and subvariants were later identified, prompting Komi to propose a more detailed classification. In this classification, types I and II correspond to the C-P and P-C variants, respectively. The various types of APBJ, their respective incidence, and association with choledochal cysts are presented below (Fig. 27.2; Table 27.2).

27.4 Clinical Presentation

About 80–85% of choledochal cysts are identified in the pediatric population. Infants (under 1 year) present distinct clinical features compared to those older than 1 year. The classical triad of jaundice, pain, and abdominal mass occurs in 0%–17% of infants. While pain is uncommon in this age group, abdominal mass and jaundice are present in 82% and 64%, respectively. Children often display at least two of the classic triad of symptoms in 85% of cases. In contrast, these symptoms are seen in only 25% of adults. In symptomatic individuals, common presenting features include abdominal pain, fever, jaundice, and vomiting. Abdominal pain is the most frequently observed symptom in adult patients, with an incidence ranging from 78% to 90%. Pain typically occurs in the epigastrium or right hypochondrium and may radiate to the back. Jaundice and cholangitis occur in 40%–50% of adult patients. Abdominal masses are rare in adults and warrant investigation for malignancy. Symptomatic cases in

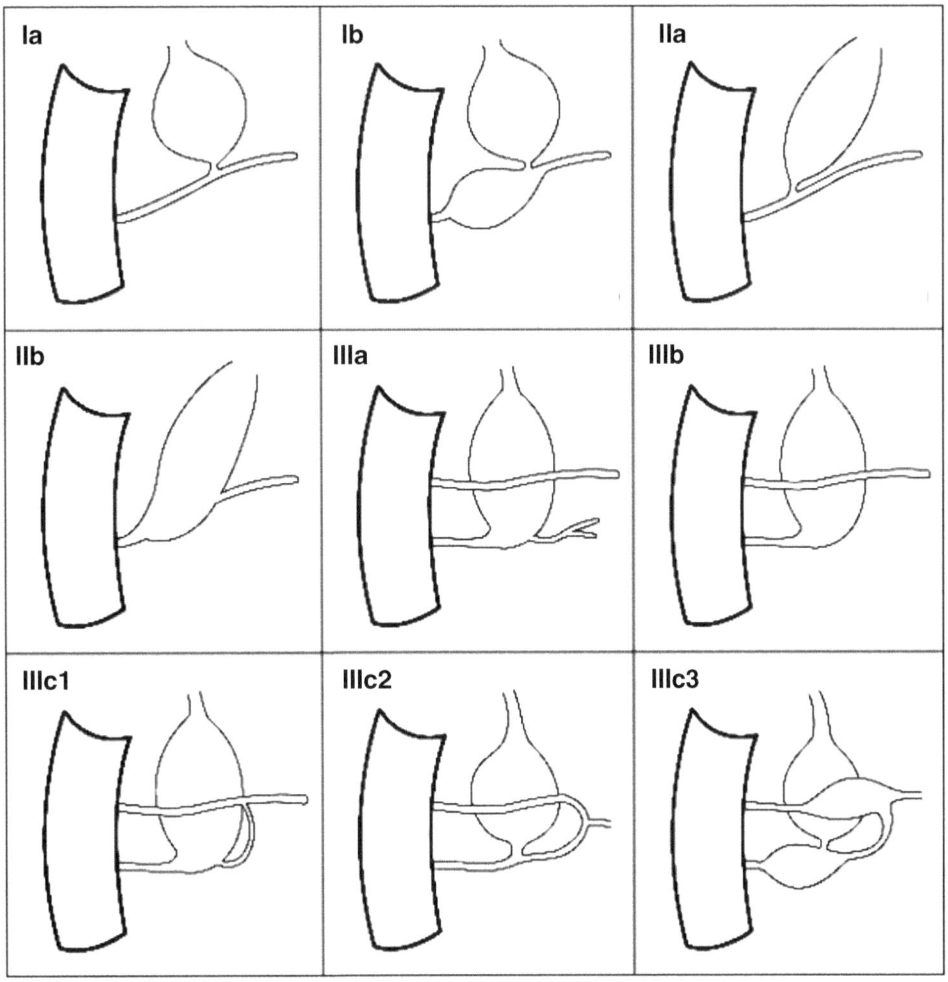

Fig. 27.2 Komi classification of APBJ. See below for details

Table 27.2 Komi classification, incidence of APBJ, and its association with choledochal cyst

Type	Features	Incidence	CC
I	Union of the BD and PD at a right angle to each other	58%	29%
a	*Without dilatation*		
b	*With dilatation of the common channel*		
II	Union of the duct BD and PD with an acute angle between them	32%	61%
a	*Without dilatation*		
b	*With dilatation of the common channel*		
III	Complex patterns of the pancreatic ductal system	6%	7%
a	*Pancreas divisum with biliary dilatation*		
b	*Absence of the Wirsung's duct*		
c 1	*Minor communication between the main duct and the accessory duct*		
c 2	*Normal communication between the common and accessory ducts*		
c 3	*Complete or partial dilatation of the ductal system*		

CC choledochal cyst, *BD* bile duct, *PD* pancreatic duct

adults often indicate underlying complications primarily related to stone formation, inflammation, and secondary infections. These complications encompass cystolithiasis, cholelithiasis, cholangitis, biliary strictures, and acute pancreatitis. Spontaneous perforation is an infrequent complication of biliary cysts. Recurrent or chronic pancreatitis is also observed in about 30% of patients. Adults with Type IV A and Caroli's disease tend to experience a complicated course with a history of multiple interventions. They may present with secondary biliary cirrhosis and signs of portal hypertension. Malignancy within the biliary system is a recognized risk, with a reported incidence ranging from 6% to 20%. This risk shows geographical variation, with higher rates reported in Japan and other Asian countries. An abdominal mass accompanied by weight loss or progressive jaundice should raise a strong suspicion of malignancy. The reported sites of malignancies and their corresponding frequencies are as follows: extrahepatic bile duct 50%–62%, gallbladder cancer 38%–46%, intrahepatic biliary tree 2%–2.5%, and liver and pancreas 0%–0.7%. Reports from Japan, however, show a higher incidence of gallbladder cancer, which is twice that of bile duct cancer (Table 27.3).

Table 27.3 Hepatobiliary and pancreatic complications of choledochal cyst

Cystolithiasis, hepatolithiasis
Calculous cholecystitis
Acute and chronic pancreatitis
Spontaneous bile duct perforation
Intrahepatic abscesses
Secondary biliary cirrhosis
Cholangiocarcinoma
Gallbladder cancer
Pancreatic cancer

27.5 Investigations

Ultrasonography (USG) A choledochal cyst is suspected when a dilated bile duct is found on screening USG in patients presenting with upper abdominal pain. USG has a sensitivity of 70%–90% in diagnosing choledochal cysts. Ultrasound may also detect associated stones and sludge. Any focal thickening of the cyst wall should raise suspicion of malignancy.

Magnetic Resonance Cholangiopancreatogram (MRCP) MRCP is the gold standard investigation for patients with choledochal cysts, exhibiting a sensitivity of 95–100% (Figs. 27.3, 27.5 and 27.6). It identifies the type of choledochal cyst, the extent of involvement in the intrahepatic and extrahepatic biliary tree, ABPJ, associated cholangiocarcinoma, as well as bile duct and intrahepatic stones. The involvement pattern of the intrahepatic biliary tree in Type IV is crucial, given the risk of recurrent cholangitis and hepatolithiasis even after excision of the extrahepatic biliary tree. Generally, fusiform dilatation of the intrahepatic biliary tree results from downstream obstruction and resolves after surgery. True intrahepatic involvement is marked by saccular dilatation of intrahepatic radicles, characterized by at least a 50% change in the caliber of the duct. Identifying these saccular Type IV A and V choledochal cysts on MRCP is essential, as they carry significant long-term prognostic implications.

Endoscopic Retrograde Cholangiopancreatogram (ERCP) ERCP is no longer used as a diagnostic tool for choledochal cysts due to the risk of infection and pancreatitis. However, it may play a role in type III choledochal cysts,

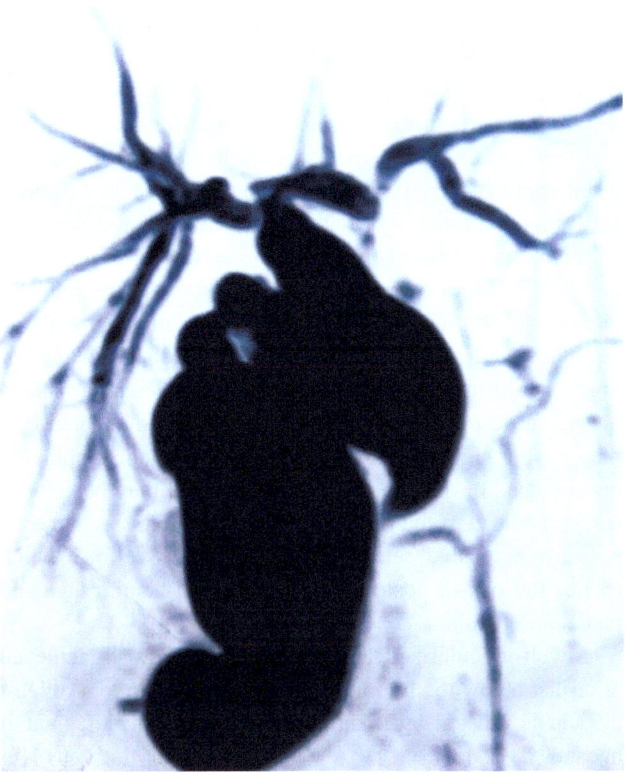

Fig. 27.3 MRCP appearance of type 1 choledochal cyst

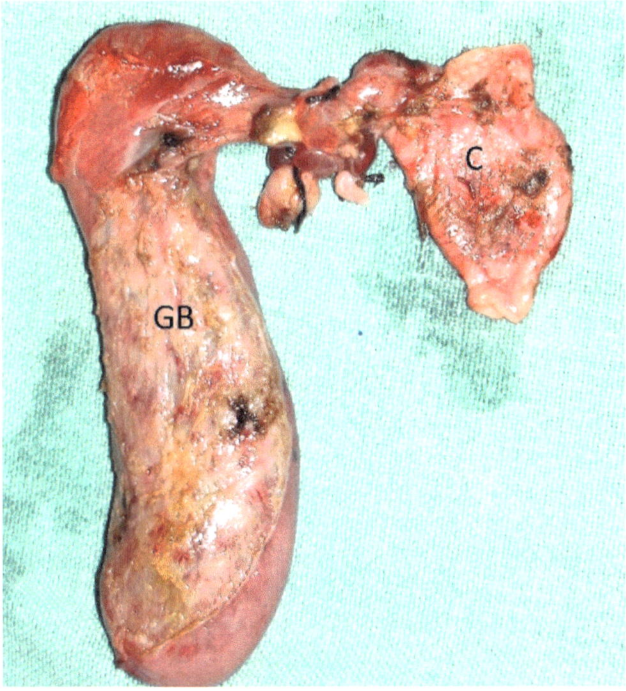

Fig. 27.4 Excised specimen. C, choledochal cyst; GB, gallbladder

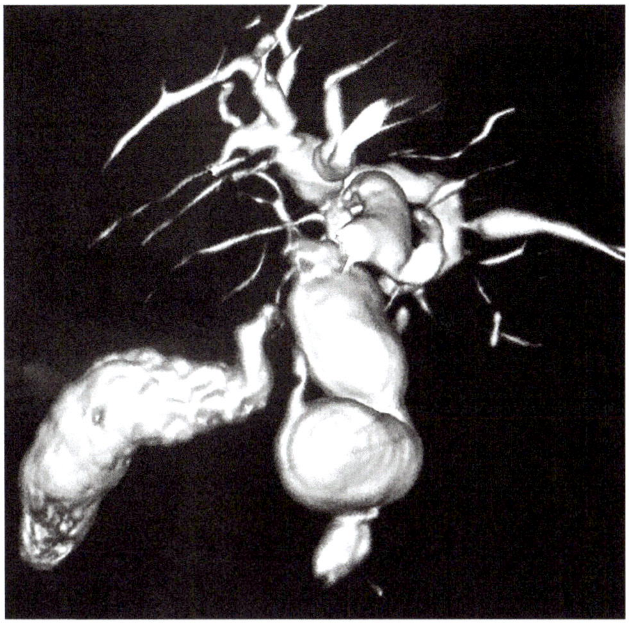

Fig. 27.5 Choledochal cyst type IVa; 3-D reconstruction of MRCP image

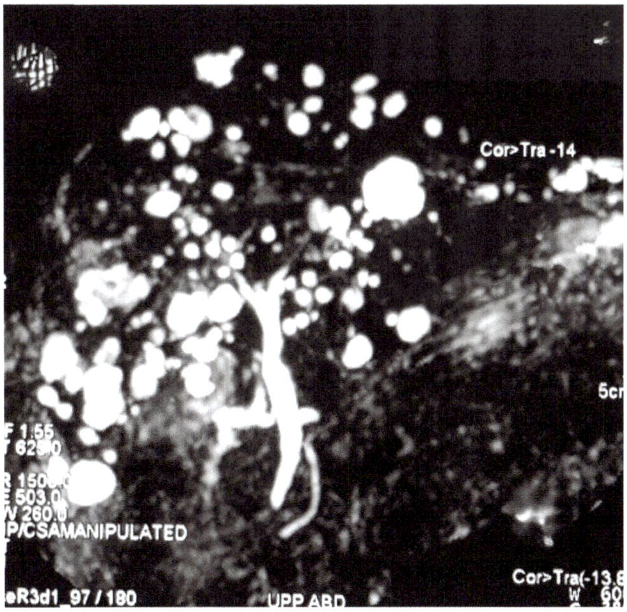

Fig. 27.6 Choledochal cyst type V (Caroli's disease). Coronal reconstruction of the MRI image

aiding in diagnosis and allowing for a therapeutic endoscopic sphincterotomy to be performed.

Endoscopic Ultrasound (EUS) EUS is useful only in choledochal cysts suspected of malignancy.

Contrast-Enhanced CT Scan A CT scan is generally not used to diagnose choledochal cysts. However, it can help in preoperative mapping of arterial anatomy variations and collateral circulation in patients with portal vein thrombosis. It is helpful for staging in patients with associated cholangiocarcinoma. For patients with Type IV and V choledochal cysts who have hepatolithiasis, it aids in identifying segmental involvement, atrophy, hypertrophy, hepatic abscesses, liver volumes, and portal vein thrombosis, which are essential for surgical planning.

27.6 Management

Once diagnosed, all choledochal cysts require treatment if the patient is a suitable surgical candidate, regardless of symptoms, due to long-term risks of recurrent pancreatitis, cholestasis, and cholangitis, which can lead to hepatic fibrosis, secondary biliary cirrhosis, and cholangiocarcinoma.

In patients with cholangitis, jaundice, or pancreatitis, surgery is usually postponed for 2–6 weeks to allow the infection and local inflammation to subside. If biliary sepsis does not improve with antibiotics, percutaneous or endoscopic biliary drainage should be performed. Rarely, patients may experience spontaneous perforation of the choledochal cyst. Laparoscopic or open lavage and T-tube drainage of the bile duct may be necessary to handle the emergency (Table 27.4).

Operative Strategies for Choledochal Cyst Laparoscopic choledochal cyst excision and bilioenteric anastomosis are considered safe alternatives to open surgery when expertise is available. The operative time is longer, and the surgery remains technically demanding. Regardless of the approach, the principles of surgery remain the same.

The more common Type 1 and Type IV choledochal cysts are treated with laparoscopic or open excision of the extrahepatic biliary segment, followed by Roux-en-Y hepaticojejunostomy (HJ). Alternatively, in suitable cases, excision and hepaticoduodenostomy can also be performed. Lateral cystoenteric anastomosis without excision is of historical interest and not recommended due to the persistent risk of malignancy, pancreatitis, and anastomotic stenosis with cholangitis. After an initial cholecystectomy, the dissection of the extrahepatic bile duct remains close to the choledochal cyst wall, avoiding injury to the hepatic artery and portal vein. In patients with dense peri-choledochal adhesions due to recurrent cholangitis, separating the posterior wall from the vascular structures may risk bleeding from the portal vein and injury to the right hepatic artery. In such cases, the posterior wall may be left intact, and the mucosa of the posterior wall is obliterated by diathermy (Lillie's modification). Complete resection of the intrapancreatic cyst is important due to the risk of dysplasia and malignancy in the remnant bile duct lining. The junction of the pancreatic duct with the bile duct needs to be correlated with the preoperative imaging to avoid intraoperative injury to the pancreatic duct. In the pediatric population, a large type 1 A choledochal cyst may have a significant retropancreatic component splaying out the head of the pancreas; in this case, it may be safer to resect the head of the pancreas (pancreatectomy) rather than perform extensive retro/intrapancreatic dissection, which carries the risk of postoperative pancreatic hemorrhage and pancreatic fistula.

A well-vascularized, tension-free anastomosis is achieved at or just below the hilum. An adequate HJ stoma of at least 2.5 cm is created by opening the extrahepatic left duct if needed. Even in Type IV A with intrahepatic duct involvement, a wide anastomosis that ensures proper bile flow is more important for preventing long-term complications than a radical excision of the dilated right and left ducts completely. Type IV choledochal cysts in children are often linked with membranous bile duct stenosis at or just above the hilum in one-third of cases. Since this stenosis is located above the proposed anastomosis, it is crucial to identify and remove this membrane.

Type II choledochal cyst (diverticular type) does not require bile duct excision. Removing the diverticular part and closing the bile duct, either directly or over a T-tube, is enough. Data show that en bloc bile duct excision and reconstruction offer no advantage over cyst excision alone.

The anatomical location of a type III choledochal cyst (choledochocele) requires a pancreaticoduodenectomy, which carries its own risks. Because malignant transformation in these cysts is very rare, endoscopic sphincterotomy or surgical sphincteroplasty is the preferred treatment. ERCP has the advantage of being less invasive and offers better visualization of the pancreatic duct anatomy, helping to prevent pancreatic duct injury.

Managing type IV cysts with saccular intrahepatic dilatations presents a challenge. Patients with this condition often develop multiple intrahepatic stenoses, recurrent cholangitis, hepatic abscesses, and eventually intrahepatic cholangiocarcinoma and secondary biliary cirrhosis. If the disease is

Table 27.4 Surgical management of choledochal cyst

Type I: Bile duct excision with roux-en-Y hepaticojejunostomy
Type II: Excision of diverticulum without bile duct excision
Type III: Endoscopic sphincterotomy or surgical sphincteroplasty
Type IV: Excision of extrahepatic bile duct with roux-en-Y hepaticojejunostomy
Type IVb & V: *Unilobar*-liver resection, *bilobar*-liver transplantation
Type VI: Cholecystectomy with complete excision of the dilated cystic duct

localized to one half of the liver, a hemi hepatectomy of the involved segment, along with extrahepatic bile duct excision and a Roux-en-Y HJ to the remnant liver, is preferred (Fig. 27.7).

Managing type IV choledochal cysts with bilobar liver involvement and type V choledochal cyst (Caroli's disease) is challenging. One approach involves removing the extrahepatic biliary tree, using cholangioscopic retrieval for intrahepatic stones, then performing hepaticojejunostomy with an access loop or hepaticoduodenostomy. The access loop or duodenal access makes future endoscopic reinterventions easier. An alternative is hepaticojejunostomy with external drainage through bilateral percutaneous transhepatic biliary drainage (PTBD) catheters to enhance drainage. These procedures aim to reduce the risk of cholangitis and prevent or delay secondary biliary cirrhosis. However, these options often become ineffective over time, leaving liver transplant as the only viable solution.

Type VI choledochal cyst (isolated cystic dilatation of the cystic duct) is treated with cholecystectomy along with complete excision of the dilated cystic duct.

Forme fruste choledochal cyst: Forme fruste choledochal cyst refers to an evolving or incompletely developed cyst. When symptomatic, it presents with any of the outlined symptoms of a choledochal cyst. Biochemical evidence of biliary obstruction primarily supports the diagnosis, which is mainly based on MRCP. A normal or minimally dilated bile duct and APBJ serve as the diagnostic clinchers. Excision of the extrahepatic bile duct and hepaticojejunostomy are recommended as the treatment of choice.

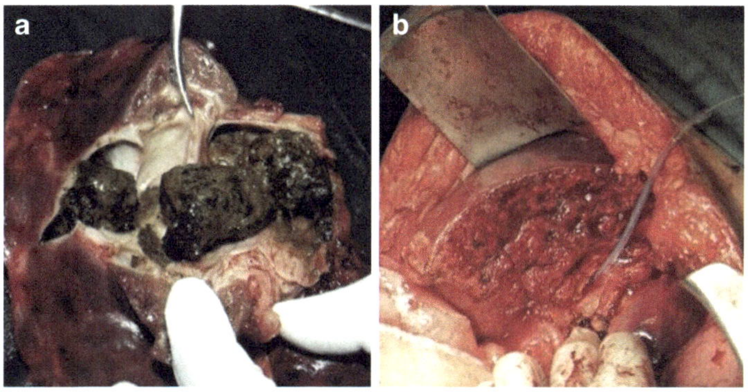

Fig. 27.7 Choledochal cyst type IVa with predominant involvement of left lobe ducts. (**a**) Left hepatectomy specimen showing dilated intrahepatic ducts with hepatolithiasis. (**b**) Residual right lobe of the liver

Key Points

- Choledochal cysts, also known as bile duct cysts, are characterized by focal or segmental dilatations of the biliary tree.
- In Todani's classification, five types of choledochal cysts are identified; types I and IV make up the majority.
- Considered to be developmental in origin, APBJ is an important predisposing factor, associated with choledochal cyst in 60%–90% of cases.
- APBJ is defined as the union of the biliary and pancreatic ducts outside the duodenal wall, resulting in a long common channel.
- Based on the configuration of the ductal union, APBJ has been classified into three main types. Type I variant is the most common, but type II variant is more frequently associated with choledochal cyst.
- The clinical presentation of a choledochal cyst typically includes a classic triad of jaundice, pain, and an abdominal mass. Children often exhibit at least two of these symptoms in 85% of cases. Conversely, these symptoms are present in only 25% of adults. Symptomatic individuals commonly present with abdominal pain, fever, jaundice, and vomiting.
- Symptomatic cases in adults often indicate underlying complications, e.g., cystolithiasis, cholelithiasis, cholangitis, biliary strictures, biliary malignancy, and pancreatitis.
- MRCP is the investigation of choice that not only delineates the cyst but also displays APBJ, presence of stones, stricture, or malignancy.
- Resection of the extrahepatic segment of the cyst is recommended.
- Multiple intrahepatic cysts (types IVa and V) are difficult to manage and may ultimately require liver transplantation.

Selected Reading

1. Edil BH, Olino K, Cameron JL. The current management of choledochal cysts. Adv Surg. 2009;43:221–32.
2. Tadokoro H, Takase M. Recent advances in choledochal cysts. Open J Gastroenterol. 2012;2:145–54. https://doi.org/10.4236/ojgas.2012.24029.
3. Ishibashi H, Shimada M, Kamisawa T, et al. Japanese Clinical Practice Guidelines for congenital biliary dilatation. J Hepatobiliary Pancreat Sci. 2017;24(1):1–16. https://doi.org/10.1002/jhbp.415.
4. Gadelhak N, Shehta A, Hamed H. Diagnosis and management of choledochal cyst: 20 years of single center experience. World J Gastroenterol. 2014;20(22):7061–6.

Cholangiohepatitis

28

Hamza Wani

Abstract

Cholangiohepatitis is a biliary disease that is being seen more often in parts of Asia, especially in China and other Southeast Asian countries. The presence of stones, strictures, infection, and inflammation creates a vicious cycle that results in disease progression. The symptoms of RPC can be nonspecific, variable, and subtle in the early stages. As the disease progresses, patients may present with intermittent mild to severe cholangitis and sepsis. MRCP is the preferred imaging test for diagnosis, classification, and management planning. Definitive surgical treatment, depending on the extent of the disease, includes stone clearance and T-tube drainage, biliary drainage with bilioenteric anastomosis with or without access-loop hepaticojejunostomy, and resection of the involved liver segment.

Keywords

Oriental cholangiohepatitis · Intrahepatic stones

Cholangiohepatitis is a biliary disease that is increasingly seen in parts of Asia, particularly in China and other Southeast Asian countries. It is characterized by low-grade infection and/or inflammation of the biliary tree, leading to biliary strictures, stones, and sludge formation, mainly near the primary biliary confluence. The biliary inflammation can eventually affect the hepatic parenchyma, often resulting in progressive liver damage, cirrhosis, and liver failure.

28.1 Epidemiology

Cholangiohepatitis was first identified by Digby in Hong Kong (1930). The term Oriental Cholangiohepatitis (OCH) was popularized by Stock and Fung (1962); the entity is also known as Hong Kong disease (Mage and Morel 1965), hepatolithiasis (Nakayama 1980), and oriental infestational cholangitis (Seel and Park 1983). The occurrence varies among different Asian populations as well. However, with the increase in global travel and migration, cases have also been reported in Western countries. In the Indian context, the incidence appears higher in the northern Himalayan regions (Jammu and Kashmir) and the eastern states (Odisha and Bengal). Given its worldwide distribution, it is more appropriate to refer to this condition as cholangiohepatitis or recurrent pyogenic cholangitis (RPC) instead of OCH.

28.2 Risk Factors and Etiopathogenesis

Parasitic Infections The most significant association in endemic areas is with parasitic infections, particularly *Clonorchis sinensis* (Chinese liver fluke) and *Opisthorchis viverrini*. These liver flukes are primarily found in freshwater fish and are common in regions where the consumption of raw or undercooked fish is frequent. Chronic infestations by these flukes can lead to bile duct inflammation, fibrosis, and cholangiohepatitis, which may advance to cirrhosis and biliary cancer. Roundworms, such as *Ascaris lumbricoides*, have also been linked to the development of this disease, particularly in the Kashmir Valley of India.

Autoimmunity and Genetic Susceptibility While parasitic infections are the most well-established cause, autoimmunity and genetic predispositions may also play a role. In particular, certain polymorphisms in genes related to immune response might make individuals more prone to chronic cholestasis and biliary inflammation. The exact genetic markers for RPC are still under investigation, but researchers are exploring how specific human leukocyte antigen (HLA) haplotypes may contribute. It is often observed that the number of mucous glands in diseased ducts increases. The combined influence of bacteria and mucus contributes to the formation

H. Wani (✉)
Government Medical College, Jammu, India

M. Ibrarullah (ed.), *Recent Concepts in Gastrointestinal (GI) Surgery*, https://doi.org/10.1007/978-981-92-1118-0_28

of intrahepatic stones. Overexpression of gel-forming apomucins (MUC2 and MUC5AC) in the biliary epithelium, caused by TNF-α and activation of protein kinase C, also plays a part. As a result, this mucin hypersecretion and mucus plug formation create a nidus for stone development.

Chronic Biliary Obstruction Some patients with RPC have a history of ongoing biliary blockage, which may result from stones, strictures, or other biliary abnormalities. This results in prolonged bile stagnation, which encourages bacterial infections (such as those caused by gram-negative organisms like *E. coli*, *Klebsiella*, and *Pseudomonas*) and inflammation of the biliary tree. The stones are mostly composed of calcium bilirubinate (75%), resulting from bacterial β-glucuronidase activity.

Biliary epithelial damage caused by Clonorchis or Ascaris is the initial event. Superimposed bacterial infection and inflammation further contribute to epithelial injury, leading to stricture formation. The β-glucuronidase activity of bacteria promotes the formation of calcium bilirubinate stones. The presence of stones, strictures, infection, and inflammation creates a vicious cycle that results in disease progression. Protein-calorie malnutrition, dietary fat deficiency, ductal abnormalities, and immune suppression are other presumed contributing factors.

28.3 Pathological Features

Histologically, RPC is characterized by several distinctive features, with the primary ones being infection accompanied by fibrosis and strictures, with or without pigmented stone formation.

Biliary Ductal Proliferation There is a significant increase in bile ducts, especially small intrahepatic ones, which may appear in clusters. The duct walls lose their parallel arrangement, with increased and irregular branching, along with abrupt terminations or "arrowhead" formations in smaller bile ducts. Repeated infections and fibrosis often lead to strictures, more commonly affecting the left-sided ductal system (40%). Bilateral involvement occurs in about 40%, while isolated right-sided disease accounts for roughly 20%. It is believed that the relatively horizontal position of the left main duct contributes to this higher occurrence. The proximal dilation that develops subsequently is likely a secondary effect.

Chronic Inflammation Inflammation characterized by persistent lymphocytic infiltration and fibrosis is mainly periportal but may extend into the pericentral zones as the disease advances.

Fibrosis and Cirrhosis As the disease progresses, fibrosis increases and may eventually lead to liver cirrhosis. The fibrosis is typically periportal but can become more widespread over time. This usually occurs after long-standing severe disease. Such patients often undergo multiple interventions, ranging from endoscopic procedures to surgery, with repeated episodes of biliary sepsis and symptoms. Along with cirrhosis, portal hypertension and bleeding esophageal varices are common consequences. In these cases, additional biliary decompression might require prior portosystemic shunting. Chronic severe disease that does not respond to medical or surgical treatment can also frequently result in liver dysfunction, potentially requiring a liver transplant.

Granulomatous Inflammation In some cases, especially when a parasitic infection is present, granulomas can form, mainly in areas of bile duct injury. These are more often histological findings in postoperative specimens.

Biliary Sludge and Stones In patients with chronic biliary stasis or parasitic infection, biliary sludge and even gallstones can develop. Stones are soft, friable, and pigmented. Removing these can be challenging due to their soft nature. Repeated flushing and often intraoperative cholangioscopy can help achieve better clearance and improve postoperative results. Cholangiography is usually avoided due to risks, including the potential for cholangitis flare-ups and proximal migration of stones or sludge. The gallbladder is diseased in up to 20% of cases, and the presence of gallstones suggests that the disease may be present elsewhere.

28.4 Clinical Feature

The clinical presentation of RPC can range from mild and asymptomatic to severe and life-threatening. It may initially appear in the emergency room with biliary sepsis or in clinics with prolonged, mild to moderate biliary symptoms. In both scenarios, early diagnosis is crucial to prevent irreversible liver damage.

28.4.1 Symptoms

The symptoms of RPC are often nonspecific, variable, and may be subtle in the early stages. Both women and men are equally affected. Some present acutely with cholangitis and sepsis, while others may show signs of end-stage liver disease. Common complaints include:

Fatigue and Malaise: General feelings of tiredness and unwellness are common early signs of the disease. This may coincide with symptoms of chronic malnutrition.

Jaundice: As the disease progresses and biliary obstruction worsens, jaundice (yellowing of the skin and eyes) becomes more noticeable due to the accumulation of bilirubin in the bloodstream. Some may also develop frank cholangitis or sepsis.

Abdominal Pain: Pain in the upper right quadrant of the abdomen is common and may be related to biliary colic or secondary cholangitis. The pain can be intermittent or persistent.

Fever and Chills: Fever and chills may occur in cases of superimposed bacterial cholangitis or active parasitic infection.

Pruritus: Intense itching is a common symptom, especially when cholestasis occurs. It is believed to be related to the accumulation of bile acids in the blood. This is typically seen with chronic biliary obstruction and worsening disease.

Weight Loss and Anorexia: In advanced stages of the disease, malnutrition and weight loss may occur due to impaired bile flow and subsequent malabsorption of fat-soluble vitamins.

28.4.2 Physical Examination

In an acute attack, physical examination reveals a restless patient who is unwell, with jaundice, fever, or even hemodynamic instability. The abdomen may exhibit signs of previous surgery, including tenderness and guarding, particularly in the right upper quadrant. On examination, patients with RPC may exhibit:

Hepatomegaly: An enlarged liver is common due to both chronic inflammation and fibrosis. It occurs in up to 60% of patients.

Splenomegaly: As cirrhosis progresses, portal hypertension can cause the spleen to enlarge, affecting about 20% of patients.

Ascites: In advanced stages, especially with cirrhosis, ascites may develop because of portal hypertension.

Signs of Chronic Liver Disease: In advanced cases, patients may show signs such as spider angiomata, palmar erythema, and symptoms of liver failure like confusion, hepatic encephalopathy, or even variceal bleeding.

28.5 Diagnosis

The diagnosis of RPC is based on a combination of clinical, radiological, serological, and histological findings.

Routine hematological and liver function tests reveal features consistent with bacteremia and biliary obstruction. As such, it is not possible to distinguish patients with RPC from those with biliary sepsis due to other causes. Leukocytosis, accompanied by an obstructive liver function test, is characteristic of cholangitis. In endemic areas, the first step in diagnosis is to screen for parasitic infections, especially *Clonorchis sinensis, Opisthorchis viverrini, or Ascaris lumbricoides*. Serological tests for specific antibodies or stool examination for ova may be diagnostic.

28.5.1 Imaging Studies

Ultrasound (US) Abdominal ultrasound used as a first-line imaging technique can identify biliary stones, ductal dilations, cholangitic abscesses, and signs of cirrhosis. Calcium bilirubinate stones, however, show the same or slightly higher echogenicity compared to the liver and produce a weaker acoustic shadow, which requires expert sonological interpretation. In cases of parasitic infection, liver flukes or Ascaris may be seen in the bile ducts or liver tissue. Other signs include segmental liver atrophy and decreased blood flow in affected segments. Pneumobilia, caused by recurrent infections or previous endoscopic procedures, may be present and can limit sonographic visualization. Doppler ultrasound provides information about portal vein blood flow. Prominent periportal echogenicity may indicate pericholangitis and periportal fibrous thickening, especially in advanced stages of RPC.

Contrast-Enhanced Computed Tomography (CECT) CECT provides better resolution and helps evaluate the extent of biliary duct involvement, liver fibrosis, and complications such as liver abscesses or portal hypertension. It can accurately distinguish intrahepatic stones from pneumobilia. Additionally, it is an effective tool for assessing liver volume redistribution and contour changes often seen in these patients. This information is valuable for planning drainage or resection procedures and for evaluating candidates who need a liver transplant. In acute cases, persistent segmental enhancement may indicate the presence of suppuration.

Magnetic Resonance Imaging/Cholangiopancreatogram (MRI/MRCP) MRI/MRCP is similar to US and CT scans in determining the volume and contour of the liver. T2-weighted MR images provide excellent visualization of the ductal system, showing ductal dilatation, strictures, and stones, as bile appears hyperintense and stones as filling defects. Therefore, compared to CT or US, MRI offers superior mapping of ductal anatomy, strictures, and stones. MRCP is also better than ERCP for visualizing intrahepatic

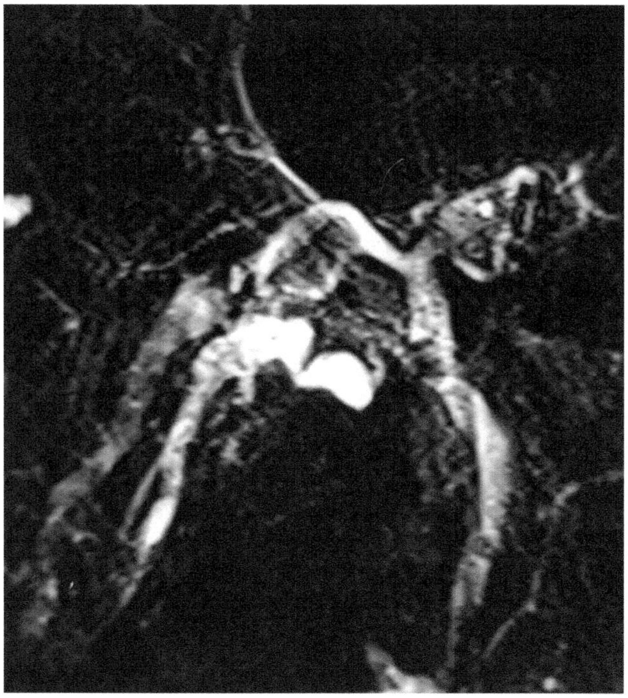

Fig. 28.1 Cholangiohepatitis affecting both lobes of the liver. Note dilatations and stones in the right hepatic segmental ducts, the left hepatic duct, and the common bile duct

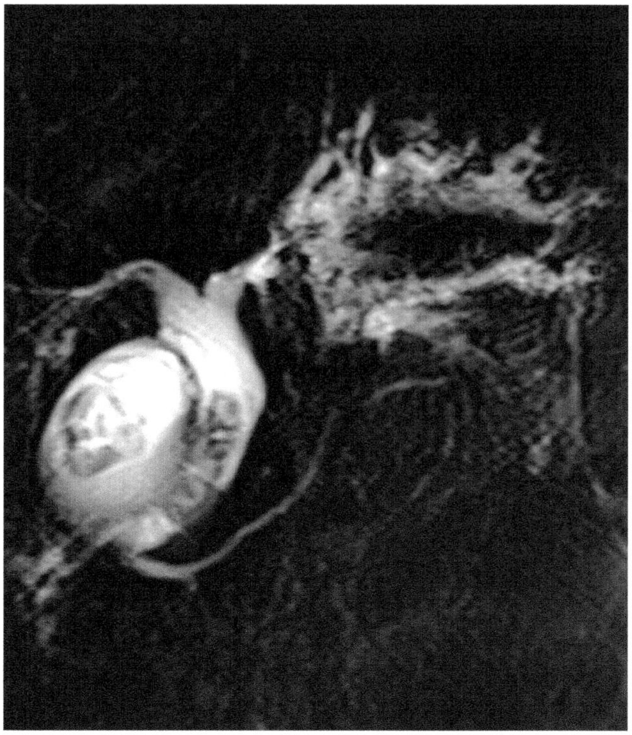

Fig. 28.2 Focal stricture involving the left hepatic duct with proximal dilatation and stones. Note the dilated common bile duct and the gallbladder containing stones

stones, as strictures can limit contrast flow to the smaller distal biliary ducts. As a purely diagnostic modality, MRCP is preferred over ERCP, which is an invasive procedure (Figs. 28.1 and 28.2).

Endoscopic Retrograde Cholangiopancreatography (ERCP) and Percutaneous Transhepatic Cholangiography (PTC) ERCP and PTC are invasive procedures that combine direct cholangiography with therapeutic intervention, providing real-time visualization of the biliary tree. Strictures can be dilated and stones extracted using either method, depending on the case and location of the strictures or stones. PTC is preferred when ERCP is limited by a prior bilioenteric bypass procedure or when a stone or stricture at the biliary confluence prevents the filling of intrahepatic ducts. ERCP is preferable in cases of extrahepatic disease when larger ducts are involved, although newer scopes and techniques, combined with cholangioscopy, further enhance the utility of ERCP.

Liver Biopsy The definitive diagnosis of RPC is usually confirmed with a liver biopsy, which shows the characteristic features mentioned earlier: biliary ductal proliferation, chronic inflammation, fibrosis, and sometimes granulomatous inflammation caused by parasitic infection. Progressive disease with cirrhosis may also require a liver biopsy.

Microbial Culture If bacterial cholangitis is suspected, culture of bile obtained via ERCP or percutaneous transhepatic cholangiography (PTC) can identify infectious organisms and guide antibiotic therapy.

28.6 Classifications

Several classification systems have been proposed to categorize disease severity and guide treatment. These mainly focus on the presence of stones and strictures.

28.6.1 Dong's Classification

Feng et al. proposed a classification method based on the location of the stones, the presence of hepatic atrophy, biliary stricture, cirrhosis, and the function of the sphincter of Oddi.

Type I: Localized stones.
- Ia: Stones in one lobe
- Ib: Stones in both lobes

Type II: Diffuse disease.
- IIa: No hepatic atrophy or bile duct stenosis

IIb: Segmental atrophy and/or biliary strictures
IIc: Biliary cirrhosis and portal hypertension

Type E: Extrahepatic stones with.
Ea: Normal sphincter of Oddi
Eb: Relaxed sphincter of Oddi
Ec: Stenosis of the sphincter of Oddi

28.6.2 Tsunoda's Classification

Type 1: Unilateral intrahepatic lithiasis *without* conduit dilatation/stenosis

Type II: Unilateral intrahepatic lithiasis *with* conduit dilatation and choledochal stenosis

Type III: Unilateral intrahepatic lithiasis with stenosis and conduit dilatation

Type IV: Bilateral intrahepatic lithiasis with stenosis and conduit dilatation

28.6.3 LHO Classification System

The most recent classification method was published by Wang et al. in 2023. They named it the LHO Classification System, where each letter represents one of three key points used to develop an effective surgical plan and standardize the treatment of patients with hepatolithiasis. "L" refers to the distribution of stones in the segmental bile ducts, the presence of hepatic atrophy, and the patient's tolerance for anatomical hepatectomy. "H" pertains to the presence or absence of stones at the hilum or hilar strictures, and "O" indicates whether there is dysfunction of the sphincter of Oddi.

With regard to the subtypes of type LHO,

L0: No obvious stones in the segmental bile ducts, no apparent atrophy of the hepatic parenchyma, and normal liver function.

L1: Presence of stones in the segmental bile ducts and/or liver parenchymal atrophy. The patient can tolerate hepatectomy.

L2: Presence of complex hepatolithiasis, which indicates diffuse disease and atrophy, without feasibility for anatomical hepatectomy of all the affected segments within the safe limits of resectability (as per the University of Zurich criteria).

H0: Absence of hilar stones or strictures.

H1: Stones visible but no strictures around the hepatic hilum.

H2: Presence of both stones and hilar strictures, including cases that are usually more challenging to manage.

O0: Normally functioning sphincter of Oddi.

O1: Presence of sphincter relaxation.

O2: Stricture of the sphincter of Oddi.

28.7 Treatment

The management of RPC is multidisciplinary, involving antiparasitic therapy, biliary interventions, and measures to control liver fibrosis. At presentation, management of all patients with acute cholangitis should include IV fluids and antibiotics, along with necessary supportive measures such as intensive care if needed for patients in septic shock. Broad-spectrum antibiotics are initiated since it is a polymicrobial infection. Biliary drainage should be the next focus after supportive care and initial assessment are complete. Severe cholangitis still has a reported mortality rate of 2.1%–14.3%.

Once focus shifts to definitive therapy, it aims for stone removal, stricture dilation if possible, and resection based on the indications. However, it is important to emphasize that failure to clear stones and manage strictures can lead to progression to biliary cirrhosis and even cholangiocarcinoma (2.1%–16%, as reported from Asian centers).

28.7.1 Endoscopic/Percutaneous Therapy

Endoscopic papillotomy with nasobiliary decompression or endobiliary stenting can be beneficial if the obstruction site is outside the liver, especially within the CBD. Purulent bile is drained, reducing the microbial load and significantly improving the patient's condition. However, it is ineffective for intrahepatic disease involving proximal stones and strictures. In such cases, a percutaneous approach with transhepatic biliary drainage under ultrasound or CT guidance is recommended. These drainage procedures greatly enhance supportive therapy and improve recovery in acute cholangitis patients with RPC. Empyema of the gallbladder should be considered alongside liver abscesses, which may require separate treatment such as drainage, cholecystostomy, or cholecystectomy. Additionally, close attention should be paid to percutaneous drainage tubes, which are relatively small and need regular aspiration and flushing with warm saline.

28.7.2 Emergency Surgery

Surgical decompression primarily aims to save the patient's life and drain the blocked biliary system with minimal operative trauma. The most common procedure involves exploring the common bile duct (CBD) and draining it via a wide-bore T-tube. After opening the CBD through a choledochotomy, thick pus is drained and collected for culture and sensitivity testing, and obstructing stones are removed. Complete clearance and stone removal must be confirmed through gentle handling of forceps and flushing of the extrahepatic biliary system. Most stones in RPC are soft bilirubinate stones, often accompanied by biliary mud or sludge. Once bile flow is established from both liver lobes, the choledochotomy is closed over the T-tube with absorbable sutures. The wide bore of the tube is essential since residual stones are found in up to 30% of cases, and this tract, besides providing effective drainage, can serve as a conduit for percutaneous manipulation postoperatively. Intrahepatic strictures, if feasible, can be dilated with graduated sounds. After dilation of these tight proximal strictures, a transhepatic tube can be placed following the same principles as a percutaneous drainage procedure under radiologic guidance, ensuring proper postoperative bile flow with ongoing monitoring and management of these drainage tubes. Since the primary goal is lifesaving biliary decompression, placing a wide-bore tube with adequate clearance to ensure effective bile flow typically results in a significant improvement in the patient's condition. Patients who are critically ill with septic shock may require extended ICU care and supportive measures to prevent death from multiorgan failure, sepsis, and coagulopathy (Fig. 28.3).

28.7.3 Definitive Management

Definitive therapy focuses on clearing the biliary system to ensure adequate drainage, which may require percutaneous access in some cases. Hepatic resection is indicated for severely diseased liver segments, and/or treatment of cholangiocarcinoma. Liver transplantation is reserved for advanced biliary cirrhosis. Accordingly, RPC cases can be categorized as either simple or complex. A "simple" case, without intrahepatic strictures, malignancy, or cirrhosis, can often be managed with cholecystectomy, CBD exploration, and choledochoscopy, with or without bilioenteric drainage (choledochoduodenostomy/hepaticojejunostomy). The "complex" cases may require stricturoplasty, hepaticocutaneous jejunostomy, partial or segmental hepatectomy, or liver transplant.

Extrahepatic Disease Disease affecting the extrahepatic bile ducts requires a graded approach to the biliary tract; nearly all procedures involve open surgery, as recurrent inflammation and fibrosis, along with the presence of portal hypertension in some cases, can complicate a minimally invasive approach. After a thorough radiological assessment and abdominal exploration, the first step is always to open the bile duct at the most prominent anterior location, avoiding the lateral vascular plexus (3- and 9-o'clock positions). The choledochotomy or hepaticodochotomy is extended vertically depending on the stone load and the location of the strictures. Such an extension becomes necessary in cases of impacted stones at the hilum or at the insertion of the posterior sectoral duct. Once wide exposure is achieved, the focus shifts to managing the stones or strictures. Because stones tend to be friable and soft, they require gentle manipulation using a combination of forceps, saline flushes, inflatable balloon catheters, and Dormia baskets. Intraoperative fluoroscopy or choledochoscopy is an essential tool to assist in stone removal and ensure complete clearance. After stone removal, a T-tube may be placed in cases of distal disease. Drainage procedures, such as choledochoduodenostomy or hepaticojejunostomy, may be necessary for patients with dilated extrahepatic ducts and multiple stones or strictures. Strictures present a different challenge; they are often difficult to manage. They may be short-segment, multiple, or long-segment strictures. Short-segment or isolated strictures—typically in the left main duct—can sometimes be managed through dilation and long-term stenting. Most extrahepatic strictures are either resected with restoration of bilioenteric continuity or entirely bypassed with a T-tube or ductoenterostomy. Cholecystectomy is indicated if cholelithiasis is present.

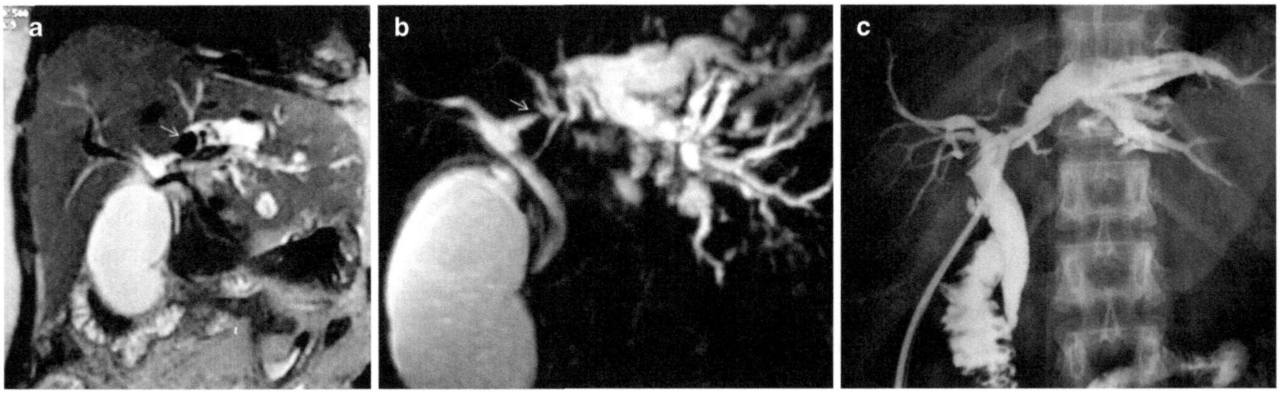

Fig. 28.3 MRCP showing (**a**) an obstructed left hepatic duct caused by a large stone (arrow) and (**b**) a focal stricture (arrow) with a grossly dilated proximal ductal system. The patient presented with acute cholangitis. (**c**) Emergency treatment involved open surgical removal of the obstructing stone and T-tube drainage of the left duct

Intrahepatic Disease Intrahepatic disease with extensive strictures affecting the smaller ducts and peripheral biliary radicles presents a significant challenge. Surgical options include biliary drainage with ductal intubation (internal or external), a novel percutaneous approach via a hepaticocutaneous jejunostomy (access-loop hepaticojejunostomy), partial liver resection for extensively damaged segments or lobes, and sometimes even a liver transplant in cases of secondary biliary cirrhosis.

Hepaticocutaneous Jejunostomy A permanent or temporary fistula is established between the bile ducts and the skin. It is usually created using a Roux-en-Y limb of jejunum. This procedure is performed for therapeutic or palliative reasons in complex biliary strictures within the deep biliary radicles, such as in RPC. Although it is seldom used today due to advances in endoscopic and radiological techniques, it remains a viable option when such expertise is unavailable. The stoma is closed, buried under the skin, and marked for future reference. Care should be taken when creating the access loop to keep it relatively straight and short from the stoma to the biliary tract to avoid redundancy, which can complicate intubation and endoscopy.

Hepatic Resection Hepatectomy, whether partial or segmental, is indicated in select cases when conservative or less invasive methods have failed. It is especially used in cases of destroyed and poorly functioning liver segments. The advantages of resection include providing definitive treatment for localized disease by removing the entire diseased segment. It is also beneficial as a method to prevent or reduce the risk of malignancy, such as cholangiocarcinoma. With advancements in preoperative and postoperative care, hepatectomies now offer a one-time, long-term feasible solution for carefully selected patients. Resections can include segmentectomies or lobectomies (most common) for localized disease, such as a left lateral segmentectomy for left-sided disease. Hemihepatectomies are considered when there is extensive unilateral involvement. Some cases can also be treated with nonanatomic resection, particularly for focal abscesses or strictures (Figs. 28.4 and 28.5).

28.7.4 Liver Transplantation

Indications for liver transplantation in cholangiohepatitis include widespread bilateral disease that cannot be removed or treated endoscopically, disease progression to cirrhosis and liver failure, and the development of cholangiocarcinoma. Prompt referral for transplant assessment is essential in patients with decompensated liver disease. Several challenges specific to RPC, such as dense and extensive adhesions from recurrent inflammation and previous surgeries, can complicate transplantation.

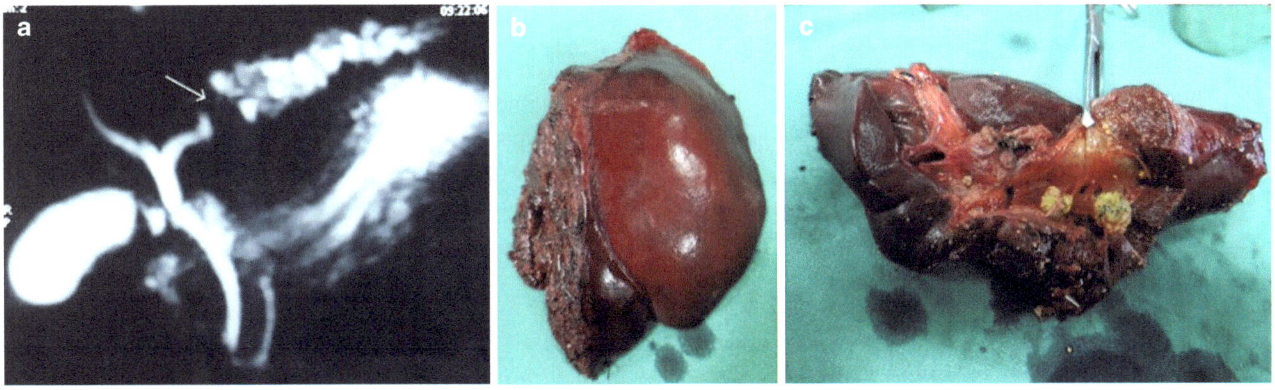

Fig. 28.4 (**a**) MRCP showing involvement of the left hepatic duct. A focal stricture (arrow) and extensive dilation of the proximal ductal system create a "Christmas-tree" appearance. (**b**) Resected the left hepatic lobe. (**c**) Opened specimen displaying dilated ducts and yellow pigment stones

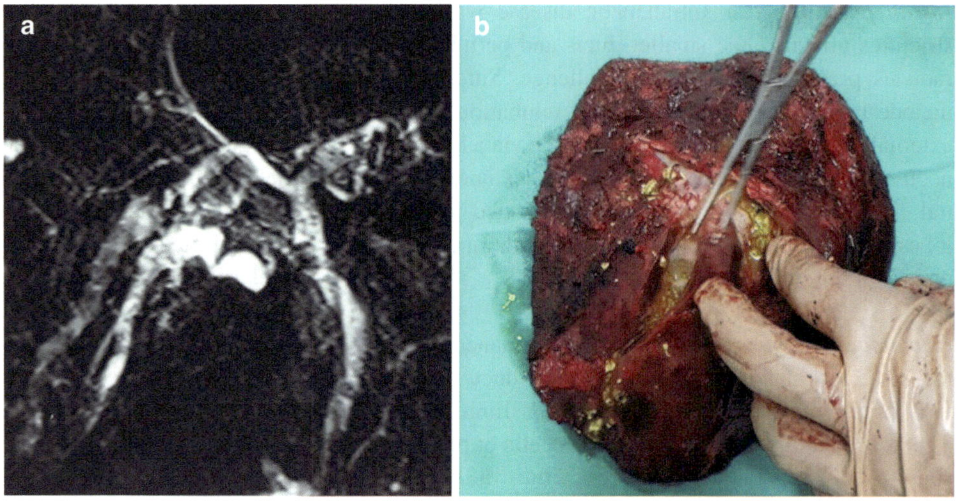

Fig. 28.5 (**a**) MRCP showing diffuse involvement of the biliary system: dilated ducts with filling defects suggestive of stones. (**b**) Treated with a formal right hepatectomy and drainage of the left and common hepatic ducts

28.7.5 Management of Cholangiohepatitis Due to Biliary Ascariasis (Table 28.1)

Table 28.1 Parray classification and management strategy

Grade	Features	Management
1	Disease limited to the extrahepatic ducts with stones/worms, no liver parenchymal disease, no strictures, and CBD size less than 1.5 cm	CBD exploration with T-tube drainage
2	Disease limited to the extrahepatic ducts with stones/worms, no liver parenchymal disease, with strictures of CBD, or CBD > 1.5 cm	CBD exploration with hepaticojejunostomy with or without access loop
3	Disease involving intrahepatic ducts, right or left, with stones/worms, with dilatable strictures, and no liver parenchymal disease	CBD exploration with clearance of intrahepatic stones and dilatation of strictures with hepaticojejunostomy with an access loop
4	Disease involving intrahepatic ducts, right or left, with stones/worms, with severe nondilatable strictures or parenchymal disease on the same side	Liver resections, left lateral segmentectomy, right or left hepatectomy
5	Disease involving both intrahepatic ducts, with stones/worms, with severe nondilatable strictures or parenchymal disease on both sides	Hepatectomy on the more affected side with clearance of contralateral ducts and dilatation of the strictures, and hepaticojejunostomy with an access loop. Or referral for liver transplant

Key Points

- Cholangiohepatitis is a biliary disease that is being seen more often in parts of Asia, especially in China and other Southeast Asian countries.
- The disease is caused by *Clonorchis sinensis* (Chinese liver fluke) and *Opisthorchis viverrini* in Southeast Asian countries, and by Ascaris in the Kashmir Valley and other parts of the Indian subcontinent.
- Epithelial damage caused by Clonorchis or Ascaris is the initial event. Superimposed bacterial infection and inflammation further contribute to epithelial injury, leading to stricture formation. The β-glucuronidase activity of bacteria promotes the formation of calcium bilirubinate stones. The presence of stones, strictures, infection, and inflammation creates a vicious cycle that results in disease progression.
- The symptoms of RPC can be nonspecific, variable, and subtle in the early stages. As the disease progresses, patients may present with intermittent mild to severe cholangitis and sepsis.
- MRCP is the preferred imaging test for diagnosis, classification, and management planning.
- Management of an acute presentation of the disease includes broad-spectrum antibiotics, supportive care, and biliary drainage.

(continued)

- Definitive surgical treatment, depending on the extent of the disease, includes stone clearance and T-tube drainage, biliary drainage with bilioenteric anastomosis with or without access-loop hepaticojejunostomy, and resection of the involved liver segment.
- Liver transplantation is indicated for patients with diffuse liver involvement, hepatic fibrosis, cirrhosis, or the development of cholangiocarcinoma.

Selected Reading

1. Parray FQ, Wani MA, Wani NA. Oriental cholangiohepatitis-Is our surgery appropriate? Int J Surg. 2014;12(8):789–93.
2. Wang W, Yang C, Wang J, et al. Hepatolithiasis classification based on anatomical hepatectomy. J Gastrointest Surg. 2023;27(5):914–25. https://doi.org/10.1007/s11605-022-05572-x.
3. Motta RV, Saffioti F, Mavroeidis VK. Hepatolithiasis: epidemiology, presentation, classification and management of a complex disease. World J Gastroenterol. 2024;30:1836–50. https://doi.org/10.3748/wjg.v30.i13.1836.

Gallbladder Cancer

29

Yashika Gupta and H. H. Nag

Abstract

Gallbladder cancer is categorized into various types: (i) Infiltrative, (ii) Nodular, (iii) Nodular-infiltrative, (iv) Papillary, and (v) Papillary-infiltrative. CECT findings in GBC include the GB lumen filled with a mass (42%), a mass replacing the GB (26%), a polypoid mass (26%), and diffuse wall thickening (6%). Simple cholecystectomy is curative in 90% of T1a tumors. Radical cholecystectomy is recommended for T1b and T2 tumors. En bloc adjacent organ resection may have to be performed with radical cholecystectomy for T3 and T4 tumors, though the prognosis may not be good.

Keywords

Gallbladder cancer · Carcinoma gallbladder

Gallbladder cancer (GBC) is the fifth most common gastrointestinal cancer. It is the most common biliary malignancy. GBC is endemic in India, Latin America, and East Asia. Although its incidence is relatively low in the USA, certain ethnic groups, such as American Indians and Alaskan Natives, face a disproportionately high risk. Females and the elderly are more frequently affected; however, in India, it is also common among the younger population (Table 29.1).

Table 29.1 Risk factors

Female sex	Cholelithiasis
Multiparity	Porcelain gallbladder
Obesity	Mirizzi syndrome
Ethanol abuse	Xanthogranulomatous cholecystitis
Tobacco abuse	True gallbladder polyps
Salmonella infection	Primary sclerosing cholangitis (PSC)
Helicobacter pylori infection	Anomalous pancreaticobiliary junction (APBJ)

29.1 Pathology

In GBC, fundus of the gallbladder (GB) is involved in 60% of cases, the body in 30%, and the neck region in 10%. Broadly, GBC can be categorized into various types: (i) Infiltrative, (ii) Nodular, (iii) Nodular-infiltrative, (iv) Papillary, and (v) Papillary-infiltrative. The infiltrative type of GBC is the most common variant. The papillary form of GBC is associated with a relatively better prognosis because it tends to be less invasive. However, if papillary GBC becomes invasive, its prognosis aligns with other histological types at similar stages. The most common histological type of GBC is adenocarcinoma. Other histologies, accounting for less than 10%, include squamous/adenosquamous carcinoma (2%–3%), neuroendocrine/oat cell carcinoma (2%–3%), as well as clear cell, sarcoma, carcinoid, lymphoma, and melanoma.

Y. Gupta · H. H. Nag (✉)
G B Pant Institute of Postgraduate Medical Education and Research (GIPMER), New Delhi, India

M. Ibrarullah (ed.), *Recent Concepts in Gastrointestinal (GI) Surgery*, https://doi.org/10.1007/978-981-92-1118-0_29

29.2 Clinical Presentation

Unsuspected GBC can present in three ways: (1) incidentally on preoperative imaging, (2) intraoperatively during cholecystectomy, and (3) postoperatively on histopathology of the GB specimen. Symptomatic primary GBC is more common in endemic areas like India and other Asian countries, whereas asymptomatic incidental GBC is frequent in the West. GBC patients may present with symptoms similar to benign biliary disease. Tumors of the GB neck, infundibulum, or cystic duct can infiltrate the porta hepatis and mimic hilar cholangiocarcinoma, causing obstructive jaundice and major vascular invasion. Persistent pain, a palpable right upper quadrant mass, anorexia, jaundice, malaise, and weight loss suggest an advanced and unresectable stage of GBC. Tumor markers are often nondiagnostic. However, both carcinoembryonic antigen (CEA) and carbohydrate antigen 19–9 (CA 19–9) may show increased secretion in GBC and can be used for surveillance of recurrence.

29.3 Investigations

Ultrasonography (USG) is the preferred initial investigation for suspected cases of GBC. A polypoid GB mass appears in 27% of cases, and an invasive lesion in 50%. Other US findings suggestive of GBC include echogenic mucosa, discontinuous GB mucosa, or submucosal echolucency. Patients without evidence of disseminated disease on USG should undergo cross-sectional imaging such as contrast-enhanced computed tomography (CECT) or magnetic resonance imaging (MRI) of the abdomen. Cross-sectional imaging serves three main purposes: it defines the local extent of the disease and evaluates nodal and distant metastasis. CECT findings in GBC include the GB lumen filled with a mass (42%), a mass replacing the GB (26%), a polypoid mass (26%), and diffuse wall thickening (6%) (Fig. 29.1). MRI of the abdomen with MR cholangiopancreatogram (MRCP) is preferred in patients with biliary obstruction and to identify small hepatic metastases and CBD involvement. Positron emission tomography (PET) scan is more sensitive for detecting metastatic disease compared to conventional imaging, according to some studies, and can influence management in up to 25% of patients deemed resectable on conventional imaging. However, because PET scan has nonspecificity for malignancy and limited effectiveness for nodal metastases, it cannot be routinely recommended for all GBC patients. PET is considered only in cases of locally advanced disease seen on CT/MRI, those requiring extended resection beyond standard radical cholecystectomy, or patients with suspected distant metastases.

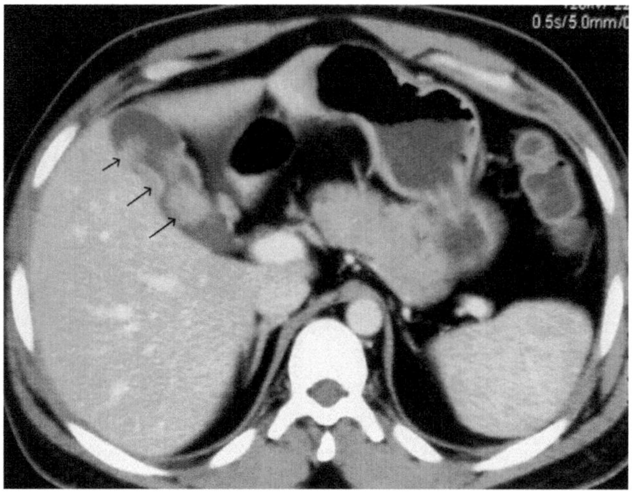

Fig. 29.1 CECT showing polypoidal tumor (arrows) in the GB

Accurately identifying lymph node metastases before surgery can be very difficult. CT detection of ring-like or heterogeneous enhancement in lymph nodes larger than 10 mm has an accuracy of 89% for detecting metastases. However, only 38% of nodal metastases are identified preoperatively by CT. Patients with visible distant nodes (celiac, superior mesenteric, and aortocaval) on cross-sectional imaging should undergo image-guided FNAC. If these nodes are involved, such patients are excluded from curative resection. Endoscopic USG can be used to assess peripancreatic and periportal lymphadenopathy.

Colonoscopy and upper gastrointestinal endoscopy are recommended for patients with suspected colonic and duodenal involvement, as determined by preoperative imaging. Significantly elevated CA 19–9 and CEA levels in the absence of biliary obstruction help predict metastatic disease.

Percutaneous core biopsy is not recommended due to the risk of needle track seeding of cancer cells. However, percutaneous fine needle aspiration cytology is safe and offers satisfactory diagnostic accuracy; it is useful in unresectable cases when nonoperative therapies are considered. Therefore, current guidelines recommend biopsy only in cases that are unresectable. Biliary cytology analysis has a suboptimal sensitivity of about 50% for identifying GBC.

29.4 Staging

The tumor stage is considered the most accurate predictor of survival outcomes in GBC. The most widely used and recognized staging system is the American Joint Committee on Cancer (AJCC) staging system. The current version of AJCC staging, namely the eighth edition, uses the standard tumor (T), nodal (N), and metastatic (M) classification. Depth of invasion is described by the T classification: T1a tumors invade the lamina propria, while T1b tumors are limited to the muscular layer. The T2 stage involves the invasion of the perimuscular connective tissue, which is further divided into T2a if it occurs on the peritoneal side and T2b if it occurs on the hepatic side of the GB. T3 tumors indicate serosal infiltration or direct invasion of the liver or adjacent organs. A T4 tumor involves the main portal vein, hepatic artery, or two or more of the adjacent organs.

Lymph node (LN) classification in TNM staging is categorized into N0 (no positive nodes), N1 (1–3 positive regional nodes), and N2 (4 or more positive regional nodes). LN involvement outside the porta hepatis, such as celiac, paraaortic, and aortocaval nodes, is designated as metastatic and labeled M1. Resection of at least six lymph nodes is considered standard for accurate pathological staging.

29.5 Management

29.5.1 Extent of Primary Resection Based on T Stage

The extent of primary resection in GBC depends on the T stage. Simple cholecystectomy is curative in 90% of T1a tumors, where the tumor is confined to the lamina propria. This stage 1 GBC is usually identified only through pathological review of the GB specimen after routine cholecystectomy. No further surgery is necessary for these patients unless there is a positive cystic duct margin, in which case re-resection becomes mandatory. However, simple cholecystectomy is considered inadequate for T1b stage tumors because it is associated with LN metastases upon reexploration in 10%–20% of cases. Therefore, radical resection is recommended for T1b tumors.

Patients with T2 tumors have a 50% risk of nodal metastases and a 40%–50% chance of positive margins after routine cholecystectomy. Therefore, extended cholecystectomy with portal lymphadenectomy is considered the preferred procedure for Stage II GBC. This increases the 5-year survival rate for these patients to 70%–90%.

The appropriate extent of resection for T3 and T4 tumors is debatable because they invade nearby organs and require en bloc removal. According to NCCN guidelines, radical cholecystectomy for these tumors includes removal of segments IVb and V, lymphadenectomy, and extended hepatic or biliary resection as needed to achieve clear margins. However, major hepatic resections combined with bile duct and/or vascular resection and reconstruction in T4 stage GBC can increase postoperative complications and death. Therefore, patients with T3 or T4N1 disease are encouraged to participate in clinical trials with neoadjuvant therapy rather than undergo aggressive initial surgery.

The standard procedure for GBC is the so-called radical or extended cholecystectomy, which comprises cholecystectomy, en bloc resection of the rim of segments IVb and V, and lymphadenectomy (including cystic, pericholedochal, periportal, and posterior pancreaticoduodenal lymph nodes, as well as local aortocaval lymph nodes). This management is reserved for resectable GBC patients with pathological stages above T1a.

29.5.2 Incidental Gallbladder Carcinoma

Incidental GB carcinoma (IGBC) is one that was not suspected before surgery and is diagnosed during or after cholecystectomy performed for a presumed diagnosis of simple GB stone disease (GSD) (Fig. 29.2). The incidence of IGBC ranges from 0.3% to 2.1% of all cholecystectomy specimens. Most IGBC cases are early-stage or pathologic T stage 1 or 2, making them suitable for treatment. When GBC is diagnosed during laparoscopy, the operating surgeon should inform the patient's relatives and either convert to open exploration for potential extended cholecystectomy or halt the surgery with plans for reexploration or referral. IGBC diagnosed through pathology is further staged as either T1a, T1b, or higher. NCCN recommends observing T1a stage tumors and assessing ≥T1b tumors for metastases using cross-sectional imaging. However, 10%–57% of patients may have radiologically occult metastatic disease, which could be detected during staging laparoscopy. Therefore, NCCN guidelines suggest considering staging laparoscopy for IGBC patients with stage ≥T1b, although it is not mandatory.

29.5.3 Nonincidental Gallbladder Carcinoma

These patients present with symptoms indicative of advanced disease, such as abdominal pain, weight loss, jaundice, and an abdominal lump. These nonincidental cancers are generally considered to predict worse outcomes compared to IGBC. Since nonincidental cancers are likely to show both disseminated disease and locally advanced unresectable disease, it is recommended to perform staging laparoscopy for all suspected GBC patients.

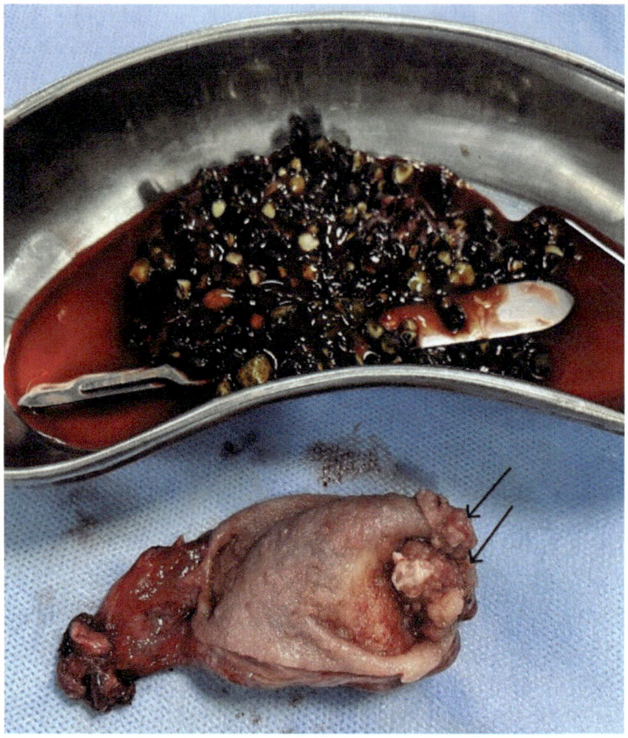

Fig. 29.2 Unsuspected polypoidal growth (arrows) in the GB fundus detected in the cholecystectomy specimen. The GB was packed with stones, obscuring the tumor

29.5.4 Indications for Major Hepatectomy

The rationale behind hepatic resection in GBC is:

- Removal of direct neoplastic invasion into the GB bed to achieve R0 resection
- Removal of micrometastatic disease to prevent local recurrence
- Prevention of potential invasion of the hepatoduodenal ligament

Although it is recommended that ≥T1b tumors undergo radical or extended cholecystectomy, the optimal extent of hepatic resection remains debated. It can range from a formal anatomic resection of segments IVb and V to a nonanatomic wedge resection or a major hepatectomy. Several retrospective studies suggest that parenchymal-sparing wedge resection has oncologic effectiveness comparable to anatomical segmental resection as long as an R0 resection is achieved. Major hepatectomy should only be performed if necessary to obtain negative margins, as R0 resection is crucial for a favorable prognosis (Fig. 29.3).

29.5.5 Bile Duct Resection

Routine bile duct excision is not linked to improved survival; therefore, it is not regarded as essential. Current indications for bile duct excision in patients without direct bile duct involvement include:

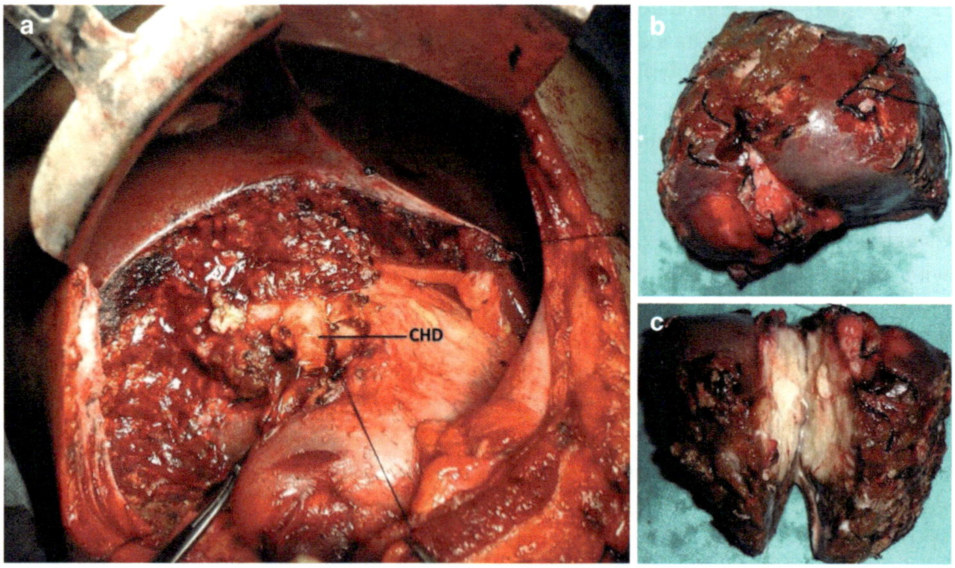

Fig. 29.3 Radical cholecystectomy. (**a**) Excision of the liver segments V, VI, IVb, and the common bile duct. (**b**) Excised liver segments with the GB tumor. (**c**) Cut-open specimen showing infiltrative growth replacing GB

- Gross lymph node enlargement near or involving the common hepatic duct or hilum
- Inflamed or fatty hepatoduodenal ligament, making nodal dissection difficult
- Positive cystic duct margin on intraoperative frozen section
- Associated ABPJ abnormality or choledochal cyst
- Synchronous bile duct malignancy
- When vascular resection or reconstruction is necessary

Malignant infiltration of the bile duct, causing jaundice, indicates advanced disease, a low chance of R0 resection, and thus a poor prognosis.

29.5.6 Portal Lymph Node Dissection

In GBC, lymph nodal involvement is reported in 12% with T1b, 31% with T2, and 45% with T3 tumors. The lymphatic plexuses present in the GB wall course through the medial and lateral walls to drain into the cystic node and pericholedochal nodes, respectively. Lymphatics from these nodes then follow one of three pathways:

- The cholecysto-retropancreatic pathway: This is the primary lymphatic pathway that converges into the retroportal LN.
- The cholecysto-celiac pathway: GB wall lymphatics travel to the left via the hepatoduodenal ligament to reach the celiac LNs.
- The cholecysto-mesenteric pathway: Some lymphatics travel anterior to the portal vein and connect with the root of the mesenteric LNs.

These three pathways ultimately converge into the Interaortocaval (IAC) lymph nodes near the left renal vein. LN metastases confer a poorer prognosis, and thus LN dissection is performed as part of radical or extended cholecystectomy to improve survival rates. Portal lymphadenectomy is the standard of care in radical cholecystectomy (Fig. 29.4).

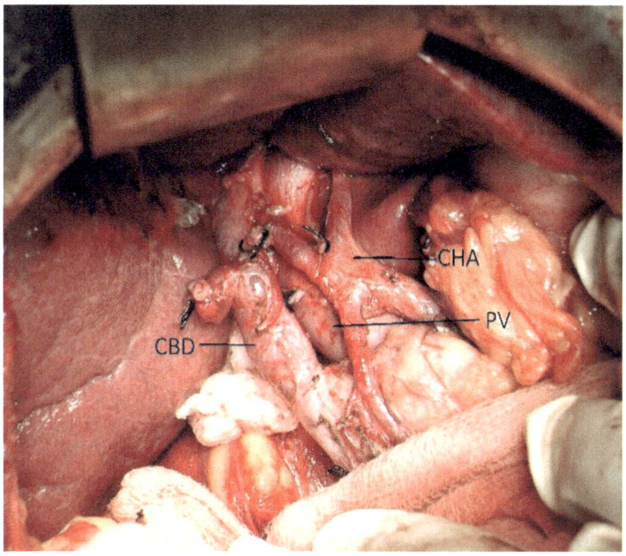

Fig. 29.4 Hepatoduodenal lymph node dissection. CBD, common bile duct; PV, portal vein; CHA, common hepatic artery

29.5.7 Port Site Resection

Port site metastases have been observed in 10% of IGBC cases after laparoscopic cholecystectomy. Port site recurrence in IGBC can result from improper extraction techniques, which often cause localized recurrence, whereas recurrence due to bile spillage is typically associated with disseminated disease. Since information about the type of extraction technique used and any intraoperative bile spillage is typically unavailable, port site recurrence is often associated with peritoneal dissemination and advanced disease. Therefore, resecting the port site as part of radical cholecystectomy is questionable. Several researchers have reported that adding port site resection does not improve survival after radical cholecystectomy; therefore, it is not considered part of radical completion cholecystectomy.

29.5.8 Adjuvant Therapy

The postoperative recurrence rate in GBC has been reported to be around 70%. Most recurrences occur at distant sites. Therefore, there is a need for adjuvant treatment with effective systemic therapies. However, GBC is highly resistant to chemotherapy, and due to its tendency for diffuse peritoneal spread, radiation therapy is generally not effective. The current indications for adjuvant therapy are:

- T stage—T2 or more
- N stage—Node-positive disease
- Resection status—R1 or R2 resection
- Histological features—Poorly differentiated tumor, lymphovascular and perineural invasion

Several studies have been conducted to compare adjuvant treatment with the best supportive care in the postoperative period. Among the major studies, the BILCAP (Biliary Treat Cancer) trial by Primrose and colleagues is the only RCT to date that has demonstrated improved outcomes in the adjuvant therapy arm (Capecitabine) for biliary tract malignancies. This trial randomized 447 patients with cholangiocarcinoma of all sites and muscle-invasive GBC after complete macroscopic resection between March 2006 and December 2014. Significantly improved overall survival has been observed in patients who received adjuvant therapy.

As a result of this trial, the currently recommended adjuvant treatment strategy for postoperative GBC patients is treatment with Capecitabine for 6 months.

29.5.9 Neoadjuvant Therapy

Neoadjuvant therapy has several benefits in the treatment of locally advanced GBC:

- Downstaging of primary tumor
- In vivo testing of chemosensitivity
- Treatment of micrometastatic disease
- Appropriate patient selection for definitive surgery, thus sparing patients with aggressive tumor biology from the postsurgery morbidity
- Borderline resectable tumors constitute a subset of patients who could benefit from neoadjuvant therapy. Borderline resectable tumors lead to a higher risk of perioperative complications because of complex surgery, increased risk of systemic recurrence due to the advanced tumor stage, and higher risk of margin positivity. However, unlike pancreatic cancer, there is a lack of consensus on the definition of borderline resectable GBC. Tata Memorial Hospital (TMH) criteria was proposed by Goel et al. as an indication for neoadjuvant chemotherapy in locally advanced/borderline resectable GBC, which resulted in curative surgical resection or disease stabilization in a significant proportion of patients (Table 29.2).

Table 29.2 Tata Memorial Hospital (TMH) criteria for locally advanced/borderline resectable GBC

Tumor (T3–T4 tumors)
Contiguous liver involvement >2 cm
Involvement of the bile duct causing obstructive jaundice (type I/II block on MRCP/ERCP/PTBD)
Radiological/endoscopic involvement of the antropyloric region of the stomach, duodenum, hepatic flexure of the colon, or small intestine
Node (N1 station)
Radiological suspicion of lymph node involvement N1
Hepatic artery (station 8)
Hepatoduodenal ligament (station 12)
Retro pancreatic/retroduodenal (station 13)
Size >1 cm in short axis, round in shape, and heterogeneous enhancement on CT/PET scan
Vascular (T4 tumors)
Impingement/involvement (<180°) of one or more of the following blood vessels:
Common hepatic artery and right & left hepatic artery
Main portal vein and right & left portal vein
For incidental GBC
Residual/recurrent mass in GB fossa/liver bed
N1 nodes as per nodal criteria
Involvement of the bile duct causing obstructive jaundice (type I/II block)

29.6 Survival Outcomes and Prognosis in Gallbladder Cancer

With improved survival after aggressive surgical resection and chemotherapy in carefully selected GBC patients, a shift from nihilism to optimism has been observed. After curative resection for GBC, recurrence has been observed at both locoregional and systemic levels. Recurrence has been mostly observed in the first 3 years after surgery; thus, patients who undergo curative surgical resection are followed up at 3-monthly intervals for 1 year, every 6 months for 2 years, and then annually. Patients on follow-up are evaluated with clinical examination, liver function tests, tumor markers (CEA and CA19–9), and ultrasonography. Current NCCN guidelines recommend radiological imaging of the chest, abdomen, and pelvis at 3–6 monthly intervals for the first 2 years, then every 6–12 months for up to 5 years or as clinically required. Survival outcomes and prognosis in GBC patients who underwent therapeutic surgical management are determined by the biology of the tumor, which in turn depends on:

- *T & N Stage*: The higher the stage, the worse the prognosis. T1a patients have an excellent prognosis, while complete resection of T1b lesions to negative margins also confers a similarly excellent outlook. Survival in T2 lesions has been linked to nodal status; thus, 5-year survival has increased from 20% to over 60% with advancements in radical resection. The 5-year survival for patients with T3 lesions is less than 20%, while those with T4 tumors have survival measured in months.
- *M Stage*: Metastatic disease at presentation has shown a median survival of 13 months.
- *Histological Features*: Lymphovascular invasion, perineural invasion, and pericapsular invasion are associated with poorer survival.
- *Resection Status*: Patients with R0 resection have better survival than those who underwent R1 or R2 resection.
- *Inflammatory Markers*: Patients with preoperative cholecystitis, cholangitis, and those with elevated neutrophil-lymphocyte ratio have worse survival.

As most GBC patients present with advanced disease, the overall survival of GBC remains <15%.

Key Points

- Gallbladder cancer (GBC) is endemic in India, Latin America, and East Asia.
- Cholelithiasis, porcelain gallbladder, Mirizzi syndrome, xanthogranulomatous cholecystitis, true gallbladder polyps, primary sclerosing cholangitis (PSC), and anomalous pancreaticobiliary junction (APBJ) are some of the risk factors associated with GBC.
- GBC can be categorized into various types: (i) infiltrative, (ii) nodular, (iii) nodular-infiltrative, (iv) papillary, and (v) papillary-infiltrative.
- Unsuspected GBC can present in three ways: (1) incidentally on preoperative imaging, (2) intraoperatively during cholecystectomy, and (3) postoperatively on histopathology of the GB specimen.
- CECT is the preferred investigation of choice for diagnosis and staging.
- CECT findings in GBC include the GB lumen filled with a mass (42%), a mass replacing the GB (26%), a polypoid mass (26%), and diffuse wall thickening (6%).
- TNM staging is used for planning treatment and prognostication.
- Simple cholecystectomy is curative in 90% of T1a tumors.
- Radical cholecystectomy is recommended for T1b and T2 tumors.
- En bloc adjacent organ resection may have to be performed with radical cholecystectomy for T3 and T4 tumors, though the prognosis may not be good.
- Routine bile duct excision is recommended only in specific circumstances, either to achieve R0 resection or to facilitate nodal clearance.
- Port site resection is not routinely recommended for completion cholecystectomy in case of incidental GBC after laparoscopic cholecystectomy.
- Currently recommended adjuvant treatment strategy for postoperative GBC patients is treatment with Capecitabine for 6 months.
- T1a patients have an excellent prognosis, while complete resection of T1b lesions to negative margins also confers a similarly excellent outlook. Survival in T2 lesions has been linked to nodal status; thus, 5-year survival has increased from 20% to over 60% with advancements in radical resection. The 5-year survival rate for patients with T3 lesions is less than 20%, while those with T4 tumors have a survival rate measured in months.

Selected Reading

1. Zhou Y, Yuan K, Yang Y. Gallbladder cancer: current and future treatment options. Front Pharmacol. 2023;14:1183619. https://doi.org/10.3389/fphar.2023.1183619.
2. Aloia TA, Jarufe N, Javle MM, Maithel SK, Roa JC, et al. Gallbladder cancer: expert consensus statement. HPB Oxf. 2015;17(8):681–90. https://doi.org/10.1111/hpb.12444.
3. Alrawashdeh W, Kamarajah SK, Gujjuri RR, et al. Systematic review and meta-analysis of survival outcomes in T2a and T2b gallbladder cancers. HPB Oxf. 2022;24(6):789–96. https://doi.org/10.1016/j.hpb.2021.12.019.

Cholangiocarcinoma

30

Bramhadatta Pattnaik, Sunita Gupta, Ranjan Patel, and Siba Narayan Padhi

Abstract

Cholangiocarcinoma (CCA) is categorized into three types: intrahepatic (10%), perihilar (70%), and distal (20%). Extrahepatic CCA presents with painless, progressive cholestatic jaundice. The type and extent of liver resection for hilar CCA depend on the Bismuth–Corlette classification. Most hilar CCAs require caudate lobectomy along with major liver resection because of the proximity and drainage of the caudate ducts with the biliary confluence. Neo-adjuvant chemo-radiotherapy followed by liver transplantation is emerging as a potential treatment in selected cases of CCA.

Keywords

Cholangiocarcinoma · Klatskin's tumor · Bile duct cancer

Cholangiocarcinoma (CCA) develops from the cholangiocytes lining the biliary tract. Anatomically, it can be classified into three types: intrahepatic (10%), hilar (70%), and distal (20%). A tumor located proximal to the secondary confluence of the hepatic ducts is known as intrahepatic CCA. In contrast, one distal to the cystic duct–common hepatic duct junction is referred to as the distal CCA. A tumor arising from the intervening portion of the biliary tree is referred to as hilar CCA. The Bismuth–Correlate classification is the most widely used system for further classifying the hilar CCA, also known as Klatskin tumors (Fig. 30.1; Table 30.1).

30.1 Pathogenesis

Most cases of CCA occur sporadically, but several factors are known to contribute to its development. Chronic inflammation of the bile ducts and bile stasis are common among these factors. The most common identifiable cause is primary sclerosing cholangitis (PSC), which has a lifetime risk of 5%–20% for CCA. Caroli's disease, Type I and IV biliary cysts increase CCA risk by up to 30 times, although cyst removal can reduce, but not completely eliminate, this risk.

30.2 Pathology

30.2.1 Intrahepatic Cholangiocarcinoma

Primarily, adenocarcinomas with biliary differentiation can arise from the bile duct of any segment of the liver. Histologically, intrahepatic CCA shows peripheral tumor cells with central desmoplastic stroma and sparse tumor cells.

30.2.1.1 Macroscopic Pattern

According to the macroscopic appearance, the Liver Cancer Study Group of Japan has subdivided ICC into four categories:

1. Mass-Forming type (MF) (65%)—Well-delineated, firm, non-encapsulated mass within the liver with no macroscopic communication with a bile duct.
2. Periductal Infiltrating type (PI) (6%)—Spreads along intrahepatic portal tracts.
3. Intraductal-Growing type (IG) (4%)—Polypoid or papillary mass within the bile duct.
4. Mixed pattern (25%).

B. Pattnaik (✉) · S. Gupta · R. Patel · S. N. Padhi
All India Institute of Medical Sciences, Bhubaneswar, Odisha, India

M. Ibrarullah (ed.), *Recent Concepts in Gastrointestinal (GI) Surgery*, https://doi.org/10.1007/978-981-92-1118-0_30

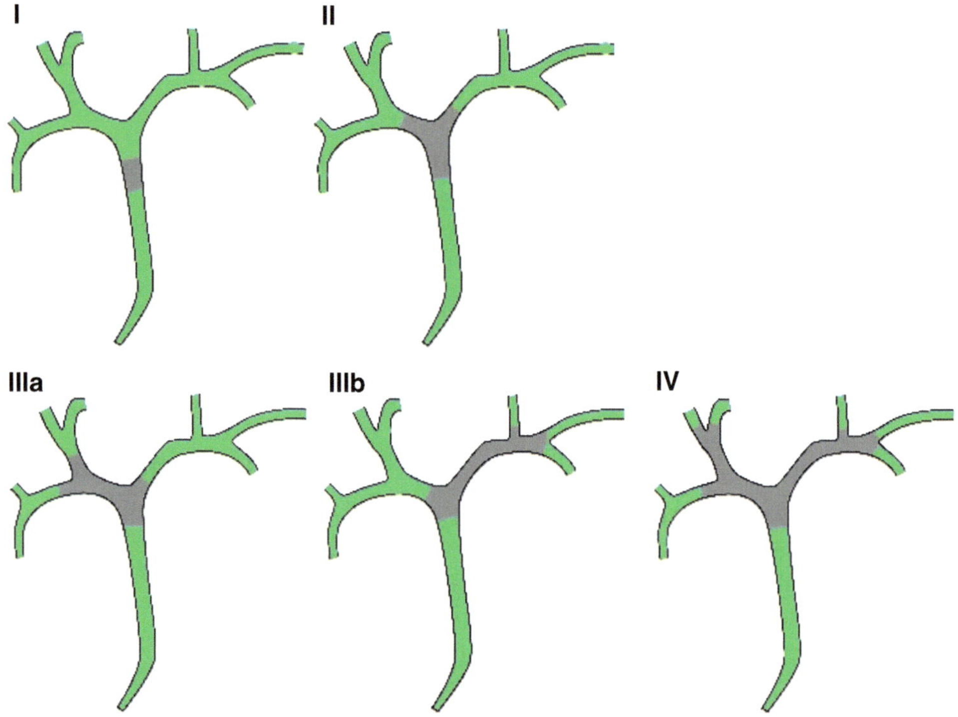

Fig. 30.1 The Bismuth–Corlette classification of the hilar tumor

Table 30.1 The Bismuth–Corlette classification of hilar tumors

Type	Description
1	Tumor below the confluence of the right and left hepatic ducts
2	Involvement of the primary confluence
3	Extension to the right or left hepatic duct (a) *Involvement of primary confluence and the right hepatic duct* (b) *Involvement of the primary confluence and the left hepatic duct*
4	Involvement of bilateral secondary confluences

Table 30.2 Predisposing factors for cholangiocarcinoma

Inflammatory diseases
Primary sclerosing cholangitis
Hepatolithiasis
Liver fluke infestation (Opisthorchis viverrini, Clonorchis sinensis)
Congenital diseases
Caroli's disease
Choledochal cysts (types I and IV)
Chemical agents
Thorotrast
Toxins (dioxins, polyvinyl chloride)
Viral infection
HBV, HCV
Others
Chronic liver disease
Diabetes mellitus, obesity
Chronic alcohol use (>80 g/day), tobacco

30.2.1.2 Microscopic Pattern

Typically, intrahepatic CCA is a mucin-producing adenocarcinoma and has three major architectural patterns:

1. Well Differentiated
2. Moderately Differentiated
3. Poorly Differentiated

30.2.2 Extra-Hepatic Bile Duct Carcinoma (EBDC)

30.2.2.1 Macroscopic Pattern

According to their macroscopic appearance, EBDC may also be further divided into four categories:

1. Sclerosing (Scirrhous) Constricting type—(Most common)—Diffuse wall thickening due to extensive tumor infiltration and fibrosis.
2. Polypoid type.
3. Nodular type.
4. Diffusely Infiltrating type—Usually spreads linearly along the bile duct wall.

30.2.2.2 Microscopic Pattern

Hilar CCA tends to microscopically extend longitudinally beyond the visible macroscopic disease. This hidden microscopic extension is usually observed up to 10 mm (invasive) to 20 mm (non-invasive) along the bile duct. Four microscopic patterns have been described.

1. Adenocarcinoma of biliary type—Most common
2. Adenocarcinoma of foveolar type
3. Adenocarcinoma of intestinal type
4. Squamous cell carcinoma—Rarest pattern

30.3 Clinical Presentation

The most common presentations of hilar CCA or distal CCA include painless, progressive jaundice, often accompanied by cholestasis symptoms such as pruritus and clay-colored stools. Cholangitis occurs in about 10% of patients. Abdominal palpation may reveal a lump, often caused by enlargement of one lobe, especially in the context of an atrophy–hypertrophy complex or in cases of a large intrahepatic CCA. Patients often report significant weight loss, partly due to malabsorption of fat-soluble vitamins. In contrast, most patients with intrahepatic CCA experience non-specific symptoms, including abdominal discomfort, loss of appetite, and cachexia. Rarely, these tumors present with symptoms of biliary obstruction, particularly when they compress the hepatic hilum. Notably, 19–43% of intrahepatic CCA cases are found incidentally.

30.4 Diagnosis

30.4.1 Laboratory Investigations

In addition to routine blood tests, tumor markers should be performed in all cases of CCA. CA 19–9 and CEA are the most commonly used markers; they not only help differentiate CCA from benign mimickers but also play an essential role in follow-up after surgical resection. Elevated serum levels of Ca 19–9 should be interpreted with caution in patients with cholestasis. The serum level should be compared after biliary drainage is achieved. Some correction factors are suggested in the literature for CA 19–9 levels in cholestatic patients, such as the actual CA 19–9 level = CA 19–9 level/total serum bilirubin. In patients with intrahepatic CCA, serum AFP should also be checked to rule out the possibility of hepatocellular carcinoma (HCC), which has a worse prognosis than intrahepatic CCA.

30.4.2 Tissue Diagnosis

Histological diagnosis can be challenging and is not always necessary for managing hilar CCA, which often appears as biliary thickening and stricture on imaging. When needed, various tissue sampling methods include endoscopic or percutaneous trans-hepatic brush biopsy, forceps biopsy, and cholangioscopic-guided biopsy. The sensitivity of a single method is often inadequate; therefore, combining multiple approaches increases the likelihood of obtaining a positive diagnosis. Currently, cholangioscopic-guided biopsy (Spyglass) allows sampling with direct visualization of the abnormal area, achieving a sensitivity of 71%–100% and a specificity of 96.7%–100%. Intrahepatic mass-forming CCA is often accessible for tissue biopsy under ultrasound or CT guidance.

30.4.3 Radiological Imaging

Since surgical resection is the only potentially curative option, imaging plays a vital role in determining preoperative staging and surgical resectability. Each imaging modality contributes uniquely to the evaluation of CCA. Consequently, a multimodal imaging approach is often used (e.g., multiphasic CECT, MRI with MRCP, PET) to provide a comprehensive assessment. Additionally, invasive techniques such as ERCP, choledochoscopy, and intraductal US are performed on a case-by-case basis for histologic diagnosis and tumor extent evaluation, depending on availability (Table 30.3).

Table 30.3 Advantages and limitations of various imaging modalities used in the evaluation of cholangiocarcinoma

Imaging	Technique	Advantages	Disadvantages
Contrast-enhanced computed tomography (CECT)	Dual-phase CT (arterial + venous) Delayed phase at 3–5 min to differentiate intrahepatic CCA from HCC/metastasis	Images extent of the tumor, local HA, and PV involvement MPR & MIP further aid in the evaluation of tumor extension and vascular involvement MinIP aids in the assessment of biliary obstruction and longitudinal tumor extension	Underestimation of longitudinal tumor extent along the bile ducts
Magnetic Resonance Cholangiopancreatogram (MRCP) ± dynamic post-contrast magnetic resonance imaging (MRI)	Heavily T2W MRCP including a 3D sequence Dynamic post-contrast MRI additionally provides multiphasic evaluation like multiphasic CT and allows simultaneous evaluation of tumor, biliary tree and vascular anatomy	MRCP provides better longitudinal tumor extension along the biliary tree in hilar or distal CCA Visualization of the entire biliary tree, even proximal to biliary stricture unlike ERC No need for contrast in heavily T2W MRCP sequence DWI provides a better detection of intrahepatic and nodal metastases	Lower spatial resolution for vascular evaluation Longer acquisition time and more prone for motion artifact
Endoscopic retrograde cholangiogram (ERC)	Choledochoscopy and intraductal US can be added to ERC	High spatial resolution imaging for evaluation of biliary strictures and intraductal lesions Tissue sampling and therapeutic biliary drainage can be done simultaneously	Invasive Precludes complete evaluation of biliary tree proximal to a high-grade stricture
FDG-PET	Whole body imaging for tumor staging	Allows detection of nodal and distant metastases	False positive results in biliary inflammation and false negative results in mucinous CCA

HA hepatic artery, *PV* portal vein, *MPR* multiplanar reformation, *MIP* maximum intensity projection, *MinIP* minimum intensity projection, *DWI* diffusion-weighted imaging, *CCA* cholangiocarcinoma

30.5 Hilar Cholangiocarcinoma

The periductal infiltrating type is the most common morphologic growth pattern. On imaging, it typically appears as a narrowed hilar biliary duct with irregular wall thickening and associated upstream biliary dilatation. Due to the desmoplastic stroma, the thickening gradually and progressively increases. Skip lesions may also be observed in some cases. These imaging findings are nonspecific and can also be seen in certain benign biliary strictures, such as primary sclerosing cholangitis, recurrent pyogenic cholangitis, eosinophilic cholangitis, and IgG4-related cholangiopathy. Therefore, a histological diagnosis may be necessary in cases with diagnostic uncertainty, although obtaining a representative tissue sample is often difficult. Additionally, clinical profiles, serum bilirubin levels, and tumor markers can help distinguish malignant from benign biliary strictures (Figs. 30.2 and 30.3; Table 30.4).

30.5.1 Intrahepatic Cholangiocarcinoma

The mass-forming type is the most common form of intrahepatic CCA, usually appearing as a well-defined hepatic mass with lobulated or irregular borders, often with capsular retraction. Nearby peripheral biliary dilation and satellite nodules near the main tumor may also be seen. On multiphasic CT or MRI, typical intrahepatic CCA shows early peripheral rim enhancement during the arterial phase, with incomplete progressive centripetal enhancement in later stages. This early peripheral rim enhancement indicates hypercellularity at the tumor's outer edge, which may exhibit

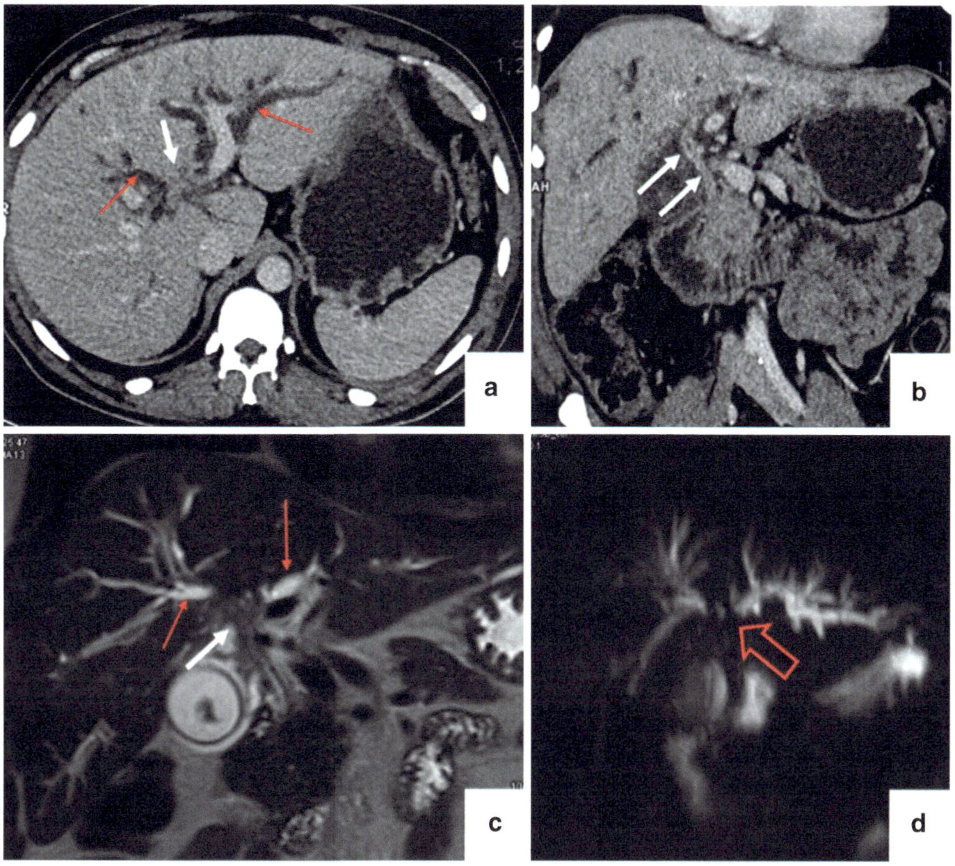

Fig. 30.2 CECT and MRI in periductal infiltrating hilar cholangiocarcinoma (Type 2). (**a**, **b**) Axial and coronal venous phase CT images show enhancing thickening involving CBD and CHD and extending to the primary confluence (white arrows **a**, **b**) with upstream bilobar biliary dilatation (red arrows **a**, **c**). (**c**) The coronal T2W image reveals biliary thickening and stricture (white arrow **c**). (**d**) The 3D MRCP image depicts hilar separation (open red arrow **d**) with bilobar biliary dilatation, and the secondary confluence is free on both sides. CECT, contrast-enhanced computed tomography; MRCP, magnetic resonance cholangiopancreatography; CBD, common bile duct; CHD, common hepatic duct

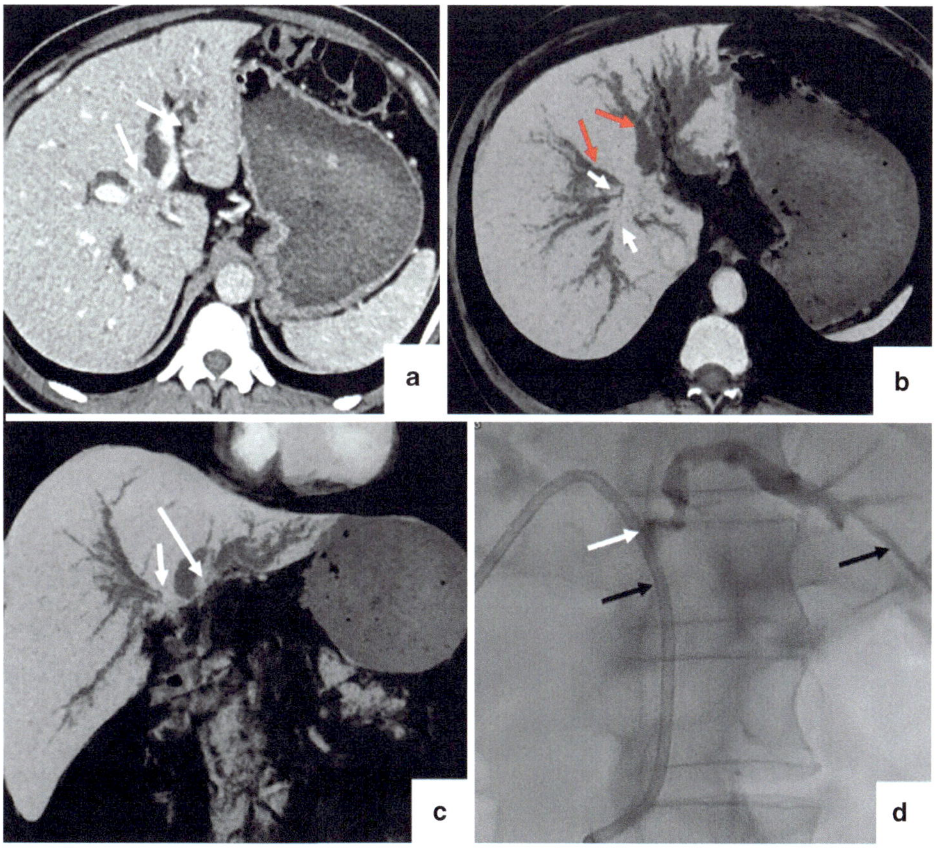

Fig. 30.3 Periductal infiltrating hilar cholangiocarcinoma (Type 4) (**a**) axial venous phase CT image shows enhancing thickening at the primary confluence, also extending to the right and left secondary confluence (white arrows). (**b**, **c**) Axial and coronal MinIP images show bilobar biliary dilatation with separation of right (short white arrows) and left secondary confluence. (**d**) Bilateral PTBD was done for hyperbilirubinemia. MinIP, minimum intensity projection; PTBD, percutaneous transhepatic biliary drainage

Table 30.4 Imaging features to differentiate benign from malignant strictures

	Benign	Malignant
Morphology	Smooth, symmetric border	Irregular, asymmetric stricture
Margin	Tapered	Shouldered
Stricture	Usually, short	Long
Upstream dilatation	Less	More
Portal venous phase enhancement	Less common	More common

washout in the delayed phase. DWI displays peripheral hyperintensity and central hypointensity, also called the "target sign" or "target appearance." Importantly, the scirrhous subtype of HCC (tumor with central fibrous stroma) can resemble typical intrahepatic CCA on imaging (Fig. 30.4).

Hepatocholangiocarcinoma is a variant where both HCC and CCA components coexist. As a result, it exhibits mixed imaging features of HCC and CCA. When the diagnosis is uncertain, histological evaluation is crucial for proper management.

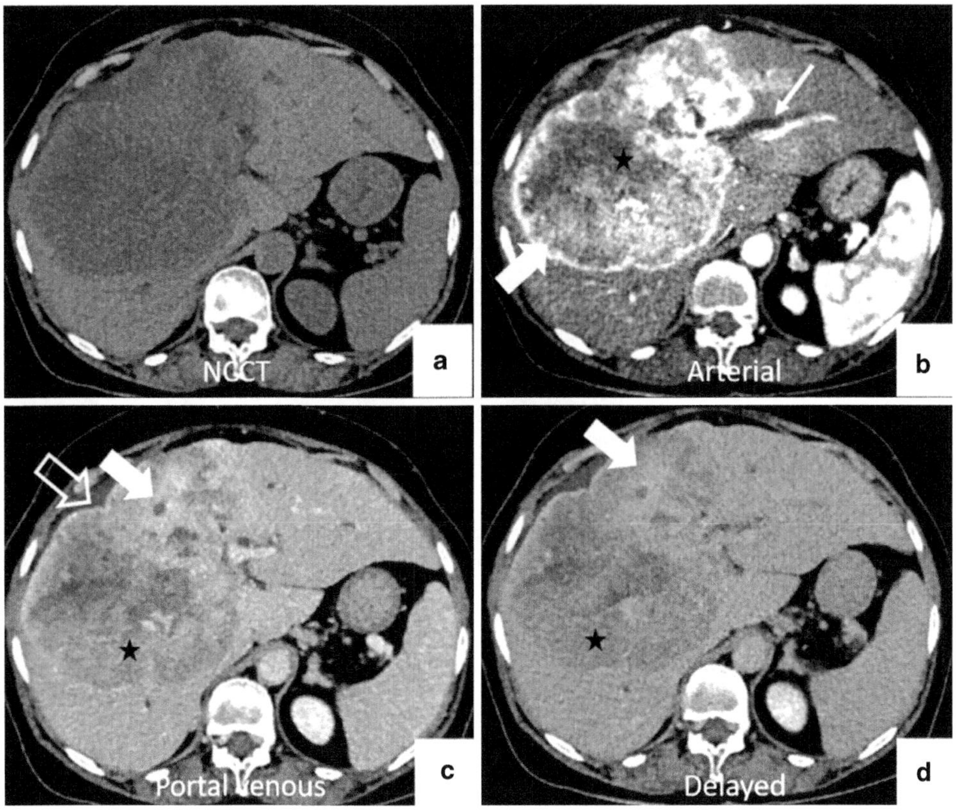

Fig. 30.4 Intrahepatic cholangiocarcinoma. (**a**) Non-contrast CT shows a large hypodense hepatic mass. (**b**) After contrast injection, the tumor exhibits early peripheral rim enhancement (thick white arrow) with central hyperenhancement during the arterial phase. Note the adjacent biliary dilatation (thin white arrow). (**c**, **d**) There is incomplete and progressive centripetal enhancement (thick white arrows) in the portal venous and delayed phases. Also, note the associated capsular retraction (open white arrow)

30.6 Management

Curative surgery involving R0 resection remains the cornerstone of treatment for cholangiocarcinoma. However, only about 25% of cases are deemed resectable at the time of diagnosis.

30.6.1 Preoperative Management

30.6.1.1 Biliary Drainage

Preoperative biliary drainage (PBD) is an integral part of preoperative care, aimed at improving liver function and reducing postoperative complications. Biliary drainage for hilar CCA can be performed as either curative or palliative treatment. The goal of the first is to lower serum bilirubin to 3.0 mg/dl before major liver resections. Biliary drainage methods are classified as endoscopic (ERCP/EUS/ENBD) or percutaneous (PTBD). Endoscopic drainage is preferred for distal obstructions. In proximal blocks, the choice depends on the center's expertise and resources. In hilar blocks, draining the future liver remnant (FLR) is crucial because it directly influences liver regeneration after major resections. Often, draining the FLR alone is sufficient to achieve the required bilirubin level for intervention radiology procedures and surgery. If bilirubin levels do not decrease as expected, remaining segments can be drained. The rate of bilirubin decrease after PBD depends heavily on liver quality and the integrity of the primary confluence. All infected segments should be drained in patients with cholangitis. Cholestasis caused by biliary obstruction inhibits proper hypertrophy of the FLR. In patients with PTBD or ENBD, bile should be refed whenever possible. This significantly restores the patient's nutritional status, immunity, and electrolyte balance.

30.6.1.2 Prehabilitation

Preoperative optimization remains an underrated aspect that significantly influences outcomes after major hepato-pancreato-biliary procedures. This involves nutritional enhancement, cardio-pulmonary exercises, and psychological interventions. Focused nutritional protocols, combined with rigorous physical exercises, boost immunity and support liver regeneration, becoming especially critical in challenging postoperative scenarios, such as sepsis or small-for-size situations. Branch chain amino acids, such as leucine, isoleucine, and valine, may also play a role in promoting liver regeneration during the postoperative period.

30.6.1.3 Assessment of Resectability

In hilar CCA, a properly timed triphasic CT is incredibly helpful in assessing local tumor extension, nodal involvement, vascular involvement, FLR volume, relevant vascular and biliary anatomical variants, and detecting distant metastasis. The longitudinal tumor extension along the biliary tree in cases of hilar CCA is one of the most critical aspects that impact planning the type of liver resection. Although triphasic CT can reasonably predict this, MRCP with dynamic post-contrast MRI has the advantage of better detecting wall thickening on either side of the tumor along the duct. However, in patients with a stent in place, this particular interpretation becomes more challenging, and it's wiser to overestimate the length of involvement rather than compromise oncological safety.

PI and IG-type CCA tend to extend into the submucosal and mucosal layers, respectively. As a result, the microscopic tumor margin might extend beyond the visible tumor margin. Therefore, it is recommended to resect at least 20 mm beyond the macroscopic tumor margin for IG or MF types and at least 10 mm beyond for PI types of CCA to achieve a negative surgical margin. Intraoperative frozen section examination can help guide the hepatic surgeon regarding a negative proximal or distal duct margin, but in patients with a stent in place or a history of cholangitis, it is especially challenging for a pathologist to distinguish between inflammation-related dysplasia and malignancy.

The resectability in hilar CCA should be assessed very carefully, preferably by a surgeon well-experienced in liver resections and an experienced radiologist. It depends upon the following anatomical factors:

- Tumor extent on the left and right hepatic duct (minimum 10 mm margin)
- Segment IV duct involvement
- Extent of distal CBD involvement
- Hepatic artery involvement
- Main portal vein involvement
- Contralateral vascular structure involvement to that of the tumor site

The traditional anatomical criteria for unresectability in hilar CCA are (a) type IV hilar block, (b) type III block with contralateral atrophy or vascular involvement, and (c) invasion of the central portal vein or common hepatic artery. However, with advances in surgical techniques and perioperative management over the past two decades, the scope of surgery has expanded considerably. For example, a Type IV BC (Bismuth-Corlette) block may be resectable if a patient has an adequate extrahepatic biliary stump proximal to the right or left secondary confluence. There is substantial literature supporting favorable outcomes after resection for type IV CCA, especially when combined with portal vein or hepatic artery reconstructions.

30.6.2 Liver Resection for Hilar CCA

The type and extent of liver resection depend on the Bismuth-Corlette classification of CCA. Most hilar CCAs require caudate lobectomy along with major liver resection due to the proximity and drainage of the caudate ducts with the biliary confluence. Extended right and extended left hepatectomy are preferred for type IIIA and IIIB tumors, respectively. For type II and IV tumors, there is sufficient evidence supporting both right and left extended hepatectomy. It is important to be familiar with the course of the right hepatic artery, which typically runs behind the common hepatic duct just below the hilum. This artery is often involved by the tumor regardless of the hilar CCA type, prompting surgeons to favor right liver resection. However, when both right and left liver resections are anatomically feasible, left liver resection may result in better postoperative morbidity profiles and is preferred by many hepatobiliary surgeons due to a larger FLR.

30.6.3 FLR Assessment and Augmentation

The liver has a unique ability to regenerate after resections (Table 30.5).

Assessing the FLR is crucial when planning major hepatic resections. Patients with inadequate FLR face higher risks of postoperative hepatic failure, increasing morbidity and mortality. The minimum FLR needed for major liver resections in a cholestatic liver is 40%. The FLR is calculated pre-operatively using CECT, either manually or with dedicated software such as Myrian. If the FLR is insufficient, the patient requires FLR augmentation. Portal vein embolization (PVE) is a method for FLR augmentation, where the portal flow is blocked at the resection site to divert blood to the FLR, promoting hypertrophy. The revised FLR volume is measured 3–4 weeks post-PVE. The average FLR growth rate after PVE is 10%–12%. If adequate hypertrophy does not occur despite PVE, hepatic vein embolization may be considered. Both portal vein and hepatic embolization are referred to as dual vein embolization (DVE) or hepatic venous deprivation (HVD), and this technique has been shown to produce greater FLR hypertrophy than PVE alone (Fig. 30.5).

Table 30.5 Factors influencing the regeneration of the liver

Age	Cholangitis
Co-morbidities	Liver fibrosis or cirrhosis
Nutritional status	Portal hypertension
Prior chemotherapy	Need for resection of additional organ
Cholestasis	Need for vascular reconstruction

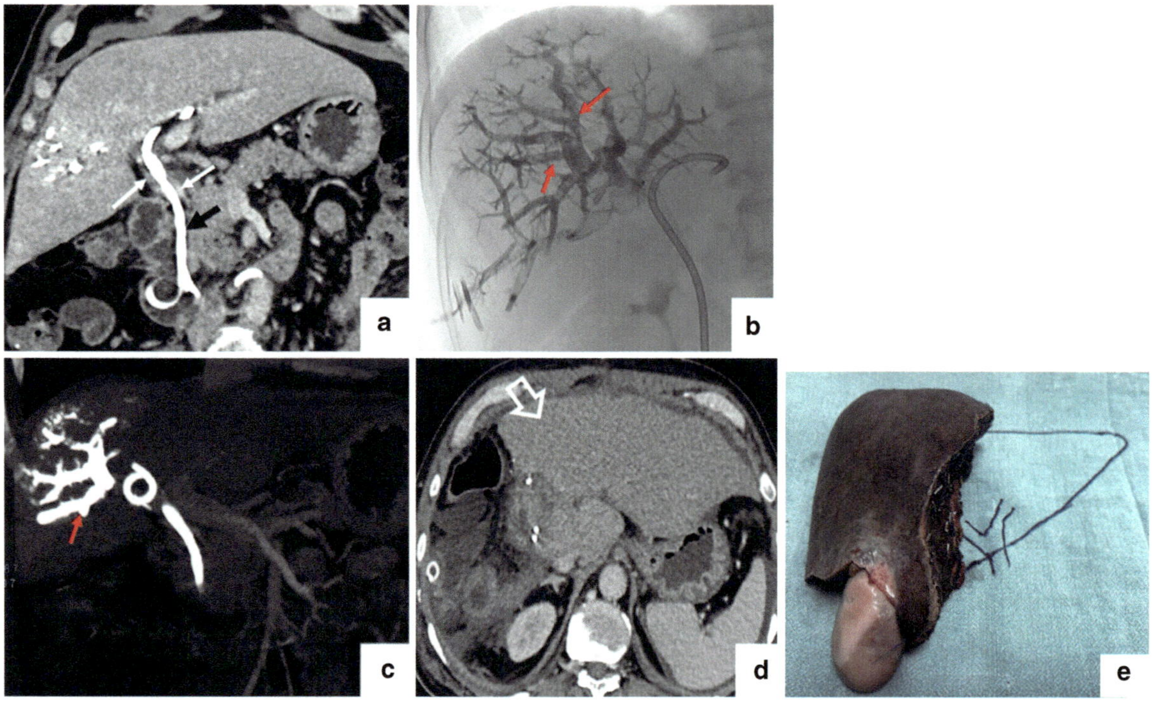

Fig. 30.5 Right modified extended hepatectomy for Type 2 hilar CCA. (**a**) Coronal venous phase CT image shows enhancing CHD and proximal CBD thickening (white arrows). ERCP stent is seen in situ (thick black arrow). The proximal extent of the tumor is not well-delineated due to the post-stenting status. Initial standardized FLR was 27%. (**b**, **c**) Portal vein embolization was performed using a 20% glue-lipiodol mixture. A glue cast is seen within the portal vein radicles (red arrows). FLR hypertrophy (from 27% to 41%) was noticed at the 4-week follow-up scan. (**d**) Postoperative CT scan following Right modified extended hepatectomy. Hypertrophied FLR is marked with an open white arrow. (**e**) The resected specimen. CBD, common bile duct; CHD, common hepatic duct; ERCP, endoscopic retrograde cholangiopancreatography; FLR, future liver remnant

30.7 Postoperative Morbidity and Mortality

Post-Hepatectomy Liver Failure (PHLF) is the most feared complication after major liver resections, occurring in about 10%–30% of cases. Despite advances in surgical techniques and critical care, PHLF remains the leading cause of morbidity and death following major liver resections. Insufficient FLR plays a key role in the development of PHLF. It usually presents with a triad of hyperbilirubinemia, coagulopathy, and hepatic encephalopathy. The 50–50 Criteria, which is rarely used nowadays, include the following parameters: serum bilirubin level greater than 50 μmol/L (2.9 mg/dL) and prothrombin time less than 50% (INR > 1.7) on day 5. International Study Group of Liver Surgery (ISGLS) grading is currently the most widely adopted and dynamic system for assessing PHLF (Table 30.6).

Some other common complications after major liver resections include intra- or postoperative bleeding, bile leaks, strictures, and superficial or deep space infections. Any source of infection during the postoperative period will hinder liver regeneration. Early initiation of enteral feeding with a high protein content is crucial for addressing postoperative sepsis and liver failure. Preventing ileus by correcting potassium and magnesium levels and avoiding opioids is essential. Excessive drain output should be compensated with intravenous albumin infusion.

Table 30.6 Grading of Post-Hepatectomy Liver Failure (PHLF) by International Study Group of Liver Surgery (ISGLS)

	Grade A	Grade B	Grade C
Clinical status	Deterioration in LFT	Deviation from the normal postoperative course without invasive procedures	Multi-organ dysfunction requiring invasive treatment
Symptoms	None	Ascites Weight gain Confusion Encephalopathy	Large volume ascites Renal failure Respiratory failure Hemodynamic instability
Urine output	> 0.5 ml/kg/hr	≤ 0.5 ml/kg/hr	≤0.5 ml/kg/hr
Blood urea nitrogen	< 150 mg/dl	<150 mg/dl	≥150 mg/dl
O_2 saturation	> 90%	<90% despite O_2 supplement	≤85% despite high fraction of inspired oxygen support
INR	< 1.5	≥1.5 and <2.0	≥2.0
Point of care	Surgical ward	HDU/ICU	ICU
Treatment	None	*Non-invasive* FFP Albumin Diuretics NIV	*Invasive* Intubation Hemodialysis Vasopressor support Extra-corporeal liver support

30.8 Adjuvant Therapy

Several clinical trials have recently been published regarding the role of adjuvant chemotherapy in biliary tract cancers. The BILCAP study, a randomized controlled trial conducted in the United Kingdom, compared Capecitabine to simple observation following curative surgery. The per-protocol analysis revealed a significantly longer overall survival for the Capecitabine group compared to the observation group (53 months versus 36 months; $p = 0.02$), suggesting that Capecitabine could be considered the standard of care following curative surgery.

Another phase 3 randomized study, the PRODIGE-12/ACCORD-18 trial from France, compared Gemcitabine and Oxaliplatin (GEMOX) to simple observation in patients with biliary tract cancers who had undergone curative resection. This study found no significant difference in median survival between the GEMOX group and the observation group (75.8 months versus 50.8 months; $p = 0.74$). Additionally, adjuvant S-1 therapy has been explored in patients with resected biliary tract cancer. S-1 is an oral anti-cancer drug consisting of tegafur, 5-chloro-2,4-dihydroxypridine, and potassium oxonate. The ASCOT trial demonstrated that adjuvant therapy with S-1 significantly improved overall survival and progression-free survival compared to the observation group.

30.9 Palliative Procedures

In cases of unresectable CCA, patients may experience symptoms of cholestasis. The primary goal of optimal palliative therapy is to relieve these symptoms while minimizing perioperative morbidity and mortality, with a strong focus on patient comfort and quality of life. The choice of a palliative procedure depends on the nature of the obstructive symptoms and an assessment of the medical risks associated with the procedure, taking into account the patient's expected survival. Biliary decompression can be achieved through endoscopic or percutaneous stenting of the obstructed segment. Additionally, via the PTBD routes, brachytherapy and photodynamic therapy may be performed with palliative intent (Fig. 30.6).

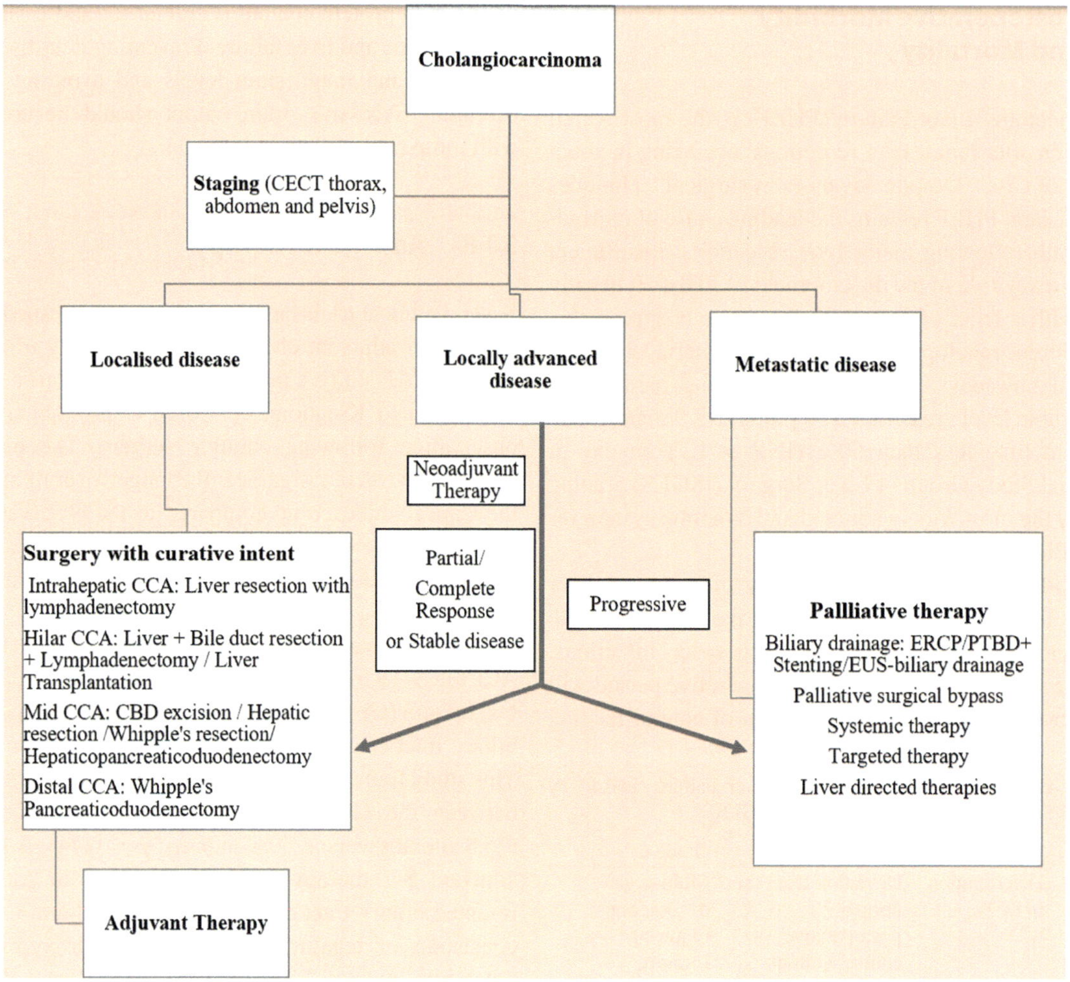

Fig. 30.6 The algorithm for management of cholangiocarcinoma

30.10 Long-Term Outcomes

Achieving a negative resection margin is the key prognostic indicator for long-term survival, with lymph node involvement also significantly affecting outcomes. Five-year survival rates range from 20% to 50%, although in carefully selected patients who undergo complete resection with N0 status, 5-year overall survival rates may improve to 54%–62%. The main concern for CCA patients is the high likelihood of recurrence, which typically occurs within the first year after resection. Other prognostic factors include tumor invasion depth, extent of surgical intervention, patient comorbidities, and treatment-related complications.

30.11 Liver Transplantation

The role of liver transplantation (LT) in hilar CCA is still developing. Early results of LT for hilar CCA were disappointing, with a high rate of recurrence. "The Mayo protocol," introduced in 1993 and offering LT for unresectable hilar CCA, is considered a major breakthrough because it incorporates neo-adjuvant chemo-radiotherapy as a key component. The criteria for the Mayo protocol are as follows: (1) Mass no larger than 3 cm in diameter. (2) Not extending below the cystic duct insertion. (3) No intrahepatic or distant metastasis. Patients who had a prior transcutaneous biopsy or cytology attempt were excluded due to the high risk of tumor seeding. The diagnosis was based on cross-sectional imaging, positive cytology or biopsy, elevated Ca 19–9, and polysomy on FISH. All patients received neo-adjuvant chemo-radiotherapy followed by a staging procedure a few days before the scheduled LT. Using this strict protocol, they reported an overall 5-year survival rate of about 50%. Currently, there is debate about whether to offer LT to patients with resectable hilar CCA as well.

Key Points

- Cholangiocarcinoma (CCA) is categorized into three types: intrahepatic (10%), perihilar (70%), and distal (20%).
- Perihilar CCA, also called hilar CCA, is further classified based on the Bismuth-Corlette classification.
- Sclerosing (Scirrhous) constricting type is the most common extrahepatic variant of CCA.
- Extrahepatic CCA presents with painless, progressive cholestatic jaundice.
- A multimodal imaging approach is often employed (e.g., multiphasic CECT, MRI with MRCP, PET) to provide a comprehensive assessment of the tumor. Additionally, invasive techniques such as ERCP, choledochoscopy, and intraductal US are conducted on a case-by-case basis for histologic diagnosis and evaluation of tumor extent.
- The type and extent of liver resection for hilar CCA depend on the Bismuth-Corlette classification. Most hilar CCAs require caudate lobectomy along with major liver resection because of the proximity and drainage of the caudate ducts with the biliary confluence.
- Extended right and extended left hepatectomies are preferred for type IIIA and IIIB tumors, respectively. For type II and IV tumors, there is sufficient evidence supporting both right and left extended hepatectomies.
- When both right and left liver resections are anatomically feasible, left liver resection may lead to better postoperative morbidity outcomes and is preferred because of a larger future liver remnant (FLR).
- The minimum FLR required for major liver resections in a cholestatic liver is 40%. If the FLR is inadequate, the patient needs FLR augmentation.
- Portal vein embolization (PVE) is a technique used to increase the future liver remnant (FLR) by blocking blood flow at the resection site, redirecting blood to the FLR to induce hypertrophy. If sufficient hypertrophy does not occur after PVE, hepatic vein embolization may be considered.
- Post-Hepatectomy Liver Failure (PHLF) is the most feared complication after major liver resections, occurring in about 10%–30% of cases.
- The International Study Group of Liver Surgery (ISGLS) grading is currently the most widely used and adaptable system for assessing PHLF.
- Different trials have recommended Capecitabine and S-1 therapy as adjuvant treatment after resection.
- Neo-adjuvant chemo-radiotherapy followed by liver transplantation is emerging as a potential treatment in selected cases of CCA.

Selected Reading

1. Vogel A, Bridgewater J, Edeline J, et al. Biliary tract cancer: ESMO Clinical Practice Guideline for diagnosis, treatment and follow-up. Ann Oncol. 2023;34:127–40.
2. Rushbrook SM, Kendall TJ, Zen Y, et al. British Society of Gastroenterology guidelines for the diagnosis and management of cholangiocarcinoma. Gut. 2024;73:16–46.
3. European Association for the Study of the Liver. EASL Clinical Practice Guidelines on the management of extrahepatic cholangiocarcinoma. J Hepatol. 2025;3:211–38.

Part VI

Pancreas

Surgical Anatomy of the Pancreas and the Ampulla of Vater

31

Murugappan Nachiappan

Abstract

The pancreas is a complex retroperitoneal organ with intricate anatomical relationships that are of paramount importance in surgical practice. A thorough understanding of the surgical anatomy of the pancreas is essential for safe operative intervention, accurate radiological interpretation, and effective management of pancreatic diseases. This chapter reviews the gross anatomy, embryology, vascular supply, lymphatic drainage, and ductal anatomy of the pancreas, with particular emphasis on surgically relevant landmarks and anatomical variations. Understanding these anatomical principles forms the foundation for reducing operative morbidity and improving outcomes in pancreatic surgery.

Keywords

Pancreas anatomy · Ampulla of Vater

The pancreas is a retroperitoneal organ that extends between the duodenum on the right and the spleen on the left. It is divided into the head, neck, body, tail, and uncinate process. The head sits within the curve formed by the C-loop of the duodenum, while the neck is positioned in front of the portal vein. The body extends to the left of the portal vein, and the tail reaches the splenic hilum or ends within the leaves of the splenorenal ligament. The uncinate process extends medially from the lower part of the head, lying posterolateral to the superior mesenteric vein and sometimes the artery.

The superior border of the pancreatic body is related to the celiac artery and its branches; the hepatic artery runs along the right side of this border, while the tortuous splenic artery follows the superior border towards the spleen. The inferior mesenteric vein runs along the inferior border and may join the superior mesenteric vein (42% of cases), splenic vein (34%), or portal vein trifurcation (24%). The middle colic artery arises from the superior mesenteric artery beneath the lower border of the pancreas, coursing between the leaves of the transverse mesocolon.

The tail is the lateral-most part of the pancreas, extending either to the hilum of the spleen or stopping short within the splenorenal ligament. The Japan Pancreas Society defined the left margin of the abdominal aorta as the border between the pancreatic head and tail. In approximately half of individuals, the tail reaches the center of the splenic hilum, while it reaches the upper part in 8% and the lower part in 42%. During splenectomy, the tail of the pancreas, if extending to the splenic hilum, may be at risk of injury, potentially resulting in a pancreatic fistula. The splenic vessels are the posterior relations of the pancreatic tail. Depending on the branching pattern of the splenic vessels, either magistral or distributed, the tail may be related to individual vessels or multiple branches and tributaries of the splenic artery and vein. The left gastroepiploic artery, the largest branch of the splenic artery, originates near the pancreatic tail, close to the splenic hilum, and runs within the layers of the gastrosplenic ligament to reach the gastrocolic ligament.

The uncinate process is an inferior extension of the head of the pancreas, located between the aorta and the superior mesenteric artery. It has a distinct embryological development compared to the rest of the pancreas (see details below). The uncinate process extends variably behind the superior mesenteric vein and artery. Classification systems have been proposed to standardize the extent of the uncinate process. Preoperative imaging is essential to assess the extent of the uncinate process before a pancreaticoduodenectomy for optimal surgical planning.

The tissue between the pancreas and major arteries is called the mesopancreas. Gockel et al. first used this term to describe the firm fibrovascular structure along Treitz's fusion fascia. Also known as the retroportal lamina, PA (pancreas-major

M. Nachiappan (✉)
Valluvanad Hospital, Ottapalam, Palakkad, India

M. Ibrarullah (ed.), *Recent Concepts in Gastrointestinal (GI) Surgery*, https://doi.org/10.1007/978-981-92-1118-0_31

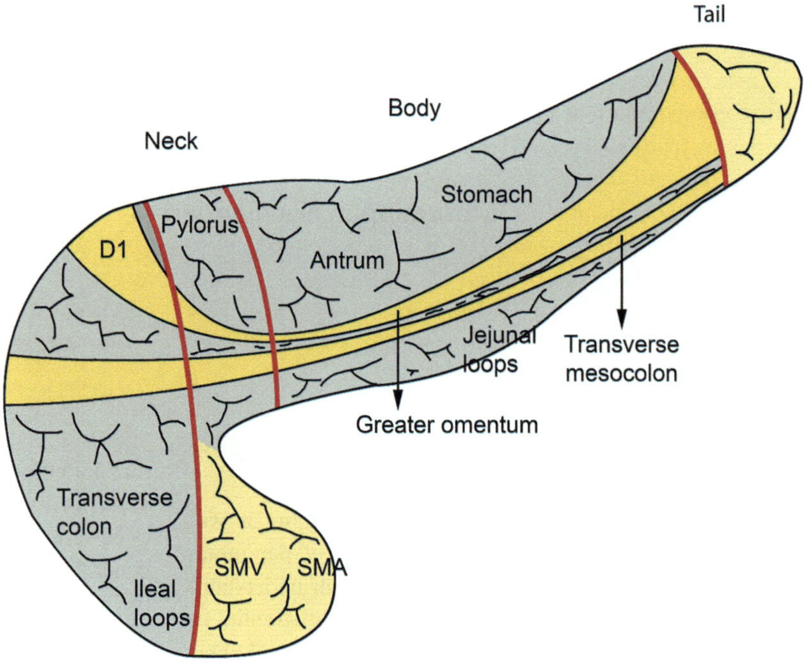

Fig. 31.1 Anterior relations of the pancreas

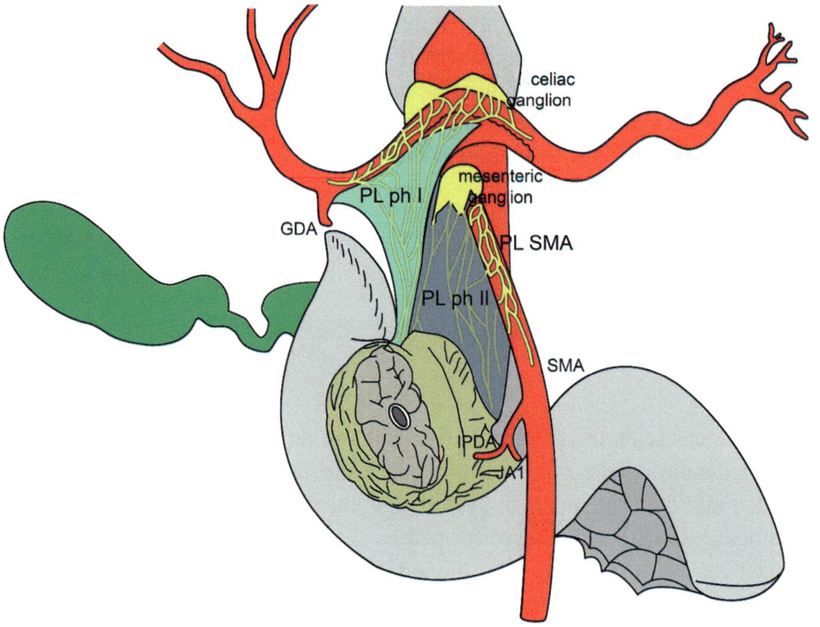

Fig. 31.2 Mesopancreas, the tissue between the pancreas and major arteries. Japan Pancreas Society has divided this area into PLph I (Area shaded green) i.e., nerve plexus between the pancreatic head and the celiac artery and PLph II (Area shaded red) i.e., nerve plexus between the pancreatic body and the superior mesenteric artery

artery) ligament, or pancreatic head plexus, the mesopancreas includes connective tissue, lymphatic tissue, and nerve plexuses originating from the celiac trunk and the superior mesenteric artery. It is bounded medially by the right border of the SMV and SMA, laterally by the pancreatic head and uncinate process, superiorly by the celiac trunk and hepatic artery, posteriorly by the left renal vein, and inferiorly by the mesenteric root. Resection of the mesopancreas is recommended to achieve an R0 resection in cases of pancreatic ductal adenocarcinoma. The Japan Pancreas Society has divided this area into two regions: PLph I, the nerve plexus between the pancreatic head and the celiac artery, and PLph II, the nerve plexus between the pancreatic body and the superior mesenteric artery (Fig. 31.2). Recognizing the concept of the mesopancreas and advocating for total mesopancreatic excision—similar to total mesorectal excision in rectal cancers to achieve radical resection—has prompted the artery-first approach. This technique enables early assessment of resectability, effective lymphatic clearance, reduced risk of IPDA bleeding through early ligation, and higher rates of R0 resections.

31.1 Developmental Anatomy

The pancreas develops from buds originating in the duodenal endodermal lining and extends into the ventral and dorsal mesentery. The ventral bud, a smaller outgrowth with two components, arises lower than the dorsal bud and shares its origin with the hepatic outgrowth. The ventral bud forms the lower part of the pancreatic head and the uncinate process, while the dorsal bud forms the rest of the gland. During development, the duodenum rotates, bringing the ventral anlage to a dorsal position, slightly below its dorsal counterpart, thereby contributing to the formation of the inferior aspect of the pancreatic head and the uncinate process. Failure of the right and left components of the ventral bud to fuse properly, combined with opposite migration of the left component, can lead to annular pancreas. In rare cases (1%–2%), abnormal migration may cause circumportal pancreas, a condition in which pancreatic tissue encircles the portal vein or superior mesenteric vein, posing a potential surgical challenge if present.

As the pancreas moves to a retroperitoneal position from its developmental origins in the ventral and dorsal mesenteries, the membrane covering the pancreatic tissue fuses with that over the inferior vena cava and aorta, forming what is known as the fusion fascia. This fascia is called the fusion fascia of Treitz in the head region and the fusion fascia of Toldt in the body and tail regions of the pancreas. These loose connective tissues create bloodless surgical dissection planes used during pancreatic resections. The superior mesenteric artery penetrates this fascia shortly after arising from the aorta, passing close to the uncinate process of the pancreas. The posterior superior pancreatoduodenal vein runs from the ampulla behind the common bile duct to join the portal vein, enclosed by the fusion fascia of Treitz. Additionally, the anterior inferior and posterior inferior pancreatoduodenal arteries, which arise from the inferior pancreatoduodenal artery (a branch of the superior mesenteric artery), course between the pancreatic parenchyma and the fusion fascia in the head region. Preserving these vessels and their arcades is possible during a duodenum-preserving pancreatic head resection.

In the body and tail regions, the transverse pancreatic vein and its small tributaries run between the parenchyma and the fusion fascia of Toldt, draining into the splenic vein. Blood vessels, their arcades, and the pancreatic neural plexus located in the posterior aspect of the pancreas are situated between the parenchyma and the fusion fascia.

31.2 Pancreatic Ductal Anatomy

After the dorsal and ventral pancreatic buds fuse, their ductal systems also merge, though this process can lead to significant variations. Usually, the main pancreatic duct (MPD) is formed by the distal part of the dorsal duct (duct of Wirsung) and the entire ventral pancreatic duct, opening into the duodenum through the major papilla (Papilla of Vater) on the medial wall of the second part of the duodenum, alongside the bile duct (see below). The proximal part of the dorsal duct, called the accessory pancreatic duct (duct of Santorini), opens slightly proximally through the minor papilla. In about 10% of individuals, the ducts do not fuse and open separately into the duodenum, a condition known as pancreas divisum.

Variations can also occur in the MPD or its drainage pattern. The MPD may follow a descending course (the most common, seen in about 50% of people), a vertical path, a sigmoid shape, or a looped pathway. Typically, the duct is located near the upper border and posterior aspect of the pancreas at the neck, which is the most anterior part of the gland. The most common drainage pattern is a bifid configuration with a dominant Wirsung duct (60%). Other arrangements include a bifid pattern with a dominant Santorini duct, an absence of the Santorini duct, and Ansa Pancreatica, where the Santorini duct forms a reverse S-shape before joining the Wirsung duct as a side branch.

31.3 Ampulla of Vater

Duodenal papilla, commonly known as the ampulla of Vater, is a nipple-like projection situated on the posteromedial aspect of the second part of the duodenum, marking the end of the CBD. Endoscopically, it appears as a longitudinal mucosal fold, accompanied by a horizontal mucosal fold at

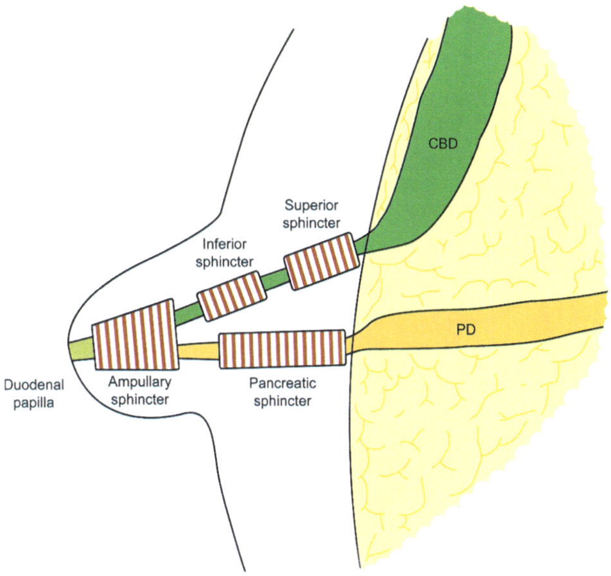

Fig. 31.3 Sphincter complex of Ampulla. See text for details. CBD Common bile duct, PD Pancreatic duct

the papilla. The intramural segments of the common bile duct and pancreatic duct contain a complex sphincter system, with lengths ranging from 6 mm to 30 mm depending on the duct's orientation. This system includes two sphincters on the CBD (superior and inferior), one pancreatic sphincter, and an ampullary sphincter for the common channel (Fig. 31.3).

Based on the formation of the ampulla and ductal openings, three anatomical types are identified: type 1 (an ampulla is present, which may or may not be dilated), type 2 (the ducts open separately on the papilla), and type 3 (the ducts open at separate points on the duodenum).

An anomalous pancreatobiliary ductal union (APBDU) occurs when the pancreatic duct and CBD join outside the wall of the second part of the duodenum, creating an elongated common channel. This anomaly is found in approximately 1-3% of the population and is linked to clinical conditions such as choledochal cysts, gallbladder cancer, and recurrent acute pancreatitis. Classification systems for APBDU include the Komi classification (Fig. 31.4 and Table 31.1) and a more simplified classification developed by the Japanese Study Group on Pancreatobiliary Maljunction (JSPBM) (Fig. 31.5; and Table 31.2).

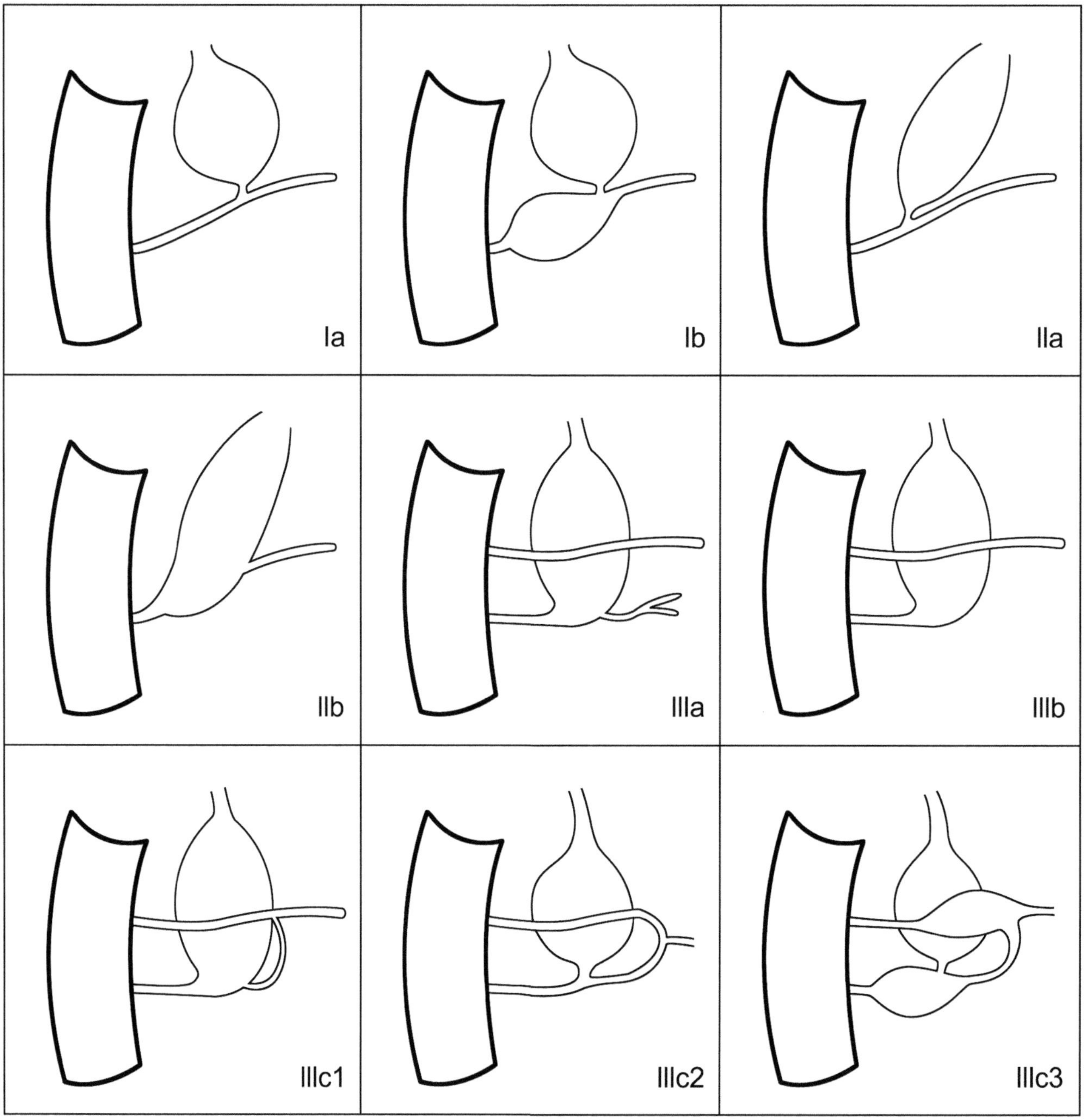

Fig. 31.4 Komi classification of APBDU (see Table 31.1 for details)

Table 31.1 Komi classification of APBDU

Type	Features	Incidence
I	Union of the BD and PD at a right angle to each other	58%
a	*Without dilatation*	
b	*With dilatation of the common channel*	
II	Union of the duct BD and PD with an acute angle between them	32%
a	*Without dilatation*	
b	*With dilatation of the common channel*	
III	Complex patterns of the pancreatic ductal system	6%
a	*Pancreas divisum with biliary dilatation*	
b	*Absence of the Wirsung's duct*	
c 1	*Minor communication between the main duct and the accessory duct*	
c 2	*Normal communication between the common and accessory ducts*	
c 3	*Complete or partial dilatation of the ductal system*	

BD bile duct, *PD* pancreatic duct

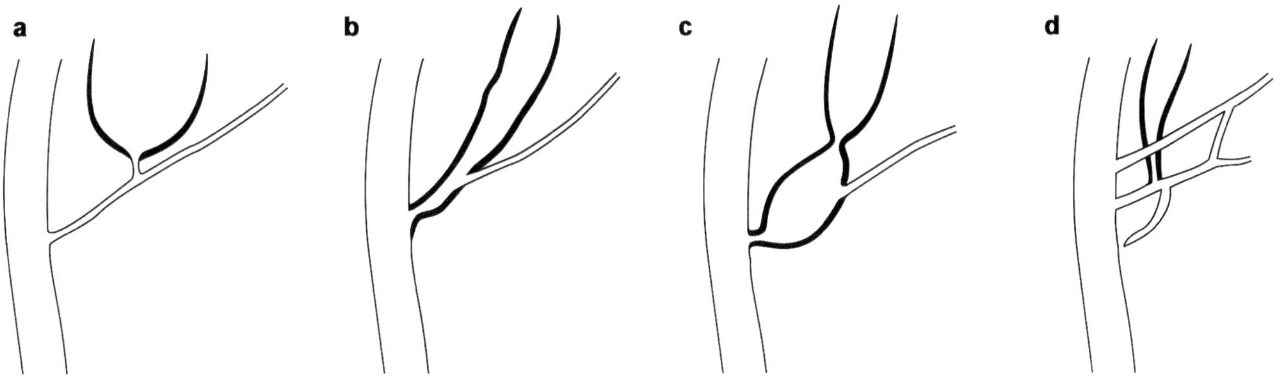

Fig. 31.5 Classification of APBDU by the Japanese Study Group on Pancreatobiliary Maljunction (JSPBM) (see Table 31.2 for details)

Table 31.2 Classification of APBDU by the Japanese Study Group on Pancreatobiliary Maljunction (JSPBM)

Types	Features
A (stenotic type)	Dilatation of the common bile duct (CBD), a stenotic or narrow segment of the distal CBD joins the common channel
B (non-stenotic type)	Normal caliber distal CBD joins the common channel. No focal dilatation of the common channel
C (dilated channel type)	The narrow segment of the distal CBD joins the dilated common channel
D (complex type)	APBJ associated with annular pancreas, pancreas divisum, or other complex duct systems

31.4 Arterial Supply of the Pancreas

The pancreas, originating from both a ventral and a dorsal bud (with the ventral bud positioned slightly lower), receives a dual blood supply from both foregut and midgut arteries. This includes prominent named vessels as well as numerous smaller, unnamed vessels. The head of the pancreas, along with the uncinate process, is richly supplied by branches of the celiac trunk and the superior mesenteric artery (Fig. 31.6).

The anterior superior pancreatoduodenal artery is the terminal branch of the gastroduodenal artery. It courses anteriorly, approximately 1.5 cm below the papilla of Vater, and then turns posteriorly to anastomose with the anterior inferior pancreatoduodenal artery—a branch of the inferior pancreatoduodenal artery—on the posterior aspect of the pancreas.

Similarly, the posterior superior pancreatoduodenal artery, which is also a branch of the gastroduodenal artery, originates at the upper border of the duodenum, anterior to the common bile duct and the portal vein. It runs along the posterior aspect of the pancreatic head, supplying the papilla of Vater, the lower part of the common bile duct, and the second part of the duodenum through the artery of the papilla of Vater. Preserving this blood supply is crucial for maintaining proper vascularity during limited resections.

The inferior pancreatoduodenal artery occurs in about 80% of people, either sharing a common origin with the first jejunal artery (in roughly two-thirds of cases) or originating separately from the superior mesenteric artery in the remaining one-third. This artery divides into anterior and posterior branches at the lower border of the pancreatic head, which then anastomose with branches of the gastroduodenal artery to form the pancreatoduodenal arcades. These arcades create a strong vascular network that supplies the pancreatic head, uncinate process, duodenum, and adjacent structures.

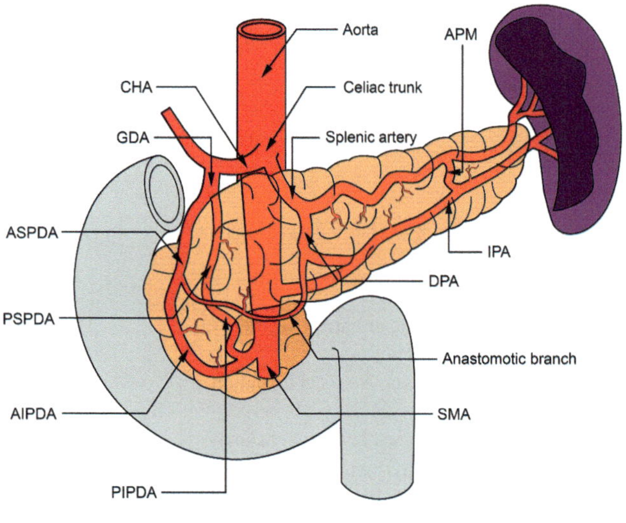

Fig. 31.6 Artery supply of the pancreas. CHA, common hepatic artery; GDA, gastroduodenal artery; ASPDA, anterosuperior pancreaticoduodenal artery; PSPDA, posterosuperior pancreaticoduodenal artery; AIPDA, anteroinferior pancreaticoduodenal artery; PIPDA, posteroinferior pancreaticoduodenal artery; SMA, superior mesenteric artery; DPA, dorsal pancreatic artery; IPA, inferior pancreatic artery; APM, artery pancreaticomagna

The pancreatic body and tail receive blood supply from numerous small, unnamed arteries and larger, named vessels, primarily originating from the splenic artery. Key named vessels include the dorsal pancreatic artery, which typically arises from the splenic artery but can also originate from the superior mesenteric artery, the middle colic branch of the superior mesenteric artery, or the hepatic artery. The dorsal pancreatic artery divides into right and left branches: the left branch, also known as the transverse or inferior pancreatic artery, runs along the pancreas's inferior border and anastomoses with other named arteries, while the right branch extends to connect with the anterior superior pancreatoduodenal artery, forming the prepancreatic arterial arch.

Additionally, the greater pancreatic artery (arteria pancreatica magna), a branch of the splenic artery, provides a substantial blood supply to the pancreatic body. The artery to the tail of the pancreas (arteria caudae pancreatis) originates from either the left gastroepiploic artery or the splenic artery and supplies the pancreatic tail.

Along with these named vessels, small, unnamed arteries run along the borders of the pancreas, penetrating at right angles to supply the parenchyma. Together, these anastomoses form a comprehensive vascular network that supports the pancreatic body and tail.

31.5 Venous Drainage of the Pancreas

The head of the pancreas is drained by the posterior superior pancreatoduodenal vein, which runs from the papilla of Vater, posterior to the CBD, to empty into the portal vein. The posterior inferior pancreatoduodenal vein, with a horizontal course, accompanies its artery and drains into the superior mesenteric vein (SMV) or occasionally into the first jejunal vein. Anteriorly, the head of the pancreas drains into the gastrocolic trunk via the anterior superior pancreatoduodenal vein (see below), which anastomoses with the anterior inferior pancreatoduodenal vein on the anterior surface of the pancreas (note: there is no posterior arcade). This anterior inferior vein drains into the SMV. The uncinate process drains directly into the SMV via small tributaries. The body and tail

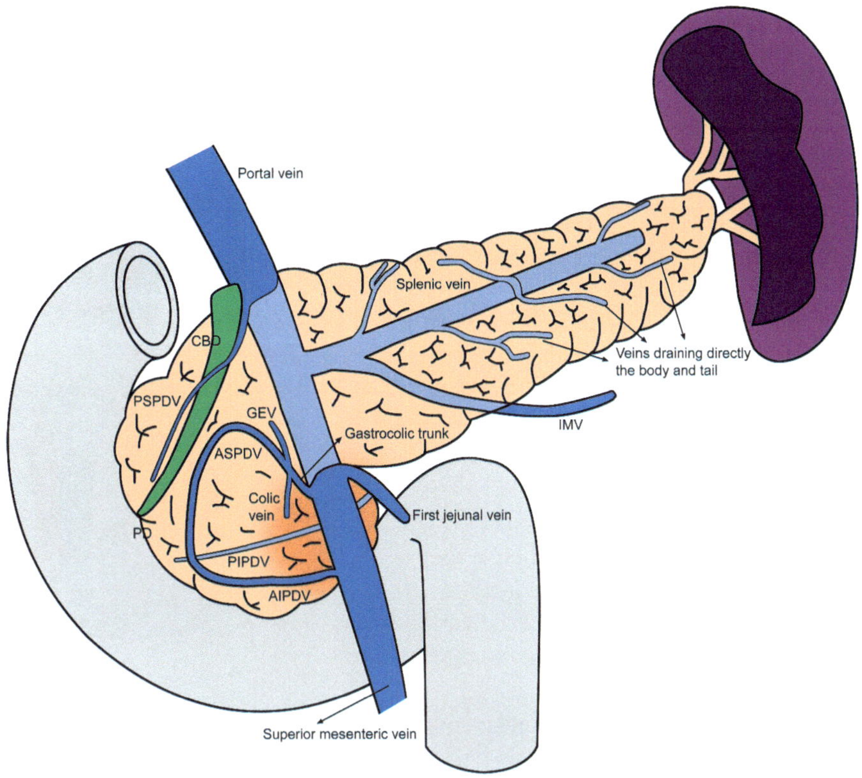

Fig. 31.7 Veins of the Pancreas. See text for details. AIPDV Anterior Inferior Pancreatoduodenal vein, ASPDV Anterior Superior Pancreatoduodenal vein, CBD Common bile duct, GEV Right Gastroepiloic vein, IMV Inferior Mesenteric vein, PD Pancreatic duct, PIPDV Posterior Inferior Pancreatoduodenal vein, PSPDV Posterior Superior Pancreatoduodenal vein

are drained by multiple small veins that open directly into the splenic vein along the posterior aspect of the pancreas. Venous connections exist between the pancreas and the retroperitoneal and lumbar veins, which may become clinically significant in cases of portal hypertension (Fig. 31.7).

The portal vein is formed by the joining of the SMV and the splenic vein, positioned behind the neck of the pancreas. The gastrocolic trunk—comprising the right gastroepiploic vein, colic, and pancreatic tributaries—drains into the SMV at the lower border of the pancreatic neck. Then, the SMV receives the splenic vein behind the neck of the pancreas, forming the portal vein. In about one-third of cases, the inferior mesenteric vein joins this confluence. The SMV is located to the right of the superior mesenteric artery.

At the superior border of the pancreas, the portal vein receives tributaries from the posterior superior pancreatic vein, as well as the right gastric and coronary veins. Within the hepatoduodenal ligament, the portal vein is flanked by the common bile duct on the right and the proper hepatic artery on the left. The gastroduodenal artery branches off from the common hepatic artery at the superior border of the pancreas, anterior to the portal vein. Dividing this artery reveals the suprapancreatic segment of the portal vein above the upper border of the pancreas. Separating the gastroepiploic vein while preserving the colic branches at the lower border exposes the infrapancreatic portion of the SMV. Further blunt dissection facilitates creating a tunnel behind the neck of the pancreas, in front of the SMV and portal vein.

31.6 Lymphatic Drainage of the Pancreas

The pancreas has an extensive lymphatic drainage system, following the paths of its arterial supply. Lymphatic drainage from the head, uncinate process, and neck of the pancreas flows toward the nodes along the pancreatoduodenal, hepatic, and superior mesenteric arteries. Drainage from the body and tail of the pancreas, however, proceeds to the mesocolic nodes, pancreatosplenic nodes, or directly to the pre-aortic nodes. These lymph nodes subsequently drain into the celiac nodes, left lumbar nodes (which include the paraaortic nodes), and phrenic nodes (Fig. 31.8).

According to the Japanese Pancreas Society, specific regional lymph node stations are designated for pancreatic tumors based on the tumor's location. For tumors in the head of the pancreas, the relevant lymph node stations include stations 6, 8a, 8p, 12a, 12b, 12p, 13, 14t, and 17. For tumors in the body of the pancreas, the stations are 8a, 8b, 9, 10, 11p,

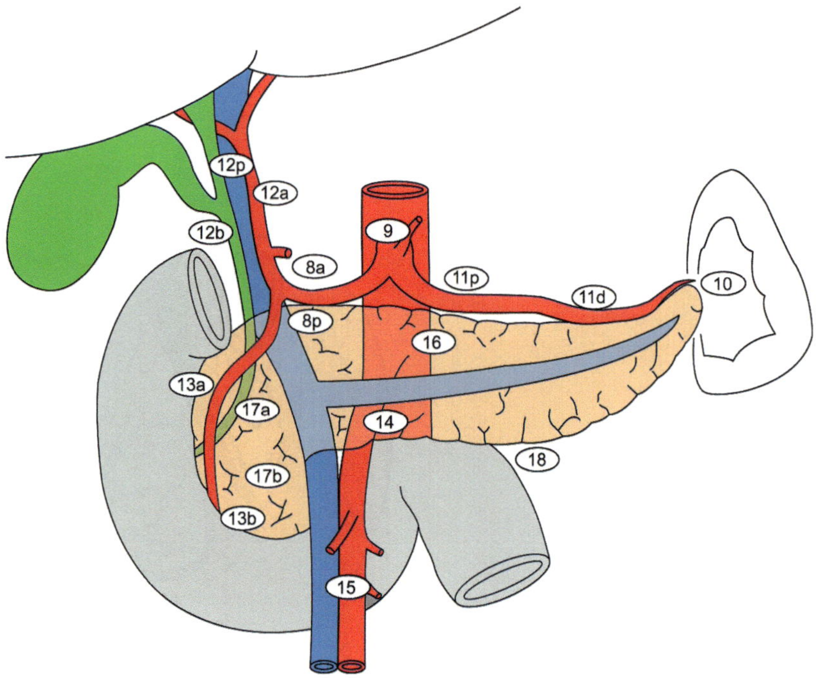

Fig. 31.8 Lymph nodes stations related to the Pancreas, from Japan Pancreas Society. Stations mentioned in yellow are posterior in location. Station 14 is classified as 14t and 14op based on the tumor location

11d, 14t, and 18. For tumors in the tail of the pancreas, the regional lymph node stations include stations 8a, 9, 10, 11p, 11d, and 18. This lymphatic mapping is crucial for staging and surgical planning in pancreatic cancer.

31.7 Nerve Supply of the Pancreas

The pancreas is innervated by sympathetic fibers from the splanchnic nerves and parasympathetic fibers from the vagus nerves. The celiac ganglion, located on either side of the aorta at the origin of the celiac artery, contains pre- and postganglionic sympathetic fibers, preganglionic parasympathetic fibers, and afferent pain fibers from the pancreas. Plexus fibers that cross both above and below the celiac artery contribute to this complex innervation network.

For pain management in chronic pancreatitis or advanced malignancy, relief can be achieved through a celiac plexus blockade for temporary pain relief or by neurolysis, which involves permanent destruction of nerve fibers for longer-term relief. Neurolysis may be performed under imaging or endoscopic ultrasound (EUS) guidance or through an open surgical approach. In surgical settings, the celiac artery can be located by palpating the splenic and common hepatic arteries with the index and middle fingers of the left hand, allowing for targeted neurolytic injection on either side of the celiac axis.

Alternatively, bilateral thoracic splanchnicectomy, or splanchnic nerve denervation, may be considered. The choice of procedure is tailored to the patient's specific clinical condition, indication, and the required duration of pain relief.

31.8 Surgical Approach to the Pancreas

The approach to the pancreas is tailored to the specific indications. For pancreatic necrosectomy or drainage of walled-off pancreatic necrosis, a transgastric or mesocolic approach may be utilized. In most cases, however, pancreatic exploration is performed through the gastrocolic omentum. Other approaches include complete detachment of the greater omentum from the transverse colon or, less commonly, access through the gastro-hepatic ligament.

During procedures involving the head of the pancreas, the approach is achieved through a series of key steps. First, a Cattell–Braasch maneuver and complete Kocherization are performed to identify the left renal vein and the superior mesenteric artery via a posterior approach. This enables an artery-first approach, allowing the surgeon to assess the resectability of the lesion early in the procedure. The choice of approach for assessing the involvement of the superior mesenteric artery varies depending on tumor location.

The posterior approach is suited for periampullary tumors or posteromedial tumors extending to the portal vein or superior mesenteric vein. For tumors along the inferior border of the pancreas, an anterior approach (inferior supracolic) is preferred. In contrast, the superior approach is chosen for tumors at the superior border of the pancreas. Tumors of the uncinate process may require a medial uncinate approach, left posterior approach, or a mesenteric (inferior infracolic) approach.

To expose the anterior aspect of the pancreas, entry into the lesser sac is made by dividing the gastrocolic omentum below the gastroepiploic arcade. As dissection proceeds toward the head of the pancreas, the fused planes between the layers of the greater omentum and the mesocolon must be carefully separated, remaining within the embryonic plane to avoid bleeding from vessels on either side. It is essential to consider anatomical variations of the gastrocolic trunk and avoid excessive traction by assistants retracting the colon, which could lead to unintended bleeding.

The gastrocolic trunk commonly receives the anterior pancreaticoduodenal vein (referred to as the anterior inferior or anterior superior pancreaticoduodenal vein), the superior right colic vein, one or more right colic veins, and the right gastroepiploic vein. Careful dissection and ligation of the right gastroepiploic vein and the pancreatic branches of the gastrocolic trunk, while preserving colic branches and detaching the mesocolon from its fused area over the head of the pancreas, provide full exposure of the pancreas's anterior surface. For surgeries involving the body and tail of the pancreas, mobilizing the splenic flexure and distal transverse colon is necessary to access the inferior border.

Key Points

- The pancreas develops from buds originating in the duodenal endodermal lining. The ventral bud forms the lower part of the pancreatic head and the uncinate process, while the dorsal bud forms the rest of the gland.
- The main pancreatic duct (MPD) is formed by the distal part of the dorsal duct (duct of Wirsung) and the entire ventral pancreatic duct, opening into the duodenum through the major papilla (Papilla of Vater). The proximal part of the dorsal duct, called the accessory pancreatic duct (duct of Santorini), opens slightly proximally through the minor papilla.
- In about 10% of individuals, the ducts do not fuse and open separately into the duodenum, a condition known as pancreas divisum.
- Based on the formation of the ampulla and ductal openings, three anatomical types are identified: type 1 (an ampulla is present, which may or may not be dilated), type 2 (the ducts open separately on the papilla), and type 3 (the ducts open at separate points on the duodenum).
- An anomalous pancreatobiliary ductal union (APBDU) occurs when the pancreatic duct and CBD join outside the wall of the second part of the duodenum, creating an elongated common channel. This is linked to clinical conditions such as choledochal cysts, gallbladder cancer, and recurrent acute pancreatitis. Classification systems for APBDU include the Komi classification and a more simplified classification developed by the Japanese Study Group on Pancreatobiliary Maljunction (JSPBM).
- The tissue between the pancreas and major arteries is called the mesopancreas. The mesopancreas includes connective tissue, lymphatic tissue, and nerve plexuses originating from the celiac trunk and the superior mesenteric artery.
- The main artery to the pancreas comes from the superior and inferior pancreaticoduodenal arteries, the dorsal pancreatic artery, and the splenic artery.
- Splenic vein and superior mesenteric veins joining to form the portal vein provide the main venous drainage to the pancreas.
- According to the Japanese Pancreas Society, specific regional lymph node stations are designated for pancreatic tumors based on the tumor's location. The pancreas is innervated by sympathetic fibers from the splanchnic nerves and parasympathetic fibers from the vagus nerves.

Selected Reading

1. Zhu C, Ma L, Jia Z, Shi H, Jin J, Lou W, et al. Novel morphological classification of the normal pancreatic uncinate process based on computed tomography. J Int Med Res. 2020;48:300060520957453.
2. Gockel I, Domeyer M, Wolloscheck T, Konerding MA, Junginger T. Resection of the mesopancreas (RMP): a new surgical classification of a known anatomical space. World J Surg Oncol. 2007;5:44.
3. Ishida M, Fujii T, Kishiwada M, Shibuya K, Satoi S, Ueno M, et al. Japanese classification of pancreatic carcinoma by the Japan Pancreas Society: eighth edition. J Hepatobiliary Pancreat Sci. 2024;31:755–68.
4. de Souza MFE, Strobel O, Girão C, Moraes-Junior JMA, Torres OJM. What do surgeons need to know about the mesopancreas? Langenbeck's Arch Surg. 2021;406:2621–32.
5. Türkvatan A, Erden A, Türkoğlu MA, Yener Ö. Congenital variants and anomalies of the pancreas and pancreatic duct: imaging by magnetic resonance cholangiopancreaticography and multidetector computed tomography. Korean J Radiol. 2013;14:905–13.
6. Komi N, Udaka H, Ikeda N, Kashiwagi Y. Congenital dilatation of the biliary tract; new classification and study with particular reference to anomalous arrangement of the pancreaticobiliary ducts. Gastroenterol Jpn. 1977;12:293–304.
7. Kimura W. Surgical anatomy of the pancreas for limited resection. J Hepato-Biliary-Pancreat Surg. 2000;7:473–9.

Acute Pancreatitis

32

Peeyush Varshney, Sanjamjot Singh, and Tashmeen Kaur Sethi

Abstract

The revised Atlanta classification is used to categorize the severity and complications of AP. Initial management of AP includes fluid resuscitation, analgesics, and monitoring for organ dysfunction. Early cholecystectomy is recommended for uncomplicated biliary pancreatitis to prevent recurrence of the condition.

Keywords

Acute pancreatitis · Pancreatic necrosis · VARD

Acute pancreatitis (AP) is one of the most common abdominal emergencies that requires hospitalization. The reported annual incidence varies from 4.9 to 35 per 100,000 people. The risk of AP is similar for males and females and tends to increase with age. The global rise in AP cases may be connected to higher rates of obesity and related gallstones. Gallstones and alcohol are the two leading causes of AP. About 80%–85% of patients have mild disease, with symptoms that usually resolve within a week. Around 15%–20% of patients develop severe disease, which may include organ failure and/or necrotizing pancreatitis. The death rate in severe pancreatitis ranges from 15% to 30%, compared to less than 1% in mild cases.

32.1 Definition

Acute pancreatitis is characterized as a distinct episode of cellular injury and inflammation in the pancreas, usually presenting with symptoms such as abdominal pain, nausea, and vomiting. It is typically accompanied by elevated serum amylase or lipase levels and radiographic evidence of pancreatic inflammation, edema, or necrosis. Although the pancreas may seem to recover quickly after an episode, complete recovery might not occur if the damage is severe. Repeated episodes can lead to a progression from acute inflammation, necrosis, and apoptosis to chronic inflammation and fibrosis, which are characteristic of chronic pancreatitis. In some cases, distinguishing between acute pancreatitis and a flare of chronic pancreatitis can be challenging.

32.2 Classification (Tables 32.1 and 32.2)

Table 32.1 Pancreatitis Severity Classification based on the Revised Atlanta 2012 Consensus criteria

Mild acute pancreatitis (MAP)	No organ failure No local/systemic complication
Moderately severe acute pancreatitis (MSAP)	Organ failure that resolves within 48 h (transient organ failure) &/or local/systemic complications without organ failure
Severe acute pancreatitis (SAP)	Persistent organ failure (>48 h)

P. Varshney (✉) · S. Singh · T. K. Sethi
All India Institute of Medical Sciences, Jodhpur, India
e-mail: varshneyp@aiimsjodhpur.edu.in

M. Ibrarullah (ed.), *Recent Concepts in Gastrointestinal (GI) Surgery*, https://doi.org/10.1007/978-981-92-1118-0_32

Table 32.2 Revised Atlanta Classification based on cross-sectional imaging

Collection	Duration since pain	Pancreatitis subcategory	Location	Imaging feature
Acute peripancreatic fluid collection (APFC)	≤4 weeks	Interstitial edematous pancreas	Extrapancreatic	Homogeneous, fluid attenuation conforms to retroperitoneal structures, no wall
Acute necrotic collection (ANC)	≤4 weeks	Necrotizing pancreatitis	Intra/extrapancreatic	Inhomogeneous, non-liquefied component, no wall
Pseudocyst	>4 weeks	Interstitial edematous pancreas	Extrapancreatic	Homogeneous fluid, circumscribed, encapsulated with a wall
Walled-off necrosis (WON)	>4 weeks	Necrotizing pancreatitis	Intra- and/or extrapancreatic	Inhomogeneous, non-liquefied components, encapsulated with a wall

Table 32.3 Acute pancreatitis—etiology, presumed mechanism, and risk of chronicity

Risk factors for acute pancreatitis	Presumed mechanism	Risk for chronicity
Alcohol abuse	Dose-dependent cell injury	High
Smoking	Dose-dependent cell toxicity	High
Gallstones	Pancreatic duct obstruction	–
Hypertriglyceridemia	Blood viscosity, local tissue ischemia	High (in familial)
Endoscopic procedures (ERCP)	Cell injury, increased duct pressure	–
Abdominal trauma	Pancreatic tissue damage	High (disrupted duct syndrome)
Drugs	Cell toxic or metabolic effects	–
Autoimmune diseases	Immune cell infiltration	High
Dominant PRSS1 mutation	Elevated trypsin activity	Very high
Predisposing genetic mutation	Protease activation, ER stress	High
Infections	Direct tissue injury	–

32.3 Etiology (Table 32.3)

32.3.1 Gallstones

Gallstones and alcohol abuse are the most common causes of acute pancreatitis, each accounting for 30%–50% of cases. Biliary pancreatitis occurs more often in women. In 1901, Ernest L. Opie proposed the common channel theory of acute pancreatitis, which states that a gallstone can trigger acute pancreatitis by blocking the pancreatic duct at the ampulla.

32.3.2 Alcohol

Chronic alcoholism can trigger an episode of acute pancreatitis and increase the risk of developing chronic pancreatitis. The highest occurrence of alcohol-related acute pancreatitis occurs between the third and fifth decades of life. Drinking 50–80 g, or 4–7 drinks a day, has been linked to pancreatitis, although individual differences and susceptibility vary. While epidemiological data support the connection between alcohol and pancreatitis, only a small percentage of alcoholics develop either acute or chronic pancreatitis. This suggests that alcohol consumption alone might not be the sole cause of pancreatitis; instead, it could make the pancreas more vulnerable to other factors like a high-fat diet, infectious agents, or tobacco smoke. Ethanol and its metabolites induce complex cellular changes in pancreatic acini, including shifts in intracellular calcium levels, endoplasmic reticulum stress, increased mitochondrial permeability, impaired autophagy, and the co-localization and activation of lysosomal and pancreatic digestive enzymes, ultimately leading to a pancreatitis attack.

32.3.3 Hypertriglyceridemia

The incidence of acute pancreatitis is linked to elevated triglycerides in about 10% of cases. It is believed that high plasma levels of triglycerides and chylomicrons increase blood viscosity, leading to local tissue ischemia. During ischemia, metabolism shifts from aerobic to anaerobic, causing cells to depend on anaerobic glycolysis, which produces L-lactate. This local ischemia results in increased lactate levels and acidosis; the acidosis enhances the toxicity of free fatty acids and promotes the autoactivation of trypsinogen. Along with other risk factors like alcohol, tobacco, or medications, ischemia can trigger acute pancreatitis. Patients with familial lipoprotein lipase deficiency face a unique risk of recurrent acute pancreatitis episodes. Similarly, pregnant women have an inherent risk of hypertriglyceridemia-induced pancreatitis due to hormone-driven increases in cholesterol and triglyceride levels. Differences have been observed between primary and secondary hypertriglyceridemia. The Fredrickson classification identifies five types of primary hyperlipidemia, with types I, IV, and V associated with a higher risk of acute pancreatitis. Type I primarily involves elevated chylomicrons, similar to lipoprotein lipase deficiency; Type IV shows increased very-low-density lipoproteins (VLDLs); and Type V involves elevated levels of both VLDL and chylomicrons. Primary hypertriglyceridemia results from genetic abnormalities with recessive inheritance in Type I and dominant inheritance in Types IV and V. Secondary hypertriglyceridemia is linked to obesity, pregnancy, poorly controlled diabetes, medications, or chronic and acute alcohol abuse. According to the Atlanta classification system, a diagnosis of hypertriglyceridemia-induced acute pancreatitis requires serum triglyceride levels above 1000 mg/dL. The risk of experiencing at least one episode of acute pancreatitis increases by 20% in individuals with triglyceride levels exceeding 1000 mg/dL.

32.3.4 Endoscopic Procedures

Pancreatitis is the most common complication after endoscopic retrograde cholangiopancreatography (ERCP), with an incidence of 2%–15%. In 1%–2%, the attack can be severe, leading to death in 0.1% of patients. The identified risk factors include younger age (under 60 years), female sex, sphincter of Oddi dysfunction, a history of pancreatitis, difficult cannulation, pancreatic sphincterotomy, balloon dilation of the sphincter, osmolarity, pH, contrast medium composition, and increased pressure during contrast injection.

32.3.5 Trauma

The incidence of abdominal trauma in polytraumatized patients in Germany is 20%, with 95% of these cases involving blunt force trauma. Typically, parenchymatous organs such as the liver and spleen are affected, while traumatic injury to the pancreas is rare (6%) because of its retroperitoneal location. However, there is no correlation between the force applied and the extent of pancreatic damage. Common outcomes of pancreatic trauma include pancreatitis, fissures, lacerations, a disconnected duct, or a combination of these, which underscores the complexity of managing such injuries. Abdominal trauma carries a high mortality rate due to potential severe bleeding, septic complications, and an increased risk of multi-organ failure.

32.3.6 Rare Causes

Drug-induced acute pancreatitis is rare, occurring in 0.1%–2% of cases. Its pathogenesis includes sphincter spasm, cytotoxic and metabolic effects, hypersensitivity reactions, localized angioedema, or arteriolar thrombosis. Some commonly prescribed drugs associated with acute pancreatitis are angiotensin-converting enzyme inhibitors (which can cause localized angioedema), statins (which can cause direct toxicity and accumulation), oral contraceptives or hormone replacement therapy—especially estrogen—diuretics, antiviral therapy (for HIV), valproic acid, and antidiabetic agents like GLP-1 mimetics.

32.4 Clinical Presentation

- Sudden onset of epigastric pain after a heavy meal or alcohol that peaks within 12–24 h. The pain is persistent, often radiates to the back, shoulders, or iliac fossa, and then spreads across the entire abdomen. It usually worsens with walking and lying on the back, but improves when sitting and leaning forward.
- Nausea and vomiting.
- Severe pancreatitis may present with septic shock, fever, hypotension, and ARDS.
- Mild icterus.
- Guarding, rigidity, and distention of the abdomen.
- Abdominal tenderness is more marked in the epigastrium.
- Severe, advanced cases may cause bruising and discoloration in the left flank (Grey Turner's sign due to tissue breakdown of Hb) and around the umbilicus (Cullen's sign due to hemoperitoneum). These are rare and late signs of extensive pancreatic damage.

32.5 Diagnosis

AP is diagnosed when two of the following three criteria are met:

- Abdominal pain consistent with AP.
- Serum lipase or amylase level is at least three times above the upper limit of norma.
- Characteristic features of AP on cross-sectional imaging—computed tomography (CT) or magnetic resonance imaging (MRI).

32.5.1 Blood Investigations

Serum Amylase A threefold or more increase in the level of serum amylase indicates acute pancreatitis. Levels may return to normal after 48–72 h. Raised serum amylase has also been reported in chronic renal failure, duodenal perforation, bowel ischemia, ruptured ectopic pregnancy, narcotics abuse, salivary gland inflammation, and liver cirrhosis.

Serum Lipase Raised serum lipase is a more reliable and specific indicator because elevated levels can be detected up to 7–14 days after an acute pancreatitis attack, and because it is less prone to false positivity (Table 32.4).

Full Blood Count Leucocytosis as a prognostic marker in Ranson's criteria.

Liver Function Test To assess the cause of pancreatitis/obstructive jaundice.

Blood Urea and Serum Electrolyte Levels To determine hydration status.

Random Blood Glucose Damage to beta cells can cause hyperglycemia, especially in severe cases.

Serum Calcium To evaluate the cause of high serum calcium.

Lipid Profile To rule out hypertriglyceridemia as the cause.

Lactic Dehydrogenase (LDH) Markedly elevated LDH (>500 U/dL) suggests a poor prognosis.

Table 32.4 Temporal pattern of serum amylase and lipase levels in acute pancreatitis

	Amylase	Lipase
Rising trend	4–8 h	4–8 h
Peak	12 h	24 h
Return to normal	3–4 days	8–14 days

C-Reactive Protein (CRP) Serial assessment indicates disease progression.

32.6 Imaging

32.6.1 X-Ray Abdomen and Chest

In acute pancreatitis, common findings on abdominal X-rays include generalized or localized ileus (sentinel loop), a colon cut-off sign, and calcified gallstones. Chest X-rays in severe cases may reveal diffuse alveolar shadowing, as seen in acute respiratory distress syndrome. Left-sided pleural effusion is also typical of acute pancreatitis (Fig. 32.1).

32.6.2 Abdominal Ultrasonography (USG)

USG is the preliminary screening investigation in acute pancreatitis that may show.

- Enlarged pancreas suggestive of an edematous gland
- Hypoechoic foci in the pancreas indicating necrosis
- Peripancreatic fluid and inflammation, with ascites and pleural effusion
- Biliary pathology, such as gallstones and dilated CBD with or without stones (Fig. 32.2)

32.6.3 Computed Tomography (CT) Scan

Contrast-enhanced CT scan (CECT), obtained with pancreatic protocol, is the most important imaging modality for

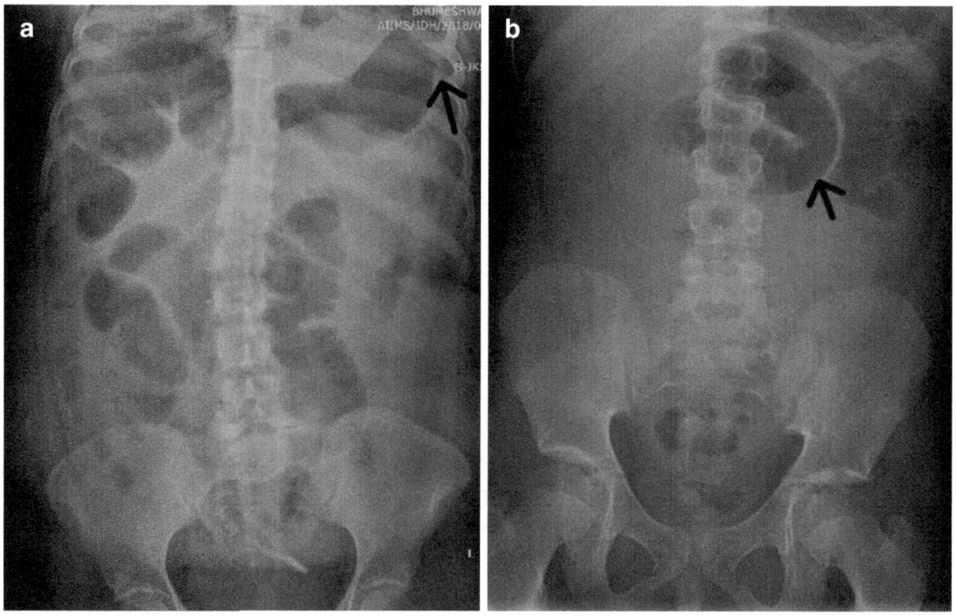

Fig. 32.1 X-ray abdomen showing (**a**) colon cut-off (arrow) and (**b**) sentinel loop (arrow)

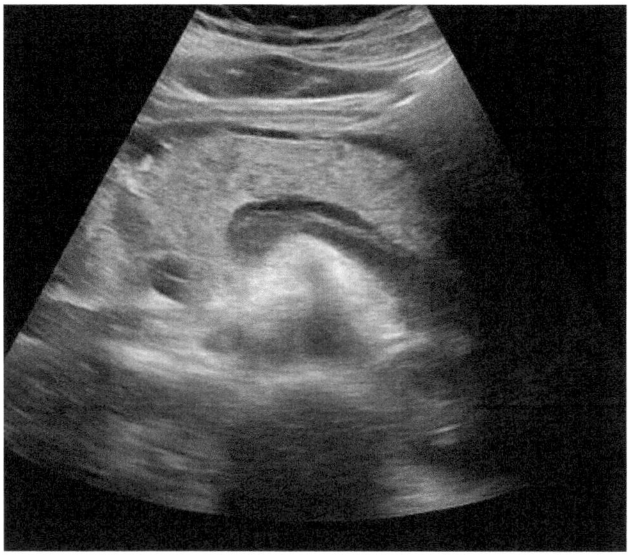

Fig. 32.2 USG Showing an Enlarged Pancreas Suggestive of Acute Pancreatitis

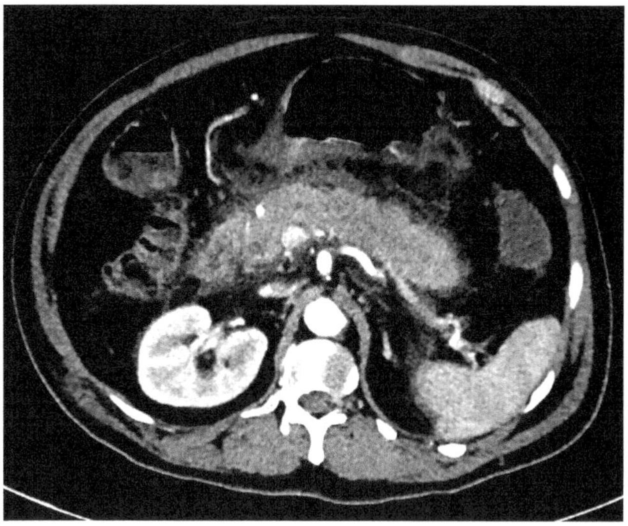

Fig. 32.3 CECT appearance of acute interstitial edematous pancreatitis. The entire gland is enlarged but well-enhanced with contrast

diagnosing, assessing severity, and monitoring the progression of acute pancreatitis for management purposes. The ideal timing for a CT scan is 3–5 days after symptom onset; if the patient does not improve or worsens, a follow-up scan should be performed after 2 weeks. Abnormalities that may be seen include the folllowing:

- Focal or diffuse parenchymal enlargement.
- Changes in density because of edema.
- Indistinct pancreatic margins with surrounding retroperitoneal fat stranding.
- Pancreatic and peripancreatic fluid collection.
- Pancreatic necrosis suggested by lack of parenchymal enhancement on contrast injection.
- The presence of gas bubbles indicates infected necrosis.
- Circumscribed fluid collection indicating pancreatic pseudocyst.
- Hemorrhage appearing as high-attenuation fluid in the retroperitoneum or peripancreatic tissues (Figs. 32.3, 32.4, 32.5, 32.6 and 32.7).

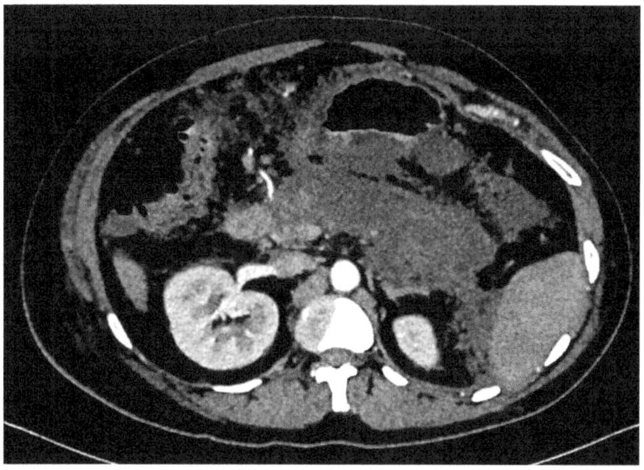

Fig. 32.4 Pancreatic necrosis. Non-enhancing, enlarged gland

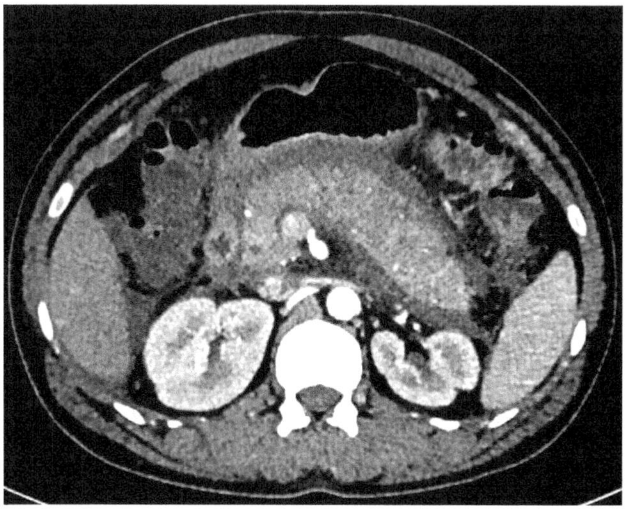

Fig. 32.5 Peripancreatic fluid collection around a well-enhancing gland

32.6.4 Magnetic Resonance Imaging (MRI)

- MRI provides all the information obtained with CECT and offers better soft tissue contrast resolution. However, in clinical practice, CT scans are more popular due to familiarity and easier interpretation for the average clinician.
- In necrotizing pancreatitis, the necrotic area displays hypointensity on T1WI and hyperintensity on T2WI.
- Acute peripancreatic fluid collections (APFCs) are homogeneously hypointense on T1WI and hyperintense

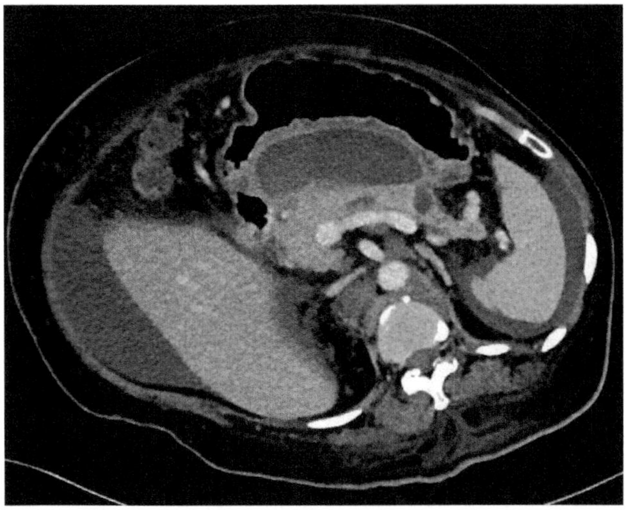

Fig. 32.6 Peripancreatic fluid collection anterior to the gland, in the perisplenic and perihepatic region

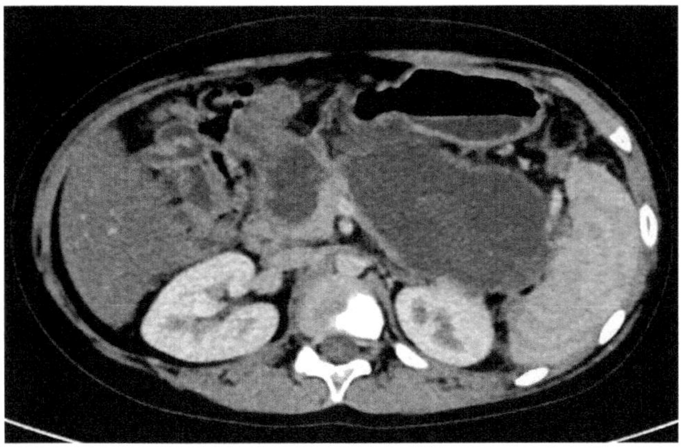

Fig. 32.7 Walled-off pancreatic necrosis

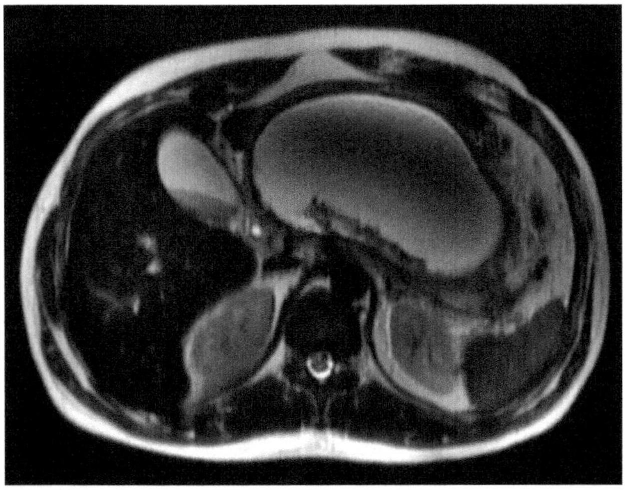

Fig. 32.8 Walled-off pancreatic necrosis on MRI

on T2WI, with no cystic walls and no solid components.

- Pancreatic pseudocysts have a thin, smooth wall, homogeneous intensity on T1WI and T2WI of the liquid content, and no solid component or debris in the fluid.
- Disruption of the pancreatic duct is better appreciated on MRI.
- Biliary pathology is better diagnosed on MR Cholangiopancreatogram (MRCP) (Fig. 32.8).

32.7 Scoring Systems and Stratification of Severity of Acute Pancreatitis (Table 32.5, 32.6, 32.7 and 32.8)

Table 32.5 Ranson's scoring system

Ranson's criteria	Acute pancreatitis	Acute biliary pancreatitis
Upon admission		
Age	>55 years	>70 years
WBC	>16,000/mm3	>18,000/mm^3
Glucose	>200 mg/dl	>220 mg/dl
LDH	>350 IU/L	>400 IU/L
AST	>250 IU/L	>440 IU/L
Within 48 h		
Drop in HCT	>10%	>10%
Serum calcium	<8 mg/dL	<8 mg/dl
Base deficit	>4 mE/L	>4 meq/L
Increase BUN	>5 mg/dL	>2 mg/dl
Fluid deficit	>6 L	>6 L
Arterial PO2	<60 mmHg	<60 mmHg

A score of 0–2 is considered mild, and ≥3 is severe pancreatitis with a mortality of <2% and > 15%, respectively

Table 32.6 Variables in the APACHE system

1. Body temperature	7. Na (mmol/l)
2. Mean arterial pressure	8. K (mmol/l)
3. Heart rate	9. Creatinine (mg/100 ml)
4. Respiratory rate	10. Hematocrit
5. Oxygenation (mmHg)	11. Total leucocyte count
6. pH	12. Glasgow coma score

Table 32.7 Modified CT Severity Index (CTSI)

Prognostic indicator	Points
Pancreatic inflammation	0
Pancreatic abnormalities +/− peripancreatic inflammation	2
Pancreatic or peripancreatic fluid collection or fat necrosis	4
Pancreas necrosis	
None	0
<30%	2
>30%	4
Extra-pancreatic complications (pleural effusion, ascites, parenchymal complications, GI tract involvement)	2

CTSI >7 is considered severe pancreatitis

Table 32.8 Bedside Index for Severity in Acute Pancreatitis (BISAP)

1. Blood urea nitrogen >25 mg/dl
2. Impaired mental status such as disorientation, lethargy, somnolence, coma, or stupor
3. Systemic inflammatory response syndrome (SIRS)
4. Age > 60 years
5. Pleural effusion detected on imaging

32.8 APACHE (Acute Physiology Score and the Chronic Health Evaluation) Scoring System

The APACHE scoring system is the first major attempt to quantify the severity of illness in ICU patients. It consists of 12 continuous variables. The main advantage of this scoring system is that it can be used to monitor the patient's response to therapy, whereas the Ranson criteria is mainly designed for assessment at presentation. A score of more than eight points predicts severe pancreatitis, which is associated with a mortality rate of 11% to 18%.

One point is assigned for each variable within 24 hours of presentation. Incremental increases in the BISAP score (3 or more) have been shown to correlate with an increased risk of organ failure, pancreatic necrosis, and mortality.

32.9 Management

32.9.1 Intensive Care Management

All patients except those with mild pancreatitis should be managed in the intensive care unit (ICU) with strict monitoring of their vital parameters and organ function.

32.9.2 Fluid Therapy

Early and adequate fluid resuscitation within the first 24 h of admission is expected to minimize necrosis and the incidence of SIRS and MOD in acute pancreatitis. On the contrary, overhydration may increase the risk of pulmonary complications due to fluid overload, necessitating strict monitoring of fluid administration. The recommendation for initial fluid resuscitation in acute pancreatitis is crystalloid, preferably Ringer's lactate. Optimum fluid therapy should be based on the following parameters: heart rate < 120/min, mean arterial pressure between 65 and 85 mmHg, urine output >0.5–1 ml/kg/h.

32.9.3 Analgesics

The primary symptom of AP is abdominal pain, often severe and persistent, which requires effective management. Pain control is a pivotal element in the multidisciplinary management of AP; however, no single analgesic strategy has been universally accepted as superior in terms of efficacy and safety.

Opioids: Opioids provide potent analgesia and are particularly effective in managing severe pain associated with AP. Their rapid onset of action and efficacy in reducing visceral pain make them a preferred choice in many clinical scenarios. Although opioids are effective, they are associated with a risk of respiratory depression, constipation, and potential for dependence.

NSAIDs and Acetaminophen: NSAIDs and acetaminophen, especially intravenous formulations like dexketoprofen, diclofenac, and paracetamol, provide an alternative to opioids. Their anti-inflammatory properties may also offer additional advantages in managing pancreatitis. However, caution is advised when using them in patients with renal impairment, gastric ulcers, or those at risk of bleeding.

Epidural analgesia: Thoracic epidural analgesia has been tested for pain control in patients with AP admitted to the ICU. It is linked to lower mortality rates in a multicenter retrospective propensity analysis. The advantages include better pancreatic blood flow and reduced AP severity, with no significant increase in adverse events related to epidural analgesia in ICU patients with severe AP.

32.9.4 Preventing Infectious Complications

Intravenous antibiotic prophylaxis is not recommended during the initial stages of AP. Several guidelines suggest using antibiotics to treat infected necrosis, which occurs in about 30% of patients with SAP and significantly increases the risk of death. The American Gastroenterological Association Institute guidelines state that carbapenems, quinolones, and metronidazole, which are known for their ability to penetrate pancreatic necrosis, may be beneficial in patients with infected pancreatic necrosis. These antibiotics can sometimes help delay or avoid surgery and may reduce both morbidity and mortality.

32.9.5 Nutritional Support

Oral feeding in predicted mild pancreatitis can resume once abdominal pain subsides and inflammatory markers improve. In severe acute pancreatitis, enteral nutrition is preferred over parenteral nutrition. This is achieved through nasojejunal or nasogastric tube feeding using either elemental or polymeric enteral nutrition formulations. Parenteral nutrition is reserved for those who cannot tolerate tube feeding.

32.9.6 In-Hospital Course

Patients with mild pancreatitis usually recover in 7–10 days. Persistence of clinical symptoms, signs of sepsis, and organ dysfunction indicates the onset of complications that require confirmation by blood tests and imaging (preferably CECT). Once confirmed, complications of acute pancreatitis should be managed according to the need, which may include continuation in the ICU and therapeutic interventions—radiological, endoscopic, or surgical. After recovery from mild pancreatitis, the goal should be to prevent recurrence by identifying and treating the underlying cause.

32.9.7 Specific Management of Biliary Pancreatitis

Biliary pancreatitis is suspected when alanine aminotransferase levels rise within the first 48 hours. An abdominal ultrasound confirms the presence of gallstones. A CT scan is usually performed between the third and fifth days and may be repeated based on clinical and laboratory findings. Management of acute biliary pancreatitis depends on its severity. For mild cases, cholecystectomy should be performed during the same hospital stay, before discharge. For moderately severe and severe cases, treatment includes resuscitation, early continuous enteral feeding, and management of complications. An interval cholecystectomy is scheduled for later. Endoscopic retrograde cholangiopancreatography with sphincterotomy should be performed in emergencies for choledocholithiasis with cholangitis or within 72 hours for persistent biliary obstruction.

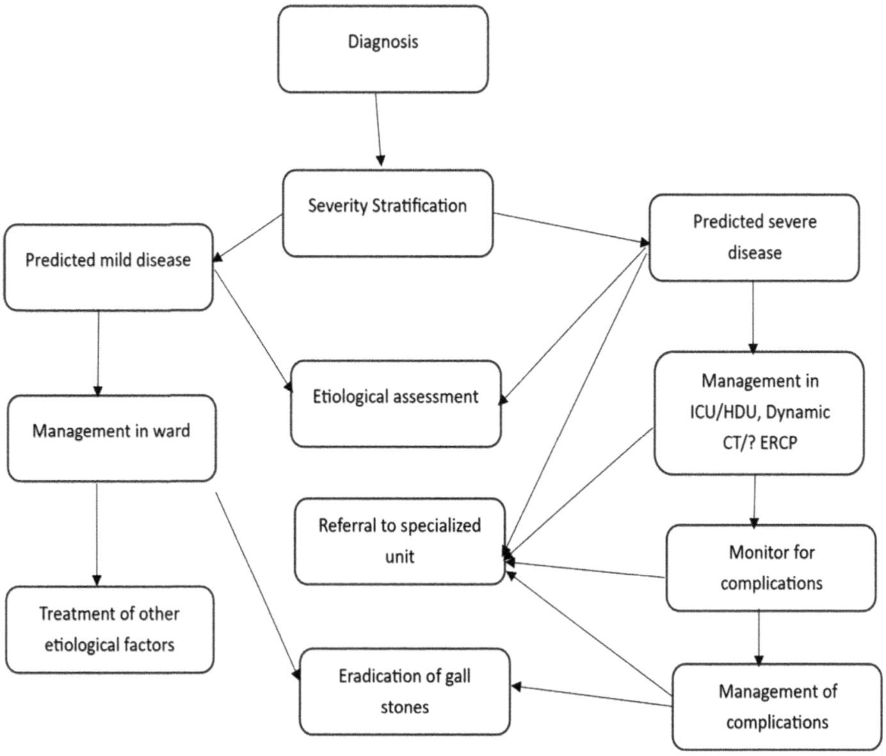

Fig. 32.9 Management of acute pancreatitis

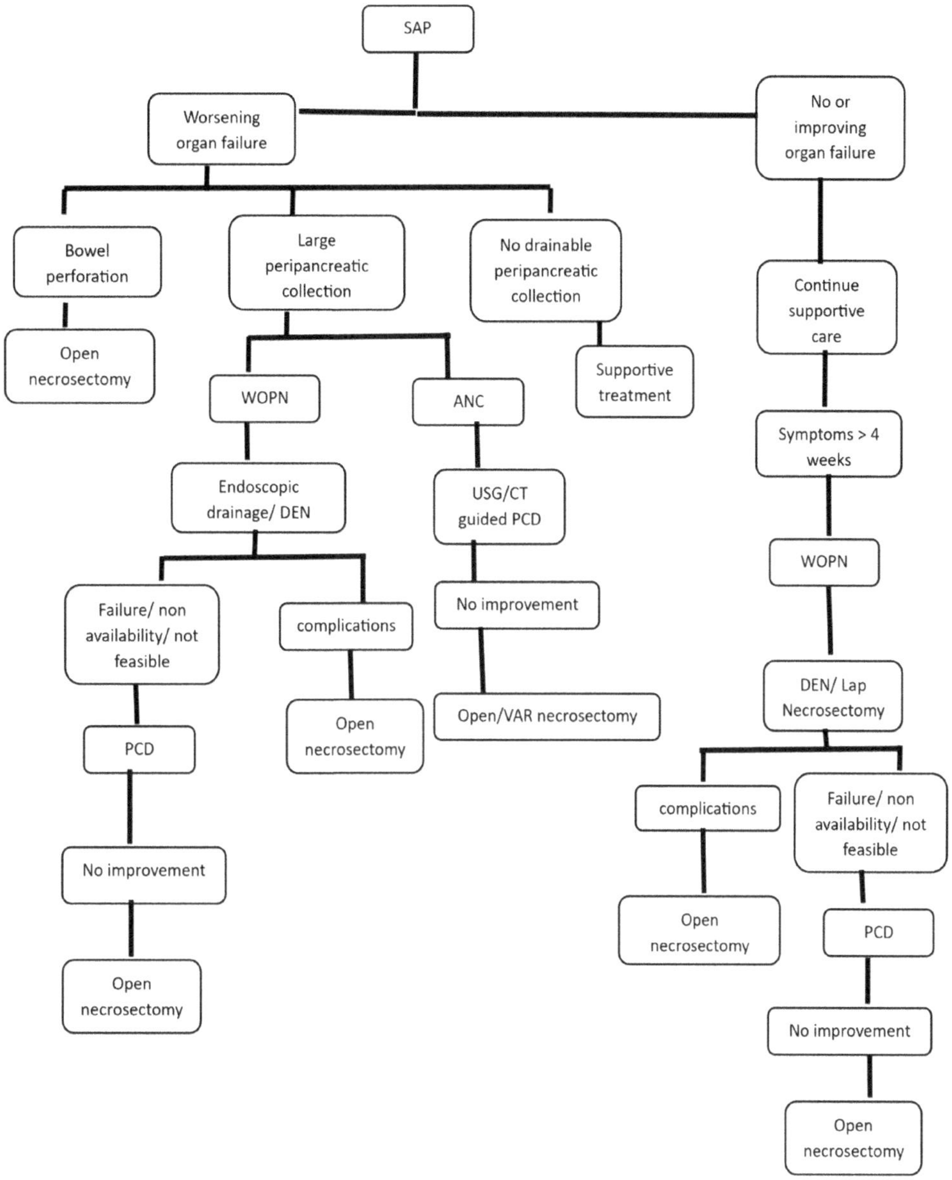

Fig. 32.10 Management of severe acute pancreatitis (SAP)

Key Points

- Acute pancreatitis (AP) is one of the most common abdominal emergencies worldwide, with gallstones and alcohol responsible for most cases.
- Diagnosis of AP relies on clinical signs, increased serum amylase and lipase levels, and imaging results.
- The revised Atlanta classification is used to categorize the severity and complications of AP.
- Risk stratification relies on various scoring systems such as Ranson, APACHE, and BISAP scores.
- Initial management of AP includes fluid resuscitation, analgesics, and monitoring for organ dysfunction.
- Antibiotics are not recommended in the early stages of AP.
- Enteral nutrition is preferred over parenteral nutrition.
- Early cholecystectomy is recommended for uncomplicated biliary pancreatitis to prevent recurrence of the condition.

Selected Reading

1. Banks PA, Bollen TL, Dervenis C, Gooszen HG, Acute Pancreatitis Classification Working Group, et al. Classification of acute pancreatitis—2012: revision of the Atlanta classification and definitions by international consensus. Gut. 2013;62:102–11. https://doi.org/10.1136/gutjnl-2012-302779. Epub 2012 Oct 25. PMID: 23100216.
2. Vege SS, DiMagno MJ, Forsmark CE, Martel M, Barkun AN. Initial medical treatment of acute pancreatitis: American Gastroenterological Association Institute Technical Review. Gastroenterology. 2018;154:1103–39.
3. Crockett SD, Wani S, Gardner TB, Falck-Ytter Y, Barkun AN, American Gastroenterological Association Institute Clinical Guidelines Committee. American Gastroenterological Association Institute Guideline on initial management of acute pancreatitis. Gastroenterology. 2018;154:1096–101.

Local Complications of Acute Pancreatitis

33

Phani Krishna Ravula and Suresh Sepuri

Abstract

Pseudocyst and WOPN are sequelae of interstitial pancreatitis and necrotizing pancreatitis, respectively. Intervention is recommended only when symptoms persist or there is evidence of infection. Delayed intervention after 4–6 weeks has a better outcome than early intervention. A step-up approach with less invasive measures like PCD, followed by endoscopic, MIS, or VARN, is the current gold standard of treatment.

Keywords

Acute pancreatitis · Pancreatic necrosis · Pancreatic pseudocyst

Acute pancreatitis (AP) is a systemic illness characterized by features of systemic inflammatory response syndrome (SIRS), such as fever, tachycardia, tachypnea, leukocytosis, and varying degrees of multiorgan dysfunction depending on the severity of pancreatitis. After the first 2 weeks, local complications of pancreatitis begin to manifest and significantly contribute to prolonged hospital stay, increased morbidity, and mortality.

AP is classified into two main subtypes based on the presence or absence of necrosis: interstitial edematous pancreatitis (IEP), which lacks necrosis, and necrotizing pancreatitis (NP), characterized by varying degrees of pancreatic and peri-pancreatic tissue necrosis. The severity, complication rate, and mortality are significantly lower in IEP compared to necrotizing pancreatitis (mortality <1% vs. 10%–15%). Common outcomes of IEP include acute pancreatic fluid collections (APFC) and pseudocysts. APFC usually occurs outside the pancreas, has minimal or no necrosis, and lacks a well-formed wall. After 4 weeks, it progresses to a pseudocyst, which develops a well-defined wall. In contrast, necrotizing pancreatitis (NP) can lead to acute necrotic collections (ANC) and walled-off pancreatic necrosis (WOPN), depending on the duration and whether a well-formed wall has developed. This distinction has important clinical and therapeutic implications. Intervention is best performed after 4 weeks, when the collection is encapsulated and clearly delineated, to minimize the risks of bleeding and bowel fistula. Managing WOPN differs from pseudocyst treatment because of the varying amounts of solid tissue present (Table 33.2).

Table 33.1 Local complications of acute pancreatitis

Pseudocyst and walled-off pancreatic necrosis (WOPN)
Portal vein thrombosis
Pseudoaneurysm and hemorrhage
Biliary obstruction
Gastric outlet obstruction
Bowel ischemia and fistula

P. K. Ravula (✉) · S. Sepuri
Pace Hospitals, Hyderabad, India

M. Ibrarullah (ed.), *Recent Concepts in Gastrointestinal (GI) Surgery*, https://doi.org/10.1007/978-981-92-1118-0_33

Table 33.2 Pancreatic fluid collections and necrosis: definitions and imaging features (Atlanta Classification 2016)

Collection	Duration since onset of AP	Pancreatitis subcategory	Location	Imaging features
APFC	≤4 weeks	IEP	Extra pancreatic	Homogeneous, fluid attenuation, no wall. Conforms to RP structures
ANC	≤4 weeks	NP	Intra and/or extra pancreatic	Non-homogeneous, non-liquified components, absent wall
Pseudocyst	>4 weeks	IEP	Extra pancreatic	Homogenous, fluid-filled, encapsulated with a wall
WOPN	>4 weeks	NP	Intra &/or extra pancreatic	Non-homogeneous, non-liquified components encapsulated with a wall

AP acute pancreatitis, *APFC* acute pancreatic fluid collection, *IEP* interstitial edematous pancreatitis, *ANC* acute necrotic collection, *NP* necrotizing pancreatitis, *WOPN* walled-off pancreatic necrosis

Table 33.3 Imaging features detectable on CECT in acute pancreatitis

Extent of pancreatic necrosis—CT severity index
Size and location of collection/s
Demarcation and wall formation
Contents of collection (solid[a]/liquid/ air)
Bowel erosion/fistulation
Hemorrhage/pseudoaneurysm formation
Portal/splenic vein thrombosis

[a]Solid contents are better imaged on ultrasonography

33.1 Diagnosis of Complications

In patients diagnosed with acute pancreatitis, persistent symptoms such as abdominal pain, distension, fever, tachycardia, signs of inflammation, and new-onset organ dysfunction beyond 2 weeks indicate the development of local complications. Although ultrasonography is used as a screening tool and for follow-up to monitor the size of collections, contrast-enhanced CT scan (CECT) is the preferred investigation. CECT performed within the first 48–72 h may underestimate the extent of necrosis. When repeated after a week, it provides a clearer picture for assessing the CT severity index, which has both therapeutic and prognostic implications (Table 33.3).

Magnetic resonance imaging (MRI) can serve as an alternative to CECT and offers better visualization of pancreatic duct integrity and its communication with pseudocysts, if present. It also detects related biliary conditions such as gallstones and common bile duct stones. However, gadolinium contrast used in MRI may cause kidney injury in patients with impaired renal function. Another drawback of MRI is that it can be time-consuming and difficult for patients who are claustrophobic or severely ill. MRI is especially useful in distinguishing APFC from pseudocysts or WOPN based on the presence or absence of a capsule. Peripancreatic fluid collections appear hypointense on T1-weighted images and hyperintense on T2-weighted images. Patients with necrosis show mixed signals on both T1- and T2-weighted images. The exact nature of the collections, whether solid or liquid, is better visualized with MRI than with a CT scan or an ultrasound.

Endoscopic ultrasound (EUS) with a linear probe (5–12 Hz) plays a vital role in diagnosing and managing local complications of AP. In biliary pancreatitis, it helps identify bile duct stones, sludge, and other biliary issues. EUS can detect collaterals in the gastric wall and determine whether pancreatic collections are solid or liquid, aiding in safe and effective drainage. EUS-guided fluid analysis and biopsy are also valuable for distinguishing between pancreatitis-related pseudocysts and cystic neoplasms.

Fine needle aspiration cytology (FNAC): FNAC of WOPN can accurately identify infected pancreatic necrosis to guide further treatment. However, the usefulness of FNAC has become questionable for several reasons. First, FNAC alone does not determine the need for intervention; it has a false positive rate of 15% and a false negative rate of 15%, and the decision to intervene is primarily based on the clinical picture of persistent sepsis, worsening or new-onset organ dysfunction, and imaging features such as air bubbles in the cyst cavity. Second, the increasing role of percutaneous drainage as the first intervention has made FNAC less necessary, as PCD provides fluid for culture and supports the step-up approach.

33.2 Indications for Therapeutic Intervention

Pseudocyst Pseudocysts larger than 6 cm that last more than 6 weeks and are associated with chronic pancreatitis are unlikely to resolve on their own. However, in current clinical practice, intervention can be delayed regardless of size and duration as long as the patient remains asymptomatic. An exception is made in cases of total pancreatic duct disruption—disconnected pancreatic duct syndrome (DPDS)—where intervention is necessary because cyst resolution is unlikely.

Generally, intervention is necessary if a pseudocyst remains symptomatic and enlarges beyond 4 weeks. It can be treated with endoscopy or laparoscopy. The choice depends on available expertise, as well as the cyst's size and location. Cysts near the pancreatic head or body that bulge into the lesser sac may indent the posterior wall of the stomach and the C-loop of the duodenum. These can be managed with cystogastrostomy or cystoduodenostomy, respectively, using either laparoscopic or endoscopic techniques. Cysts mainly protruding into the mesocolon are better treated with open or laparoscopic cysto-jejunostomy. Lesions in the pancreatic tail with peri-splenic pseudocysts can be managed through drainage or distal pancreatectomy with splenectomy.

Walled-Off Pancreatic Necrosis WOPN, a complication of necrotizing pancreatitis, may require intervention in about one-third of cases. Indications for intervention include documented infection with clinical and biochemical signs of sepsis, new onset organ dysfunction, or evidence of infection on CT scan (gas bubble) or positive fluid culture (Fig. 33.1).

Delayed Intervention Early (<4 weeks) interventions are associated with high morbidity, such as worsening sepsis, bowel fistula, and hemorrhage, which lead to higher mortality (15%–20%). Therefore, it is recommended to delay intervention for at least 4–6 weeks or until the clinical condition remains stable. Waiting allows necrosis to become well demarcated and liquefy, making drainage more effective.

Step-Up Approach The step-up approach uses a more cautious strategy by initially performing decompression through percutaneous drainage (PCD) or endoscopic drainage to reduce sepsis risk. About one-third of patients resolve with PCD alone. For those with worsening symptoms or no improvement, additional procedures such as endoscopic, retroperitoneoscopic, or laparoscopic necrosectomy are used to minimize the physiological impact. Major surgery is reserved for non-responders with persistent collections within the step-up protocol. Along with the PANTER trial, multiple subsequent studies and meta-analyses have demonstrated that adopting the step-up approach can decrease the risk of serious complications and death, establishing it as the standard of care in managing pancreatic necrosis.

Resection or aggressive debridement of pancreatic necrosis carries a high risk of bowel fistulization, hemorrhage, and death. Using a more conservative step-up approach for pancreatic necrosis allows for decompression and removal of easily separable necrosis, instead of performing aggressive debridement. Gradually increasing catheter size in patients managed with PCD and employing high-volume irrigation (1–2 l/day) are recommended to remove residual necrosis rather than attempting an extensive and aggressive necrosectomy all at once.

Intervention for WOPN involves a multidisciplinary team of radiologists, endoscopists, and surgeons. The choice of intervention depends on several factors, including the time since diagnosis, the location and nature of necrosis, the patient's clinical and nutritional status, and the available expertise.

Percutaneous Drainage (PCD) PCD is the first step in the "step-up" approach. Using CT guidance, drainage catheters are inserted into the necrotic cavity. The optimal entry point is the retroperitoneal space between the colon and the left kidney, as it offers access to the entire lesser sac. The catheter track enables further invasive procedures such as retroperitoneoscopic or video-assisted necrosectomy (VARD). Proactive upsizing, re-interventions, or multiple PCDs with irrigation have been shown to reduce the need for subsequent necrosectomy.

Direct Endoscopic Necrosectomy (DEN) DEN is the preferred procedure for centrally located WOPN. The technique is effective in 40%–50% of cases and depends on the amount of

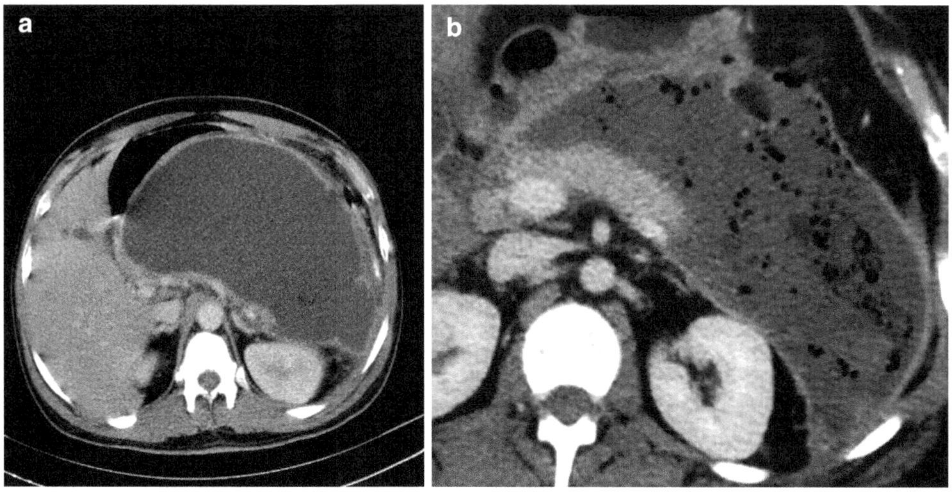

Fig. 33.1 (**a**) Pancreatic pseudocyst on CT scan. (**b**) Infected WOPN on CT scan. Note the gas bubbles in the necrotic cavity

liquefied debris in the cavity. Fully covered self-expanding metallic stents (FCSEMS) and lumen-apposing metal stents (LAMS) are used to facilitate drainage. These stents should be removed within 1–3 months to prevent complications such as bleeding, buried stent syndrome, and failed removal. To prevent recurrence in cases of complete disruption of the pancreatic duct (DPDS) and major ductal leaks, endoscopic placement of pancreatic duct stenting is recommended at the time of metallic stent removal. The endoscopic approach is associated with a lower incidence of pancreatic fistula and a shorter hospital stay. However, the major complication rates and mortality are similar to those of the surgical step-up approach.

Minimally Invasive Retroperitoneal Pancreatic Necrosectomy (MIRPN) or Video-Assisted Retroperitoneal Drainage (VARD) Retroperitoneal necrosectomy is performed when CT-guided PCD fails to fully resolve necrosis and clinical symptoms. The retroperitoneoscopic approach is preferred when lateral necrosis extends along the paracolic gutters or central necrosis extends to the lateral abdominal wall. Existing PCD can serve as a guide to access the necrotic cavity. Once the drain's position is confirmed on the CT scan, the tract is serially dilated over a stiff guidewire, preferably under fluoroscopic guidance, and a sheath is secured in place. A rigid endoscope, similar to a nephroscope, is introduced through the sheath, and debridement is performed using a grasper and continuous saline lavage. This method is associated with a decreased incidence of pancreatic fistula and new-onset organ failure. Multiple re-interventions may be necessary in patients with extensive necrosis and can be performed through the same tract under sedation.

Video-assisted retroperitoneal necrosectomy (VARN) is preferred for necrosis with significant solid contents. Similar to retroperitoneoscopy, pre-existing PCD is used as a guide, and the collection is accessed through a flank incision made at the drain's entry site. The lumbar access is created along and posterior to the drain to avoid colon injury. Using S-shaped retractors to visualize the cavity and under laparoscopic camera guidance, large necrotic casts, pus, and loose necrotic tissue are removed with blunt instruments like sponge-holders (Figs. 33.2 and 33.3).

Laparoscopic transgastric or transjejunal drainage is performed based on the location of necrosis, similar to the approach for pseudocysts. Internal drainage decreases the risk of postoperative pancreatic fistula. Transperitoneal laparoscopic necrosectomy can be done in patients with more extensive necrosis along both paracolic gutters and the root of the mesentery. The technique of necrosectomy is similar to that of open surgery. However, intolerance to prolonged pneumoperitoneum and a distended bowel may limit conventional laparoscopic access for necrosectomy.

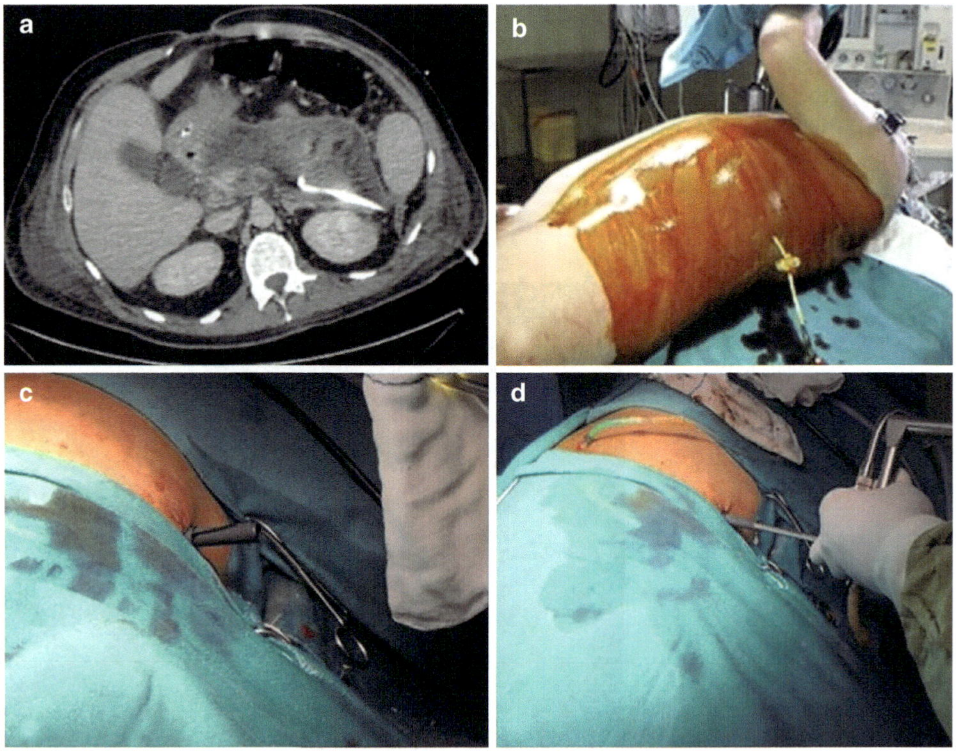

Fig. 33.2 VARD: (**a**, **b**) CT-guided PCD. (**c**) After serial dilation, a sheath (cannula) remains in the PCD tract for instrumentation. (**d**) Necrosectomy is performed using a nephroscope through the sheath

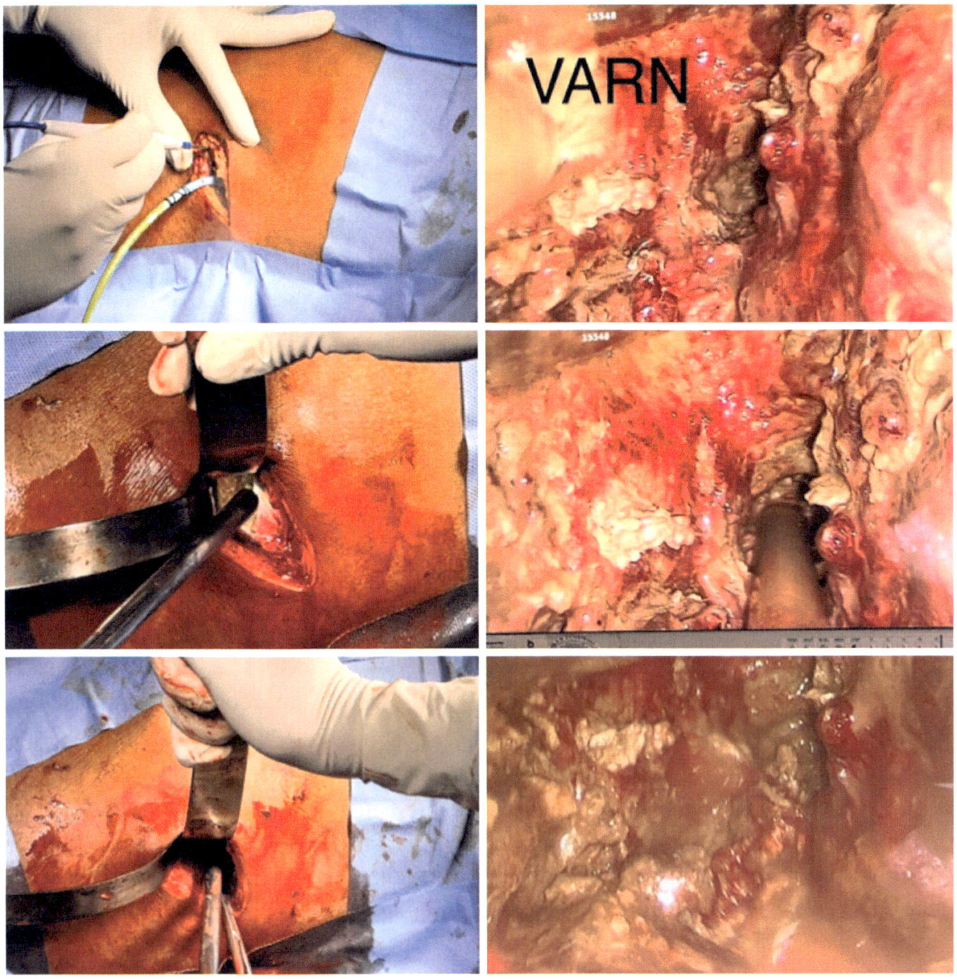

Fig. 33.3 VARN: The PCD tract is incised and opened to access the necrosis

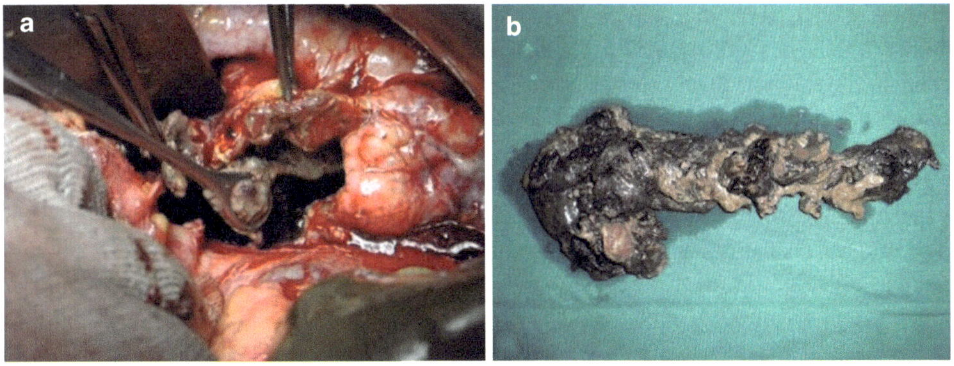

Fig. 33.4 (**a**) Open necrosectomy through the lesser sac. (**b**) Necrotic pancreas removed by gentle finger dissection

Open Necrosectomy The indications for open necrosectomy are as follows:

- Extensive necrosis
- Necrosis extending along the root of the mesentery and areas not accessible by video endoscope
- Associated bowel complications
- Salvage procedure in step-up algorithm

Open necrosectomy, once a standard procedure, is associated with serious complications such as bowel fistula, pancreatic fistula, hemorrhage, and mortality rates of up to 20%–30%. Currently, its role is limited to being a last resort in the "step-up" approach, and the mortality rates have decreased to less than 10%. A closed approach is preferred over ventral open packing. In this approach, after necrosectomy, the abdomen is closed, and the necrotic cavity is managed postoperatively with continuous irrigation through catheters placed during surgery (Fig. 33.4).

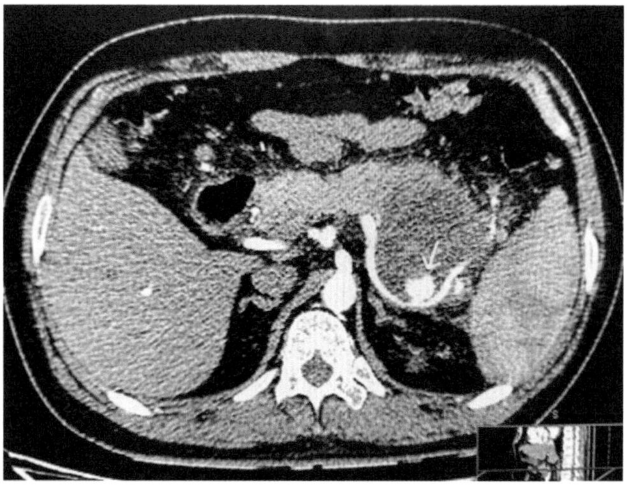

Fig. 33.5 Splenic artery pseudoaneurysm (arrow). Pancreatic necrosis involving the distal pancreas

Pseudoaneurysm Pseudoaneurysm and bleeding are seen in around 5%–10% of patients with pancreatitis. It forms due to weakening of the arterial wall caused by leaking pancreatic enzymes. The splenic artery is the most commonly affected. Bleeding from a pseudoaneurysm may occur into the gastrointestinal (GI) tract, necrotic cavity, or intraperitoneal space. It is crucial to identify and treat pseudoaneurysms before draining the collection, as the resulting bleeding can be fatal. The pseudoaneurysm is either embolized or bridged with vascular stents, placed under radiological guidance (Fig. 33.5).

Splanchnic Vein Thrombosis The splenic vein, portal vein, and rarely the superior mesenteric vein, are prone to thrombosis in acute pancreatitis, with a reported incidence ranging from 5% to 36%. Predisposing factors include a hostile environment, systemic inflammatory response, ileus, and systemic dehydration. It may present with ascites, GI bleeding, intestinal ischemia, or frank venous gangrene. Diagnosis is confirmed with CECT and CT angiography. Most patients can be successfully managed with anticoagulant therapy. The drug of choice is a therapeutic dose of low molecular weight heparin. Surgical intervention is necessary for patients with intestinal gangrene. Long-term sequelae include portal hypertension and hypersplenism in patients with portal vein thrombosis, and left-sided portal hypertension with gastric varices in patients with isolated splenic vein thrombosis.

Disconnected Pancreatic Duct Syndrome (DPDS) DPDS is a condition where there is complete disruption of the pancreatic duct due to acute necrotizing pancreatitis, chronic pancreatitis, or trauma. Studies have shown that DPDS can complicate 16%–20% of necrotizing pancreatitis cases. It can be diagnosed with a CT scan showing necrosis of at least 2 cm of the pancreas, with viable pancreatic tissue upstream. Complete ductal disruption can be demonstrated on MRCP or by extravasation of contrast material injected into the pancreatic duct during ERCP. It can present as pancreatic ascites, WOPN, or pseudocyst. Diagnosing DPDS is important because the resulting collection or pancreatic fistula is unlikely to resolve with conservative management. Endoscopic stenting of the pancreatic duct to bridge the disruption may successfully treat this condition. Internal drainage by pancreaticogastrostomy or pancreaticojejunostomy, and distal pancreatectomy are the two main surgeries recommended for DPDS when non-surgical methods fail.

Biliary and Duodenal Obstruction Duodenal obstruction is a rare complication of acute pancreatitis. Groove pancreatitis or underlying duodenal or peri-ampullary malignancies should be ruled out in patients presenting mainly with duodenal or biliary obstruction. These patients can be managed conservatively, endoscopically, or rarely through surgery. If the biliary or duodenal obstruction results from external compression, drainage of the pseudocyst or WOPN may be enough to relieve symptoms. Surgery is reserved for patients who do not improve with conservative measures. Gastrojejunostomy and bilio-enteric anastomosis are recommended for patients with duodenal or biliary obstruction, respectively.

Bowel Complications The GI tract is affected in 10%–12% of patients with necrotizing pancreatitis. Possible mechanisms include direct erosion of nearby organs by the WOPN or venous thrombosis leading to ischemic necrosis of the colon or small bowel. Colonic fistulae (60%) are the most common, followed by duodenal fistulae (20%). Colonic necrosis has a serious prognosis and presents with sudden clinical deterioration. Sometimes, spontaneous resolution of WOPN occurs after fistulation into the stomach or duodenum. For patients scheduled for necrosectomy, especially when imaging shows large air pockets in WOPN or signs of obstruction, a CT cologram with rectal contrast is essential to rule out colonic involvement. Management depends on the patient's clinical condition. Since most patients are ill and tissues fragile, primary closure or anastomosis is usually avoided in favor of diversion stoma/stomas. Restoring gut continuity with a definitive procedure is typically delayed for 3–6 months.

Key Points

- Pseudocyst and WOPN are sequelae of interstitial pancreatitis and necrotizing pancreatitis, respectively.
- Intervention is recommended only when symptoms persist or there is evidence of infection.
- Delayed intervention after 4–6 weeks has a better outcome than early intervention.
- A step-up approach with less invasive measures like PCD, followed by endoscopic, MIS, or VARN, is the current gold standard of treatment.
- Decompression is recommended instead of aggressive surgical debridement.
- Central or lateral location of necrosis, amount of solid debris, and local expertise are key factors in choosing the procedure.

Selected Reading

1. van Brunschot S, van Grinsven J, Voermans RP, et al. Transluminal endoscopic step-up approach versus minimally invasive surgical step-up approach in patients with infected necrotising pancreatitis (TENSION trial): design and rationale of a randomised controlled multicenter trial. BMC Gastroenterol. 2013;13:161. https://doi.org/10.1186/1471-230X-13-161.
2. van Santvoort HC, Besselink MG, Bakker OJ, et al. A step-up approach or open necrosectomy for necrotizing pancreatitis. NEJM. 2010;362:1491–502. https://doi.org/10.1056/NEJMoa0908821.
3. Onnekink AM, Boxhoorn L, Timmerhuis HC, et al. Endoscopic versus surgical step-up approach for infected necrotizing pancreatitis (extension): long-term follow-up of a randomized trial. Gastroenterology. 2022;163:712–22.
4. Minami K, Horibe M, Sanui M, Sasaki M, et al. The effect of an invasive strategy for treating pancreatic necrosis on mortality: a retrospective multicenter cohort study. J Gastrointest Surg. 2020;24:2037–45.
5. Baron TH, DiMaio CJ, Wang AY, Morgan KA. American gastroenterological association clinical practice update: management of pancreatic necrosis. Gastroenterology. 2020;158:67–75.
6. Heckler M, Hackert T, Hu K, Halloran CM, et al. Severe acute pancreatitis: surgical indications and treatment. Langenbeck's Arch Surg. 2020;406(3):521–35.
7. Rahnemai-Azar AA, Sutter C, Hayat U, et al. Multidisciplinary management of complicated pancreatitis: what every interventional radiologist should know. Am J Roentgenol. 2021;217:921–32.

Chronic Pancreatitis

34

Pothugunta Sai Krishna, Biju Pottakkat, Paresh Sharma, Manmohan Rajpoot, and Ajay Sharma

Abstract

Chronic pancreatitis (CP) is characterized by recurrent inflammation resulting in progressive and irreversible disease of the pancreas. Abdominal pain is the predominant symptom attributable to ductal hypertension, inflammation, nerve ischemia, and entrapment. Diagnosis is based on imaging studies like USG, CECT, and MRI-MRCP. CT scan and MRI provide complete morphology of the gland and the pancreatic duct, a prerequisite to planning surgery. Management of CP is directed at the control of pain and the management of complications. Medical management precedes interventional management and comprises analgesics and antioxidants. Interventional treatment, endoscopic or surgical, is required in 40–75% of patients. Endoscopic treatment is contraindicated in multiple or long pancreatic duct strictures. It comprises transpapillary dilatation of MPD strictures, stone extraction, and stenting. Lithotripsy may be required to fragment large stones to facilitate extraction. Surgery provides better long-term outcomes than endoscopic treatment.

Keywords

Chronic pancreatitis · Chronic calcific pancreatitis

Chronic pancreatitis (CP) is characterized by recurrent inflammation that leads to progressive and irreversible damage to the pancreas. The replacement of pancreatic tissue with fibrosis and the gradual decline in endocrine and/or exocrine pancreatic function significantly affect patients' survival and quality of life.

P. S. Krishna · B. Pottakkat (✉)
Jawaharlal Institute of Post-Graduate Medical Education and Research (JIPMER), Puducherry, India

P. Sharma · M. Rajpoot · A. Sharma
Mahatma Gandhi University of Medical Sciences and Technology (MGUMST), Jaipur, India

34.1 Classification and Severity Assessment (Table 34.1)

34.2 Etiology and Pathogenesis

Alcohol accounts for nearly one-third of all cases of CP. The disease is idiopathic in the remaining cases, with potential genetic, metabolic, or environmental causes. Family history of CD and diabetes mellitus, in 2% and 13% respectively, suggests a genetic predisposition.

34.2.1 Alcohol Consumption

Alcohol consumption plays a crucial role in CP because its metabolites have been reported to cause damage to acinar cells and activate pancreatic stellate cells (PSC). Individuals who consume more than four drinks per day are at an increased risk of developing CP and experiencing its progression, compared to non-drinkers. Acetaldehyde, a by-product of ethanol in higher quantities, damages acinar, mesenchymal, or ductal cells, leading to apoptosis or necrosis. Macrophages destroy these damaged cells through phagocytosis, releasing cytokines like transforming growth factor beta 1 (TGF-β1). This triggers the transformation of PSC into myofibroblast-like cells, which secrete collagen types III and I, along with fibronectin, damaging and replacing parenchymal cells, and causing a progressive loss of exocrine and endocrine functions.

34.2.2 Smoking

Nicotine consumption was previously thought to be a co-causative factor in the development of CP, but recent evidence considers smoking as an independent factor that causes acinar cell changes, leading to cellular degeneration and, ultimately, fibrosis. Nicotine has been reported to induce

M. Ibrarullah (ed.), *Recent Concepts in Gastrointestinal (GI) Surgery*, https://doi.org/10.1007/978-981-92-1118-0_34

Table 34.1 Classification systems for chronic pancreatitis

Classification year	Criteria	Description	Merits	Pitfalls
Manchester 2006	Based on disease severity classification and clinical correlation	*Mild disease* Radiological evidence of CP Abdominal pain Preserved endocrine and exocrine function No regular analgesia No peri-pancreatic complications *Moderate disease* Radiological evidence of CP Abdominal pain Impaired endocrine and exocrine function Regular analgesia No peri-pancreatic complications *End stage* Radiological evidence of CP One or more complications—biliary stricture, portal hypertension, duodenal stenosis One or more of the following: Diabetes, steatorrhea	The first classification for disease severity	Not all the clinical parameters are included

M-ANNHEIM 2007	Based on clinical symptoms, function assessment, complications and imaging	*Diagnostic criteria*
		Definite CP—one or more of the following
		Pancreatic calcifications
		Moderate or marked ductal lesions
		Marked or persistent exocrine insufficiency—steatorrhea responding to enzyme supplementation
		Morphological changes on microscopy
		Probable CP—one or more of the following
		Mild ductal alterations
		Recurrent or persistent pseudocysts
		Abnormal exocrine function on fecal elastase-1 or secretin-pancreaozymin test
		Endocrine insufficiency
		Borderline CP—Typical history of pancreatitis without any additional criteria mentioned above
		Imaging criteria—Dilatation of the duct proximal to the occlusion
		Severity grading—Asymptomatic
		Symptomatic
		  Without pancreatic insufficiency
		  With partial pancreatic insufficiency
		  Painful & complete pancreatic insufficiency
		  Stage of secondary painless disease
			Detailed classification system on Etiology
			Symptomatology
			Disease severity
			Imaging features
				Clinical correlation of disease severity with management outcomes is not described

(continued)

Table 34.1 (continued)

Classification year	Criteria	Description	Merits	Pitfalls
Milosaljevic 2010	Based on clinical symptoms, function assessment, and complications	*Stage A* Pain of any type or degree Pain attacks of any frequency No exocrine or endocrine abnormalities No complication *Stage B* Complications are present No exocrine or endocrine abnormalities *Stage C* End-stage functional impairment with or without complications C1—Endocrine impairment C2—Exocrine impairment C3—Endocrine/exocrine impairment and/or complications	A comprehensive classification of disease severity that can be applied easily	Radiological findings are not taken into consideration

cytoplasmic swelling, vacuolization, and damage to the exocrine pancreas through oxidative stress and lipid peroxidation of acinar cells. Nitrosamine ketone (NNK), a derivative of nicotine that structurally resembles beta-adrenergic receptors, activates these receptors, resulting in increased intracellular cyclic adenosine monophosphate (cAMP). This increase causes zymogen activation and secretion, ultimately leading to persistent inflammation, recurrent attacks, and disease chronicity.

34.2.3 Genomics and Genetic Alterations

The genetic mechanism in the pathogenesis of CP includes the following:

Mechanism 1—Premature activation of proteases

The crucial genes involved in activating and preventing the degradation of trypsinogen are PRSS1 and PRSS2, while the serine protease inhibitor Kazal type (SPINK) gene prevents trypsin activation. The PRSS1 mutation reduces chymotrypsin C (CTRC) dependent degradation of trypsinogen, leading to auto-activation of trypsinogen and pancreatitis. SPINK, also called pancreatic secretory trypsin inhibitor (PSTI), is found in the pancreas and in the mucus layer of the intestinal tract, where it promotes cell repair after injury. SPINK inhibits trypsinogen activation by forming covalent bonds with the enzyme, thus preventing activation. The pN34S mutation is a loss-of-function (LOF) mutation in SPINK, causing increased activation of acinar cells and resulting in recurrent acute pancreatitis and CP.

Mechanism 2—Endoplasmic reticulum (ER) stress theory

Increased degradation of trypsin, lipase, and carboxypeptidase 1 leads to the accumulation of byproducts in cells, causing damage to the endoplasmic reticulum, apoptosis, and cell death. Genetic mutations in PRSS1, carboxy-ester lipase (CEL), and pancreatic lipase (PNLIP) are involved in the ER stress theory. Single-base deletions in CEL and PNLIP genes can cause lipase to accumulate within cells, resulting in increased activation that leads to acinar loss and exocrine dysfunction.

Mechanism 3—Ductal pathway dysfunction

The function of ductal cells is in the selective absorption and secretion of various compounds, which helps maintain the homogeneity of pancreatic juice. This function is regulated by genes such as CLDN2, cystic fibrosis transmembrane conductance regulator (CFTR), and calcium-sensing receptor (CaSR). The pR117H allele mutation of the CFTR gene disrupts the normal coding of this gene for a transmembrane protein involved in the expression of the cAMP-derived chloride channel on the surface of epithelial cells. This reduction in chloride secretion causes chloride to become trapped within ductal and acinar cells, leading to a decrease in pH. Consequently, intracellular protein coagulation damages the epithelial barrier, causing auto-activation of cells and resulting in pancreatitis.

Mechanism 4—Inflammatory pathway dysfunction

The genes involved in the inflammatory pathway cascade leading to persistent inflammation and CP are Alpha-1 antitrypsin (a1AT), Tumor necrosis factor alpha (TNFα), and Gamma-glutamyl transpeptidase 1 (GGT1). Mutations in a1AT and TNFα cause polymorphisms in the promoter regions, resulting in increased expression of these pro-inflammatory factors. This causes continuous activation of neutrophils, leading to acinar cell apoptosis and eventually fibrosis.

34.3 Tropical Chronic Pancreatitis

Tropical pancreatitis (TCP), reported from the Indian subcontinent, accounts for nearly 4% of all cases of CP. It is characterized by the following:

- Early age of onset (<30 years).
- Malnourished patients (BMI < 18 kg/m^2.
- Large main pancreatic duct (MPD) calculi predominantly in the pancreatic head.
- Insulin-dependent and ketosis-resistant diabetes.

34.4 Pathogenesis of Pain in Chronic Pancreatitis

Pain is the most common symptom, reported in 60–90% of patients with CP. The causes of pain can be multifactorial. Some of the proposed mechanisms are as follows:

- Ductal and tissue hypertension due to obstructive calculus or stricture.
- Inflammatory irritation of the nerve fibers.
- Ischemia of the nerve fibers due to fibrosis and entrapment.
- Neuropathic pain: peripheral and central nervous system sensitization.

34.4.1 Peripheral Pain Mechanism

Pain signals from the pancreas are transmitted by the sympathetic neurons of the celiac ganglia, which have their cell bodies in the dorsal root ganglia (DRG). The afferent nerves from the DRG project into the dorsal horn of the spinal cord. The vanilloid receptors, such as transient receptor potential vanilloid (TRPV1), play a crucial role in mediating peripheral pain in CP. When these receptors are activated—either by physical stimuli (heat), acidification, or endogenous peptides like prostaglandins—they increase the flow of calcium and sodium into the cells, leading to depolarization and the release of substance P (SP) and calcium gene-related peptide (CGRP). These substances cause vasodilation, fluid extravasation, and neutrophil infiltration, resulting in inflammation around nociceptive neurons and pain.

34.4.2 Central Sensitization

Cellular mechanism: Microglial cells, the counterparts of tissue macrophages in the brain, are activated by the excitation of nociceptive neurons. CCL2 and CCR2 on microglial cells are reported to be involved in their activation. P38, a mitogen-activated protein kinase, acts as a co-stimulatory factor with microglial cells, leading to the persistence of visceral pain caused by nociception. Activation of astrocytes by inflammatory neuropeptides, prostaglandins, and cytokines like IL1B, IL16, and TNF-alpha also plays a role in central pain mechanisms.

Reorganization Several observational studies noted that pain in CP exhibits a phenomenon called reorganization in the viscera, caused by increased afferent signaling from gut neurons. In this process, there is an increased perception of pain due to distension of the hollow viscus, resulting from reduced evoked potential in the CNS.

34.5 Pathogenesis of Pancreatic Stone Formation

Pancreatic stones are the most common imaging finding in patients with CP and are observed in up to 90% of cases. Morphologically, a pancreatic stone consists of a core matrix composed of mucopolysaccharides, acids, and neutral glycoproteins. The outer sheath surrounding the matrix is mainly made of calcium carbonate (>90%). Pancreatic stones undergo several developmental stages, from the pre-calcified to the calcified phase, as they progress from nucleation to precipitation and ultimately to crystal formation. Within the same affected pancreatic tissue, these stones may be at different stages. Current evidence regarding the mechanism of stone formation includes three hypotheses: the calcium binding hypothesis, the pancreatic juice stabilization hypothesis, and the adsorption hypothesis (Fig. 34.1).

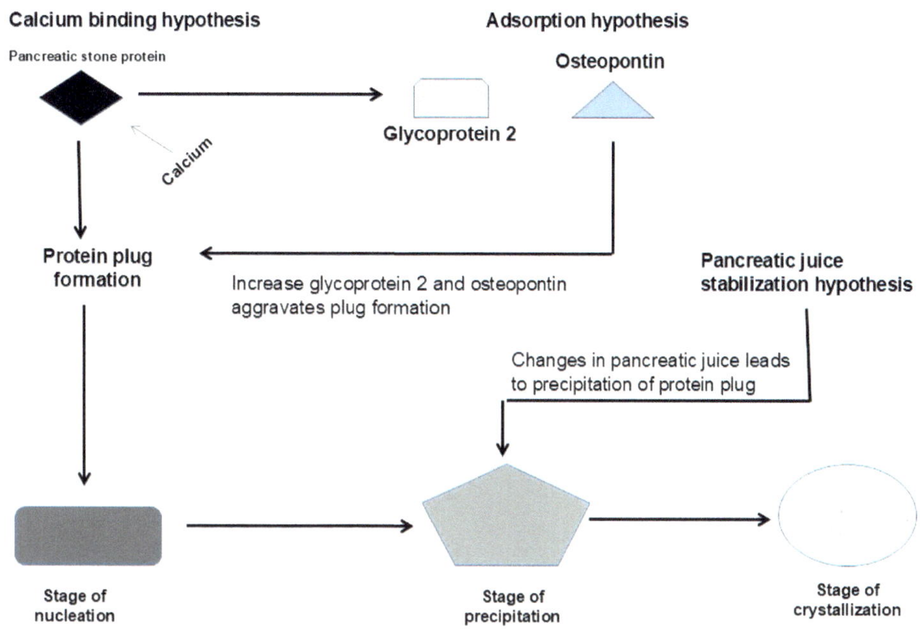

Fig. 34.1 The process of pancreatic stone formation

34.6 Clinical Presentation

34.6.1 Abdominal Pain

Upper abdominal pain radiating to the upper back is a classic clinical feature of CP and occurs in 60 to 90% of patients. The pain is usually felt in the epigastric region, worsened by eating and relieved by bending forward, prompting patients to sit in the "pancreas position." Another feature is the episodic nature of the pain, which lasts for several days and is associated with nausea, vomiting, and fatigue. The time between pain episodes tends to decrease as the disease advances. After five years, nearly half of the patients with CP become pain-free due to a "burnt out" pancreas. However, it is not possible to identify this subgroup of patients prospectively from a treatment perspective.

34.6.2 Endocrine Insufficiency

Diabetes mellitus (DM) in CP occurs in about 60 to 70% of patients. Pancreatic inflammation that leads to a gradual loss of islet cells is the main cause of type 3c diabetes. It requires the destruction of at least 65% of beta cells for DM to manifest. It is typically insulin dependent in 50%, manageable with oral hypoglycemic agents in 34% and diet modification in the remaining 16% of patients.

34.6.3 Exocrine Insufficiency

Pancreatic exocrine insufficiency (PEI), also known as "pancreatic maldigestion," results from decreased pancreatic enzyme activity in the intestine caused by progressive destruction of acinar cells in CP. The reduced levels of protease and lipases in the small intestinal lumen impair the digestion of carbohydrates and fats, leading to maldigestion. Main symptoms of PEI include abdominal fullness, anorexia, intolerance to fatty foods, passage of greasy stools, and eventual weight loss. Steatorrhea is often accompanied by diarrhea in most patients due to decreased intestinal transit and accelerated gastric emptying. Although only 10–15% of patients present with steatorrhea initially, about 40–48% may have subclinical PEI. It typically develops later in the disease course and is reported to occur 10 to 20 years after a diagnosis of DM. Lipase secretion is affected early on because of its high susceptibility to the acidic pH of pancreatic juice. Patients may also experience vitamin deficiencies due to impaired absorption of fat-soluble vitamins A, D, E, and K.

In addition to the above clinical presentation, a subset of patients may present with complications of recurrent inflammation in CP. The various complications and the respective incidences are listed in the table below (Table 34.2).

Table 34.2 Complications of chronic pancreatitis

Pseudocyst	16%
Jaundice	8–10%
Pancreatic cancer	4–12%
Pancreatic fistula, ascites	5%
Portal hypertension	3%
GI bleeding	2%
Pseudoaneurysm	2%
Duodenal obstruction	2%
Colonic obstruction	2%

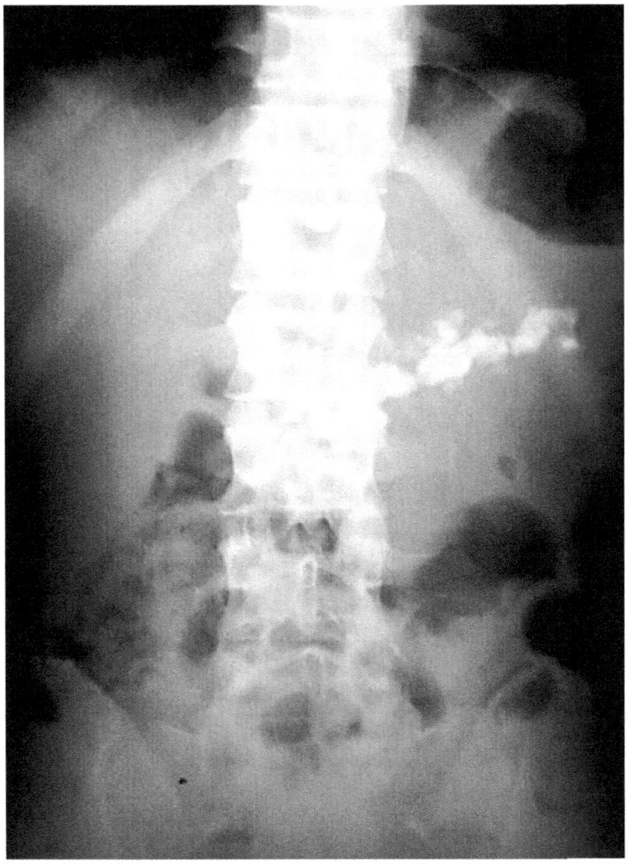

Fig. 34.2 Plain X-ray abdomen—pancreatic calcification along the MPD

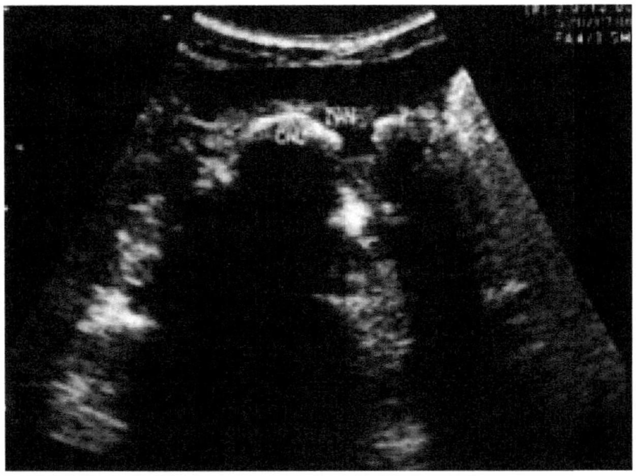

Fig. 34.3 USG—dilated pancreatic duct and calculi inside, casting posterior acoustic shadows

34.7 Diagnosis

Diagnosis of CP is made on clinical suspicion and confirmed on imaging studies (Figs. 34.2, 34.3, 34.4, and 34.5; Table 34.3).

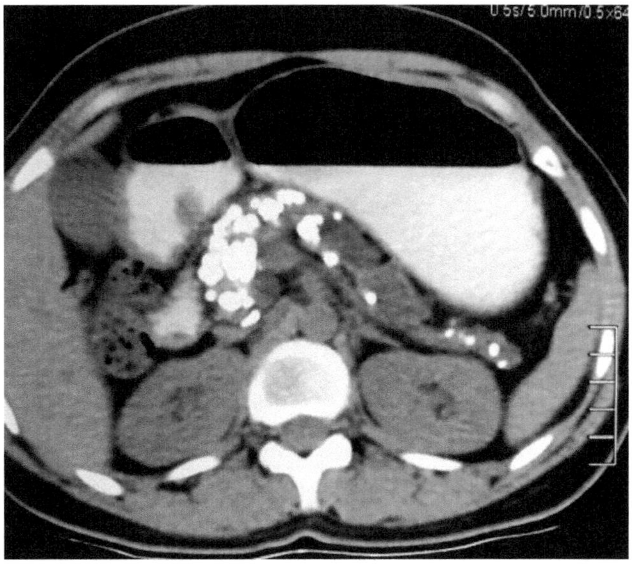

Fig. 34.4 CECT abdomen—atrophic pancreas. Calcifications predominantly in the head region

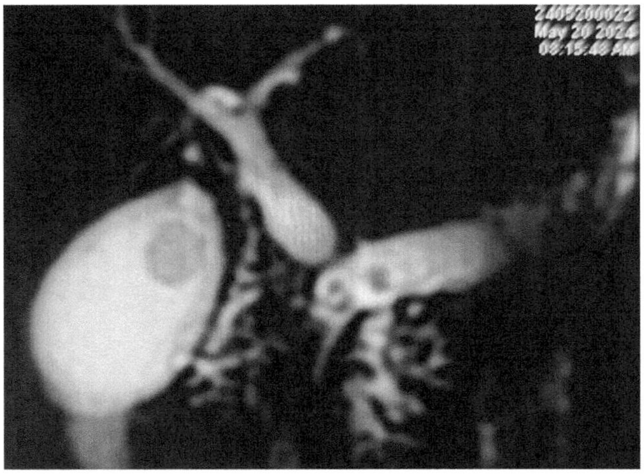

Fig. 34.5 MRCP: Dilated MPD containing calculi. Note the dilated CBD and stone inside the distended gallbladder

Table 34.3 Imaging in chronic pancreatitis

Imaging	Sensitivity/ specificity (%)	Findings	Limitations
USG	64 /98	*Used as a screen modality* Hyperechoic areas with post-acoustic shadowing s/o stones Altered echo-texture of the pancreas Iso or hypoechoic soft tissue mass s/o inflammatory mass Linear hypoechoic lines s/o pancreatic duct Hypoechoic homo-heterogeneous well-defined cavities s/o pseudocyst/necrotic collection	Difficulty in imaging in obese patients and in the presence of bowel gas shadows Inter-observer variability Decreased accuracy in analyzing peri-pancreatic vessels
CECT	75/91	*Most reliable investigation for diagnosis, study of the ductal morphology, and detection of complications* Pancreatic ductal dilatation, calcifications, parenchymal atrophy, bile duct dilatation, peripancreatic fat standing in acute exacerbation, hypodense mass, *Uncommon findings—* Pseudoaneurysm of arteries and venous thrombosis, fluid or necrotic collections	Low accuracy in determining ductal anatomy compared to MRI/MRCP.
MRI/ MRCP	78/96	*Accurate for studying ductal morphology and cystic lesions* T1 weighted phase— Hypointense due to decreased protein content (fibrosis) T1 contrast—Reduced enhancement T2 weighted phase—Fluid collection/pseudocyst and necrosis—Hyper-intense Intra-ductal calcifications—Signal void Early stage—Branch duct dilatation and clubbed appearance Late stages—MPD dilatation, narrowing, irregular contour, and filling defects	Difficulty in assessing findings in the presence of calcifications Contraindicated in the presence of metal implants, a pacemaker device, and claustrophobia
EUS	81/90	*Indicated to detect early changes of CP, evaluate head mass, and cystic lesions* Hyperechoic foci/strands, lobularity, cysts Main duct irregularities/dilatation Side branch irregularities/dilatation Parenchymal atrophy	Invasive investigation Operator dependent
CE-EUS	93/89	Homogeneous enhancement of parenchyma in the arterial phase with delayed washout Malignant lesions—Hypovascular	Invasive investigation Inter-observer variability Availability
ERCP	82/94	Largely given up as a diagnostic modality. Used as an adjunct to therapeutic interventions	Invasive investigation High risk of morbidity (up to 30%) Can only assess the ductal abnormalities of chronic pancreatitis The severity of ductal abnormality may not correlate with clinical findings

USG ultrasonogram, *CECT* contrast-enhanced computed tomography, *MRCP* magnetic resonance cholangiopancreatography, *MPD* main pancreatic duct, *EUS* endoscopic ultrasound, *CE-EUS* contrast-enhanced EUS, *ERCP* endoscopic retrograde cholangiopancreatography

34.8 Management

The disease process in CP, by definition, is progressive and irreversible. Therefore, the management of CP can only be considered palliative, focusing on alleviating pain, treating exocrine and endocrine deficiencies, and managing complications. Managing CP requires a multidisciplinary approach that includes radiologists, endoscopists, surgeons, and experts in pain management, nutrition, and psychological support. Withdrawal of causative factors like alcohol and smoking should be strictly enforced. A significant proportion of patients with CP respond to medical management. Interventional treatments, either endoscopic or surgical, are needed in about 40–75% of patients. The superiority of any particular intervention remains a matter of ongoing debate, although current evidence suggests that surgery is the definitive approach in managing CP and offers better pain control compared to endoscopic methods.

34.8.1 Medical Management

Pain being the most important presenting symptom, its management presents the greatest challenge. A stepwise escalation of analgesics is recommended for optimal pain control. Pancreatic enzyme supplements, in both enteric-coated and uncoated forms, have shown mixed results for pain relief. Recent developments in pain management include the use of

Table 34.4 Pharmacotherapy of chronic pancreatitis

Medication	Dosage	Common side effects
Non-opioid analgesic		
Paracetamol	325 to 650 mg every 4–6 hrs, maximum 4 gm/day	Dyspepsia High doses—hepatotoxicity
Opioid analgesic		
Tramadol	50 to 100 mg 12 hrly, maximum dose of 400 mg/ day	Constipation, drowsiness, nausea, and vomiting
Codeine	15–60 mg orally, every 4–6 hrs, maximum 360 mg/day	Constipation, drowsiness
Morphine	10–20 mg orally, every 4–6 hrs, maximum 150 mg /day	Urinary retention, constipation, dependence, and respiratory depression
Centrally acting analgesic		
Amitriptyline	10—25 mg at bedtime, maximum dose of 300 mg/day	Dry mouth, urinary retention, orthostatic hypotension, and blurring of vision
Pregabalin	75 mg 12 hrly, maximum 600 mg/day	Somnolence, xerostomia, peripheral edema
Antioxidants		
Selenium, methionine, vitamin A, C, and E	Organic selenium—600 micrograms Ascorbic acid—0.5 gm Methionine—2 gm Alpha tocopherol—270 IU Beta carotene—9000 IU	Headache, abdominal discomfort

pregabalin and antioxidants. The latter appears promising, providing pain relief in nearly one-third of patients compared to placebo. The various pharmacological agents used in the escalation ladder are summarized in Table 34.4.

34.8.2 Pancreatic Enzyme Replacement Therapy (PERT), Diet, and Lifestyle Modification

PERT includes the initiation of lipase at 30000 to 40,000 IU with each meal and 15,000 to 20,000 IU with each snack. The response to PERT should involve clinical improvement, such as fewer and more consistent stools, no fat droplets in the stools, and weight gain. If patients remain symptomatic after confirming compliance, the PERT dose can be doubled, and adding proton pump inhibitors (PPIs) may be helpful. The diet for patients with CP should include adequate protein (50 to 75 grams) and supplementation of medium-chain triglycerides if steatorrhea continues.

34.8.3 Diet and Lifestyle Modification

Malnutrition is one of the most common and underestimated complications of CP. A concerning observation is that malnutrition worsens as the disease advances. The causes of malnutrition are multifactorial, but the primary reason is enzyme deficiency, particularly lipase, leading to impaired absorption of triglycerides and fat-soluble vitamins. Other contributing factors include decreased oral intake due to pain and changes in blood glucose levels.

34.8.4 Endoscopic Management

Endoscopic management aims to clear ductal stones, dilate strictures, and place stents in the main pancreatic duct (MPD) to decompress and facilitate drainage. The procedure is contraindicated in patients with multiple and/or long strictures that are not suitable for endoscopic dilation. Larger and/or peripheral stones may require fragmentation through lithotripsy. Options include extracorporeal shock wave lithotripsy (ESWL) and single-operator pancreatography with intraoperative lithotripsy (SOPIL). Long-term stent placement to treat ductal stenosis can be achieved using multiple plastic stents or fully covered self-expanding metallic stents. The overall treatment process is lengthy, repetitive, and consequently expensive. With a long-term success rate of less than 20% in most published reports, this procedure is considered a poor alternative to surgery and is usually only an option for patients who are unfit or unwilling to undergo surgery.

34.8.5 Surgical Management

Recent advances in understanding the pathophysiology of pain indicate an effective treatment window for pain in CP, particularly within the first three years of onset. Delaying treatment can cause central sensitization of pain, which is a major reason for surgical failure. Therefore, the notion of considering surgery only as a last resort after medical and endotherapy options fail should be reconsidered in favor of early surgical intervention. Evidence suggests that early decompression of MPD can slow the progression of CP and potentially improve endocrine and exocrine functions. Although still hypothetical, early decompression might even prevent the development of pancreatic cancer. All these points support early drainage for dilated MPD with stones or strictures, even in the absence of symptoms or complications (Table 34.5).

Table 34.5 Indications of surgery in chronic pancreatitis

Intractable pain, frequent, interfering with normal lifestyle, not responding to medical management, and/or requiring opiate analgesics
Failure of endotherapy to relieve pain
Complications of the disease
Pseudocyst
Biliary obstruction
Pseudoaneurysm
Duodenal/colonic obstruction
Suspicion/superimposed malignancy
Relative indication
Dilated MPD with stones/ strictures.

34.8.5.1 Principles of Surgery in Chronic Pancreatitis

- To clear the duct of stones.
- To lay open the duct across the stricture/s.
- To excise or resect the pacemaker of the pancreas (pancreatic head).
- To resect any mass suspicious of malignancy.
- To treat complications of CP.

34.8.5.2 Surgical Procedures

The following factors guide the choice of the surgical procedure:

- MPD diameter.
- Presence and distribution of stones and strictures.
- Presence of an inflammatory mass.
- Complications of CP-like biliary obstruction, duodenal or colonic stenosis, pseudoaneurysm, or venous thrombosis.

The surgical procedures are broadly classified into drainage, resection, and hybrid procedures (Fig. 34.6 and Table 34.6).

34.8.6 Outcomes of Surgery

When properly applied, each surgical procedure described above provides pain relief in about 90% of patients, complete relief in 70–75%, and partial relief in 10–15%. Long-term pain relief is observed in approximately 35–50% of patients. Recurrence or lack of pain relief can be caused by several factors discussed later in this chapter.

The major long-term consequences of pancreaticoduodenectomy include metabolic issues such as new-onset DM, pancreatic enzyme insufficiency (PEI), and steatohepatitis. These effects can be linked to the removal of pancreatic tissue and the duodeno-jejunal region, as well as biliopancreatic and gastric diversion. After duodenectomy, hormones like insulin, pancreatic polypeptides, and gastric inhibitory polypeptides, which regulate glucose metabolism, are significantly reduced. Additionally, duodenectomy results in the disconnection of the duodeno-pancreatic neural axis, disrupting the relationship between interdigestive gastrointestinal hormone release and insulin secretion. All these changes may eventually lead to DM. PEI is associated with a marked decrease in gut and pancreatic hormones such as CCK, secretin, motilin, and gastrin, due to antrectomy, duodenojejunal excision, and diversion (gastrojejunostomy). The development of steatohepatitis after PD is not well understood, but it may be caused by dysregulation of adipokines and hormones, increased insulin resistance, and alterations in the upper gut microbiome. Studies suggest that these issues can be minimized by preserving the duodenum and proximal jejunum, as seen in various types of duodenum-preserving pancreatic head resection (DPPHR) (Table 34.7).

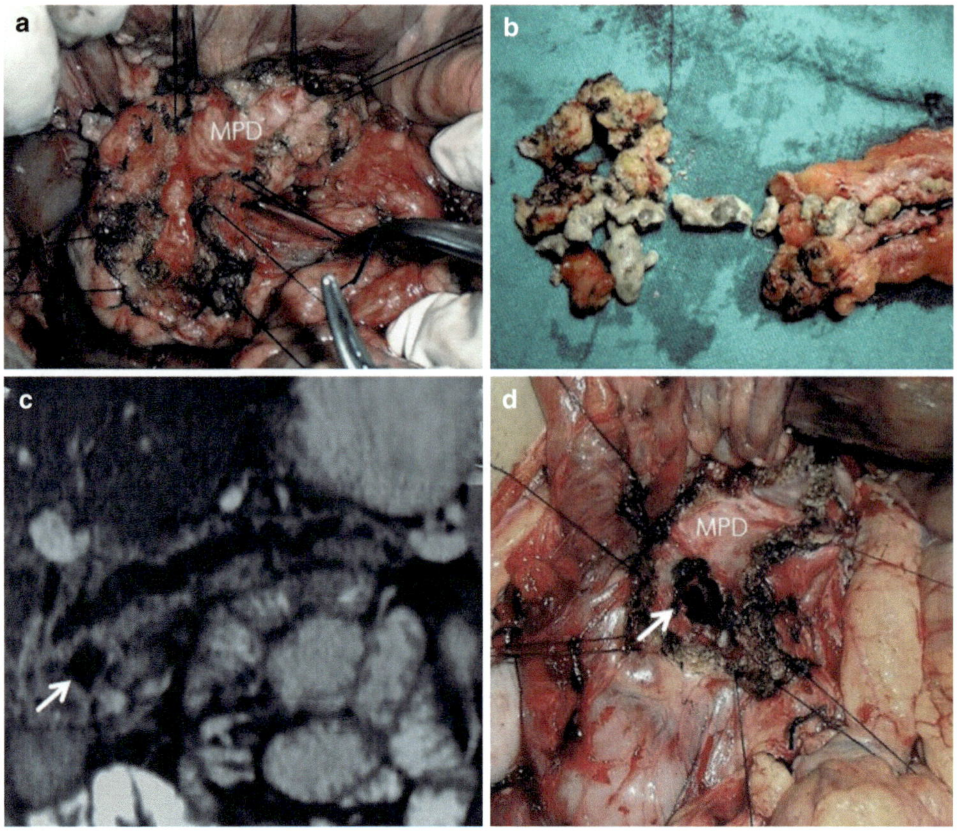

Fig. 34.6 (**a**) Head coring. Note that only a thin rim of pancreatic tissue remains along the C loop of the duodenum. The MPD is laid open in its entire length. (**b**) Distal pancreatectomy and head coring. The distal pancreas is atrophic and fibrotic, replaced by fat. Stones from the MPD and the fibrotic tissue cored out are seen in the picture. (**c**) CT scan coronal image showing dilated MPD and a small pseudocyst (arrow). (**c'**) MPD is laid open along with the pseudocyst (arrow)

Table 34.6 Indications and techniques for various surgical procedures in chronic pancreatitis

Procedure	Indication	Technique
Drainage procedures		
Partington & Rochelle modification of Puestow's operation	Dilated MPD containing stones and strictures. No gross disease in the pancreatic head	MPD opened along its entire length, lateral pancreato-jejunostomy (LPJ)
Izbicki procedure	Undilated MPD (≤2 mm) with normal pancreatic head	Longitudinal V-shaped excision of the ventral pancreas along the entire length of MPD, LPJ
Hybrid (resection and drainage) procedures		
Frey's procedure	Enlarged and diseased pancreatic head with stones. Dilated MPD with stones and strictures	Pancreatic head cored out, leaving behind the posterior capsule and a thin rim of parenchyma along the duodenal margin. MPD laid open, LPJ incorporating the cored-out head
Hamburg procedure (modified Frey's)	More extensive disease of the head	Subtotal excision of the pancreatic head, including the uncinate process + LPJ. The extent of the head excision is comparable to the Beger procedure while avoiding the transection of the gland over the mesenteric-portal axis
Livocado procedure	End-stage severe CP with vascular involvement by the inflammation and fibrosis	In-situ near total pancreatectomy. Duodenum-preserving pancreatic resection, leaving behind the fibrous capsule to protect the vessels and for LPJ
Near-total pancreatic head resection	Extensive disease in the pancreatic head (inflammatory mass/ extensive calcifications) with ductal lesions	Near total resection of the pancreatic head, leaving only the posterior pancreatic capsule. The duct is opened along its entire length. Single anastomosis—Longitudinal pancreato-jejunostomy, and the jejunum is sutured to the posterior pancreatic capsule and duodenal serosa medially

(continued)

Table 34.6 (continued)

Procedure	Indication	Technique
Resection procedures		
Beger's procedure	Extensive disease in the pancreatic head (inflammatory mass/ extensive calcifications) with no ductal lesions	The head is completely resected, including the posterior pancreatic capsule, leaving a rim of tissue on the medial aspect of the duodenum. The transected body of the pancreas and the excised head are anastomosed with the jejunum
Berne's modification of Beger's procedure	Extensive disease in the pancreatic head (inflammatory mass/extensive calcifications) with no ductal lesions	The head is resected without dissection of the mesenteric-portal axis. Single pancreato-jejunostomy with the edges of the resected pancreatic tissue
Whipple's Pancreatoduodenectomy / pylorus-preserving pancreaticoduodenectomy	Inflammatory head mass with suspicion of malignancy or proven malignancy	Resection of pancreatic neck at the level of PV/SMV junction, duodenal resection, resection of distal CBD, distal gastrectomy +/− pylorus preservation, and resection of proximal jejunum. Reconstruction includes pancreatico-jejunostomy, hepatico-jejunostomy, and gastro-jejunostomy
Total pancreatectomy with islet auto-transplantation	Hereditary chronic pancreatitis with no risk of malignancy, preferably in younger patients	The pancreas is totally removed, followed by enzymatic degradation of the pancreas and isolation of islet cells. Islet cells are injected (0.25 ml/kg) into the portal vein

Table 34.7 Long-term metabolic consequences following pancreaticoduodenectomy (PD) versus duodenum-preserving pancreatic head resection (DPPHR)

	DPPHR	PD
New onset DM	05%	16%
New onset PEI	07%	44%
Steatohepatitis	03%	24%

34.9 Management of Complications of Chronic Pancreatitis

34.9.1 Biliary Obstruction

The incidence of biliary obstruction (BO) in CP ranges from 3% to 46%, with clinical jaundice occurring in 8% to 10%. Silent BO presents as elevated serum alkaline phosphatase (SAP), dilated CBD on imaging, or delayed excretion on biliary scintigraphy. The mechanism of biliary obstruction, its presentation, cholangiographic appearance, and management are listed below (Fig. 34.7 and Table 34.8).

34.9.2 Pseudocyst

Acute pseudocysts are managed conservatively. Endoscopic or percutaneous drainage may be necessary for persistent and symptomatic cysts. Cysts caused by chronic pancreatitis are more often small and communicate with the MPD. During surgery, the MPD is opened along with the cysts and drained into the jejunal loop.

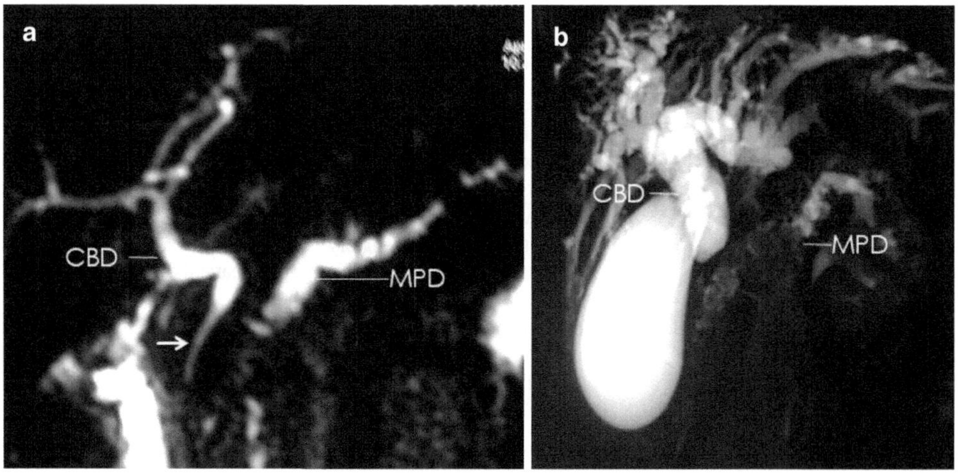

Fig. 34.7 Biliary obstruction in chronic pancreatitis. (**a**) Long stricture (benign) involving intrapancreatic CBD (arrow). (**b**) Complete obstruction by malignant mass in the pancreatic head. Note dilated MPD with calculi

Table 34.8 Biliary obstruction in chronic pancreatitis

Mechanism	Presentation	Cholangiogram	Management
Acute exacerbation of CP, ampullary edema	Transient jaundice	Dilated CBD till ampulla	Conservative
Compression by inflammatory mass/ pseudocyst	Intermittent/low-grade persistent jaundice	Smooth compression of the intrapancreatic CBD	Endoscopic stenting/ decompression by head-coring
Obstruction of the ampulla by pancreatic stone (rarely)	Intermittent jaundice	Dilated CBD, stone at ampulla	Endoscopic papillotomy & stone extraction
Fibrosis due to recurrent inflammation	Persistent jaundice. SAP elevation two times or more for more than four weeks	Long intrapancreatic CBD stricture	Choledocho-jejunostomy
Malignant mass in the pancreatic head	Progressive jaundice	Irregular stricture (short or long) of the intrapancreatic segment of CBD/ CBD, showing complete cut-off at the suprapancreatic level	Pancreaticoduodenectomy if resectable

34.9.3 Duodenal/Colonic Obstruction

The reported incidence of luminal obstruction is 1–2%. The obstruction is more often caused by external compression from an inflammatory mass or pseudocyst, and less commonly by fibrosis or malignant infiltration (Fig. 34.8). Duodenal obstruction, depending on its level, can be treated with duodeno- or gastrojejunostomy. Colonic obstruction generally requires excision of the stricture and reconstruction.

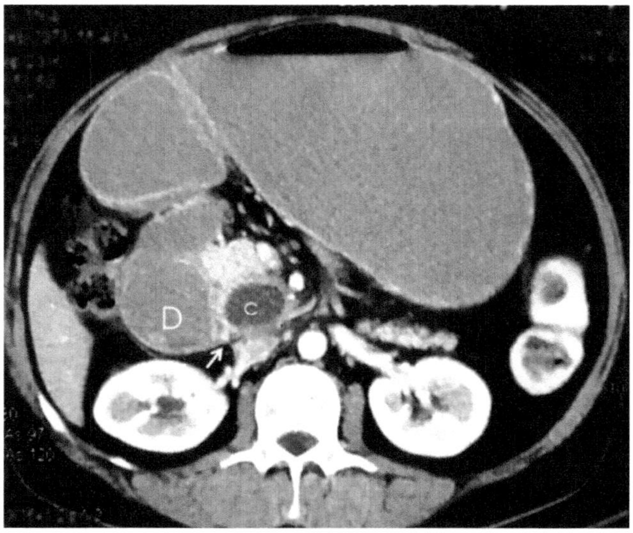

Fig. 34.8 CECT abdomen—duodenal (D) obstruction (arrow) by a pseudocyst (C) in the pancreatic head

34.9.4 Superimposed Malignancy

The incidence of superimposed malignancy in CP ranges from 4% to 12%, while concomitant malignancy in an "inflammatory pancreatic head mass" occurs in 18–40%. The predictors of malignancy in CP are listed below (Fig. 34.9; Table 34.9).

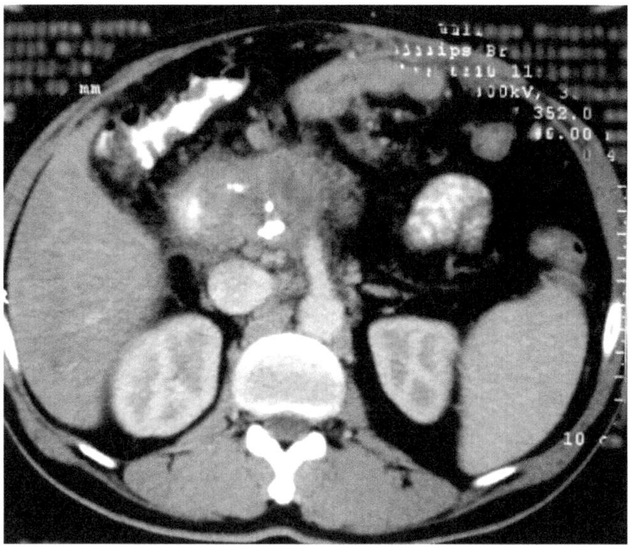

Fig. 34.9 Malignant pancreatic head mass showing calcifications and vessel encasement

34.10 Persistent Pain After Surgery

Approximately 15–20% of patients still experience pain after surgery, and another 20–30% develop recurrent pain at varying times post-surgery. The predictors of poor outcomes following surgery are as follows:

- Surgery >3 years of symptoms.
- Patients on opioids preoperatively.
- More than five endoscopic interventions before surgery.
- Persistent pain pattern with high Izbicki pain score at initial presentation.
- Postoperative complications.

Table 34.9 Factors predicting malignancy in chronic pancreatitis

Old age
Jaundice, serum bilirubin >5.8 mg/dL
Recent worsening abdominal pain.
Recent onset or worsening of pre-existing DM
Duodenal obstruction
Significant weight loss
CA 19–9 > 127 U/mL
Main pancreatic duct >11.5 mm
Common bile duct >14.5 mm

The most common cause in these patients is a mistaken diagnosis, such as a non-pancreatic cause of pain, or inappropriate or inadequately performed pancreatic surgery (Table 34.10).

A revision drainage or resectional procedure can be selected based on the evaluation. However, nearly 10% of patients continue to experience pain despite having undergone appropriate and adequately performed revision surgery. Such patients should undergo a neuropsychiatric assessment to address neural sensitization as the cause of ongoing pain. The interventional procedures recommended as last resorts for these patients are as follows:

EUS-guided celiac ganglion block.

Total pancreatectomy.

Total pancreatectomy + Islet auto transplantation (TP-IAT).

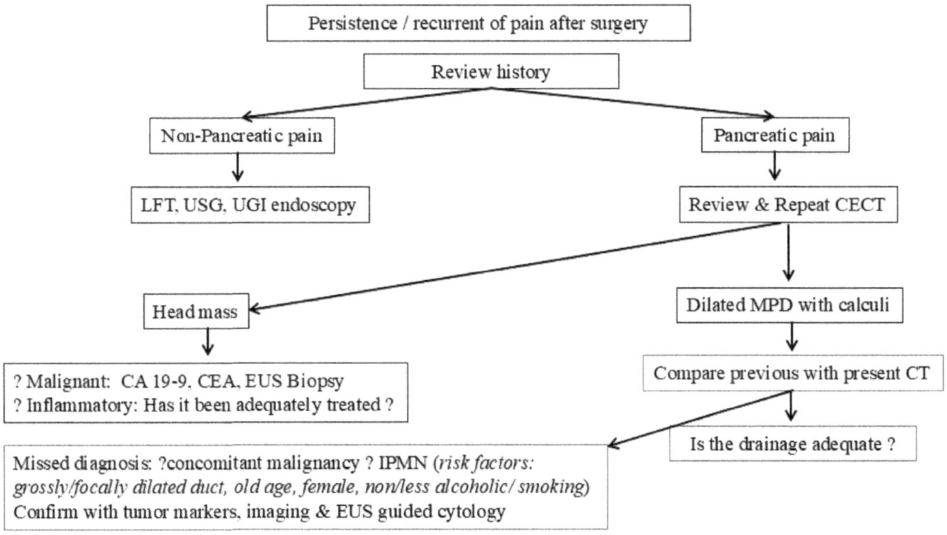

Table 34.10 Assessment of patients with ongoing or recurring pain following surgery

Key Points

- Chronic pancreatitis (CP) is characterized by recurrent inflammation resulting in progressive and irreversible disease of the pancreas. Its aetiology includes a complex relationship of environmental and genetic factors.
- Abdominal pain is the predominant symptom attributable to ductal hypertension, inflammation, nerve ischemia, and entrapment. Central and peripheral nervous system sensitization for pain may occur in longstanding symptoms and may be the reason for continued pain even after ductal drainage.
- Diagnosis is based on imaging studies like USG, CECT, and MRI-MRCP.
- CT scan & MRI provide complete morphology of the gland and the pancreatic duct, a prerequisite to planning surgery.
- Management of CP is at best palliative, directed at control of pain and management of complications.
- Medical management precedes interventional management, comprises analgesics and antioxidants.
- Interventional treatment, endoscopic or surgical, is required in 40–75% of patients.
- Endoscopic treatment is contraindicated in multiple or long pancreatic duct strictures. It comprises transpapillary dilatation of MPD strictures, stone extraction, and stenting. Lithotripsy may be required to fragment large stones to facilitate extraction.
- Surgery provides better long-term outcomes than endoscopic treatment.
- Surgical procedures are categorized into drainage procedures, resections, or a combination of both.
- Most commonly performed surgical procedures include Frey's procedure for head-dominant disease with dilated MPD, Beger's duodenum-preserving pancreatic head resection for inflammatory head mass, and pancreaticoduodenectomy for suspicion or superimposed malignancy.
- Immediate pain relief is reported in up to 90% of patients after surgery, but this drops to 35–50% on long-term follow-up.
- Inappropriate and inadequate surgery is the most common cause of failure.
- Recurrence or ongoing pain after surgery requires a thorough evaluation to determine if revision surgery is necessary.
- Despite all efforts, 10% of patients still experience pain and may be candidates for total pancreatectomy with islet auto-transplantation.

Selected Reading

1. Abdallah AA, Krige JEJ, Bornman PC. Biliary tract obstruction in chronic pancreatitis. HPB (Oxford). 2007;9:421–8.
2. Balakrishnan V, Unnikrishnan AG, Thomas V, et al. Chronic pancreatitis. A prospective nationwide study of 1086 subjects from India. JOP. 2008;9:593–600.
3. Singh VK, Yadav D, Garg PK. Diagnosis and management of chronic pancreatitis: a review. JAMA. 2019;322:2422–34.
4. Beyer G, Habtezion A, Werner J, et al. Chronic pancreatitis. Lancet. 2020;396:499–512.
5. Kichler A, Jang S. Chronic pancreatitis: epidemiology, diagnosis, and management updates. Drugs. 2020;80:1155–68.
6. Issa Y, Kempeneers MA, Bruno MJ, et al. Effect of early surgery vs endoscopy-first approach on pain in patients with chronic pancreatitis – the ESCAPE Randomized Clinical Trial. JAMA. 2020;323(237–2):47.
7. Cohen SM, Kent TS. Etiology, diagnosis, and modern management of chronic pancreatitis: a systematic review. JAMA Surg. 2023;158:652–61.
8. Maoa SH, Zou WB, Mao XT, Li ZS, Liao Z. A comprehensive review of recent advances in chronic pancreatitis. J Pancreatol. 2024;7:1. https://doi.org/10.1097/JP9.0000000000000016.
9. van Veldhuisen CL, Leseman CA, De Rijk FEM. Surgery for chronic pancreatitis across Europe (ESCOPA): prospective multicentre study. BJS. 2025;znaf068 https://doi.org/10.1093/bjs/znaf068.

Evaluation of Pancreatic Head Mass

35

S. Sankar, Govind K. Purushothaman, and Neha Sharma

Abstract

Inflammatory mass in chronic pancreatitis and adeno carcinoma (PDAC) are the two most important causes of pancreatic head mass. Anorexia, weight loss, new onset or worsening of diabetes mellitus, and elevated CA 19-9 levels indicate the development of PDAC. Imaging modalities are the mainstay of diagnosis. EUS evaluation has additional benefits of cytology and/or biopsy of the mass.

Keywords

Inflammatory head mass · Pancreatic head mass

A pancreatic head mass can be benign, inflammatory, or neoplastic in origin, and may be solid or cystic. Although a preoperative biopsy is not always necessary before planning a resection if malignancy is suspected, the surgery can be technically challenging, associated with higher morbidity, and often unnecessary in cases of inflammatory masses. Therefore, obtaining an accurate preoperative diagnosis is essential for appropriate management (Table 35.1).

However, it should be noted that in patients with chronic pancreatitis (CP), the inflammatory head mass and malignancy can coexist in about 18–40% of cases. The assessment of a pancreatic head mass begins with a thorough history-taking and clinical examination. Pancreatic ductal adenocarcinoma (PDAC), intraductal papillary mucinous neoplasm (IPMN), and serous cystadenoma (SCN) are generally more common after age sixty. Cystic neoplasms are more frequently seen in females. A history of ethanol consumption is significant for CP. Chronic pain combined with endocrine and exocrine insufficiency indicates CP. The typical profile of PDAC includes a male patient over sixty years old, who is a smoker, presenting with progressive jaundice, weight loss, and recent onset of diabetes mellitus or sudden worsening of pre-existing diabetes. Functioning neuroendocrine tumors (NETs) are characterized by symptoms related to the hormone they secrete.

Table 35.1 Common causes of pancreatic head mass

Benign/inflammatory	Neoplastic
Inflammatory head mass in CP	Pancreatic ductal adenocarcinoma
Groove pancreatitis	pNET
Focal autoimmune pancreatitis	Cystic neoplasm
Pseudocyst or true cyst	Pancreatic lymphoma
Tuberculosis	Metastatic deposit
Lymphangioma	

CP chronic pancreatitis, *pNET* pancreatic neuroendocrine tumor

Table 35.2 Assessment of the pancreatic head mass

A. Tumor markers
B. Biochemical markers
C. Pancreatic imaging
Pancreatic protocol CT scan
Magnetic resonance imaging (MRI)
Endoscopic ultrasound (EUS) and biopsy
PET scan
Intraoperative ultrasound (IOUS)
D. Intraoperative biopsy & frozen section

S. Sankar (✉)
Sri Ramachandra Medical College, Chennai, Tamil Nadu, India

G. K. Purushothaman
Paalana Institute of Medical Sciences, Palakkad, Kerala, India

N. Sharma
Max Institute of Cancer Care, Vaishali, Ghaziabad, Uttar Pradesh, India

M. Ibrarullah (ed.), *Recent Concepts in Gastrointestinal (GI) Surgery*, https://doi.org/10.1007/978-981-92-1118-0_35

35.1 Tumor Markers

- Carbohydrate antigen 19-9 (CA 19-9): Elevated CA 19-9 levels are found in nearly 80% of PDAC cases. However, it is neither specific nor diagnostic for pancreatic cancer. It can be elevated in conditions such as cholangitis, cholestasis, cirrhosis, pancreatitis, and other gastrointestinal tract-related malignancies. It may also yield a false negative result in non-secretors (those who are negative for the Lewis antigen). A corrected CA 19-9 (after biliary decompression) value greater than 500 U/ml may suggest metastatic disease. Serial monitoring is useful for assessing tumor response or progression.
- Carcinoembryonic antigen (CEA): It may be elevated in PDAC, but it is less specific.
- CA 125: May be elevated in pancreatic cancer, but its specificity is low.
- MIC-1 (Macrophage Inhibitory Cytokine-1): It is a new marker being studied for early detection and prognosis, but it has not yet been widely used in clinical practice.
- Chromogranin A (CgA): This glycoprotein serves as a tumor marker for pancreatic NETs and also helps monitor treatment response.

35.2 Biochemical Markers

Serum amylase may be persistently elevated in a pseudocyst of the pancreas associated with acute pancreatitis. Rarely, the elevation may be due to tumor-associated pancreatitis.

35.3 Pancreatic Protocol CT

The pancreatic protocol CT is a specialized imaging technique used to examine the pancreas and surrounding structures. In brief, this protocol includes: high-resolution images with very thin slices (1–2 mm) to capture critical details of the pancreas and nearby blood vessels. Intravenous contrast is administered using a power injector at a rate of 3–5 ml per second. Besides the plain images, additional scans are taken at specific times to obtain necessary information. Early arterial phase: acquired 20 seconds after contrast injection, effectively functioning as a CT angiogram to provide details of the arterial anatomy, which is vital for preoperative planning. Late arterial or pancreatic parenchymal phase: acquired 45 seconds after contrast administration. Since PDACs are usually hypovascular, they are best detected at this stage against the enhanced pancreatic tissue. Conversely, NETs are highly vascular and show bright enhancement during the arterial phase. A small NET might even resemble a vascular structure. Portal venous phase: Images are captured at 70 seconds. In PDAC, the primary tumor and liver metastases appear hypodense. Because primary and metastatic NETs are highly vascular, they demonstrate enhancement in both the arterial and venous phases (Figs. 35.1 and 35.2).

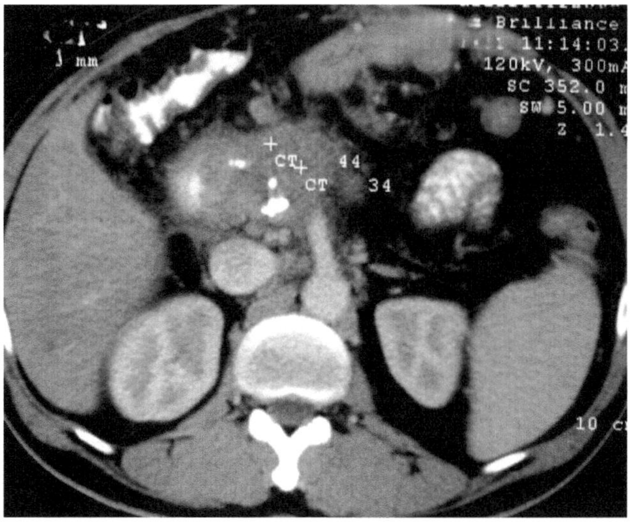

Fig. 35.1 CT scan showing pancreatic head mass in chronic calcific pancreatitis. Note the vessel encasement suggestive of superimposed malignancy

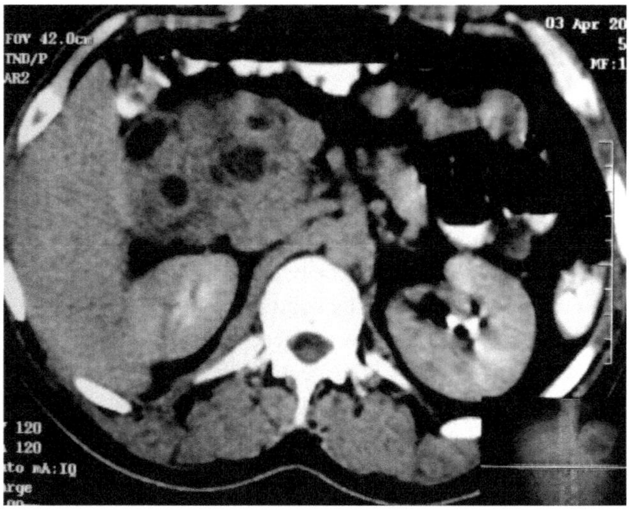

Fig. 35.2 Inflammatory mass in the head of the pancreas. Note the multiple cystic spaces inside the mass

35.4 Magnetic Resonance Imaging

The distinct advantages of MRI over CT scans are that MRI provides better soft tissue differentiation. Especially in cystic neoplasms, the septa and mural nodules are more clearly visualized with MRI. The morphology of both biliary and pancreatic ducts is better delineated for diagnosis and management. The nature of the lesion is better appreciated on diffusion-weighted imaging (Fig. 35.3).

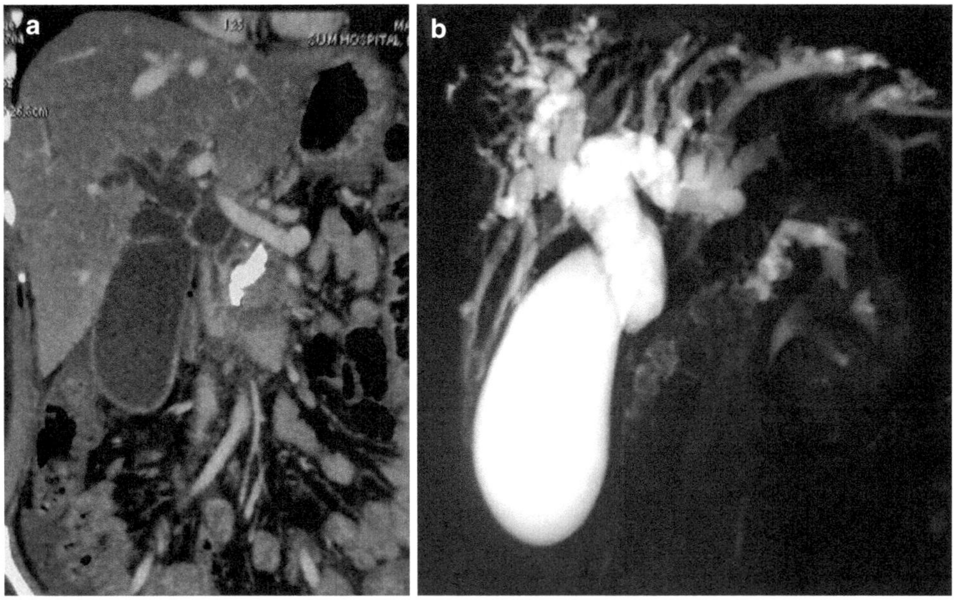

Fig. 35.3 (a) CT scan, coronal view showing calculi in the MPD. Head mass causing compression of the duodenum and the bile duct. (b) MRCP image of the same. Pancreatic duct calculi and the dilated MPD can be seen. Note the dilation of the proximal biliary tree in both images

35.5 Endoscopic Ultrasound

EUS, when available, is considered the preferred method for managing pancreatic head masses. In addition to providing more precise and more detailed images, EUS-guided needle aspiration for fluid analysis, cytology, and/or biopsy offers the well-known advantages of this approach. Image quality can be improved with the use of contrast agents like SonoVue, which contains Sulfur Hexafluoride that releases microbubbles after intravenous injection. EUS elastography is an advanced imaging technique that evaluates tissue stiffness. It provides real-time imaging during EUS, creating a color-coded elastogram (blue, green, red, and yellow) that reflects tissue stiffness, aiding in the differentiation of benign from malignant lesions.

35.6 Positron Emission Tomography Scan

PET scan is more effective in detecting metastatic disease than the primary tumor in the head of the pancreas. FDG PET can be considered a valuable option for differentiating an inflammatory mass from PDAC when chronic pancreatitis is "burned out" and lacks signs of acute inflammation. When a pancreatic protocol scan suggests NET, it is essential to stage the disease with a Gallium DOTA PET scan. Well-differentiated and low-grade NETs are best assessed with Gallium DOTA PET. However, poorly differentiated NETs may not express somatostatin receptors; in such cases, FDG PET may be the preferred investigation. Gallium DOTA and FDG PET complement each other. Since NETs are heterogeneous tumors, dual PET protocols are recommended for select cases to evaluate their biological aggressiveness in the metastatic setting. Dual imaging also aids in determining treatment options, such as peptide receptor radionuclide therapy (PRRT), chemotherapy, or a combination of both.

35.7 Fibrinogen Activation Protein Inhibitor PET (FAPI PET)

PDAC is a desmoplastic tumor characterized by abundant tumor stroma containing cancer-associated fibroblasts. FAPI PET targets this feature and is becoming a valuable tool in evaluating pancreatic head masses. Its advantages include improved tumor detection, differentiation from chronic pancreatitis, assessment of tumor extent, prognostication, and guiding therapy. A key benefit of FAPI PET is its ability to detect tumors with higher stromal content and lower metabolic activity, which may be missed on FDG PET.

35.8 Intraoperative Ultrasound

IOUS is one of the essential tools in managing functioning NET, both in terms of localization and ruling out occult lesions not detected by other modalities.

35.9 Role of Biopsy in Pancreatic Head Mass

With the advent of EUS, percutaneous biopsy with the possibility of needle track seeding is now rarely performed. However, when EUS is unavailable, an intraoperative transduodenal Tru-Cut needle biopsy of the mass can be performed for tissue cytology and frozen-section analysis. The

Table 35.3 Inflammatory head mass versus cancer head of pancreas

Criteria	Inflammatory mass	Cancer head of pancreas
Old age, anorexia, weight loss	Less common	More common
Worsening / new onset diabetes	Less likely	More likely
Serum bilirubin>10 mg/dL	Less likely	More likely
CA 19-9 > 300 IU/ml	Less likely	More likely
Imaging	Dilatation of the side branches of the pancreatic duct. *Duct penetrating sign*—smooth narrowing of the pancreatic duct and no abrupt cut-off as it traverses the pancreatic head	Peripheral migration of calcification Abrupt cut-off of the pancreatic duct Grossly dilated pancreatic duct and CBD *Double duct sign*—Simultaneous dilatation of both pancreatic and common bile ducts Vessel encasement Duodenal obstruction

positive and negative predictive values of the biopsy are approximately 95% and 50%, respectively. Differentiating PDAC in the context of chronic pancreatitis can be challenging.

35.10 Groove Pancreatitis (GP)

In groove pancreatitis (GP), the pancreato-duodenal groove is affected by chronic inflammation. It may present with pain, duodenal obstruction, biliary obstruction, or recurrent pancreatitis. Different morphological variants of GP are as follows:

- Cystic variant: Characterized by multiple tiny cystic lesions in the pancreato-duodenal groove.
- Fibrotic variant: Dense fibrotic tissue in the pancreato-duodenal groove mimics malignancy.
- Mixed variant.
- Cystic dystrophy of the duodenum: Heterotopic pancreatic tissue in the duodenal wall develops cystic dystrophy, leading to intramural cystic lesions in the duodenum.

35.11 Autoimmune Pancreatitis (AIP)

Two types of AIP have been described. Type 1 AIP is a form of IgG4-related disease that affects various organs, including the salivary glands, thyroid, kidneys, liver, biliary tract, and retroperitoneum. IgG4 levels are elevated in the blood and tissues. Type 2 AIP is associated with inflammatory bowel disease.

35.12 HISORt Criteria for Diagnosis of AIP

H—Histology.
  Presence of lymphoplasmacytic infiltrate
  Fibrosis and/or inflammatory cell infiltration.
I—Imaging.
  Typical features on CT/MRI.
  Diffuse or focal pancreatic enlargement.
  Low-density mass in the pancreas.
  Enhanced capsule-like rim.
S—Serology.
  Elevated levels of IgG4, ANA (antinuclear antibodies), and anti-lactoferrin antibodies.
O—Other organ involvement.
R—Response to steroid therapy.
  Clinical and radiological improvement within 2–4 weeks after steroid treatment.
t—Time-course of the disease.
  s

Each category is given one point. Definite diagnosis of AIP is considered with a score of 4–6.

Key Points

- Inflammatory mass in chronic pancreatitis and adenocarcinoma are the two most important causes of pancreatic head mass.
- Anorexia, weight loss, new onset or worsening of diabetes mellitus, and elevated CEA levels indicate the development of PDAC.
- Imaging modalities are the mainstay of diagnosis.
- EUS evaluation has additional benefits of cytology and/or biopsy of the mass.

Selected Reading

1. Sidharth Harindranath S, Sundaram S. Approach to pancreatic head mass in the background of chronic pancreatitis. Diagnostics. 2023;13:1797. https://doi.org/10.3390/diagnostics13101797.
2. Kirkegård J, Mortensen FV, Cronin-Fenton D. Chronic pancreatitis and pancreatic cancer risk: a systematic review and meta-analysis. Am J Gastroenterol. 2017;112:1366–72.
3. Al-Hawary MM, Kaza RK, Azar SF, et al. Mimics of pancreatic ductal adenocarcinoma. Cancer Imaging. 2013;13:342–9.

Carcinoma Pancreas

36

Aditya R. Kunte, Saneya Pandrowala, Rajesh S. Shinde, and Shailesh V. Shrikhande

Abstract

Tumors in the pancreatic head often present early with obstructive jaundice, while those in the neck and central body tend to present later and have a poorer prognosis. New-onset diabetes or unexplained, unintended weight loss should raise clinical suspicion and prompt further investigation. A contrast-enhanced CT scan (CECT) of the abdomen and pelvis is the preferred initial investigation for diagnosis and staging; MRCP is useful for cystic lesions, and FDG-PET-CT is suited for high-risk metastatic disease. Management depends on the stage of the disease (resectable, borderline resectable, locally advanced, or metastatic), with complete surgical resection offering the best chance of cure for resectable cases.

Keywords

Pancreatic cancer · Malignant obstructive jaundice · Pancreaticoduodenectomy

Approximately 170,000 new cases of pancreatic cancer are diagnosed worldwide each year, accounting for roughly 2.1% of all cancer diagnoses. Pancreatic cancer ranks as the fifth leading cause of cancer deaths among both men and women in Western countries, with over 80% of cases occurring in individuals aged 60 to 80 years. The highest incidence of pancreatic cancer in men has been reported among New Zealand Maoris, Native Hawaiians, and Black Americans, while those in India and Nigeria have the lowest rates of this disease. A diagnosis of pancreatic cancer indicates a very poor prognosis, with over 80% of cases diagnosed at an advanced, unresectable stage. The estimated 5-year survival rate for pancreatic cancer is less than 5%.

36.1 Pathogenesis and Risk Factors

Most PDAC cases originate from microscopic pancreatic intraepithelial neoplasia (PanIN), a small growth in the pancreatic ducts that is less than 5 mm. A smaller portion of PDAC cases (< 10%) develop from intraductal papillary mucinous neoplasms (IPMNs), which are larger cystic lesions within the pancreatic duct system. Precancerous pancreatic lesions are quite common, and most low- to intermediate-grade lesions do not progress to invasive cancer. However, up to 20–30% of high-grade precursor lesions (PanIN-3) can advance to invasive cancer if not removed.

The mutational landscape of PDAC includes key driver mutations and significant genetic diversity. The most frequently mutated gene in PDAC is KRAS, with activating mutations in over 90% of cases, causing abnormal cell signaling and growth. TP53 mutations, present in about 75% of pancreatic cancers, disrupt cell cycle regulation and contribute to genomic instability. Other common mutations involve the inactivation of CDKN2A and SMAD4, which are observed in approximately 30–60% of cases. Additionally, PDAC exhibits complex chromosomal rearrangements, structural alterations, and copy number variations, all of which promote its aggressive behavior and resistance to therapy. Mutations in DNA repair genes, such as BRCA1, BRCA2, and PALB2, occur in a smaller subset, particularly among cases with a family history, providing unique vulnerabilities to treatments like PARP inhibitors. Overall, the diverse mutational profile of PDAC drives its progression and presents therapeutic challenges, highlighting the importance of identifying targetable mutations for personalized treatment approaches (Table 36.1).

A. R. Kunte · S. Pandrowala · R. S. Shinde · S. V. Shrikhande (✉)
Tata Memorial Hospital, Mumbai, India

M. Ibrarullah (ed.), *Recent Concepts in Gastrointestinal (GI) Surgery*, https://doi.org/10.1007/978-981-92-1118-0_36

Table 36.1 Risk factors for pancreatic ductal adenocarcinoma

Low risk (<5-fold increase in risk)	Moderate risk (5–10-fold increase in risk)
Alcohol use (>4 drinks/day)	BRCA2 gene carrier
BMI ($\geq$30 kg/m^2)	Chronic pancreatitis
BRCA1 carrier gene	Cystic fibrosis
Chlorinated hydrocarbon exposure	Family history of pancreatic cancer in two first degree relatives
Diabetes mellitus (type 2 $\geq$ 5 years)	*High risk (more than ten-fold increase in risk)*
Familial adenomatous polyposis	Familial atypical multiple mole melanoma syndrome (FAMMM)
Family history of pancreatic cancer in one first degree relative	Family history of pancreatic cancer in at least three first, second, or third degree relatives
Hereditary non-polyposis colorectal cancer	Hereditary pancreatitis
Polycyclic aromatic hydrocarbon exposure	Peutz-Jeghers syndrome
Tobacco use	

Table 36.2 Clinical presentation of pancreatic cancer

Symptom	Pancreatic head (%)	Pancreatic body & tail (%)
Weight loss	92	100
Jaundice	82	07
Abdominal pain	72	87
Anorexia	64	33
Dark urine	63	–
Acholic stools	62	–
Nausea	45	43
Vomiting	37	37
Weakness	35	42
Constipation	–	27

36.2 Clinical Presentation (Table 36.2)

Physical examination in a patient with obstructive jaundice is usually unremarkable, except for a palpable gallbladder and signs of obstructive jaundice itself. Classic signs of advanced or metastatic disease, such as the Sister Mary Joseph's node, Virchow's node, or Blumer's shelf, are uncommon. The surgeon should look for features on physical exam that could influence further management, such as the presence of fever, significant weight loss, BMI, pallor, and tests for cardiopulmonary fitness and performance status. Pancreatic cancers linked to familial syndromes may have unique physical findings that need to be noted.

36.3 Investigations

The investigative work-up is broadly categorized into diagnostic, staging, and physical fitness evaluation pathways. Diagnosis is based on radiological imaging and imaging-guided biopsy. However, a tissue biopsy is not always necessary in all pancreatic tumors, except in certain specific clinical scenarios. Suspicion of malignancy on imaging should lead to a full metastatic work-up before beginning treatment.

Table 36.3 Pancreatic protocol CT

Parameters	Details
Scan type	Helical (preferably 64-multidetector row scanner or more)
Slice thickness	Thinnest possible (<3 mm). Preferably submillimeter (0.5–1 mm) if possible
Interval	Same as slice thickness (no gap)
Oral contrast agent	Neutral contrast (positive oral contrast may compromise the three-dimensional [3D] and maximum intensity projection [MIP] reformatted images
IV contrast	Iodine-containing contrast agents (preferably high concentration [>300 mg I/L] at an injection rate of 3–5 ml/sec. Lower concentration contrast can be used if a low Kv setting is applied
Scan acquisition timing	Pancreatic parenchymal phase at 40–50 sec and portal venous phase at 65–70 sec, following the commencement of contrast injection
Image reconstruction and display	Axial images and multiplanar reformats (in the coronal and per institutional in sagittal plane) at a 2–3 mm interval reconstruction MIP or 3D volumetric thick section for vascular evaluation (arteries and veins)

36.3.1 CT Scan

A contrast-enhanced CT scan (CECT) of the abdomen and pelvis is the initial investigation of choice for diagnosis and staging of pancreatic tumors. A pancreatic protocol CT is most helpful in delineating the pancreatic lesion and its locoregional extent (Table 36.3).

Pancreatic cancers are usually hypodense, poorly defined lesions. In contrast, neuroendocrine tumors, being highly vascular, display intense enhancement during the arterial phase. Features of locally advanced or metastatic disease include blood vessel infiltration, liver metastasis, sclerotic or lytic skeletal lesions, omental thickening or nodularity, ascites, and enlarged non-regional lymph nodes. Additional imaging features that could influence management include intrahepatic biliary dilation, cholangitic liver abscesses, liver parenchymal disease, pancreatic duct size, and the nature and size of the pancreas.

36.3.2 MRCP

MRCP is generally not part of the standard work-up for PDAC. It may be performed for the initial evaluation of obstructive jaundice before biliary stenting. MRCP plays a

Table 36.4 Indications for biliary drainage in pancreatic cancer

High serum bilirubin level (arbitrarily >15 mg/dL)
Presence of coagulopathy
Acute cholangitis
Severe malnutrition requiring optimization before surgery: Serum albumin <3 g/dL or albumin/globulin ratio reversal
Neoadjuvant therapy
Palliative: In the setting of unresectable or metastatic disease

clear role in evaluating cystic pancreatic neoplasms and IPMN specifically, where assessing the pancreatic ductal anatomy is crucial. Additionally, MRI is a superior modality for monitoring small branch-duct IPMNs.

36.3.3 PET Scan

An FDG-PET-CT has been shown to have higher sensitivity for detecting metastatic disease compared to a PET or CT scan alone. Its role in evaluating pancreatic cancer is still evolving, and it is not routinely recommended as part of the standard work-up. However, studies indicate that it influences clinical management in approximately 11% of patients, making it a useful supplement to a high-quality CT scan for those at high risk of metastatic disease. Indicators of high risk include equivocal or indeterminate imaging findings, markedly elevated CA 19-9 levels, large primary tumors, sizable regional lymph nodes, significant weight loss, and severe pain. In the neoadjuvant setting, a PET/CT scan can be considered both before and after therapy starts to assess response to systemic treatment and for restaging. Recently, FAPI-PET scans have been evaluated in pancreatic cancer imaging, with early studies showing higher sensitivity than FDG-PET scans for detecting the primary tumor, nodal disease, and metastatic lesions.

36.3.4 Biomarkers

Several biomarkers, such as carcinoembryonic antigen (CEA), pancreatic anti-oncofetal antigen, tissue polypeptide antigen, CA 125, and CA 19-9, have been studied for use in pancreatic adenocarcinoma. Among these, CA 19-9 is the most validated and clinically useful biomarker, with applications in diagnosis, prognosis, monitoring treatment response, and surveillance for recurrence. CA 19-9 is a good diagnostic marker, with sensitivity ranging from 79% to 81% and specificity from 80% to 90% in symptomatic patients. Its use in screening for pancreatic cancer is limited due to a low positive predictive value. Post-resection CA 19-9 levels have been shown to have prognostic value, with levels below 180 U/mL associated with significantly better survival. Additionally, postoperative CA 19-9 levels below 90 U/mL have been reported to predict greater benefit from adjuvant gemcitabine-based chemotherapy. Notably, about 30% of pancreatic cancers do not secrete CA 19-9, making these markers less useful in detecting recurrence for such tumors.

36.3.5 Endoscopy

Routine endoscopy is rarely needed for managing pancreatic cancers. However, certain clinical situations, like duodenal infiltration or obstruction, can be identified through routine or side-viewing endoscopy, along with therapeutic transpapillary biliary stenting for obstructive jaundice.

36.3.6 Endoscopic Ultrasound (EUS)

EUS is primarily used for diagnosis and obtaining tissue biopsies from tumors. A biopsy is indicated when there is suspicion of benign conditions like IgG4 pancreatitis or in more advanced tumors that require a trial of neoadjuvant therapy before surgical resection.

36.4 Management

36.4.1 Staging

Management of pancreatic cancers depends on the stage at diagnosis. The NCCN-based definitions regarding resectability of pancreatic cancer are essential for initial decision-making and planning treatment strategies. The first step in staging pancreatic cancer is to rule out metastases, which indicates stage IV disease. Non-metastatic pancreatic cancer is divided into three groups based on local extent and resectability: resectable, borderline resectable (BRPC), and locally advanced pancreatic cancer (LAPC). Although these stages have subtle differences, broadly speaking, resectable pancreatic cancer has no vascular involvement or minimal portal vein involvement, BRPCs have significant portal vein involvement and/or early arterial involvement, and LAPCs are unresectable tumors with extensive portal vein and hepato-mesenteric arterial involvement. Achieving complete surgical resection of locoregional disease offers the greatest chance of cure in pancreatic cancer. However, it more often requires multimodal management, including surgery, chemotherapy, and radiotherapy. Decisions regarding adjuvant therapy are based on the AJCC Staging Manual (8th edition).

Table 36.5 Definitions of grades of resectability in pancreatic cancer

Definition	Resectable	Borderline resectable	Locally advanced
AHPBA/ SSAT/SSO/ NCCN	No arterial tumor contact with CA, SMA, or CHA. No tumor contacts with the SMV or PV or ≤180° contact without vein contour irregularity.	Pancreatic head/uncinate process: Solid tumor contact with CHA without extension to CA or hepatic artery bifurcation allowing for safe and complete resection and reconstruction. Solid tumor contact with the SMA of ≤180°. Solid tumor contact with variant arterial anatomy, such as accessory RHA, replaced RHA, replaced CHA, and the origin of the replaced or accessory artery, and the presence and degree of tumor contact should be noted if present, as it may affect surgical planning. Pancreatic body/tail: Solid tumor contact with the CA of ≤180°. Solid tumor contact with the SMV or PV of >180°, contact of ≤180° with contour irregularity of the vein or thrombosis of the vein, but with a suitable vessel proximal and distal to the site of involvement allowing for safe and complete resection and vein reconstruction. Solid tumor contact with the IVC.	Head/uncinate process: Solid tumor contact >180° with the SMA or CA. Pancreatic body/tail: Solid tumor contact of >180° with the SMA or CA. Solid tumor contact with the CA and aortic involvement. Unreconstructible SMV/PV due to tumor involvement or occlusion (can be due to tumor or bland thrombus).
Alliance A021101		BR-PV (SMV/PV): Tumor–vessel interface 180 degrees or more and/or reconstructable occlusion BR-A (SMA, CA) tumor–vessel interface <180. CHA: Reconstructable, short-segment tumor–vessel interface of any degree	
JPS	MV/PV: No tumor contact or contact of <180° without occlusion SMA, CA, CHA: No tumor contact/invasion	BR-PV (SMV/PV): Tumor contact/invasion of ≥180/occluf the duodenum. SMA, CA, CHA: No tumor contact/invasion BR- A SMA, CA: Tumor contact/invasion of <180° without showing stenosis/deformity. CHA: Tumor contact/invasion without showing tumor contact/invasion of the (PHA) and/or CA. (in case of contact/invasion of both PV and peripancreatic arteries, it was graded as BR-A.)	SMV/PV: Tumor contact/invasion of 180 or more degree/occlusion, exceeding the inferior border of the duodenum. SMA, CA: Tumor contact/ invasion of 180 or more degree. CHA: Tumor contact/invasion showing tumor contact/invasion of the PHA and/or CA. AO: Tumor contact or invasion
IAP consensus	SMV/PV: No tumor contact or unilateral narrowing SMA, CA, CHA: No tumor contact	BR-PV SMV/PV: Tumor contact ≥180° or bilateral narrowing/occlusion, not exceeding the inferior border of the duodenum. SMA, CA, CHA: No tumor contact/invasion BR-A SMA, CA: Tumor contact of <180 without showing deformity/ stenosis. CHA: Tumor contact without showing tumor contact of the PHA and/or CA. Involvement of the aorta is categorized as unresectable. The presence of variant arterial anatomy is not taken into consideration.	SMV/PV: Bilateral narrowing/ occlusion, exceeding the inferior border of the duodenum. SMA, CA: Tumor contact/ invasion of ≥180 CHA: Tumor contact/invasion showing tumor contact/invasion of the PHA and/or CA. AO: Tumor contact or invasion

AHPBA Americas Hepato-Pancreato-Biliary Association, *SSAT* Society for Surgery of the Alimentary Tract, *SSO* Society of Surgical Oncology, *NCCN* National Comprehensive Cancer Network, *IAP* International Association of Pancreatology, *JPS* Japan Pancreas Society, *CA* Celiac Axis, *SMA* Superior Mesenteric Artery, *CHA* Common Hepatic Artery, *RHA* Right Hepatic Artery, *PHA* Proper Hepatic Artery, *AO* Aorta, *IVC* Inferior Vena Cava, *SMV* Superior Mesenteric Vein, *PV* Portal Vein, *BRPC* Borderline Resectable Pancreatic Cancer, *LAPC* Locally Advanced Pancreatic Cancer

36.5 Surgery

Surgery is the preferred treatment for resectable pancreatic cancer. Tumors involving the pancreatic head typically require a pancreatoduodenectomy, also known as a Whipple procedure. Those involving the body and tail require a distal pancreatectomy, radical antegrade modular pancreatosplenectomy (RAMPS), or, in some cases, a total pancreatosplenectomy.

36.5.1 Staging Laparoscopy

Pancreatic cancer, especially those of the body and tail, is associated with a high rate of occult peritoneal metastases. Staging laparoscopy can identify occult metastases in 15% to 50% of patients, depending on the selection criteria. It is recommended to use staging laparoscopy selectively in those with a higher risk for occult metastases. Suggested criteria include a preoperative CA 19-9 level of ≥150 U/mL or a primary tumor larger than 3 cm.

36.5.2 Pancreatoduodenectomy

A pancreatoduodenectomy involves surgical resection of the pancreatic head and uncinate process, as well as the duodenum, common bile duct, and proximal jejunum, along with regional lymph nodes. The distal stomach may or may not be removed depending on whether the pyloric sphincter is preserved.

36.5.2.1 Artery-First Approach

The "artery-first" or "SMA-first" approach to a pancreatoduodenectomy was devised to allow early assessment of resectability by dissecting the pancreatic head and uncinate process away from the SMA as one of the initial steps in the procedure. Separating from the SMA guarantees resectability without requiring any irreversible steps during the operation. Six common approaches to the SMA are described as follows (Fig. 36.1 and Table 36.6):

36.5.2.2 Pancreatic Anastomosis

Reconstruction of the pancreatic remnant can be performed using pancreatogastrostomy or pancreatojejunostomy, with the latter being the standard approach. Several techniques for pancreatojejunostomy have been described over the years, but no specific technique has proven to be superior.

36.5.2.3 Distal Pancreatosplenectomy/RAMPS

A distal pancreatectomy involves resection of the pancreas to the left of the gastroduodenal artery, along with the spleen, and closing the remaining pancreatic stump. Steven Strasberg and colleagues described a more extensive procedure to reduce local recurrence in distal pancreatic cancers, which involves removing all the peripancreatic tissue in front of the left renal vein and to the left of the SMA. Unlike the lateral-to-medial approach used in a distal pancreatosplenectomy, a RAMPS starts with early exposure of the left border of the SMA and division of the pancreatic neck; the subsequent dissection proceeds from medial to lateral. The procedure is called an anterior RAMPS when the left adrenal gland is preserved, and a posterior RAMPS when it is resected.

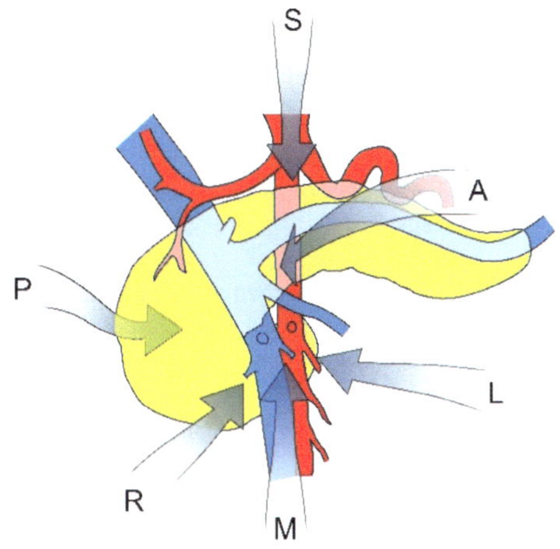

Fig. 36.1 Artery-first approaches to pancreatoduodenectomy. S: Superior approach, P: Posterior approach, R: Right/ Medial uncinate approach, M: Mesenteric approach, L: Left-posterior approach, A: Anterior approach

36.5.2.4 Extent of Lymphadenectomy

The regional lymph node basin of the pancreatoduodenal region has been divided into lymph node stations according to the Japanese classification to standardize the terminology. A standard lymphadenectomy for a pancreatoduodenectomy involves the removal of lymph node stations 5, 6, 8a, 12b1, 12b2, 12c, 13a, 13b, 14a right lateral side, 14b right lateral side, 17a, and 17b. Adequate lymph node clearance requires excising at least 15 lymph nodes. A standard template for lymphadenectomy during distal pancreatectomy involves removing lymph node stations 9, 10, 11, and 18, with a minimum of 6 lymph nodes dissected to ensure proper nodal clearance (Fig. 36.2).

36.5.3 Extended Pancreatectomy

A pancreatoduodenectomy that involves removing additional organs beyond those included in a standard pancreatoduodenectomy is called an extended pancreatoduodenectomy (Table 36.7).

Table 36.6 Artery-first approaches to pancreatoduodenectomy

Approach	Technique	Indication	Features
Posterior approach	Wide Kocher's maneuver Exposure of the SMA at its origin superior to the left renal vein. Early dissection of the posterior pancreatic capsule.	Tumors located in the posteromedial part of the head and neck.	Early identification of an anomalous RHA. Difficult in patients with peripancreatic inflammation and adhesions around the pancreatic head, and in obese patients.
Inferior supracolic/ anterior approach	SMA is approached at the inferior border of the pancreatic neck to the left of the SMV. Dissection proceeds along the right side of the SMA and abdominal aorta.	Tumors of the lower edge of the pancreas.	Facilitates retroperitoneal dissection, especially after neoadjuvant therapy. No-touch technique.
"Hanging maneuver"	Combination of the posterior and anterior technique. A tape is passed around the SMA from its origin in the aorta to its exit point in the mesentery, thus lifting the peripancreatic tissue.	Preoperative suspicion of involvement of the SMA Patients receiving neoadjuvant therapy for locally advanced disease obese patients Aberrant RHA from SMA	Constant traction and exposure of the SMA leaves both hands of the surgeon free to control the bleeding.
Inferior infracolic/ mesenteric approach	The left border of the SMA is exposed after taking down the DJ flexure. The posterior part of the SMA is dissected, with an effort to preserve the nerves on the left side. The SMV and SMA are identified from an infra-mesocolic position, and the dissection continued cranially.	Locally advanced tumors and suspected infiltration of the SMA at the origin of the aorta.	Facilitates early ligation of IPDA. Difficult to perform in obese patients, and if the origin of the SMA is high.
Right/ medial uncinate approach	The proximal jejunum is dissected, and the first jejunal loop is moved to the right of the mesenteric root. Retrograde dissection of the pancreatic head in the caudo-cranial direction. Pancreatic transection performed as the last step.	Uncinate tumors Cases with suspected involvement of the SMV or SMA.	Early ligation of the IPDA Does not allow early identification of an anomalous RHA.
Left-posterior approach	Extended Kocherization of the duodenum. Counterclockwise axial rotation of the superior mesenteric pedicle by applying leftward traction on the proximal jejunum. Ligation of the first and second jejunal arteries at the origin of the SMA. Counterclockwise rotation exposes the posterior and right faces of the SMA, allowing early ligation of the IPDA. The first jejunal vein is ligated, and the SMV is dissected. The proximal jejunum is then moved to the right of the mesenteric pedicle for the remaining dissection on the anterior side of the SMA.	Tumors of the posterior part of the pancreatic head or the uncinate process	En bloc dissection of the superior mesenteric pedicle. Early detection of aberrant RHA. Predicts the involvement of the margins in the SMA level before performing PD.
Superior approach	The hepatoduodenal ligament is dissected to expose the CHA and the gastroduodenal artery. The superior border of the pancreas is retracted caudally, and dissection proceeds caudally as far as the celiac trunk and the origin of the SMA.	Resection of tumors on the upper edge of the pancreas. Involvement of the common HA (CHA), or of the surrounding lymph nodes.	This technique is challenging to perform in patients presenting with a low origin of the SMA.

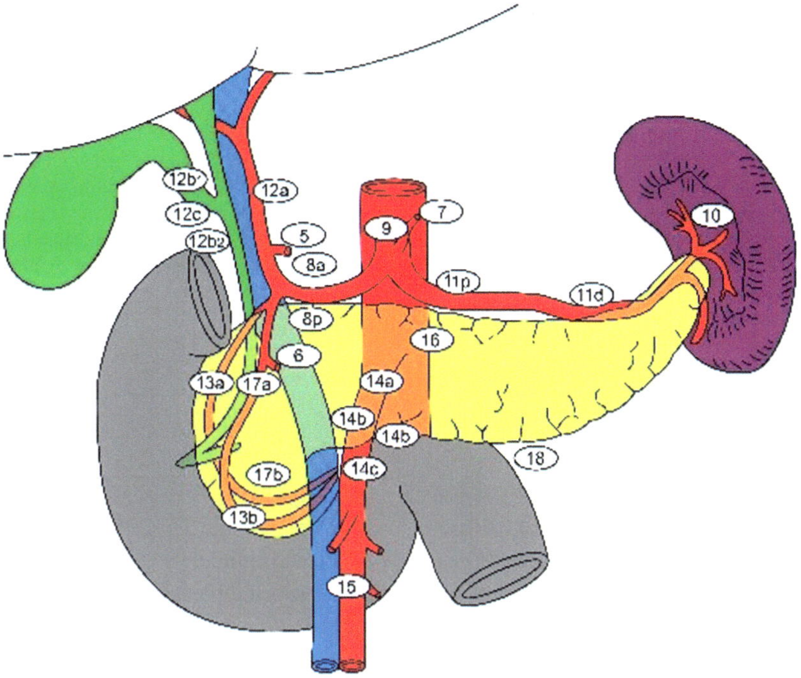

Fig. 36.2 Japanese classification of lymph node stations in pancreatic cancer

Table 36.7 The International Study Group on Pancreatic Surgery (ISGPS) definitions of standard and extended pancreatectomies

Standard procedure	Extended procedure
Pancreatoduodenectomy Resection of: Head of the pancreas and uncinate process Duodenum and the first segment of the jejunum Common bile duct and gallbladder Lymphadenectomy as per the standard template Sometimes pylorus and/or the antrum of the stomach Sometimes, elements of the transverse mesocolon, excluding relevant vasculature (e.g., limited soft tissue contiguous to the tumor but not including the colon itself).	*Pancreatoduodenectomy* Standard pancreatoduodenectomy and resection of any of the following contiguous organs: More than the antrum or distal half of the stomach Colon and/or mesocolon with relevant vascular structures of the transverse mesocolon (ileocolic, right, or middle colic vessels) Small bowel beyond the first segment of the jejunum Portal, superior mesenteric, and/or inferior mesenteric vein Hepatic artery, celiac trunk, and/or superior mesenteric artery Inferior vena cava Right adrenal gland Right kidney and/or its vasculature Liver Diaphragmatic crura
Distal pancreatectomy Resection of: Body and/or tail of the pancreas Spleen, including splenic vessels Lymphadenectomy according to the standard template Sometimes fascia of Gerota Sometimes elements of the transverse mesocolon excluding relevant vasculature (e.g., limited soft tissue adjacent to the tumor, but not including the colon itself).	*Distal pancreatectomy* Standard distal pancreatectomy plus any of the following organs involved in continuity: Any gastric resection; Colon and/or relevant vascular structures of the transverse mesocolon (middle or left colic vessels) Small bowel Portal, superior mesenteric, and/or inferior mesenteric vein Hepatic artery, celiac axis, and/or superior mesenteric artery Inferior vena cava Left adrenal gland Left kidney and/or its vasculature Diaphragmatic crura and/or diaphragm Liver

(continued)

Table 36.7 (continued)

Standard procedure	Extended procedure
Total pancreatectomy Resection of: Head, neck, body, and tail of the pancreas Duodenum and the first segment of the jejunum Common bile duct and gallbladder Spleen including splenic vessels Lymphadenectomy Sometimes the pylorus and/or the antrum Sometimes the fascia of Gerota Sometimes elements of the transverse mesocolon Exclusive of relevant vasculature (e.g., limited soft tissue adjacent to the tumor but not including the colon itself).	*Total pancreatectomy* Standard total pancreatectomy plus any of the following organs involved in continuity: More than the antrum or the distal half of the stomach; colon and/or relevant vascular structures of the transverse mesocolon (ileocolic, right, middle, or left colic vessels); small bowel beyond the first segment of the jejunum; portal, superior mesenteric, and/or inferior mesenteric veins; hepatic artery, celiac trunk, and/or superior mesenteric artery; inferior vena cava; right and/or left adrenal gland; kidney and/or its vasculature; diaphragmatic crura and/or diaphragm; liver.

36.5.3.1 Postoperative Care and Complications

The postoperative management of patients who have undergone a pancreatoduodenectomy is guided by the principles of early recovery after surgery (ERAS), which focus on early ambulation, resumption of oral feeding, and removal of invasive lines, tubes, and catheters as soon as possible. The possible complications after a pancreatoduodenectomy are as follows.

Postoperative pancreatic fistula (POPF).
Post-pancreatectomy hemorrhage.
Bile leak.
Delayed gastric emptying.
Chyle leak.
Postoperative acute pancreatitis.

Detailed management of complications following pancreatic surgery has been presented in another chapter.

36.6 Adjuvant Therapy

Adjuvant therapy is currently recommended after complete surgical resection of pancreatic cancer that is stage pT2 or higher, or involves regional lymph nodes. The most effective and preferred chemotherapy is a modified FOLFIRINOX regimen, which includes 12 cycles of 5-fluorouracil, irinotecan, and oxaliplatin. The updated 5-year results of the PROGIDE-24 trial demonstrated a median overall survival of 53.5 months with 12 cycles of adjuvant mFOLFIRINOX. Adjuvant chemoradiation is not routinely advised, as some studies have indicated a survival disadvantage. However, it may be considered if there is a positive resection margin.

36.6.1 Neoadjuvant Therapy

Neoadjuvant therapy, such as chemotherapy or chemoradiation, is indicated for borderline resectable and locally advanced pancreatic cancer. Currently, a common practice is to give four cycles of NACT, preferably FOLFIRINOX, to all BRPCs, followed by re-evaluation with imaging and tumor markers. Surgical resection is then planned after an additional 2–4 cycles of chemotherapy for tumors that show regression or remain stable. If tumors exhibit interim local disease progression, switching to a Gemcitabine-based regimen can produce a favorable response in about 30% of patients. Surgical resection is not recommended for patients with ongoing disease progression despite neoadjuvant therapy.

36.6.2 Total Neoadjuvant Therapy

Recent evidence has shown the benefits of prolonged neoadjuvant therapy, especially in locally advanced pancreatic cancers (LAPC), aiming to complete 8–12 cycles of neoadjuvant chemotherapy along with stereotactic body radiotherapy (SBRT) in select cases before surgery. Trial resection is attempted in patients with responding or stable disease who are healthy enough to undergo a major extended pancreatic resection with complex arterial and venous reconstruction.

Table 36.8 Algorithmic approach to pancreatic cancer

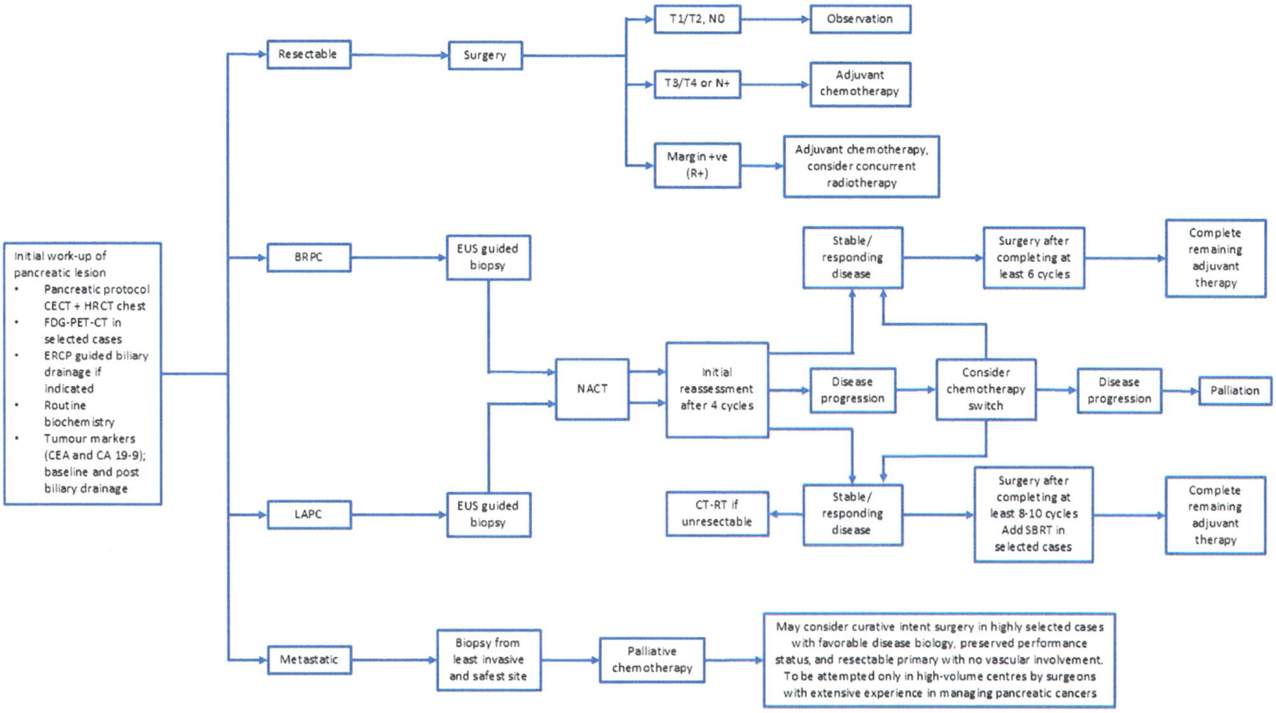

36.7 Palliation

36.7.1 Palliative Chemotherapy

Single or double agent regimens with a focus on minimizing toxicity and improving quality of life are recommended for patients with metastatic disease (Table 36.9).

36.7.2 Pain Management

One of the main symptoms of advanced pancreatic cancer is intractable pain, often caused by the tumor directly infiltrating the coeliac neural plexus. This pain can frequently be relieved through minimally invasive procedures, such as endoscopic or laparoscopic coeliac plexus neurolysis. A dedicated multidisciplinary team—including a palliative care specialist, medical oncologist, pain specialist, and pharmacist—should be involved to ensure the best possible palliative care for patients with advanced disease.

Table 36.9 Approved chemotherapy regimens for advanced pancreatic cancer

mFOLFIRINOX
NALIRIFOX
Gemcitabine + nab-paclitaxel
Gemcitabine + cisplatin
Gemcitabine
Gemcitabine + Erlotinib
Gemcitabine + Capecitabine
Gemcitabine + nab-paclitaxel + cisplatin
5-fluorouracil + Oxaliplatin
Capecitabine + Oxaliplatin
Entrectinib (if NTRK gene fusion-positive)
Larotrectinib (if NTRK gene fusion-positive)
Repotrectinib (if NTRK gene fusion-positive) 21
Selpercatinib (if RET gene fusion-positive)
Pembrolizumabj,22 (if MSI-H, dMMR, or TMB-H [≥10 Mut/Mb])
Dabrafenib + trametinib (if BRAF V600E mutation-positive) (category 2B) 19,

36.7.3 Jaundice

Obstructive jaundice caused by locally unresectable disease should be relieved by inserting metal stents because they have better patency rates than plastic stents. Relieving obstructive jaundice is essential to prevent cholangitis and to allow for palliative chemotherapy.

36.7.4 Duodenal Obstruction

Although endoscopic stenting may be attempted across the obstruction, it often proves inadequate both technically and functionally to relieve the obstruction. A surgical bypass, such as a triple bypass (gastrojejunostomy, cholecysto/choledocho-jejunostomy, and jejuno-jejunostomy), often offers significant palliation for both duodenal and biliary obstructions.

36.7.5 Bleeding

Actively bleeding tumors may be managed endoscopically with local ablation or adrenalin injection in cases of surface mucosal bleeding. However, endoscopy alone rarely achieves lasting hemostasis in such tumors, and invasive angiography with embolization is often necessary. Hemostatic radiotherapy is also a viable option in these cases. Surgical intervention for palliative resection of the bleeding tumor is generally not recommended but may be considered as a last resort in highly selected patients.

36.8 Emerging Therapies

36.8.1 Intraoperative Radiotherapy

Intraoperative radiotherapy (IORT) is a specialized treatment method that provides a single, high dose of radiation directly to the tumor bed during surgery. IORT is given immediately after tumor removal or, in unresectable cases, directly to the tumor while protecting surrounding healthy tissues. The purpose of IORT is to enable precise delivery of a high radiation dose to the tumor bed, targeting local microscopic disease and thereby reducing the risk of local recurrence. Studies show that IORT improves local control rates compared to surgery alone, with reductions in local recurrence ranging from 20 to 30%. Advantages of IORT include the following:

- Targeted Delivery: Enables precise radiation to the tumor bed with minimal exposure to surrounding structures like the duodenum, stomach, and spinal cord.
- Dose Escalation: Allows for higher radiation doses than external beam radiotherapy (EBRT) alone.
- Timing: Eliminates the delay caused by postoperative wound healing before starting radiotherapy.
- Palliation: IORT effectively relieves pain, with symptom control reported in up to 80% of patients with unresectable cases.

The limitations of IORT are as follows:

- Complexity: Requires specialized equipment and expertise.
- Limited effectiveness for distant metastases: Pancreatic cancer often spreads systemically, reducing the impact of local control on overall survival.
- Potential toxicity: Even with shielding, there is a risk of damage to nearby tissues, which can lead to complications like gastrointestinal ulcers or fistulas.

36.8.2 Irreversible Electroporation (IRE)

Irreversible electroporation (IRE) is an innovative, minimally invasive technique that utilizes high-voltage electrical pulses to create permanent pores in cell membranes, resulting in cell death while preserving surrounding structures, such as blood vessels and ducts. This makes it especially suitable for treating pancreatic cancer, particularly locally advanced, unresectable tumors. Mechanism of action includes the following:

- Electroporation: High-voltage, short-duration electric pulses disrupt the cell membrane, causing apoptosis or necrosis.
- Non-Thermal Effect: Unlike traditional thermal ablation techniques (e.g., radiofrequency or microwave ablation), IRE does not depend on heat, thus preserving critical structures such as blood vessels and bile ducts.
- Immune Modulation: IRE may trigger an anti-tumor immune response by releasing tumor antigens.

Studies show that local progression-free survival (PFS) lasts 6–12 months, with lower local recurrence rates after IRE. Median overall survival (OS) in LAPC ranges from 17 to 27 months when IRE is combined with chemotherapy. It also effectively relieves pain and improves the quality of life in many patients.

IRE can be performed percutaneously or during laparotomy. It spares vital structures, making it suitable for anatomically challenging pancreatic tumors. It may also boost systemic anti-tumor immune responses. However, IRE addresses local disease but does not impact distant metastatic spread, requires specialized training, and precise imaging guidance. Known complications include vascular thrombosis, pancreatitis, bile leak, or perforation. Rare but serious events comprise cardiac arrhythmias caused by proximity to major vessels.

Key Points

- Pancreatic cancer has a low 5-year survival rate (less than 5%), with over 80% of cases diagnosed at an advanced, unresectable stage.
- Tumors in the pancreatic head often present early with obstructive jaundice, while those in the neck and central body tend to present later and have a poorer prognosis. New-onset diabetes or unexplained, unintended weight loss should raise clinical suspicion and prompt further investigation.
- A contrast-enhanced CT scan (CECT) of the abdomen and pelvis is the preferred initial investigation for diagnosis and staging; MRCP is useful for cystic lesions, and FDG-PET-CT is suited for high-risk metastatic disease.
- CA 19-9 is the most clinically useful biomarker for diagnosing, predicting, monitoring treatment response, and surveillance of recurrence in pancreatic adenocarcinoma.
- Management depends on the stage of the disease (resectable, borderline resectable, locally advanced, or metastatic), with complete surgical resection offering the best chance of cure for resectable cases.
- Neoadjuvant therapy (chemotherapy or chemoradiation) is recommended for borderline resectable and locally advanced pancreatic cancer to enhance resectability and improve outcomes.
- Palliation for advanced pancreatic cancer focuses on managing symptoms like pain (often with celiac plexus neurolysis), jaundice (stenting), and other issues, with various chemotherapy regimens available.
- Emerging therapies like Intraoperative Radiotherapy (IORT) and Irreversible Electroporation (IRE) aim to improve local control in challenging cases by providing targeted delivery and non-thermal ablation, respectively, although they have limitations concerning distant metastases.

Selected Reading

1. National Comprehensive Cancer Network. NCCN Clinical Practice Guidelines in Oncology. Pancreatic Adenocarcinoma. NCCN. Available athttps://www.nccn.org/professionals/physician_gls/pdf/pancreatic.pdf. Version 1.2024 — December 13, 2023.
2. Tempero MA. NCCN guidelines updates: pancreatic cancer. J Natl Compr Canc Netw. 2019;17(5.5):603–5.
3. Cancer of the Pancreas Treatment Recommendations. European Society for Medical Oncology. Available athttps://www.esmo.org/guidelines/guidelines-by-topic/gastrointestinal-cancers/pancreatic-cancer/eupdate-cancer-of-the-pancreas-treatment-recommendations. March 15, 2019.

Neuroendocrine Tumors of the Pancreas

37

Prashant Kumar and Sadiq S. Sikora

Abstract

Pancreatic neuroendocrine tumors (pNETs) represent a highly heterogeneous group of endocrine tumors that develop from the islet cells of the pancreas. MEN1, ATRX, DAXX, and mTOR pathway genes are involved in the pathogenesis of pNETs. On histology, the tumor is classified as well-differentiated or poorly differentiated and graded according to mitotic figures and the Ki-67 index. Functioning tumors are rarely malignant, release hormones, and manifest with hormone-based symptoms. CECT, MRI, EUS, PET-CT, and octreotide scintigraphy are used for diagnosis, evaluation of tumor characteristics, resectability, metastasis, and functional status. Incidentally detected tumors less than 2 cm in diameter are managed expectantly. Symptomatic and large tumors over 2 cm require formal resection.

Keywords

NET pancreas · Neuroendocrine tumor

Neuroendocrine tumors of the pancreas (pNETs) are a highly diverse group of endocrine tumors that originate from the islet cells of the pancreas. They display a wide range of biological behaviors, histological features, and responses to treatment. pNETs are a common type of neuroendocrine tumor and fall under the broader category of gastro-entero-pancreatic neuroendocrine tumors (GEP-NETs). It is important to note that pNETs should not be confused with primitive neuroectodermal tumors (PNETs).

P. Kumar · S. S. Sikora (✉)
Sakra World Hospital, Bangalore, India

37.1 Epidemiology

pNETs account for about 2% of all pancreatic cancers. Although they are relatively uncommon, the number of pNET cases has been steadily increasing over time. Data from the Surveillance, Epidemiology, and End Results (SEER) Program in the United States (2000–2016) shows that the annual incidence rate rose from 0.27 to 1.00 per 100,000 people. The median overall survival (OS) for patients with pNETs has also improved significantly. According to SEER data, the median OS was 68 months, with 5-year OS rates of 83%, 67%, and 28% for localized, regional, and metastatic disease, respectively. Notably, survival has improved across all stages compared to the past decade. In India, data from a multicenter longitudinal NET registry (2016) indicates that most patients with pNETs are symptomatic, with only 24% of cases being asymptomatic. Recently, detection rates of pNETs have increased, likely due to greater awareness, better imaging techniques, and the implementation of preventive healthcare programs. Early detection has played a crucial role in improving outcomes for patients with pNETs.

37.2 Genetics and Pathogenesis

Recent gene-sequencing studies have shed light on the oncogenic pathways involved in the development of pancreatic neuroendocrine tumors (pNETs) and pancreatic neuroendocrine carcinomas (pNECs). These studies have advanced research into identifying potential therapeutic targets and clarifying prognoses (Table 37.1).

Mutations in the ATRX and DAXX genes cause a phenotype known as alternative lengthening of telomeres (ALT), which results in increased cell proliferation. Mutations in DAXX also reduce TP53 levels, further promoting tumor growth. pNETs with ATRX and DAXX mutations are linked to intermediate and high-grade tumors and tend to have a poor prognosis. The hypoxia-inducible factor-1 (HIF-1) pathway is a key regulator of these genes and is often abnormal in pNETs.

M. Ibrarullah (ed.), *Recent Concepts in Gastrointestinal (GI) Surgery*, https://doi.org/10.1007/978-981-92-1118-0_37

Table 37.1 Genes involved in the pathogenesis of pNETs

MEN1: A tumor suppressor gene encoding the menin protein
ATRX: A chromatin-remodeling complex gene
DAXX: A death domain-associated gene
mTOR pathway genes: PTEN, PIK3CA, and TSC2

Table 37.2 Histology of neuroendocrine tumors

Well-differentiated neuroendocrine tumors	Poorly differentiated neuroendocrine carcinomas
Clumped chromatin (salt and pepper) nuclei	Diffuse sheets or solid nests of markedly atypical malignant cells with small-cell or large-cell morphology
Cellular uniformity with central ovoid nuclei, rarely showing necrosis Organoid architecture: Ribbons, trabeculae, nesting, glandular, pseudoacinar patterns	Abundant mitoses and apoptotic bodies, frequent necrosis
Amyloid deposition: Commonly observed in insulinomas	

37.3 Histopathology

Histopathology is essential in diagnosing and classifying pNETs. It helps differentiate well-differentiated neuroendocrine tumors from poorly differentiated neuroendocrine carcinomas, which have different clinical behaviors and treatment options (Table 37.2).

Immunohistochemical (IHC) analysis is an essential part of evaluating and confirming the neuroendocrine nature of the tumor, aiding in distinguishing it from other pancreatic neoplasms. These stains usually include synaptophysin and chromogranin. The histopathological features of pNET, along with the Ki67 index, help determine the tumor grade, which is a key prognostic factor.

37.4 Classification Systems

Several classification systems for pNETs exist, and a few are discussed below (Table 37.3):

Mixed neuroendocrine-non-neuroendocrine neoplasms (MiNENs) are a rare subtype of pNETs characterized by the presence of both neuroendocrine (NE) and non-neuroendocrine (NNE) components. The NNE component is most often an adenocarcinoma, but may also include other epithelial tumors. For a diagnosis of MiNEN, each component must constitute at least 30% of the overall tumor volume (Table 37.4).

Table 37.3 The 2017 World Health Organization (WHO) classification of neuroendocrine neoplasms (NENs), based on the mitotic rates and Ki-67 index

Grade (G)	Mitotic rate (per 10 HPF)	Ki-67 index[a]
Well-differentiated NENs		
NET G 1	<2	<3
NET G 2	2–20	3–20
NET G 3	>20	>20
Poorly differentiated NENs		
NEC G 3	>20	>20
Small-cell type		
Large-cell type		
MiNEN		

HPF high-power field, *MiNEN* mixed neuroendocrine and non-neuroendocrine neoplasm

[a] Ki-67 protein exists in cells that are actively dividing. The Ki-67 index indicates the percentage of tumor cells that express this protein. This index serves as a marker of tumor cell proliferation. A higher Ki-67 index indicates a faster-growing tumor and can be linked to a worse prognosis

Table 37.4 Classification by functional characteristics

Type	Prevalence	Malignancy	Characteristics
Functioning	10–30%	Rare	Produce hormones that lead to specific symptoms. Many subtypes exist. The primary tumor is often small
Nonfunctioning	68–90%	Common	Do not produce hormones. The primary tumor is usually large

The American Joint Committee on Cancer (AJCC) 8th Edition: TNM staging system for pNETs is used to assess the extent of disease and guide treatment decisions. The system relies on the primary tumor (T), regional lymph nodes (N), and distant metastasis (M).

While most pNETs are sporadic, about 10% are caused by inherited syndromes. These include multiple endocrine neoplasia type 1 (MEN1), multiple endocrine neoplasia type 4 (MEN4), von Hippel-Lindau disease (VHL), neurofibromatosis type 1 (NF1), and tuberous sclerosis complex (TSC). The following table summarizes these syndromes.

37.5 Inherited Disorders Associated with pNETs (Table 37.5)

Table 37.5 Inherited disorders associated with pNETs

Syndrome	Associated clinical features	Chromosomal location	pNET type
Multiple endocrine neoplasia type 1 (MEN1)	Primary hyperparathyroidism, pituitary tumors	11q13	Gastrinoma, insulinoma nonfunctional tumors
Multiple endocrine neoplasia type 4 (MEN4)	Hyperparathyroidism, pheochromocytoma	12p13.1	Gastrinoma
Von Hippel-Lindau disease (VHL)	Pheochromocytomas (often bilateral), retinal and cerebellar hemangioblastomas, renal cell carcinoma	3p25–26	Various nonfunctional tumors, including cystic tumors
Neurofibromatosis type 1 (NF1)	Neurofibromas, café au lait spots, pheochromocytomas	17q11.2	Somatostatinoma, various nonfunctional tumors
Tuberous sclerosis complex (TSC)	Cardiac rhabdomyomas, renal cysts, angiomyolipoma	9q33.13 and 16p13	

37.6 Clinical Features

Nonfunctional tumors are the most common type of pNETs (25–75%). They are mostly malignant in 60% of cases and are often discovered incidentally. Nonfunctional pNETs are spread throughout the pancreas. Rarely, these tumors may cause symptoms such as weight loss, back pain, jaundice, or cachexia.

Functional tumors lead to syndromes based on hormones released by the tumor; salient points are listed in the Table 37.6.

Table 37.6 Clinical features of functioning pNETs

Tumor type	Description	Location	Malignancy	Symptoms	Diagnosis
Insulinoma	Most common functioning pNET; typically small, solitary, hypervascular	Any part of the pancreas	Usually, benign	Whipple triad: Neuroglycopenic symptoms (sweating, palpitations, confusion), low blood glucose (<45 mg/dL), and high insulin (>5 microU/L), symptom relief with glucose	72-hour fast with glucose and insulin level, elevated C-peptide (>0.7 ng/mL)
Gastrinoma	Secretes gastrin, causing Zollinger-Ellison syndrome (ZES)	Gastrinoma triangle	Mostly malignant (>50% metastatic at presentation)	Abdominal pain, diarrhea (improves with nasogastric aspiration)	Basal acid output >10 meq/h, fasting gastrin >1000 pg/mL, positive secretin test (gastrin rise >200 pg/mL)
Glucagonoma	Secretes glucagon	Body and tail of pancreas	Predominantly malignant (60–70%)	'4Ds' syndrome: Diabetes, dermatitis (necrolytic migratory erythema), depression, DVTs	Fasting glucagon >500 pg/mL
VIPoma	Secretes vasoactive intestinal peptide (VIP)	Body and tail of pancreas	Usually, benign	Verner-Morrison syndrome (WDHA): Watery diarrhea, hypokalemia, achlorhydria	WDHA syndrome; fasting VIP >60 pmol/L
Somatostatinoma	Secretes somatostatin	Head of pancreas	Often malignant (70%) with metastasis (70%)	Diabetes, cholelithiasis, hypochlorhydria, steatorrhea, anemia	Fasting somatostatin >14 pmol/L

37.7 Multiple Endocrine Neoplasia Type 1 (MEN1) and pNETs

MEN1 is a hereditary syndrome characterized by tumors developing in multiple endocrine glands, including parathyroid adenomas, pituitary tumors, and pNETs. pNETs associated with MEN1 are often nonfunctional, with gastrinomas and insulinomas being the most common subtypes. Patients with pNETs and a family history of MEN1, hyperparathyroidism, renal stones, prolactinomas, or Cushing syndrome should be evaluated for MEN1. Additionally, young patients with primary hyperparathyroidism caused by four-gland adenomas should be screened for pNETs.

In MEN1 patients with primary hyperparathyroidism and Zollinger-Ellison syndrome (ZES), surgery to treat hyperparathyroidism by removing three and a half parathyroid glands should be performed before pancreatic surgery. This approach can significantly improve the signs and symptoms of ZES. MEN1 is associated with a high risk of developing multiple pNETs throughout the pancreas. While removing all tumors was formerly recommended, current strategies focus on removing larger tumors (>2 cm) and using ablative techniques for smaller lesions. This approach helps reduce the extent of surgery and decreases potential complications. For families at high risk of developing MEN1, genetic counseling and screening programs should be offered. These programs can help identify at-risk individuals and enable early diagnosis and treatment.

37.8 Tumor Markers in pNETs

In functional pNETs, specific tumor markers related to secreted hormones can be used to evaluate disease activity. For instance, patients with insulinomas can monitor their insulin levels, while those with gastrinomas can track gastrin levels. In nonfunctioning pNETs, nonspecific tumor markers like chromogranin A (CgA), 5-hydroxyindoleacetic acid (5-HIAA), and pancreatic polypeptide (PP) are helpful for diagnosis. CgA is a secretory protein found in NET cells, with a sensitivity of 75% and a specificity of 95% for detecting pNETs. The CgA level helps evaluate treatment response and identify recurrence. Additionally, CgA levels can be affected by various factors, including somatostatin analog therapy, proton pump inhibitor (PPI) use, and renal failure. In cases of abnormal CgA levels, retesting may be needed with short-term follow-up, especially after stopping PPI intake for 2 weeks.

Table 37.7 Anatomical and functional imaging of pNETs

Anatomical studies	Functional studies
Ultrasonography (USG)	Octreoscan
Contrast-enhanced CT scan (CECT)	Gallium DOTATOC PET, DOTATATE, DOTANOC
Magnetic resonance imaging (MRI)	^{64}Cu Dotatate
Endoscopic ultrasound (EUS)	FDG PET
	Ga-68 DOTA-Exendin-4

37.9 Imaging

Imaging plays a vital role in diagnosing, staging, and monitoring pNETs. Small tumors are often incidentally found during imaging performed for other reasons. Various techniques, including CT, MRI, ultrasound, PET-CT, and octreotide scintigraphy, are used to evaluate tumor features, resectability, and metastatic spread (Table 37.7).

37.9.1 Anatomical Imaging

USG has limited sensitivity and specificity for detecting pNETs, especially small lesions. It is mainly used to identify potential liver metastases.

CECT is a widely used imaging modality for the initial detection of pNETs, with a sensitivity of up to 90%. It provides excellent spatial resolution, helping to evaluate tumor size, location, and the extent of disease. CT scans usually include non-enhanced images to identify calcifications or hemorrhage, along with post-contrast images taken during the arterial, pancreatic, and portal venous phases. On pre-contrast CT, pNETs often appear as well-rounded, isodense, or slightly hypodense lesions with a homogeneous pattern and smooth margins. During the arterial phase, they typically show hyperenhancement and display a slow washout, appearing hyperdense or isodense compared to the surrounding tissue in the portal phase. Involvement of the main pancreatic duct, accompanied by upstream duct dilation, is uncommon and may indicate the presence of adenocarcinoma. CT is crucial for staging pNETs, including the evaluation of lymph node metastases and distant metastases to organs such as the liver, peritoneum, bone, and lungs (Figs. 37.1 and 37.2).

MRI is a valuable imaging tool for detecting and characterizing pNETs, especially when CT findings are uncertain or inconclusive. With its superior soft tissue contrast and diffusion-weighted imaging (DWI) capabilities, MRI provides detailed information about tumor morphology and fea-

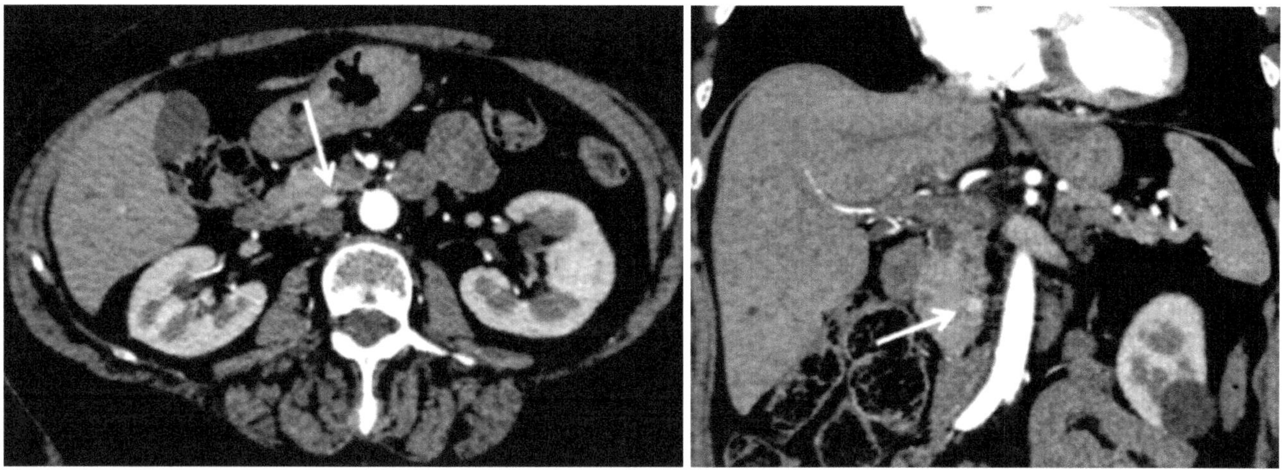

Fig. 37.1 CECT abdomen cross sectional axial view (left) and a coronal view (right) showing a small intensely enhancing tumor on arteril phase (white arrow) in the uncinate process

Fig. 37.2 CECT image. (**a**) (coronal image), (**b**) (axial image showing a large pNET (while arrow) demonstrating mixed enhancing lesion with necrosis in the head of the pancreas

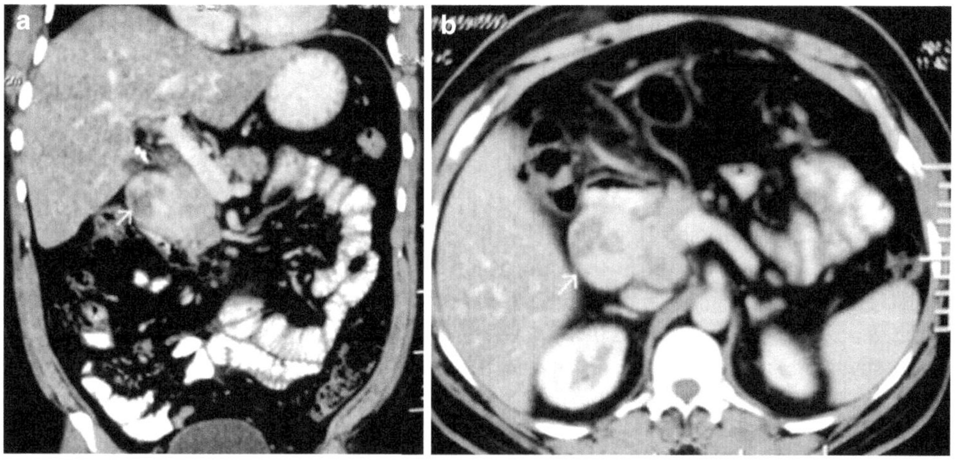

tures. It has a sensitivity of 80% and a specificity of 80–100% for detecting pNETs. On MRI, pNETs typically appear as T1 hypo-isointense lesions within the hyperintense pancreatic parenchyma. These lesions are often T2 hyperintense or less hypointense and show hyperenhancement during the arterial phase with a slow washout, similar to their appearance on CT. MRCP can assist in assessing the involvement of the pancreatic duct or common bile duct. DWI can evaluate tumor cellularity and necrosis. pNETs typically exhibit a restrictive DWI pattern, which can aid in differentiating them from other pancreatic lesions. DWI is especially useful for patients who cannot receive contrast medium. MRI may also help in monitoring patients with MEN-1 to reduce radiation exposure from repeated CT scans.

EUS is a more effective imaging technique for detecting pNETs, particularly small tumors such as insulinomas and gastrinomas. It is the preferred imaging study when other non-invasive methods are unable to diagnose pNETs. Preoperative EUS evaluation can significantly boost the detection rate of pNETs compared to CT scans. The sensitivity of EUS ranges from 70% to 90%, with nearly 100% specificity. EUS is more precise in imaging the head of the pancreas than the body or tail. False-positive results can occur due to accessory spleens and intrapancreatic lymph nodes. Typically, pNETs on EUS appear as uniformly hypoechoic masses with clear, well-defined borders. Contrast-enhanced harmonic EUS can aid in distinguishing pNETs from other lesions, as they usually show rapid and strong enhancement during the early arterial phase. Using EUS with fine-needle aspiration or biopsy is essential for obtaining tissue samples for histological confirmation. Intraoperative ultrasound (IOUS) is recommended as an additional method to locate insulinomas, which can be done laparoscopically or during open surgery. On IOUS, insulinomas generally appear as sonolucent areas compared to the echodense normal pancreas.

37.10 Functional Imaging in pNETs

Somatostatin receptors (SSTRs) are present in a significant portion of pNETs (50–80%), making them important targets for functional imaging. Nuclear imaging techniques, such as somatostatin receptor scintigraphy and positron emission tomography (PET), can be used to locate primary disease, perform presurgical staging, conduct theranostic assessments, and carry out post-treatment evaluations.

Somatostatin analogs (SSAs) bind strongly to specific SSTR subtypes, mainly sst2, sst3, and sst5. These receptors are often overexpressed on pNET cells, making them good targets for radiolabeled SSAs. In the past, somatostatin receptor scintigraphy with ^{111}In-pentetrotide (OCTREOSCAN) was the first molecular imaging technique. ^{68}Ga-labeled SSAs, combined with PET, offer better spatial resolution and sensitivity than traditional scintigraphy. PET/CT also allows for simultaneous metabolic imaging with ^{18}F-fluorodeoxyglucose (^{18}F-FDG). ^{68}Ga-DOTA-Exendin-4 PET/CT has shown high accuracy in locating insulinomas, making it a useful tool when traditional imaging cannot identify the primary tumor.

Dual-tracer imaging combining SSR PET/CT and FDG PET/CT can provide additional information about tumor features. Results may vary from lesions that are highly positive on SSR PET/CT but negative on FDG PET/CT (well-differentiated disease) to those that are negative on SSR PET/CT but highly positive on FDG PET/CT (poorly differentiated disease). For G1 and G2 pNETs, DOTA PET is recommended due to its high sensitivity in detecting these lower-grade tumors. Conversely, FDG PET is advised for G3 pNETs to assess their increased metabolic activity.

37.11 Biopsies of pNETs

Endoscopic ultrasound (EUS)-guided core biopsies are feasible for pNETs located in the head of the pancreas. Core biopsies are generally preferred over fine-needle aspiration (FNA), although cytology can provide a diagnosis in up to 97% of cases. Additionally, cytology can effectively distinguish between grade 3 and grade 1 tumors with a reliability of 83%. Biopsies serve to: i. confirm the diagnosis and grade of the tumor, aiding in choosing appropriate imaging and treatment strategies; ii. identify non-neuroendocrine components (MiNEN); and iii. Perform immunohistochemistry (IHC) for synaptophysin and chromogranin, which are markers of neuroendocrine differentiation.

Table 37.8 Factors favoring active surveillance in nonfunctioning pNETs

Less than 2 cm in size
Away from the pancreatic duct (no mass effect, 2–3 mm away from the duct)
Low grade (NET grade 1)
Elderly patients with multiple comorbidities

37.12 Treatment

Based on anatomy, tumor biology, and patient characteristics, the best treatment plan should be determined through a multidisciplinary team discussion. There is debate are debates about incidentally found pNETs smaller than 2 cm, especially when the tumor seems benign and shows slow progression. The potential risks of surgery should be carefully balanced with the possible benefits (Table 37.8).

37.12.1 Surgical Resection

Surgical resections, along with regional lymphadenectomy, remain the standard of care for pNETs, even when major vascular reconstruction is necessary. Studies have shown that surgery can significantly improve survival outcomes, even in patients with metastatic disease. Utilizing intraoperative localization techniques with IOUS—either through open or minimally invasive (laparoscopic/robotic) methods—subsequent surgeries should be performed based on lesion location.

- *Distal body and tail lesions*: Distal pancreatectomy.
- *Head lesions*: Whipple's pancreaticoduodenectomy.
- *Central body lesions:* Median pancreatectomy.

Enucleation should be considered selectively, especially for superficial pNETs. In cases of multiple lesions, the smaller ones can be managed with ablative techniques or active surveillance instead of total pancreatectomy. For functional pNETs, preoperative medical management is often necessary to address hormonal imbalances and metabolic disturbances. This may include correcting fluid and electrolyte imbalances and stabilizing blood glucose. Once these underlying conditions are controlled, surgical resection can be considered. Prophylactic cholecystectomy may be performed during surgery for pNETs to prevent biliary gallstones caused by somatostatin analogs and ischemic cholecystitis after chemoembolization. Carcinoid crisis is a rare postoperative complication, mainly linked to foregut and midgut NETs. However, it is uncommon after surgery for pNET. When it occurs, treatment with intravenous somatostatin and vasopressors is recommended.

37.12.2 Surgical Management of Metastatic pNET

The liver is the most common site of distant metastases in pNETs. The ability to surgically remove liver metastases greatly influences treatment choices. For liver metastases that can be removed, combined surgery to excise both the primary tumor and all hepatic metastases is recommended. This approach can improve survival and slow disease progression. In cases where liver metastases cannot be removed, the decision to resect the primary tumor remains. For symptomatic, advanced pNETs with liver-dominant disease, palliative resection of the primary tumor and hepatic debulking (removing up to 90% of the tumor burden) may be an option. This can relieve symptoms and prolong survival. A combination of surgery, radiologic procedures, and systemic therapies can often improve outcomes for patients with metastatic pNETs. Liver transplantation might be an option for patients with isolated neuroendocrine liver metastases, but it is not yet considered standard of care and has strict eligibility requirements (Table 37.9).

Despite surgical interventions, disease recurrence is common in patients with metastatic pNETs. Ongoing management with systemic therapies and surveillance is often necessary.

37.12.3 Interventional Radiology for pNETs

Interventional radiology techniques play a key role in managing pNETs, especially those with liver metastases. These approaches help control symptoms, enhance survival, and reduce tumor size. Needle ablation and liver-directed catheter-based treatments are commonly used to target liver metastases. With supportive care alone, the 5-year survival rate for patients with unresectable liver metastases is usually low (0–22%). However, liver-directed embolization has significantly increased 5-year survival rates to over 60%. The success of interventional radiology-based therapies is attributed to the highly vascular nature of pNET liver metastases. The hepatic arterial supply to the lesions can be targeted using various techniques:

- Bland embolization: Using embolic particles to block the tumor's blood supply.
- Classical transarterial chemoembolization: Combining chemotherapy drugs with an ethiodized oil emulsion.
- Drug-eluting bead transarterial chemoembolization: Using microspheres loaded with chemotherapy drugs.
- Radioembolization: Using yttrium-90 (^{90}Y) labeled microspheres to deliver radiation directly to the tumor.

Ablative techniques such as radiofrequency ablation, microwave ablation, cryoablation, and irreversible electroporation are commonly used for liver metastases smaller than 5 cm. Larger or multiple metastases may require catheter-based arterial treatments.

Table 37.9 Eligibility criteria for liver transplantation in isolated neuroendocrine liver metastases

Age < 55 years
Primary tumor already removed with a curative resection
Stable disease for at least 6 months before transplantation
Ki-67 < 10%
Low-grade and well-differentiated tumor (G1, G2)
Absence of extrahepatic disease
No extrahepatic combined resection

37.12.4 Somatostatin Analogs (SSA)

SSAs are synthetic derivatives of somatostatin. They are the first-line treatment for well-differentiated advanced pNETs, aimed at managing symptoms caused by hormone overexpression from these tumors.

- *Octreotide*: Available as a short-acting subcutaneous injection or a monthly long-acting repeatable (LAR) injection.
- *Lanreotide: Administered as an injectable autogel every 28 days.*

SSAs are designed to have a longer half-life than native somatostatin (1–3 minutes), enabling sustained therapeutic use. These analogs bind to somatostatin receptors, which are often overexpressed on pNET cells, leading to their inhibition. The PROMID trial demonstrated that long-acting octreotide can extend the time to tumor progression compared to placebo in patients with midgut NETs (excluding pNETs). The CLARINET study showed that lanreotide can also improve progression-free survival (PFS) in patients with well or moderately differentiated nonfunctioning NETs, including pNETs. While they may not significantly impact overall survival, they can help control tumor growth, reduce symptom severity, and improve quality of life for patients with pNETs.

37.12.5 Targeted Therapy for pNETs

Targeted therapy for pNETs aims to block specific molecular pathways involved in tumor growth and progression. Mammalian target of rapamycin (mTOR) regulates cell proliferation by participating in multiple signaling pathways. The mTOR signaling pathway, often active in tumors, regulates not only gene transcription and protein synthesis crucial for cell proliferation and immune cell differentiation but also plays a key role in tumor metabolism. The primary targets of therapy for pNETs are the mTOR pathway and the tyrosine kinase pathway. Everolimus, an oral mTOR inhibitor, has shown significant antiproliferative effects on NETs in several clinical trials. The RADIANT trials demonstrated an increase in PFS in patients with NETs treated with Everolimus compared to those treated with placebo. However, the overall survival benefit was similar to that of somatostatin analogs. Sunitinib malate is a multitargeted tyrosine kinase inhibitor that can target multiple receptors involved in tumor growth and angiogenesis. Studies have shown that sunitinib can improve PFS in patients with advanced pNETs. Overall, targeted therapies can be effective for well-differentiated pNETs that have progressed after other treatments. Nonetheless, it is important to consider the potential side effects associated with these agents.

37.12.6 Chemotherapy for pNETs

Chemotherapy is mainly recommended for poorly differentiated neuroendocrine carcinomas (NECs) and advanced or progressive pNETs. Overall survival for patients with NECs is usually poor, ranging from 5 months in metastatic cases to 38 months in localized ones. Chemotherapy can improve survival outcomes compared to best supportive care, with median survival ranging from 7 to 19 months in metastatic NECs. For GEP-NECs, platinum-based chemotherapy regimens, such as platinum and etoposide, are the most commonly used. These regimens have shown response rates of about 30% and a median survival of around 12 months. Historically, chemotherapy regimens for pNETs included streptozotocin combined with either 5-fluorouracil (5-FU) or doxorubicin. These regimens have demonstrated PFS rates of 16 to 23 months and overall response rates of 28% to 42%. More recently, temozolomide and capecitabine have become promising first-line treatments for pNETs. Studies report a median PFS of 18 months and an objective response rate of 71% with this regimen. Although several chemotherapy regimens have been approved for use in pNETs, many are not widely adopted in clinical practice due to significant side effects. Temozolomide and capecitabine offer a more effective and tolerable option compared to older regimens.

37.12.7 Peptide Receptor Radionuclide Therapy (PRRT)

PRRT is a targeted radiation therapy that employs radiolabeled peptides to deliver radiation to neuroendocrine tumors. These peptides attach to somatostatin receptors (SSTR 2), which are overexpressed on many neuroendocrine tumor cells' surfaces. PRRT is mainly used as a second-line treatment for patients with advanced or metastatic pNETs. It is an option for well-differentiated to moderately differentiated tumors that have progressed despite treatment with SSAs.

Key Eligibility Criteria for PRRT

- Somatostatin receptor expression: The tumor must express somatostatin receptors, confirmed through somatostatin receptor imaging.
- Tumor grade: Grade 1 and 2 tumors have high objective response rates compared to Grade 3 tumors.

PRRT Agents

- ^{177}Lu-DOTATATE: Emits both beta and gamma particles, enabling targeted radiation to smaller areas.
- ^{90}Y-DOTATATE: Emits beta particles, irradiating both the targeted and surrounding cells, which makes it more effective for larger tumors.

Additional Considerations

- IV infusion of amino acids (arginine/lysine): This is a critical part of ^{177}Lu-DOTATE therapy to protect the kidneys.
- PRRT has been shown to improve overall survival. The NETTER 1 trial demonstrated a estimated rate of progression-free survival at month 20 was 65.2% (95% confidence interval [CI], 50.0 to 76.8) in the 177Lu-Dotatate group and 10.8% (95% CI, 3.5 to 23.0) in the control group with Octreotide LAR alone.

Emerging Strategies for PRRT

- Neoadjuvant PRRT: Evidence indicates that PRRT may be used as a neoadjuvant therapy to reduce tumor size before surgery. Some studies show that ^{177}Lu-DOTATATE caused significant tumor shrinkage, allowing for primary tumor resection in a subset of patients.
- Salvage PRRT: Retreatment with PRRT may benefit patients who experience disease progression after initial treatment cycles with PRRT or other therapies. Current data suggest that this could extend progression-free survival. PRRT offers

a valuable therapeutic option for patients with advanced pNETs who have progressed on other treatments.

37.12.8 Recurrence and Follow-Up in pNETs

Recurrence rates for resected pNETs are relatively high, with a 12–25% recurrence at 5 years. Regular follow-up is essential for early detection of recurrence and guiding further management. Follow-up for patients who have had pNET resection typically includes clinical examination, biological markers like CgA, and radiological imaging such as CT/MRI and DOTA scan. The frequency of follow-up depends on the tumor grade and the extent of the initial resection.

- pNETs G1 or G2 with Ki-67 < 5%: Follow-up every 6 months.
- pNETs G2 with Ki-67 > 5%: Follow-up every 3 months.

This follow-up schedule should continue for at least 10 years after pancreatic resections.

Key Points

- Pancreatic neuroendocrine tumors (pNETs) represent a highly heterogeneous group of endocrine tumors that develop from the islet cells of the pancreas.
- MEN1, ATRX, DAXX, and mTOR pathway genes are involved in the pathogenesis of pNETs.
- On histology, the tumor is classified as well-differentiated or poorly differentiated and graded according to mitotic figures and the Ki-67 index.
- Functioning tumors are rarely malignant, release hormones, and manifest with hormone-based symptoms.
- Nonfunctioning tumors are more common, usually malignant, and do not release hormones.
- Tumor markers for nonfunctioning pNETs include chromogranin A, 5-hydroxyindoleacetic acid, and pancreatic polypeptide.
- CECT, MRI, EUS, PET-CT, and octreotide scintigraphy are used for diagnosis, evaluation of tumor characteristics, resectability, metastasis, and functional status.
- Incidentally detected tumors less than 2 cm in diameter are managed expectantly.
- Symptomatic and large tumors over 2 cm require formal resection.
- Several palliative treatment options are available for tumor recurrence and metastatic disease.

Suggested Reading

1. Pisegna JR, editor. Management of pancreatic neuroendocrine tumors [Internet]. New York: Springer; 2015. https://link.springer.com/10.1007/978-1-4939-1798-3
2. Ohmoto A, Rokutan H, Yachida S. Pancreatic neuroendocrine neoplasms: basic biology, current treatment strategies and prospects for the future. Int J Mol Sci. 2017;18:143. https://doi.org/10.3390/ijms18010143.
3. Pancreatic Neuroendocrine Neoplasms: 2020 Update on Pathologic and Imaging Findings and Classification | RadioGraphics. https://pubs.rsna.org/doi/abs/10.1148/rg.2020200025
4. Harris PE, Zhernosekov K. The evolution of PRRT for the treatment of neuroendocrine tumors; what comes next? Front Endocrinol. 2022; https://www.frontiersin.org/journals/endocrinology/articles/10.3389/fendo.2022.941832/full
5. Starr JS, Sonbol MB, Hobday TJ, Sharma A, Kendi AT, Halfdanarson TR. Peptide receptor radionuclide therapy for the treatment of pancreatic neuroendocrine tumors: recent insights. OncoTargets Ther. 2020;13:3545–55.
6. Das S, Al-Toubah T, Strosberg J. Chemotherapy in neuroendocrine tumors. Cancers. 2021;13(19):4872.
7. Cuthbertson DJ, Barriuso J, Lamarca A, Manoharan P, Westwood T, Jaffa M, et al. The Impact of 68Gallium DOTA PET/CT in managing patients with sporadic and familial pancreatic neuroendocrine tumours. Front Endocrinol [Internet]. 2021[cited 2025 Feb 4];12. Available from: https://www.frontiersin.org/journals/endocrinology/articles/10.3389/fendo.2021.654975/full
8. Melita G, Pallio S, Tortora A, Crinò SF, Macrì A, Dionigi G. Diagnostic and interventional role of endoscopic ultrasonography for the management of pancreatic neuroendocrine neoplasms. J Clin Med. 2021;10(12):2638.
9. Sulciner ML, Clancy TE. Surgical management of pancreatic neuroendocrine tumors. Cancers. 2023;15:2006.

Cystic Tumors of the Pancreas

38

Amit Gupta, Vivek Sanjekar, and Mohammad Ibrarullah

Abstract

Cystic neoplasms make up 10% of all pancreatic cystic lesions and 1% of all pancreatic neoplasms. SCN, MCN, IPMN, and SPEN are the most common cystic neoplasms of the pancreas. Cyst size, thickened cyst wall, contrast-enhancing mural nodule, MPD dilatation, abrupt change in pancreatic duct size, lymphadenopathy, enlarging cyst or mural nodule, acute pancreatitis, recent onset diabetes, raised serum CA 19-9, and positive cytology are essential considerations for surgical treatment.

Keywords

Cystic neoplasms · Cystic tumors · Pancreatic cyst

Pancreatic cystic neoplasms (PCNs), once thought to be rare, are now reported more frequently, mainly due to better clinical awareness and advances in imaging techniques. PCN makes up nearly 10% of all cystic lesions of the pancreas and 1% of all pancreatic neoplasms. Diagnosing PCN is important because of their malignant potential; they can range from completely benign to overtly malignant. A comprehensive diagnostic approach that includes clinical evaluation, cross-sectional imaging, endoscopic ultrasound (EUS), and fine-needle aspiration (FNA) with biochemical and cytological analysis of cyst fluid is necessary for accurate diagnosis and prognosis of these tumors (Table 38.1).

A. Gupta (✉) · V. Sanjekar
All India Institute of Medical Sciences, Rishikesh, India

M. Ibrarullah
Department of Surgical Gastroenterology, Apollo Hospitals, Bhubaneswar, Odisha, India

M. Ibrarullah (ed.), *Recent Concepts in Gastrointestinal (GI) Surgery*, https://doi.org/10.1007/978-981-92-1118-0_38

Table 38.1 Cystic lesions of pancreas: WHO Classification 2019

Epithelial		Non-epithelial	
Neoplastic	Non-neoplastic	Neoplastic	Non-neoplastic
[a]Serous cystic neoplasm (microcystic, oligocystic, macrocystic)	Lympho-epithelial cyst	Benign non-epithelial neoplasm (e.g., lymphangioma)	Pancreatic pseudocyst
Serous cystadenocarcinoma	Mucinous non-neoplastic cyst	Malignant non-epithelial neoplasms (e.g., sarcomas)	Parasitic cyst
[a]Mucinous cystic neoplasm with low/high-grade dysplasia, adenocarcinoma	Enterogenous cyst		
[a]Intraductal papillary cystic neoplasm	Para-ampullary duodenal wall cyst		
[a]Solid pseudopapillary neoplasm	Retention cyst		
Cystic neuroendocrine tumor G1–2	Endometrial cyst		
Cystic acinar cell carcinoma	Acinar cystic transformation		
Accessory-splenic epidermoid cyst	Congenital cyst		
Cystic hamartoma			
Uncommon tumors: Dermoid cyst, cystic variant of ductal adenocarcinoma/pancreatoblastoma/metastatic epithelial neoplasm			

[a]Most frequently occurring PCN

38.1 Serous Cystic Neoplasm

Serous cystic neoplasm (SCN), also known as serous cystadenoma or microcystic adenoma, accounts for 30–40% of PCN. It is characterized by a well-defined, soft mass containing multiple small cysts arranged in a honeycomb pattern. Larger cysts may be present at the periphery. A central stellate scar, which may or may not be calcified, is characteristic of SCN. Oligocystic adenomas, with an incidence of less than 10%, are characterized by one or more dominant cysts that may cause diagnostic confusion with other variants of PCN. SCN is lined by a single layer of cuboidal epithelium containing glycogen-rich, clear cytoplasm and rounded nuclei. The risk of malignancy in SCN is extremely low.

38.1.1 Clinical Presentation

SCN is more common in women, usually appearing in their 50 s to 60 s. The tumor can develop anywhere in the pancreas. It is asymptomatic in nearly 70–80% of patients. When symptoms do occur, they are typically caused by the tumor's large size pressing on surrounding structures. Common symptoms include abdominal pain, nausea, vomiting, weight loss, and sometimes jaundice. There is a strong link between SCN and von Hippel-Lindau syndrome. SCN or simple pancreatic cysts are found in 17–56% of affected individuals.

38.1.2 Diagnosis

On imaging, the SCN usually appears as a well-defined, multicystic mass with a central calcified scar in up to one-third of patients. Differentiating SCN from other cystic lesions can be difficult, especially for unilocular or oligocystic forms. Both computed tomography (CT scan) and magnetic resonance imaging (MRI) have a diagnostic accuracy of about 70%. When imaging results are inconclusive, EUS with FNA may be performed. The cyst fluid often shows low cellularity, but the presence of intracytoplasmic glycogen is characteristic. Cyst fluid analysis reveals low viscosity, with normal levels of amylase and carcinoembryonic antigen (CEA). Recent studies also indicate the potential usefulness of protein expression analysis in enhancing diagnostic accuracy.

38.1.3 Treatment

Surgery is recommended for symptomatic cysts, especially when they are larger than 4 cm in diameter or when diagnosis is difficult. A conservative procedure like enucleation can be performed for confirmed cases. When enucleation is not technically possible or if the diagnosis is uncertain, a formal resection of the tumor is advised. Follow-up surveillance is not necessary after complete resection of confirmed SCN. Non-operative management involves monitoring with serial imaging every 12–24 months for tumors less than 2 cm, and every 6–12 months for tumors measuring 2–4 cm in diameter, over 5 years (Fig. 38.1).

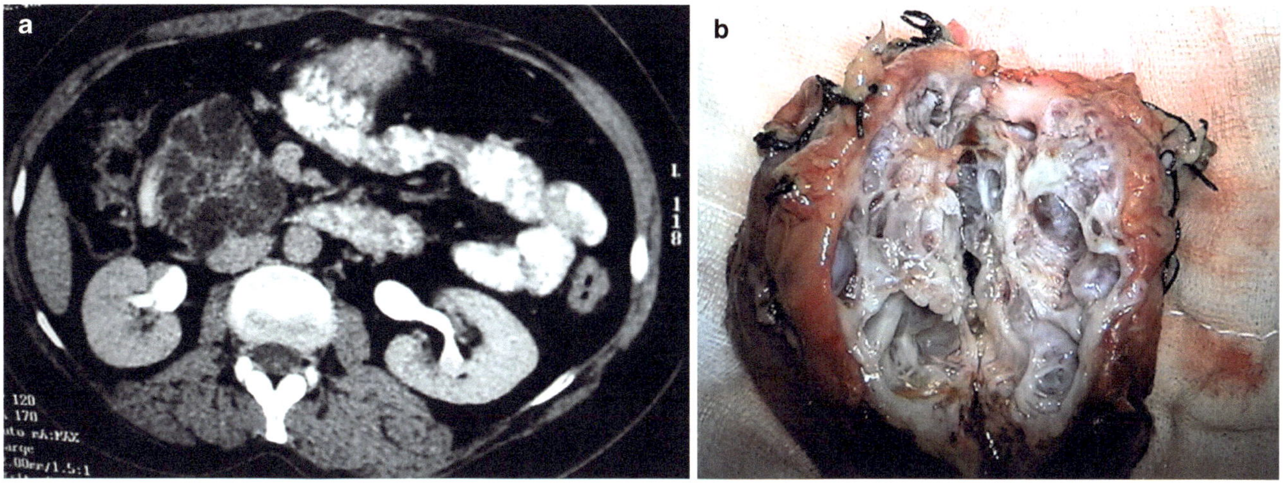

Fig. 38.1 Macrocystic SCN in the pancreatic head. (**a**) CT scan appearance. (**b**) Cut-open tumor after resection

38.2 Mucinous Cystic Neoplasm

Mucinous cystic neoplasm (MCN) accounts for about 15–30% of PCN. It is typically a thick-walled cyst that can be unilocular or septate. It is lined by tall columnar or cuboidal mucin-producing epithelium. The presence of ovarian-type stroma, characterized by dense spindle cells and elongated nuclei, is characteristic of MCN. This stroma usually expresses progesterone receptors, and in more than 60% of cases, stains positive for human chorionic gonadotropin. The similarities between MCNs and ovarian mucinous cystadenomas suggest that MCNs may arise from ovarian rests or stem cells in the pancreas. The presence of ovarian-type stroma differentiates MCN from IPMN and is considered essential for diagnosis. Nearly 70% of MCNs are benign, while 12% are invasive adenocarcinomas.

38.2.1 Clinical Features

MCN occurs almost exclusively in females between their fifth and sixth decades of life and is located in the body and tail of the pancreas. Abdominal pain or discomfort is the presenting symptom in over 70% of patients. A history of acute pancreatitis is present in 9–13% of cases, although it is less common than in IPMN. Patients with invasive carcinoma associated with MCNs typically present about 11 years later than those with non-invasive forms.

38.2.2 Diagnosis

Imaging studies and cyst fluid analysis are the main methods for diagnosis. A large unilocular tumor can be mistaken for a long-standing pseudocyst. The absence of inflammatory changes beyond the wall of the neoplasm and the lack of pancreatitis help differentiate MCN from a pancreatic pseudocyst. On imaging, MCN appears as thick-walled, septate cysts. The wall and septa show contrast enhancement. A size greater than 4 cm, irregular wall thickening, peripheral "egg shell" calcifications, the presence of mural nodules, or a mass suggest the possibility of invasive cancer. Cyst fluid analysis usually shows normal amylase levels and elevated CEA levels. When CEA levels are inconclusive, detecting a K-ras mutation in the cyst fluid can help distinguish MCN from SCN and may also indicate malignant transformation (Fig. 38.2).

38.2.3 Management

The indicators of malignancy in MCN are grouped as "risk factors." The presence of one or more of these "risk factors" is considered an indication for surgery. Larger tumors, especially those with invasive features, require formal pancreatic resection based on their location. However, extended lymphadenectomy is not beneficial in these cases. Tumors without any risk factors should undergo surveillance every six months during the first year and then annually for life for surgically fit individuals. New-onset diabetes, an increase in size by 3 mm/year, or the appearance of mural nodules or solid com-

Table 38.2 Risk factors related to MCN management

Size >3–4 cm
Presence of mural nodule or solid components
Dilated pancreatic duct >5 mm
Jaundice or acute pancreatitis secondary to the cyst
Significantly elevated serum CA 19-9
Presence of high-grade dysplasia or malignancy upon cytology

ponents calls for a thorough evaluation and consideration for resection. According to the AGA (American Gastroenterological Association) guidelines, surveillance can be discontinued after 5 years if no change in the cyst is observed or if the individual is unfit for surgery. After resection, surveillance is only needed for cysts with high-grade dysplasia or cancer. Survival outcomes are favorable for benign MCNs or those with non-invasive cancer, with a reported 100% 5-year disease-specific survival. This figure decreases to less than 25% with invasive cancer (Fig. 38.3).

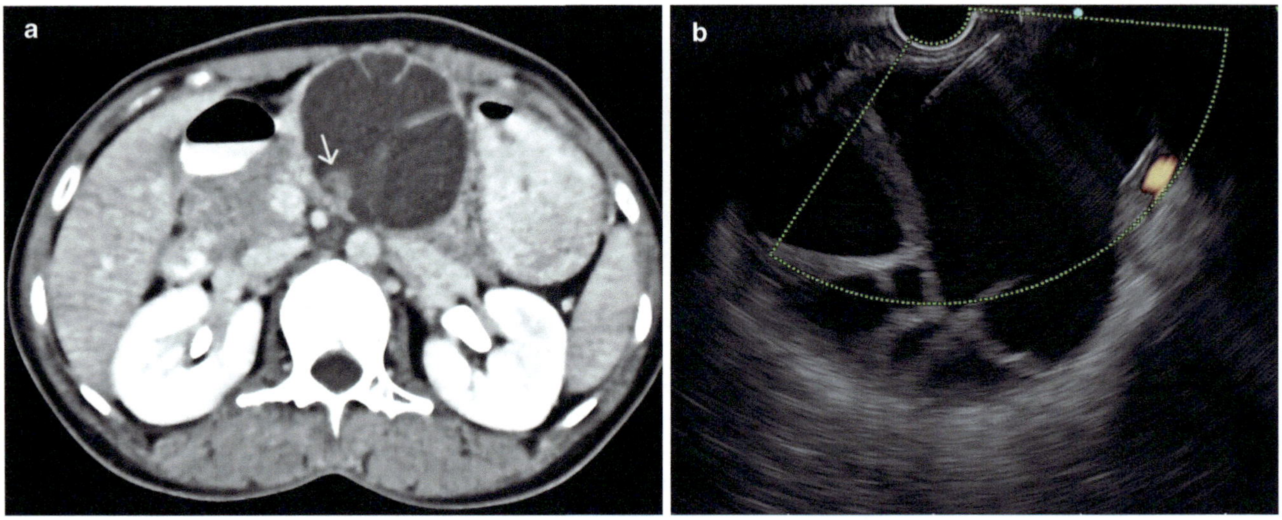

Fig. 38.2 MCN in the head of the pancreas. (A) CT scan image showing an enhancing cyst wall, multiple septa, and mural nodule (arrow). (B) EUS appearance of the same cyst. (*picture courtesy* U. Srinivasulu)

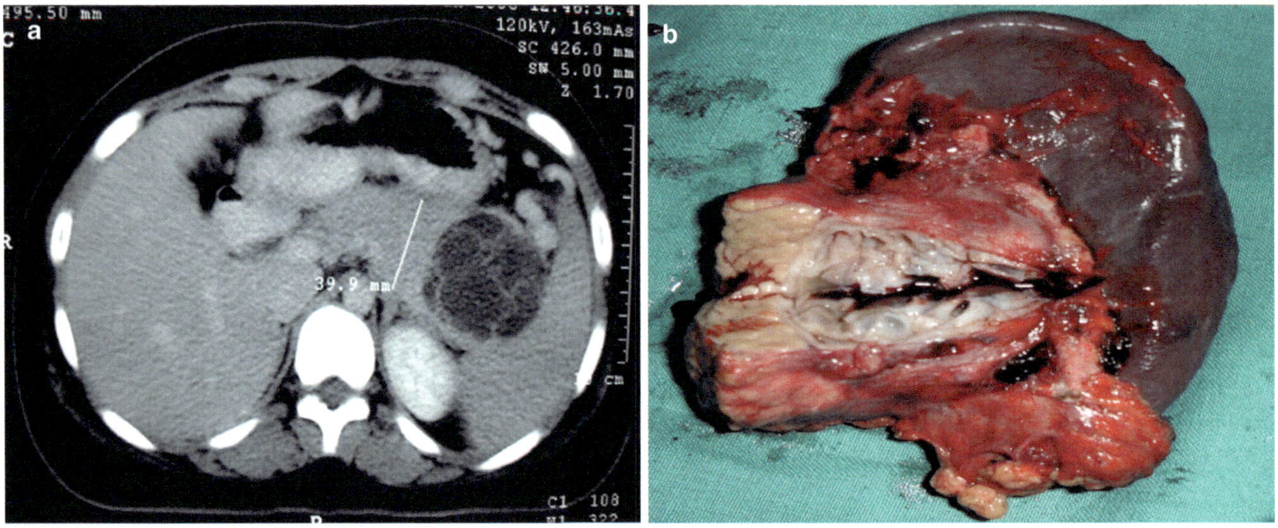

Fig. 38.3 Benign MCN. (**a**) CT scan showing a multiseptate cyst in the tail of the pancreas. (**b**) Cyst after resection

38.3 Intraductal Papillary Mucinous Neoplasm

Intraductal papillary mucinous neoplasm (IPMN) is the most common form of PCN, characterized by cystic dilation of the pancreatic duct. Depending on the segment of the duct involved, it is classified into three variants —main duct IPMN (MD-IPMN), branch duct IPMN (BD-IPMN), or mixed type (mixed-IPMN), where both main and branch ducts are affected. The cyst is lined by tall columnar epithelium, and significant mucin production is a hallmark of this disease. Considered premalignant, the reported incidence of invasive cancer is 33–60% with MD-IPMN and 11–30% with BD-IPMN; the incidence with the mixed variant is similar to that of MD-IPMN.

38.3.1 Clinical Features

IPMN occurs in the sixth to seventh decade of life with equal frequency among males and females, although some series report a slightly higher incidence in males. The pancreatic head is most commonly affected by the tumor. Benign IPMN is often an incidental finding on imaging. Ductal obstruction caused by a mucus plug can lead to acute pancreatitis in about 23% of patients. Symptoms such as anorexia, weight loss, obstructive jaundice, and new onset or worsening diabetes mellitus often indicate malignant transformation of IPMN. Additionally, patients with IPMN have an increased risk for extrapancreatic malignancies, such as colorectal and gastric cancers.

38.3.2 Diagnosis

The Ohashi triad, based on ERCP findings, such as a bulging (fish-mouth) ampulla with mucus extrusion and a dilated pancreatic duct, is considered diagnostic of IPMN. Since ERCP is now less commonly used as a diagnostic tool, these features can be demonstrated through combining side-viewing endoscopy with radiological imaging. Although contrast-enhanced CT remains the traditional imaging method for pancreatic tumors, MRI offers better detail in several areas. The relationship of the tumor to the main or branch pancreatic duct, mural nodules, and dilated pancreatic and common bile ducts is more clearly visualized on MRCP than on CT. EUS helps confirm MRCP findings and allows for cyst fluid analysis. Elevated amylase and CEA levels are useful adjuncts in diagnosing IPMN. EUS-guided aspiration cytology of the cyst fluid and mural nodules is an essential part of the treatment plan for the tumor (Figs. 38.4 and 38.5).

38.3.3 Treatment

According to the latest guideline (Kyoto 2024), the absolute and relative indications for surgery in IPMN, also known as "high-risk stigmata (HRS)" and "worrisome features (WFs)," respectively, are as follows (Table 38.3).

The presence of one or more HRS, two or more WFs, or a single WF in a young, surgically fit patient, or cases of recurrent acute pancreatitis, are considered indications for surgery. The choice of surgical procedure and the extent of pancreatic resection depend on preoperative imaging findings and intraoperative frozen section biopsy. When invasive carcinoma is suspected, a radical pancreatectomy with lymph node dissection should be performed. In the absence of suspicion, conservative resections such as middle pancreatectomy or spleen-preserving pancreatectomy can be considered.

Surveillance for non-resected IPMN or post-resection is recommended annually for patients without additional risk factors and every six months for those with high-grade dysplasia or a family history of pancreatic cancer. For non-resected BD-IPMNs, the frequency of surveillance depends on cyst size. After an initial 6-month observation, the recommended intervals are: 18 months for cysts smaller than 20 mm, 12 months for cysts measuring 20–30 mm, and 6 months for cysts 30 mm or larger. Surveillance includes imaging studies (MRI, CT scan, EUS), physical examinations, blood tests for tumor markers (CA 19-9 and CEA), and hemoglobin A1c (HbA1c). Surveillance can be discontinued for patients with BD-IPMNs smaller than 20 mm that remain stable and have no WFs after 5 years of follow-up. Considerations such as fitness for surgery and life expectancy are also important when deciding on continuing surveillance.

38.3.4 IPMN and Chronic Calcific Pancreatitis

Dilatation of the MPD in IPMN may mimic chronic pancreatitis, especially if there is additional calcification of the duct. In about 10% of IPMN cases, it is misdiagnosed as chronic pancreatitis. Conversely, IPMN coexists with 2% of chronic pancreatitis cases. While this association cannot be ignored as a mere coincidence, its exact cause remains uncertain. A probable explanation is that long-standing pancreatic duct obstruction in IPMN causes changes typical of chronic pancreatitis. However, such an association is rare and mostly anecdotal so far. Key differentiating features include the morphology of the MPD and the cyst. In IPMN, notable features are dilated MPD without stricture, a bulging ampulla, mural nodules within the duct, and a cyst that looks like a cluster of grapes with nodules inside. In chronic pancreatitis,

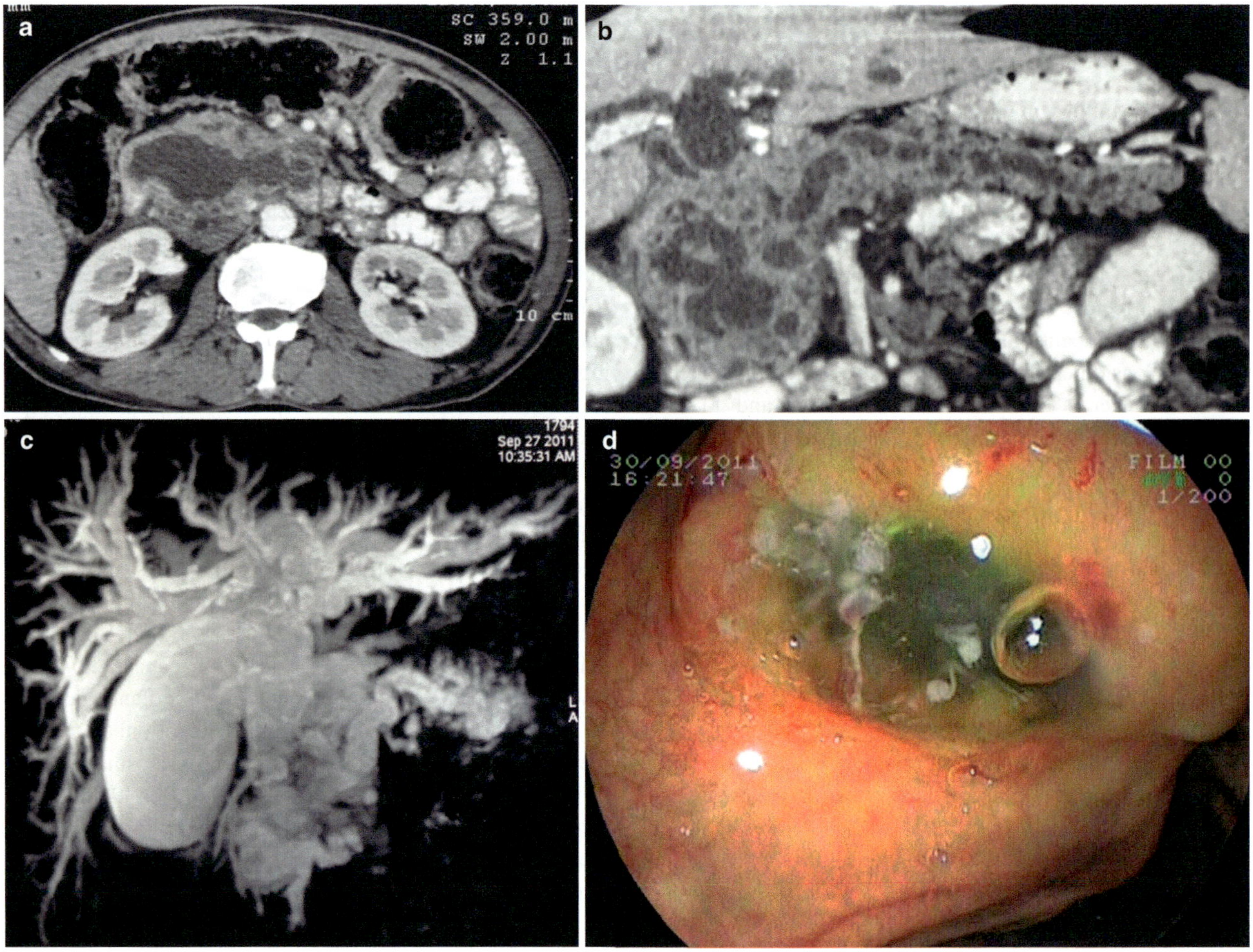

Fig. 38.4 Mixed-IPMN (**a**, **b**) CECT images showing cystic dilatation of the MPD and side branches. Dilated proximal bile duct (arrow). (**c**) Same findings on MRCP. (**d**) Appearance on side-viewing endoscopy—the tumor infiltrates the medial wall of the duodenum with an overlying adherent thick mucus plug

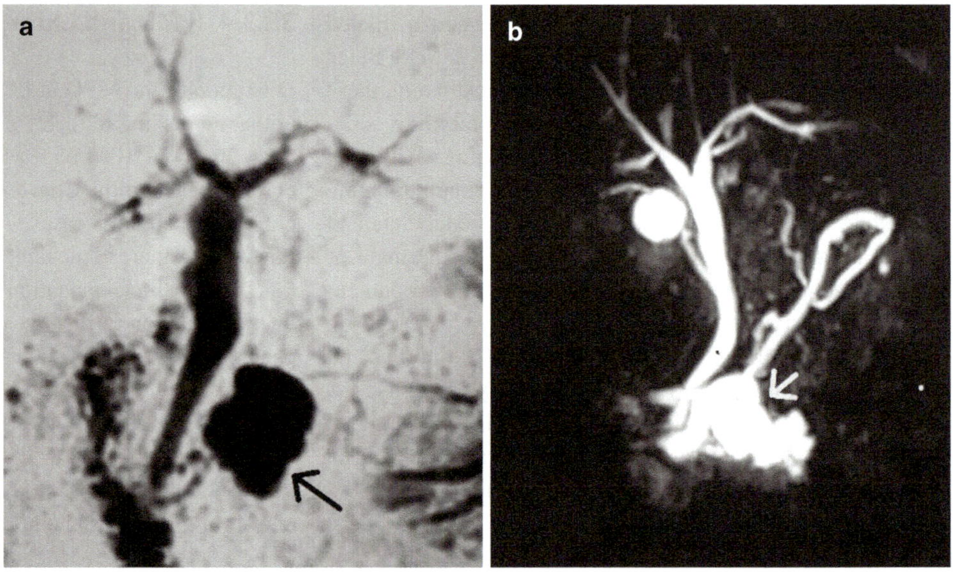

Fig. 38.5 MRCP showing (**a**) MD-IPMN (arrow), (**b**) BD-IPMN (arrow) in the proximal pancreas

the features are dilated MPD with strictures, stones within the duct, and a unilocular cyst when present. The diagnosis can be further confirmed with EUS-guided cytology of the cyst contents.

Table 38.3 Surgical indications in IPMN based on risk factors

High-risk stigmata	Worrisome features
1. Dilation of MPD ≥ 10 mm. 2. Contrast-enhancing mural nodule ≥5 mm or solid component on MRI. 3. Cytology positive for malignancy or high-grade dysplasia. 4. Obstructive jaundice caused by the cyst in the head of the pancreas.	1. Acute pancreatitis. 2. Increased level of serum CA 19-9. 3. New onset or acute exacerbation of diabetes in the past year. 4. Cyst size ≥30 mm. 5. Contrast-enhancing mural nodule <5 mm. 6. Thickened or contrast-enhancing cyst walls. 7. MPD dilation ≥5 mm and <10 mm. 8. Abrupt change in the size of the pancreatic duct with distal pancreatic atrophy. 9. Lymphadenopathy. 10. Cyst growth rate ≥2.5 mm/year.

38.4 Solid Pseudopapillary Epithelial Neoplasm

Solid pseudopapillary epithelial neoplasm (SPEN) is a rare tumor of the pancreas. It most often occurs in females in their 20 s or 30 s. The tumor size can vary from 0.5 to 35 cm, with an average of 6 cm in diameter, and it shows no specific preference for any region of the pancreas. Patients typically present with abdominal pain or a palpable lump. Most of these tumors contain pathogenic point mutations in the CTNNB1 gene, which encodes β-catenin, and they express the beta subtype of estrogen receptors (ER) and stain positive for galectin-3. Although generally benign, 10–15% may be malignant, with potential for local invasion or metastasis. On CT scans, the tumor appears well-circumscribed, oval, and often with hypodense regions caused by hemorrhage or necrosis. MRI and EUS-guided FNA are considered more accurate diagnostic tools. Surgical removal is recommended. An aggressive approach is advised even for metastatic cases, as complete resection offers a 5-year survival rate of over 95% (Fig. 38.6).

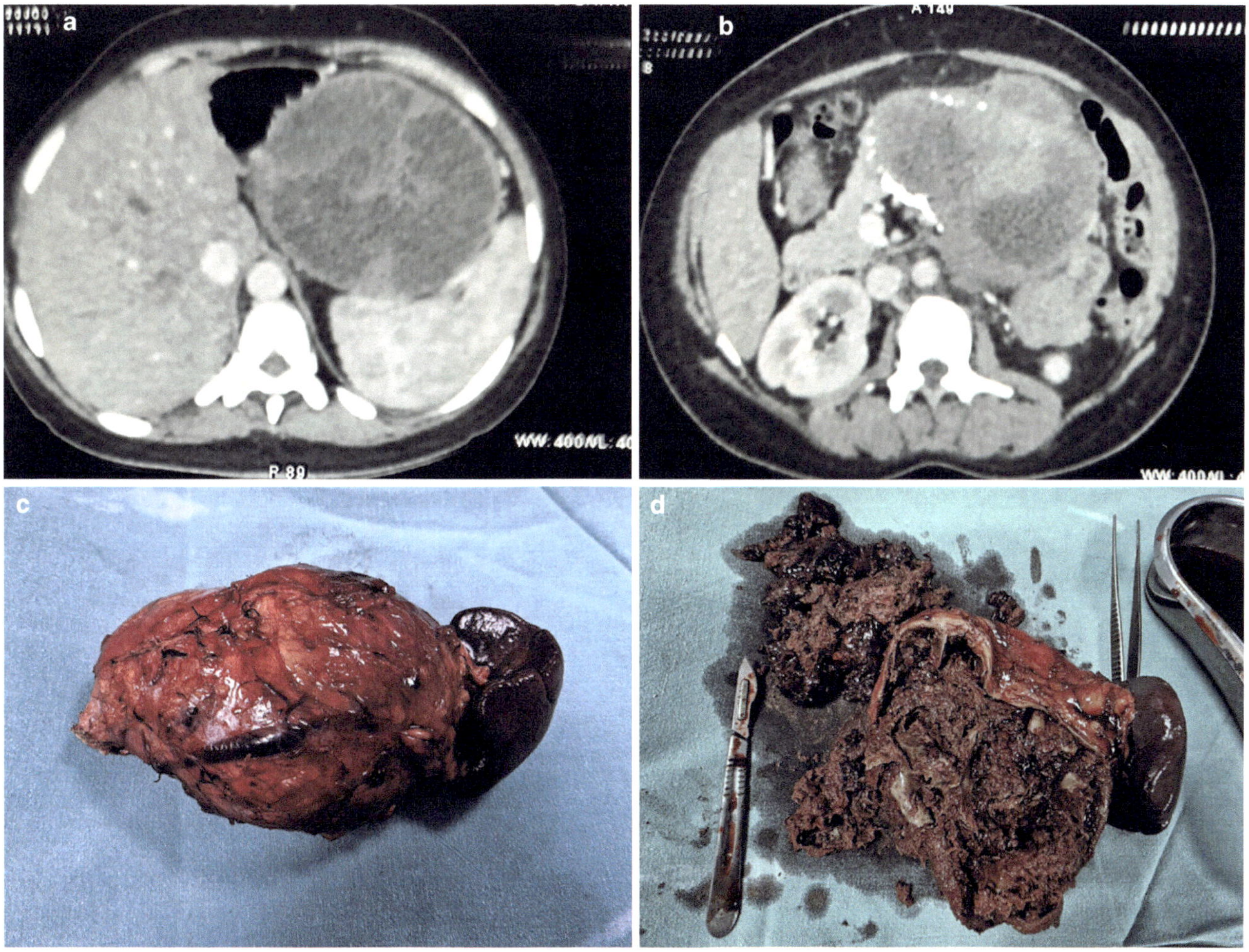

Fig. 38.6 Solid pseudopapillary epithelial neoplasm: (**a**, **b**) CT scan showing a large tumor with peripheral calcification, solid and cystic areas in the distal pancreas. (**c**) Distal pancreatectomy specimen bearing the tumor. (**d**) Cut-open specimen showing dense arborizing contents and clots

38.5 Cystic Neuroendocrine Tumor of Pancreas

The cystic variant makes up 13–17% of all pancreatic neuroendocrine tumors. Non-functional pancreatic cystic neuroendocrine tumor (C-PNET) is more common than the functional type. The former often presents with non-specific symptoms such as abdominal pain, anorexia, weight loss, or biliary obstruction if located in the pancreatic head. Functional tumors, on the other hand, present with symptoms related to the hormones they secrete. C-PNETs can be sporadic or linked to multiple endocrine neoplasia type 1 (MEN-1), which is characterized by synchronous tumors of the parathyroid glands, pancreatic islet cells, and the anterior pituitary gland. The risk of malignancy in C-PNET is approximately 20%. Diagnosis of non-functional tumors requires a CT scan, MRI, and EUS-guided FNA, while for functional tumors, it should be based on standard biochemical tests and PET scans. The management of C-PNET depends on the size and features of the lesion. Surgery is recommended for all functional tumors and non-functional tumors larger than 2 cm. Asymptomatic cysts smaller than or equal to 2 cm without evidence of malignant behavior should be monitored with EUS, MRI, or CT imaging every 6 to 12 months. Resection is advised if the cyst increases in size by 5 mm or if its final diameter exceeds 2 cm (Fig. 38.7).

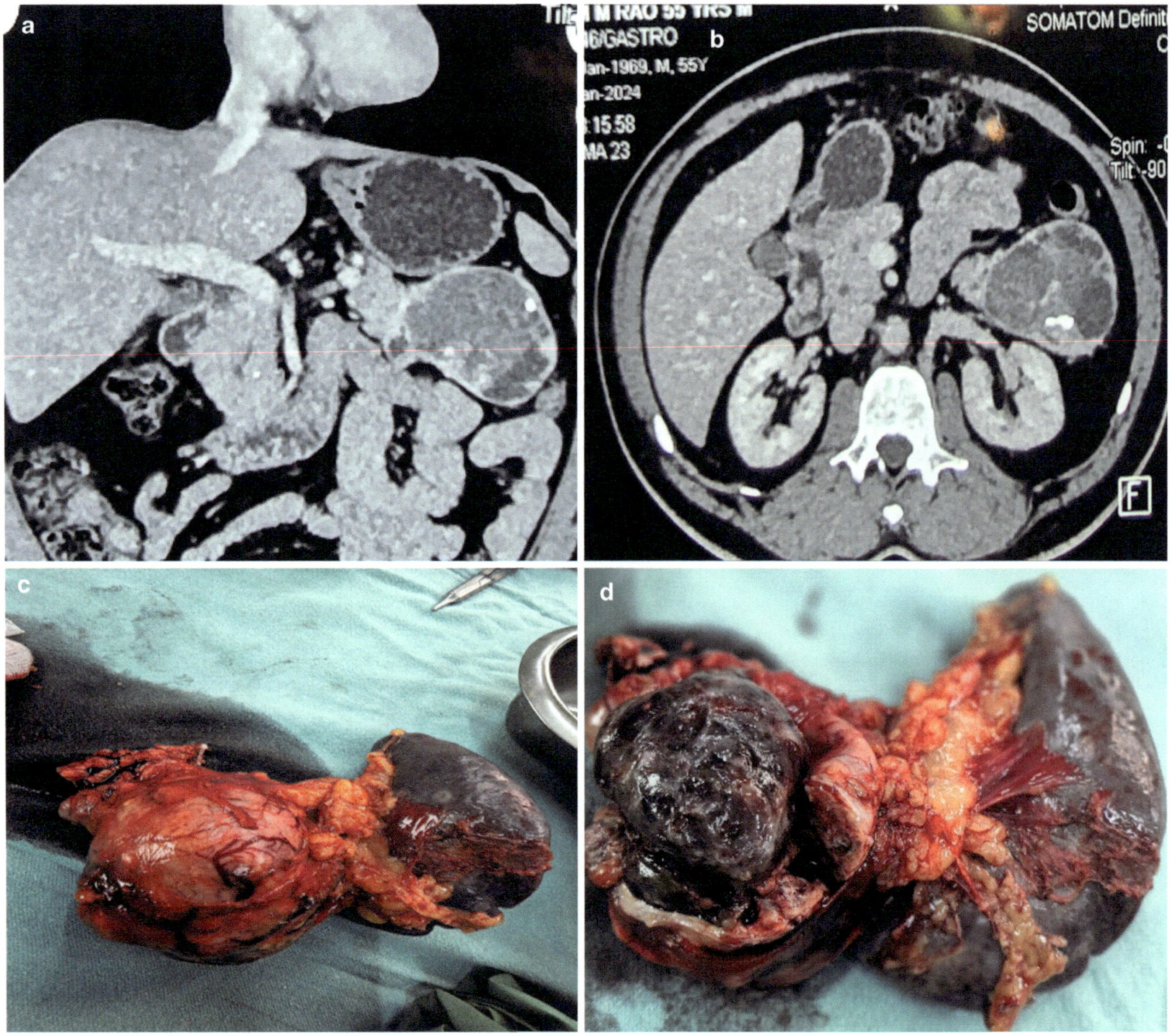

Fig. 38.7 Cystic neuroendocrine tumor of the pancreas. (**a**, **b**) CT scan showing tumor in the distal pancreas. (**c**, **d**) Tumor-bearing distal pancreatectomy specimen

38.6 Cystic Acinar Cell Neoplasms

Cystic acinar cell neoplasms are rare tumors of the pancreas with a 2:1 male predominance. Acinar cell carcinoma has better survival rates than ductal adenocarcinoma, even though it is often diagnosed at an advanced stage. These tumors can resemble IPMNs and may coexist with endocrine neoplasms in up to 40% of cases. Early symptoms are common in intraductal forms due to duct blockage. Key diagnostic indicators include immunohistochemical staining for trypsin.

38.7 Lymphoepithelial Cyst

Lymphoepithelial cyst (LEC) is an extremely rare benign pancreatic cystic tumor that is difficult to diagnose before surgery. This tumor may also have malignant potential (Fig. 38.8).

Currently, there is no reliable preoperative diagnostic method, but EUS-FNA shows promise. Surgical intervention is recommended for symptomatic patients, while a "watchful waiting" approach may be appropriate for asymptomatic cysts if the diagnosis of LECs can be confirmed nonsurgically. For uncomplicated, confirmed lesions, cyst enucleation may be considered, but definitive treatment involves resection if the diagnosis is in doubt.

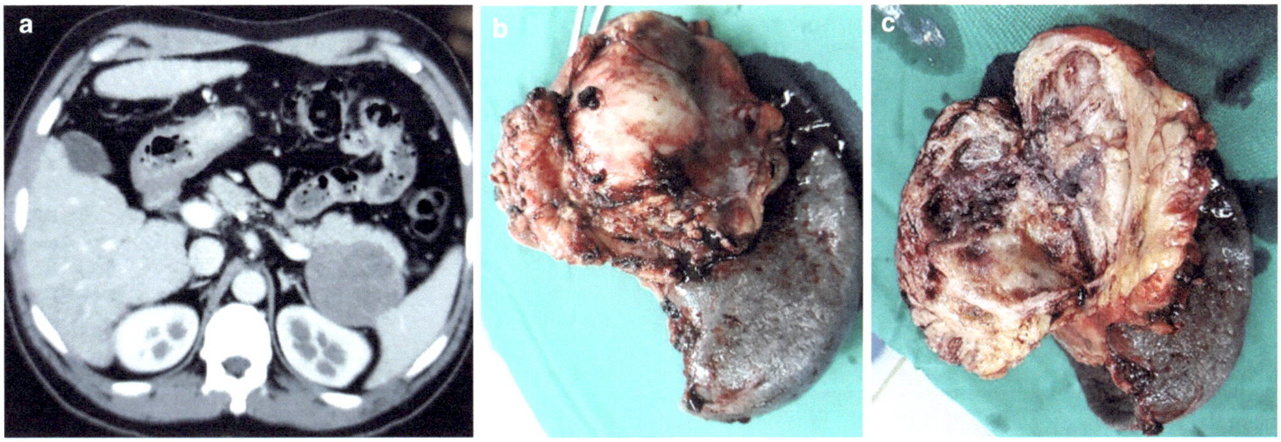

Fig. 38.8 Lymphoepithelial cyst. (**a**) CECT image showing a cyst in the distal pancreas abutting the splenic hilum. (**b**) Tumor-bearing tail of the distal pancreas and spleen after resection. (**c**) Cut-open tumor

Table 38.4 Comparative features of commonly occurring cystic lesions of the pancreas

Parameters	Pseudocyst	SCN	MCN	IPMN	SPN
Age in years	40–60	60–70	40–50	60–70	20–30
Sex	Equal	Female	Female	Equal	Female
Location	Any part	Any part	Distal body & tail	Head	Any part
Imaging	Well-circumscribed, oval or round, anechoic cyst. Inflammatory changes in & around the pancreas	Honeycomb. Central scar	Large cysts, unilocular or septate, peripheral calcification, thickened wall, enhancing mural nodule/s	Focal/segmental dilatation of the pancreatic duct. Enhancing mural nodule/s	Well-demarcated, mixed solid–cystic tumors
Communication with PD	May be present	Absent	Absent	Present	Absent
Cyst fluid amylase	Very high	Low	Low	High	Low
Cytology	Inflammatory cells and debris	Scant glycogen-rich cuboidal cells, periodic acid Schiff (PAS) stain (+)	Clusters & sheets of mucin-containing columnar cells	Tall columnar mucin-containing columnar cells with variable atypia	Papillary clusters with central capillaries, myxoid stroma, monomorphism, cercariform cells, and hyaline globules
Mucin	Negative	Negative	Positive	Positive	Negative
K-RAS mutation	Absent	Absent	Present	Present	Absent
Malignant potential	No	Extremely rare	Yes	Yes	Low-grade malignancy

Key Points

- Cystic neoplasms make up 10% of all pancreatic cystic lesions and 1% of all pancreatic neoplasms.
- SCN, MCN, IPMN, and SPEN are the most common cystic neoplasms of the pancreas.
- SCN is almost always benign, while the remaining tumors are potentially malignant.
- Diagnosis is based on clinical presentation, imaging studies, and US-guided cyst fluid analysis.
- Cyst size, thickened cyst wall, contrast-enhancing mural nodule, MPD dilatation, abrupt change in pancreatic duct size, lymphadenopathy, enlarging cyst or mural nodule, acute pancreatitis, recent onset diabetes, raised serum CA 19-9, and positive cytology are essential considerations for surgical treatment.
- Surveillance is necessary for tumors with malignant potential, whether or not resection is performed.
- Patients who are elderly, unfit for surgery, or have non-malignant resected tumors do not require additional interventions or surveillance.

Selected Reading

1. Rogowska J, Semeradt J, Durko L, Małecka E. Diagnostics and management of pancreatic cystic lesions—new techniques and guidelines. J. Clin. Med. 2024;13(16):4644. https://doi.org/10.3390/jcm13164644.
2. Ohtsuka T, Castillo CF, Furukawa T, et al. International evidence-based Kyoto guidelines for the management of intraductal papillary mucinous neoplasm of the pancreas. Pancreatology. 2024;24:255–70.

Pancreatic Surgery: Management of Complications

39

Ramkrishna Prabhu and Govindraj Dessai

Abstract

The risk of complications after pancreatic surgery is high, affecting nearly 30% to 50% of patients. Pancreatic leak and fistula (POPF), hemorrhage (PPH), delayed gastric emptying (DGE), and acute pancreatitis (PPAP) are common complications reported after pancreatectomy. Pancreatic leak is defined as any measurable volume of drain fluid on or after postoperative day 3 with an amylase level more than three times the upper limit of institutional serum amylase. PPH occurs in 1–8% of pancreatic resections and accounts for 11–38% of deaths. DGE is defined as the need to continue the nasogastric tube drainage and/or failure to resume oral intake beyond postoperative days three and seven, respectively.

Keywords

Pancreatic fistula · Pancreaticoduodenectomy

Surgeries involving the pancreas, such as pancreaticoduodenectomy (also known as Whipple's procedure), distal pancreatectomy, and total pancreatectomy, are among the most complex and high-risk procedures. Even with advancements in surgical techniques and postoperative care, the risk of complications after pancreatic surgery remains high, affecting 30% to 50% of patients and causing significant morbidity and, in some cases, death. Recognizing the types of complications, identifying risk factors, detecting issues early, and managing them effectively are essential for improving patient outcomes.

Table 39.1 Perioperative complications of pancreatic surgery

Complication	[a]Incidence %
Postoperative pancreatic leak and fistula	9–18
Intraabdominal abscess	9–10
Hemorrhage	1–8
Delayed gastric emptying	19–23
Postoperative pancreatitis	7–51
Biliary fistula	1–5
Chyle leak	Up to 10
SMV thrombosis	

[a]Following pancreaticoduodenectomy

39.1 Postoperative Pancreatic Leak and Fistula (POPF)

39.1.1 Definition and Grading

POPF remains the single most important determinant of serious postoperative morbidity and mortality related to pancreatic resection. It is defined as:

- Abnormal communication between the pancreatic ductal system and another epithelial surface that contains enzyme-rich fluid derived from the pancreas.
- Any measurable amount of drain fluid on or after postoperative day 3 with an amylase level greater than three times the upper limit of normal serum amylase at the institution.
- It includes all peripancreatic fluid collections, abscesses, leaks, or fistulas diagnosed through drain amylase levels, output, imaging, and clinical assessment.

The International Study Group of Pancreatic Surgery (ISGPS) in 2005 further clarified it and introduced a classification based on the clinical presentation of the POPF. Updated in 2016, this classification is now widely accepted for managing POPF (Table 39.2).

R. Prabhu (✉) · G. Dessai
KEM Hospital, Mumbai, India

M. Ibrarullah (ed.), *Recent Concepts in Gastrointestinal (GI) Surgery*, https://doi.org/10.1007/978-981-92-1118-0_39

Table 39.2 ISGPS grading of POPF

Grade	Presentations
Biochemical leak (*formerly known as* A)	Raised drain fluid amylase Clinically insignificant; no change in postoperative course or outcome Does not affect the postoperative hospital stay
B	Persistent drainage >3 weeks Requires a change in the postoperative management Signs of mild infection without organ failure Need to reposition the drains placed operatively, or use percutaneous or endoscopic drainage for the undrained collection Hemorrhage or pseudoaneurysm requiring transfusions and/or angioembolization
C	Requires reoperation Organ failure: Need for reintubation, hemodialysis, or ionotropic agents for respiratory, renal, and cardiac dysfunction, respectively Death attributable to pancreatic leak-related complications

Table 39.3 Type of pancreatic resection and the risk of POPF

Type of resection	Incidence of POPF
Pancreaticoduodenectomy	≈15%
Distal pancreatectomy	≈30%
Central pancreatectomy	≈40%
Duodenum-preserving pancreatic head resection	≈20%
Enucleation (tumor <3 mm from PD)	≈70%

39.1.2 Incidence and Risk Factors (Tables 39.3 and 39.4)

The occurrence of POPF varies based on the type of pancreatic resection and other factors.

39.1.3 Prevention of POPF

Anastomotic Technique A secure pancreatic anastomosis, regardless of risk factors, is crucial in preventing POPF. Among various methods, no single pancreaticojejunostomy (PJ) technique is deemed foolproof or superior in preventing pancreatic leaks. Pancreaticogastrostomy (PG), which is thought to be better than PJ because i. pancreatic juice is inactivated by gastric acid, ii. The absence of trypsin-activating enterokinase in the gastric epithelium and thus a reduced risk of leak; however, several prospective randomized trials have shown no difference in outcomes compared to PJ. Therefore, when performing pancreatic anastomosis, the only factors that should take precedence are a tension-free anastomosis with properly placed and tied sutures, a well-vascularized pancreatic stump, and an unobstructed, well-vascularized jejunal limb.

Perioperative Intravenous Fluid Management The use of goal-directed intravenous fluids during the perioperative period is crucial for caring for postpancreatectomy patients, as overhydration can cause tissue edema that may compromise any anastomosis, including PJ or PG.

Somatostatin Analogues Octreotide, a long-acting analogue of somatostatin, inhibits gastric and pancreatic exocrine secretion. The use of somatostatin analogues remains controversial, and their effectiveness in reducing POPF is inconsistent across various studies. A recent trial reported that Pasireotide, a longer-acting somatostatin analog, was able to decrease the rates of clinically relevant POPF. Therefore, it may be used prophylactically in the presence of adverse factors, such as a soft pancreas, an undilated duct, and an unsatisfactory pancreatic anastomosis.

Glues and Biological Sealants The use of fibrin sealants and acrylic glues to reduce the risk of POPF has not shown any clinical benefit.

Total Pancreatectomy When a safe pancreatic anastomosis seems difficult in unfavorable situations, total pancreatectomy can be considered a last resort. However, the benefits of the procedure must be balanced against the subsequent metabolic, endocrine, and nutritional consequences of total pancreatectomy.

39.1.4 Diagnosis and Management

The key to managing POPF includes anticipation, early recognition, and prevention of further life-threatening sequelae such as bleeding and sepsis:

- The drain fluid is assessed for its volume and nature, whether serous, seropurulent, bile mixed, or hemorrhagic.
- Drain fluid amylase estimation after 72 hours.
- Watch for signs of sepsis, e.g., fever, tachycardia, abdominal distension, and leukocytosis.
- CECT abdomen should be performed primarily to detect collections and the state of the pancreas (to diagnose postoperative pancreatitis).

Table 39.4 Risk factors for POPF

Risk factor	High incidence	Low incidence
Patient related		
Age	Old	Young
Sex	Male	Female
Obesity	High BMI	Low BMI
Comorbidity	Present	Absent
Jaundice	Present	Absent
Malnutrition	Present	Absent
Pancreas related		
Disease	Ampullary, duodenal, islet cell, or cystic neoplasm	Chronic pancreatitis, ductal adenocarcinoma
Gland texture	Soft	Firm
Pancreatic duct	Undilated	Dilated
Surgeon's experience	<10 pancreaticoduodenectomy/year	>25/year
Operative blood loss	>1000 ml	<400 ml

Table 39.5 Sequelae of POPF

Intrabdominal collection
Sepsis
Pseudoaneurysm and hemorrhage
Delayed gastric emptying

Grade A (biochemical leak) fistula does not require active intervention. However, careful daily monitoring is necessary to observe its progression or regression to later stages. Management of a Grade B fistula mainly involves draining any undrained collection, treating sepsis, ensuring proper nutrition, and addressing vascular complications as needed. Grade C fistula requires intensive care for organ dysfunction and/or reoperation, along with treatment of underlying causes such as intraabdominal sepsis, pancreatitis, or bleeding.

39.2 Postpancreatectomy Hemorrhage

Gastrointestinal or intrabdominal hemorrhage occurs in 1–8% of pancreatic resections and accounts for 11–38% of deaths. Postpancreatectomy hemorrhage (PPH), depending on the location and intensity, is characterized by bleeding from drains and nasogastric tubes, signs of hypovolemia, a drop in hemoglobin, and collections on CT scan, showing contrast enhancement. ISGPS proposed definitions and classifications for PPH to improve understanding and standardize its management (Fig. 39.1 and Table 39.6).

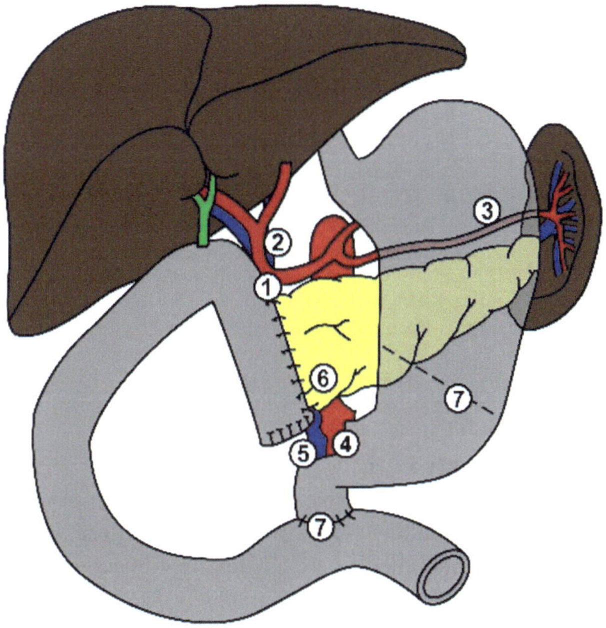

Fig. 39.1 Sites of PPH: 1—gastroduodenal artery, 2—hepatic artery, 3—splenic artery, 4—inferior pancreaticoduodenal artery, 5—portal vein tributaries, 6—pancreatic stump, and 7—gastrojejunostomy/duodenojejunostomy suture line

39.2.1 Management

Sentinel Bleed A small amount of blood appears in abdominal drains or the NG tube several hours before a major hemorrhage. This concept was introduced by Brodsky and Turnbull in 1991. It should alert the surgeon to take preemptive measures before the disaster actually happens:

- Check vital signs and shift the patient, preferably to the ICU, for close monitoring.
- Check hemoglobin and hematocrit levels.
- Reserve blood for transfusion if required.
- Contrast-enhanced CT scan (angio-CT) of the abdomen.

39.2.1.1 Early PPH

Early PPH usually occurs due to technical failure, such as inadequate hemostasis, a slipped ligature or clip, or an underlying coagulopathy. After addressing coagulopathy, if present, the patient should undergo reexploration to locate and secure the bleeding source. The same treatment approach should also be applied to any intraluminal suture line bleeding.

Table 39.6 Definition and classification of postpancreatectomy hemorrhage: ISGPS 2007

Time of onset	
Early (<24 hrs. After the index surgery)	Likely causes: Technical failure, reactionary hemorrhage, slippage of ligature or clip, perioperative coagulopathy
Late (>24 hrs. After the index surgery)	POPF or pancreatitis-induced vessel erosion or ruptured pseudoaneurysm, anastomotic ulcer bleeding
Location	
Intraluminal	Anastomotic suture lines (gastrojejunal, biliary, or pancreatic), internal rupture of pseudoaneurysm
Extraluminal	Erosion of any of the peripancreatic arteries, their branches, the mesentericoportal axis, and its tributaries
Severity of hemorrhage	
Mild	Minor bleeding through the drains and the NG tube. Drop in Hb < 3gm/dl None or mild clinical impairment Transfusion requirement: 2–3 units of packed cells in the first 24 hours at the end of surgery or 1–3 units if more than 24 hours after surgery. No need for reoperation or angioembolization
Severe	Clinical impairment (tachycardia, hypotension, oliguria) >3 units of packed cells transfused within 24 hours A drop in hemoglobin >3 gm% Need for interventional angiographic therapy Need for laparotomy

39.2.1.2 Late PPH

Late PPH is usually caused by anastomotic ulceration or vascular erosions resulting from pancreatic sepsis. Endoscopy and injection sclerotherapy are adequate for bleeding at the anastomotic suture line. CT angiography is the preferred initial investigation for bleeding suspected to be due to vessel erosion. Based on CT findings, subsequent angiographic intervention is performed.

Angiographic Intervention—Embolization or Stenting (Fig. 39.2) The most common bleeding site is the gastroduodenal artery (GDA), followed by the inferior pancreaticoduodenal artery (IPDA), hepatic artery (HA), superior mesenteric artery (SMA), and splenic artery (SA). Placing a covered stent across the pseudoaneurysm controls the bleeding without causing distal ischemia. However, in urgent situations when stenting is not feasible, coil embolization of the affected vessel may be used as a life-saving measure. Coil embolization has a success rate of 85%. The left or right hepatic artery or splenic artery can be successfully coiled without risking infarction.

Emergency laparotomy is indicated when angiographic intervention fails or is unavailable. It may also be considered in cases of exsanguinating hemorrhage when waiting for radiological intervention seems inappropriate. During laparotomy, the isolated bleeding point, if identifiable, is suture-ligated; otherwise, compression packing is applied for a relook after 24 hours.

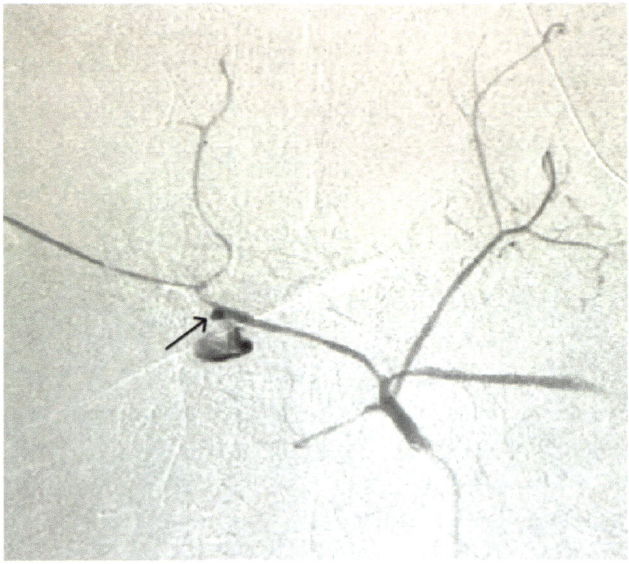

Fig. 39.2 Selective angiography showing pseudoaneurysm of the gastroduodenal artery (arrow) in a patient with POPF

39.3 Delayed Gastric Emptying

Delayed gastric emptying (DGE) is defined as the continued need for nasogastric tube (NGT) drainage and/or failure to resume oral intake beyond postoperative days 3 and 7, respectively. It is a common complication following pancreatic surgery. Although rarely life-threatening, it can lead to significant morbidity by delaying oral intake and extending hospital stay.

39.3.1 Etiology

1. The duodenal pacemaker is located in the first part of the duodenum.
2. In duodenal resection, the incidence of DGE is related to the duodenal remnant and the consequent decrease in plasma motilin levels.
3. Malignancy-induced gastroparesis, aggravated by jaundice, postoperative malnutrition, and electrolyte imbalance.
4. Extended nodal dissection along the common hepatic artery with disruption of vagal and sympathetic innervation to the antropyloric region.

5. In pylorus-preserving pancreaticodudenectomy, it is attributed to devascularization and denervation of the pylorus with subsequent pylorospasm.
6. Retrogastric inflammation and sepsis resulting from pancreatitis or leak (Table 39.7).

39.3.2 Prevention of DGE

The following measures may help in reducing the incidence of DGE following pancreatic resection:

- Minimal dissection of the antropyloric area.
- Preserve at least 2 cm of duodenum beyond pylorus.
- Antecolic gastrojejunostomy.
- Prophylactic feeding jejunostomy.

39.3.3 Management

DGE most often responds to conservative management (Table 39.8).

Table 39.7 ISGPS classification of DGE

Criteria	DGE: Gr 1	Gr 2	Gr 3
NGT removed on POD	4–7	8–14	>15
NGT reinserted after POD	3	7	14
Intolerance to solid oral diet by POD	7–13	14–20	21
Vomiting/gastric distension	+/−	+	+
Use of prokinetics	+/−	+	+
Enteral/parenteral nutritional support	+/−	+	+
Associated postoperative complications	+/−	+	+
Diagnostic evaluation: Endoscopy/CT	−	+/−	+

NGT nasogastric tube, *POD* postoperative day, *CT* computed tomography, *Gr* grade

Table 39.8 Management of DGE

Continued gastric decompression by NGT
Correct electrolyte imbalance
Correct anemia
Ensure adequate nutrition by alternative route, e.g., jejunostomy feeding or parenteral nutrition.
Rule out retrogastric sepsis by contrast-enhanced CT scan and treat if present.
UGI endoscopy is performed towards the end of the second week to exclude stomal obstruction. A nasojejunal tube may be maneuvered across the stoma into the efferent limb endoscopically under fluoroscopic guidance. This tube can be used for feeding purposes.
A gastrografin contrast study is performed toward the end of the second week to exclude efferent loop obstruction and confirm DGE.
Intravenous prokinetics, e.g., metoclopramide, Levosulpiride, erythromycin, are given towards the end of the first week.
When conventional prokinetics are ineffective, intravenous neostigmine, if not contraindicated, can be administered with cardiopulmonary monitoring. This drug often provides dramatic relief in DGE.

39.4 Postpancreatectomy Acute Pancreatitis

Postpancreatectomy acute pancreatitis (PPAP) is often an under-reported entity. Diagnosis is delayed because of its deceptive presentation. Currently, this entity is considered one of the most important causes of POPF and its sequelae.

39.4.1 Definition

The International Study Group for Pancreatic Surgery defines PPAP as elevated serum amylase levels sustained for ≥48 hours postoperatively, radiological findings consistent with acute pancreatitis, and associated clinically relevant features.

39.4.2 Incidence

The reported incidence of PPAP ranges from 7% to 51%. The series reporting a very high incidence may be due to the exclusion of radiologic features when diagnosing PPAP. Possible risk factors for PPAP include female sex, a soft pancreatic texture, a small main pancreatic duct diameter, or high C-reactive protein levels (Table 39.9).

In the immediate postoperative period, clinical signs and symptoms can be misleading. A high level of suspicion in a patient with unexplained delays in recovery or organ dysfunction should lead the clinician to consider or rule out PPAP.

39.4.3 Investigations

Serum amylase.
CECT abdomen and pelvis.

39.4.4 Management

Management of PPAP should adhere to the standard protocol for acute pancreatitis and its complications (Fig. 39.3).

Table 39.9 ISGPS grading of PPAP

Grade	Features
A	Postoperative serum hyperamylasemia; sustained rise for more than >48 hours
B	Clinically relevant change in management and radiological features of acute pancreatitis
C	Organ failure/reoperation/death

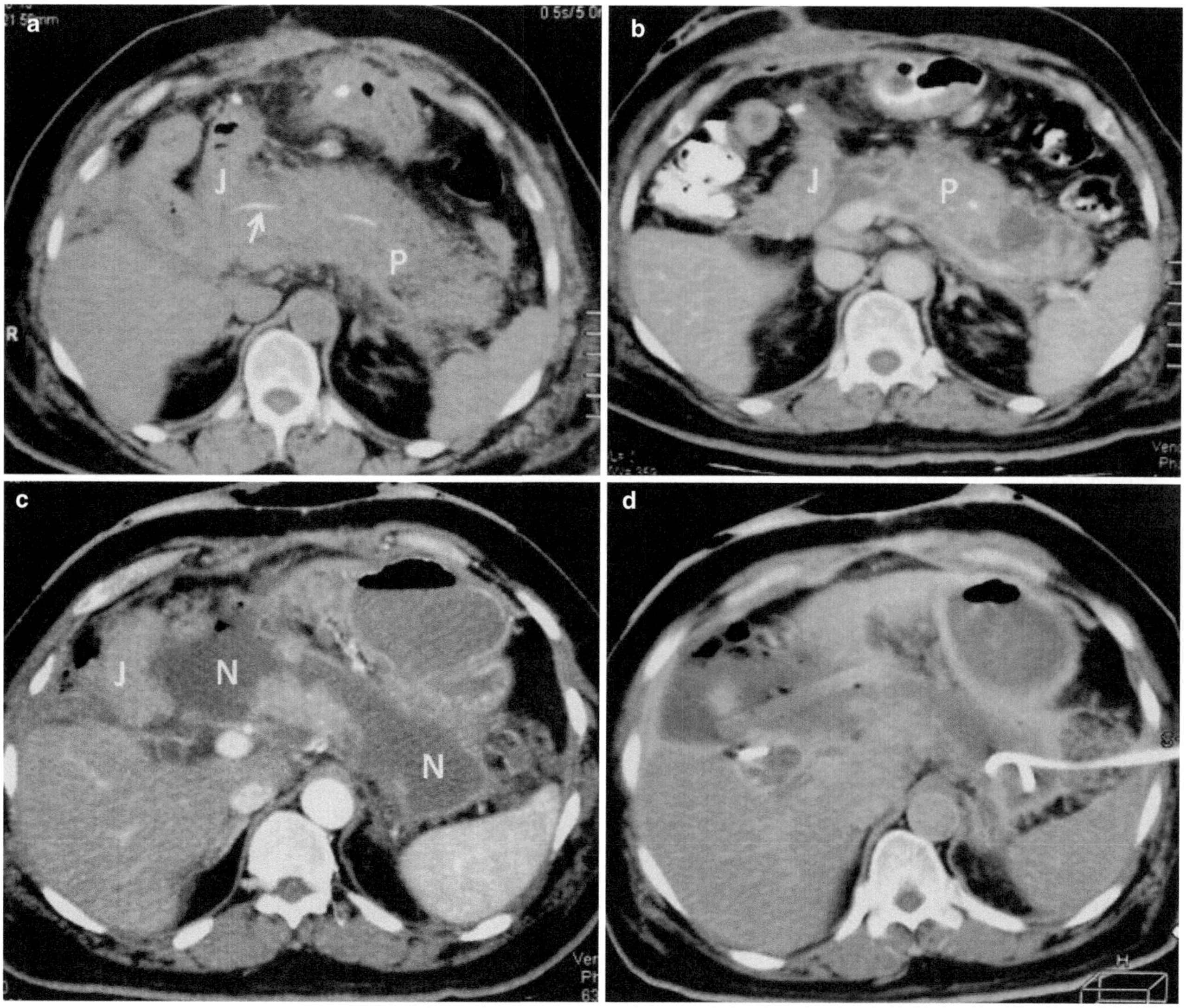

Fig. 39.3 Postpancreatectomy acute pancreatitis: (**a**) Noncontrast CT showing diffusely enlarged pancreatic stump, (**b**) contrast CT, a week later, showing patchy necrosis in the pancreas, (**c**) necrotic collection around a small enhancing pancreatic remnant seen three weeks later, (**d**) percutaneous pigtail catheter draining the necrotic collection: P-Pancreas, J-Jejunum, and N-Necrotic collection. Arrow pointing to the pancreatic stent

39.5 Postpancreatectomy Chyle Leak

Chyle leak occurs in 1–16% of patients after pancreatic surgery and is usually diagnosed around days 5–6 postoperation. The cisterna chyli and its main branches are located in front of the L1 and L2 vertebrae, which may be injured during pancreaticoduodenectomy.

39.5.1 ISGPS Consensus Definition (Table 39.10)

Chyle leak is defined as:

- Milky colored fluid from the drain or wound on or after the third postoperative day.
- Triglyceride content of the fluid >110 mg/dl.

Table 39.10 ISGPS grading of postpancreatectomy chyle leak based on therapeutic consequences

	Grade A	Grade B	Grade C
Therapeutic consequences	Good May require dietary restriction	Manageable with nasoenteral nutrition with dietary restriction of fat with/without medium-chain-triglyceride supplements. May require TPN Image-guided percutaneous catheter drainage of collection/s Maintenance of surgical drains. Octreotide treatment may be required.	Need for reoperation or radiological intervention. Admission to the intensive care unit, and/or death
Discharge with drain or readmission	No	May be	May be
Prolonged hospital stay due to chyle leak	No	Yes	Yes

39.5.2 Predisposing Factors

- Dissection of the para-aortic area, especially at the root of the superior mesenteric pedicle.
- Extensive lymph node dissection.
- Presence of retroperitoneal involvement.
- Lymphovascular invasion of the tumor.
- Neoadjuvant therapy.
- Vascular resection.
- Female sex.

39.5.3 Management

39.5.3.1 Step-Up Approach

- Dietary restrictions include limiting fat intake. Long-chain triglycerides (TGs) are replaced with medium-chain TGs.
- Total parenteral nutrition may be considered if the above proves ineffective.
- Collections, when present, are drained under image guidance.
- Therapeutic interventions such as sclerotic embolization of lymphatics, peritoneovenous shunting, lymphangiography, and operative ligation of leaking lymphatics have been described. However, there is insufficient experience to recommend their routine use.

39.6 Biliary Complications

Bile leak is observed in 1–5% of cases following pancreaticoduodenectomy. Due to its proximity to the pancreatic anastomosis, a pancreatic leak may appear bilious. This can be excluded by checking the drain fluid amylase.

39.6.1 Management

A controlled fistula requires no active management. An uncontrolled fistula and any bile collection should be drained via image-guided percutaneous intervention. In most cases, these measures suffice.

Key Points

- The risk of complications after pancreatic surgery is high, affecting nearly 30% to 50% of patients.
- Pancreatic leak and fistula (POPF), hemorrhage (PPH), delayed gastric emptying (DGE), and acute pancreatitis (PPAP) are common complications reported after pancreatectomy.
- Pancreatic leak is defined as any measurable volume of drain fluid on or after postoperative day 3 with an amylase level more than three times the upper limit of institutional serum amylase.
- Gr A POPF is a biochemical leak that is not clinically relevant. Persistence of drainage beyond three weeks is classified as a Gr B leak, which may require nonoperative therapeutic interventions such as PCD/endoscopic drainage of an undrained collection or radiological embolization of a pseudoaneurysm. Gr C is characterized by the need for reoperation, ICU care, or resulting in death.
- PPH occurs in 1–8% of pancreatic resections and accounts for 11–38% of deaths.
- Early PPH usually results from technical failure, such as inadequate hemostasis, a slipped ligature or clip, or an underlying coagulopathy. After addressing coagulopathy, if present, the patient should undergo re-exploration to locate and secure the bleeding source.
- Late PPH is usually caused by anastomotic ulceration or vascular erosions consequent upon pancreatic sepsis. CT angiography is the initial preferred investigation for bleeding suspected to be due to

(continued)

vessel erosion. Based on CT findings, subsequent angiographic intervention, such as endovascular stent placement or embolization, is performed.

- DGE is defined as need to continue the nasogastric tube drainage and/or failure to resume oral intake beyond postoperative days three and seven, respectively.
- Conservative treatment, prokinetics, and management of retrogastric sepsis are sufficient for these patients.
- PPAP is defined as elevated serum amylase levels sustained for ≥ 48 hours postoperatively, radiological findings consistent with acute pancreatitis, and associated clinically relevant features.
- The reported incidence of PPAP ranges from 7% to 51%.
- The diagnosis is based on a high index of suspicion in a patient with unexplained delays in recovery or organ dysfunction, confirmed by elevated serum amylase and CT scan results.
- PPAP is one of the most typical causes for POPF and abdominal sepsis following pancreatectomy.
- PPAP management adheres to standard guidelines for acute pancreatitis.
- Post-pancreatectomy chyle or bile leak is rare and typically responds to conservative treatment.

Selected Reading

1. Bassi C, Marchegiani G, Dervenis C, et al. The 2016 update of the International Study Group (ISGPS) definition and grading of postoperative pancreatic fistula: 11 years after. Surgery. 2017;161(3):584–91. https://doi.org/10.1016/j.surg.2016.11.014.
2. Wente MN, Veit JA, Bassi C, et al. Postpancreatectomy hemorrhage (PPH): an International Study Group of Pancreatic Surgery (ISGPS) definition. Surgery. 2007;142(1):20–5. https://doi.org/10.1016/j.surg.2007.02.001.
3. Connor S. Defining post-operative pancreatitis as a new pancreatic specific complication following pancreatic resection. HPB (Oxford). 2016;18:642–51. https://doi.org/10.12016/j.hpb.2016.05.006.
4. Marchegiani G, Barreto SG, Bannone E, Sarr M, Vollmer CM, Connor S, et al. Postpancreatectomy Acute Pancreatitis (PPAP): definition and grading from the International Study Group for Pancreatic Surgery (ISGPS). Ann Surg. 2022;275:663–72. https://doi.org/10.1097/SLA.0000000000005226.
5. Wente MN, Bassi C, Dervenis C, et al. Delayed gastric emptying (DGE) after pancreatic surgery: a suggested definition by the International Study Group of Pancreatic Surgery (ISGPS). Surgery. 2007;142(5):761–8. https://doi.org/10.1016/j.surg.2007.05.005.
6. Hanna MM, Gadde R, Allen CJ, et al. Delayed gastric emptying after pancreaticoduodenectomy. J Surg Res. 2016;202:380–8.
7. Besselink MG, Rijssen LB, Bassi C, et al. Definition and classification of chyle leak after pancreatic operation: a consensus statement by the International Study Group on Pancreatic Surgery. Surgery. 2017;161:365–72.
8. Muzzolini M, Araujo RLC, Kingham TP, et al. Incidence and risk factors for chyle leak after pancreatic surgery for cancer: a comprehensive systematic review. Eur J Surg Oncol. 2021;48:707–17. https://doi.org/10.1016/j.ejso.2021.11.136.

Pancreas and Islet Cell Transplantation

40

Venkatesh Balaraman Sundararajan, Anil Vaidya, and Senthil Muthuraman

Abstract

Pancreas transplant is primarily indicated for type 1 diabetes and select cases of type 2 diabetes. The types of transplants are simultaneous pancreas-kidney transplants, pancreas after kidney transplant, and pancreas transplant alone (PTA). Islet autotransplant (IAT) is recommended after total pancreatectomy for benign diseases and trauma. One-third of adults become insulin-free after IAT, and in a significant number, the quality of life and glycemic control improve. Results of IAT in the pediatric subgroup are better than in adults.

Keywords

Pancreatic transplantation · Islet cell transplantation

The pancreas, once thought to be mainly a "flesh" organ for cushioning the stomach, is now recognized as one of the most complex organs in the body after its endocrine and exocrine functions were discovered. The first living donor partial pancreas transplant was performed by Sutherland and his team at the University of Minnesota in 1966. Since then, over 67,000 pancreas transplants have been carried out worldwide. Over the past decade, the number of transplants has steadily increased in the East compared to the West, according to the International Pancreas Transplant Registry. Pancreas transplant is primarily done for type 1 diabetes mellitus (DM) and a select group with Type 2 DM (Table 40.1).

Table 40.1 Types of diabetes requiring transplant

DM type 1 (5%–10%): Immune-mediated destruction of beta cells, causing complete insulin deficiency
DM type 2 (75%–90%): Characterized by varying degrees of beta cell dysfunction combined with insulin resistance and metabolic syndrome (selected subset)

40.1 Types of Pancreas Transplant

1. Simultaneous pancreas-kidney transplants (SPK).
2. Pancreas after kidney transplant (PAK).
3. Pancreas transplant alone (PTA).

40.2 Indications

- Type 1 DM: Especially when complications develop that insulin therapy alone cannot adequately manage.
- End-stage renal disease (ESRD) in patients with type 1 DM is an indication for SPK.
- Hypoglycemia unawareness: Severe and frequent episodes of hypoglycemia, especially when the patient does not recognize the warning signs.

V. B. Sundararajan (✉) · A. Vaidya · S. Muthuraman
Institute of Abdominal Organ & Multivisceral Transplant CareVue Health/ MGM Healthcare, Chennai, Tamilnadu, India

M. Ibrarullah (ed.), *Recent Concepts in Gastrointestinal (GI) Surgery*, https://doi.org/10.1007/978-981-92-1118-0_40

- Brittle diabetes: Patients with type 1 DM who experience severe fluctuations in blood sugar levels (brittle diabetes).
- Complications of DM: Type 1 DM with related issues such as retinopathy, neuropathy, and vasculopathy affecting the CVS or CNS.
- Type 2 DM: Pancreas transplantation is an option in type 2 DM under specific circumstances, such as cases with low insulin production and low insulin resistance.

40.3 Contraindications

- Active sepsis.
- Incurable malignancy.
- Substance abuse or an untreated psychiatric disorder.
- Noncompliance and inability to tolerate surgery and immunosuppression.
- Cardiac: significant noncorrectable coronary artery disease, LVEF less than 50%, severe bilateral iliac vessel disease.
- Pulmonary: dependence on home oxygen, uncontrolled asthma, severe COPD, uncorrectable pulmonary hypertension, etc.

40.3.1 Relative Contraindications

- Cerebrovascular accident causing long-term impairment.
- Active hepatitis B or C infection.
- BMI > 30 kg/m^2.

40.4 Recipient Evaluation

The recipient's preoperative evaluation is similar to that of a renal transplant. The process includes a comprehensive review of medical history, physical examination, laboratory tests, viral markers, immunologic assessments, a hypercoagulability workup, abdominal CT angiography, cancer screening, prostate-specific antigen testing, and evaluations for cardiovascular, cerebrovascular, and peripheral vascular conditions.

40.5 Donor Surgery

40.5.1 Preprocurement

An ideal donor is hemodynamically stable, young (10–40 years old), ABO compatible, has a BMI under 30 kg/m^2, and is a deceased brain-dead donor (with a cause other than CVA). The Pancreas Donor Risk Index (PDRI) considers donor sex, age, race (categorized as Black or Asian), BMI, cause of death, creatinine level, height, and DCD status. A higher PDRI indicates a greater risk of graft loss. Another scoring system, called the Preprocurement Pancreas Suitability Score (P-PASS), factors in donor age, BMI, ICU stay, cardiac arrest, serum sodium, serum amylase/lipase, and vasopressor use; a score of 17 or less is deemed suitable for transplant.

40.5.2 Surgical Technique

The pancreas is visualized and examined for extensive fibrosis, calcification, intralobular fat, trauma, hematoma, and extensive edema. Only 20% of donor pancreases are retrieved. The key to a successful pancreas transplant involves a pristine procurement, precise back-benching, and perfect implantation (3Ps).

The retrieval operation starts with exposing the chest and abdomen through a long midline incision from the suprasternal notch to the pubic symphysis. After an initial inspection of the abdominal organs, right medial visceral rotation (Cattell-Brasch maneuver) and extended Kocherization are performed until the IVC, left renal vein, superior mesenteric artery (SMA), and aorta are exposed. The aorta and inferior mesenteric vein (IMV) are looped for cannulation. The gastrohepatic ligament is opened up to the porta hepatis, and the gastrocolic ligament is divided along with the division of the short gastric arteries to expose the entire pancreas up to its tail and the spleen. The lienophrenic and lienocolic ligaments are divided, and the spleen is rotated medially. The pancreas is mobilized from left to right using the spleen and tail as handles. Then, the dissection shifts to the porta hepatis. The bile duct is identified and ligated just at the level of the superior margin of the duodenum. The gastroduodenal artery (GDA) is identified and looped, followed by delineating the arterial anatomy of the common hepatic artery, left gastric artery, and splenic artery origins. The supraceliac aorta is dissected and looped. After systemic heparinization, the infrarenal aorta is cannulated. The supraceliac aorta is clamped, and the organs are flushed with a cold preservative solution while surface cooling is achieved with slush ice. The proximal duodenum distal to the pylorus is divided with a linear cutting stapler, and the distal part—the fourth part of the duodenum—is also divided. The root of the mesentery is divided 2 cm away from the inferior border of the pancreas to avoid including the inferior pancreatoduodenal artery. The GDA is divided just distal to its origin, with its distal end ligated. The splenic artery (SA) is divided distal to its origin. In case a replaced hepatic artery is present, it is divided behind the duodenum and reconstructed with the GDA stump. The portal vein is divided midway between the lower border of the liver and the upper border of the pancreas to ensure that adequate length remains with the pancreas. The SMA is divided at the level of the middle colic artery origin. The pancreas is procured, immersed in cold preservative solution, packed, and taken to the back table for benching.

40.5.3 Back Table Benching

After careful inspection for anomalies and abnormalities, the spleen is carefully removed from the pancreas tail without causing injury. The IMV is ligated, and the duodenum and jejunal loop are mobilized and shortened. The small bowel mesentery, which was previously stapled, is reinforced with 4-0 polypropylene sutures. The arterial inflow to the graft is reconstructed using donor cadaveric iliac vessels; that is, the cadaveric external and internal iliac arteries are anastomosed to the SMA and SA, respectively, along with the common iliac artery serving as a Y graft.

40.6 Recipient Surgery

Through a midline laparotomy, the peritoneal cavity is opened. The venous (endocrine) drainage of the graft pancreas (via the donor portal vein) can be directed into either the IVC, the common iliac vein (systemic circulation), the SMV, or a branch (portal circulation). The reconstructed Y arterial graft of the pancreas is anastomosed with the common iliac artery. The exocrine drainage of the pancreas can be either enteric (duodenum or small intestine) or urinary (bladder) drainage. The pancreas is mainly placed in the right iliac fossa, and the kidney is in the left iliac fossa in the case of SPK, sometimes ipsilaterally (Fig. 40.1 and Table 40.2).

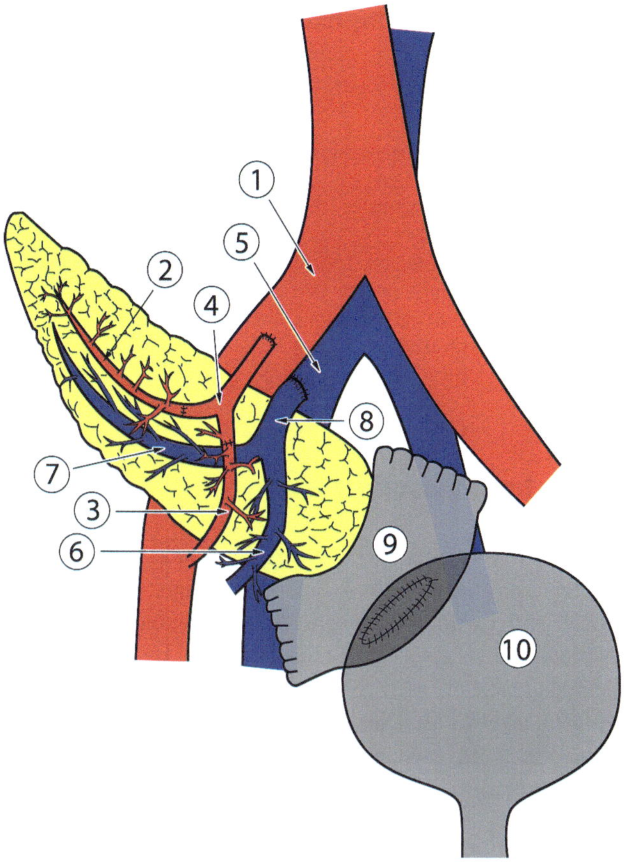

Fig. 40.1 Diagrammatic representation of pancreas transplant. 1—pancreas transplant with enteric drainage (with labels), 2—pancreas transplant with enteric drainage (with labels), 3—pancreas transplant with enteric drainage (without labels), 4—Pancreas transplant with bladder drainage (without labels), 5—post-implantation operative photograph, 6—benching operative photograph

Table 40.2 Advantages and disadvantages of various techniques

Type of drainage	Advantages	Disadvantages
Bladder exocrine and systemic venous endocrine	Early detection of dysfunction Easy access Less infection Less chances of leak, and controlling the leak is relatively easy	Fluid and electrolyte imbalance Acidosis Cystitis/urethritis/urethral stricture Reflux pancreatitis
Enteric exocrine and systemic venous endocrine	Physiological Avoids urologic complications	High incidence of pancreatitis and anastomotic leak Late detection of dysfunction Difficult access for biopsy
Enteric exocrine and portal venous	As mentioned above + Prevents postprandial hypoglycemia Better lipoprotein metabolism	Same as above+ Increased risk of graft thrombosis

40.7 Surgical Complications (Table 40.3)

Table 40.3 Postoperative complications

Complications	Early	Late
Graft parenchymal	Acute pancreatitis Necrotizing pancreatitis Fistula	Rejection Pseudocyst formation Post-transplant lympho-proliferative disease
Enteric	Anastomotic leak	Small bowel obstruction
Vascular	Venous or arterial graft thrombosis (3–10%) Bleeding	Arterial or venous pseudoaneurysm.

40.8 Immunosuppression

Current immunosuppression strategies include induction and maintenance therapy. Anti-lymphocyte serum, such as polyclonal anti-T-cell antibodies (ATG), or monoclonal anti-interleukin-2 receptor antibodies, such as basiliximab and alemtuzumab, are used for induction. Maintenance therapy typically involves a calcineurin inhibitor (Tacrolimus), an anti-metabolite (Mycophenolate Mofetil), and a steroid (Prednisone).

40.9 Results

The one-year patient and graft survival rates for SPK, PAK, and PTA are 97.4%, 97.9%, and 97%, respectively, while the five-year patient and graft survival rates for SPK are 90% and 73%. These figures are comparable to the 81% five-year kidney transplant survival rate. Immunological loss for SPK, PAK, and PTA was 1.6%, 3.7%, and 6%, respectively. Pancreas transplant significantly reduces secondary complications of diabetes, such as diabetic nephropathy and retinopathy, and lowers cardiovascular risk.

40.10 Islet Cell Transplantation

Islet cell transplantation is a promising therapeutic approach for patients with type 1 DM. The procedure involves transplanting harvested islets from a donor pancreas into a recipient to restore endogenous insulin production and improve glycemic control.

40.10.1 Historical Background

The concept of islet cell transplantation dates back to the early twentieth century. The first attempts to transplant pancreatic tissue were made in the 1890s, but significant progress was only made in the 1970s. In 1972, Paul Lacy and colleagues demonstrated the feasibility of isolating islets from the pancreas and transplanting them into diabetic rodents. The first clinical attempts in humans occurred in the 1980s, but success was limited by low islet yield and immune rejection. A breakthrough occurred in 2000 with the introduction of the Edmonton Protocol, developed by James Shapiro and colleagues at the University of Alberta. This protocol involved a steroid-free immunosuppressive regimen and the transplantation of islets from multiple donors, significantly improving outcomes. Since then, islet cell transplantation has become a viable treatment option for select patients with DM type I.

40.10.2 Indications and Patient Selection

Islet cell transplantation is primarily indicated for patients with type 1DM who experience severe hypoglycemia unawareness or brittle diabetes despite optimal medical management. Candidates usually have the following:

- Repeated severe hypoglycemic episodes.
- Reduced awareness of hypoglycemia.
- Failure of intensive insulin therapy to control blood glucose levels.

40.10.3 Contraindications

Active infections, malignancy, and significant cardiovascular disease. Psychological evaluation is also essential to ensure patient adherence to post-transplant immunosuppression.

40.10.4 Techniques of Islet Cell Transplantation

Islet isolation: The donor pancreas is digested with collagenase, and islets are separated from exocrine tissue using density gradient centrifugation. Islet purity and viability are evaluated before transplantation.

Transplantation procedure: Islets are infused into the portal vein of the recipient under radiographic guidance, allowing them to engraft in the liver. The procedure is minimally invasive and performed under local anesthesia.

Immunosuppression: The Edmonton Protocol uses a combination of immunosuppressive agents, including anti-IL-2 receptor antibodies, calcineurin inhibitors, and mTOR inhibitors. Steroid-free regimens are preferred to avoid beta-cell toxicity.

40.10.5 Results

Glycemic control: Successful islet cell transplantation can restore endogenous insulin production, reduce or eliminate the need for exogenous insulin, and improve glycemic control.

Hypoglycemia awareness: Most recipients experience a significant reduction in hypoglycemic episodes and an improved understanding of hypoglycemia.

Long-term outcomes: Although initial results are encouraging, maintaining long-term graft function remains challenging. Many recipients need repeat transplants or must resume insulin therapy within 5 years.

40.10.6 Challenges and Limitations

Donor availability: The scarcity of donor pancreases limits the widespread application of islet cell transplantation.

Immune rejection: Despite immunosuppression, immune-mediated destruction of transplanted islets remains a significant obstacle.

Islet engraftment: Poor engraftment and early loss of islets caused by hypoxia and inflammation decrease the procedure's effectiveness.

Side effects of immunosuppression: Long-term use of immunosuppressive agents raises the risk of infections, cancers, and kidney damage.

40.11 Future Directions

Alternative sources of islets, such as stem cell-derived beta cells and xenotransplantation (e.g., porcine islets), are being researched as potential solutions to donor shortages.

Immunomodulation: Strategies to induce immune tolerance, such as regulatory T cell therapy and the encapsulation of islets, are under investigation.

Bioengineering approaches: Developing bioartificial pancreas devices and 3D-printed islet scaffolds may improve islet survival and function.

Gene editing: CRISPR-Cas9 technology shows promise for creating immune-evasive islets and fixing genetic defects in beta cells.

40.12 Total Pancreatectomy and Islet Autotransplantation

Total pancreatectomy (TP) leads to type 3 DM. Achieving glycemic control without insulin or glucagon is highly challenging. Islet autotransplantation (IAT) has been proposed to address the difficulties of 'brittle diabetes' following TP. In this procedure, the patient's own islets are harvested and infused into the portal vein, where they become engrafted within the liver parenchyma. Because this is autologous tissue, such transplants do not require immunosuppression (Table 40.4).

40.12.1 Technique of Harvesting Islets

Intraductal injection of collagenase is used to break down pancreatic tissue, followed by gentle mechanical dispersion using the semiautomated Ricordi method to release islets from the exocrine tissue. The pellet containing acinar and endocrine tissue is evaluated for islet count, viability, purity, and endotoxin content. Islets are more commonly infused into the patient during the index surgery. Alternatively, islets can be cultured and infused after surgery using a percutaneous approach. Infusion into the portal system is performed by direct puncture of the portal vein, through the splenic vein, or via cannulation of the umbilical vein. During infusion, portal pressure is continuously monitored and should not exceed 25–27 cm H2O (18.4–20 mmHg). Heparin anticoagulation is recommended to prevent portal vein thrombosis.

Table 40.4 Indications and contraindications of TP-IAT

Indications	Contraindications
Chronic pancreatitis with persistent pain despite standard medical and surgical treatments	Preexisting type 1 or type 3 diabetes mellitus
Small duct disease: Chronic pancreatitis with intractable pain	Portal vein thrombosis
Idiopathic recurrent pancreatitis	Portal hypertension
Hereditary chronic pancreatitis	Steatohepatitis
Benign pancreatic tumors requiring TP	Visceral hyperalgesia/ neural sensitization of pain
TP for pancreatic trauma	Psychosocial maladaptation

40.12.2 Postprocedure Care

The islets take about 2–4 weeks to become viable and functional. Therefore, strict glycemic control with exogenous insulin is required for approximately three months. A target HbA1c level below 6.5% is desirable to lessen hyperglycemic stress on the islets. Weaning from insulin then begins.

40.12.3 Results

One-third of the patients become insulin-free, and another third require insulin supplements after IAT. Overall glycemic control and quality of life tend to improve following transplant. Children generally have better outcomes than adults, with an approximately 80% success rate; nearly 50% are insulin-free.

Key Points

- Pancreas transplant is primarily indicated for type 1 diabetes and select cases of type 2 diabetes.
- The types of transplants are: simultaneous pancreas-kidney transplants, pancreas after kidney transplant, and pancreas transplant alone (PTA).
- P-PASS score (based on donor age, BMI, ICU stay, cardiac arrest, serum sodium, serum amylase/lipase, and need for vasopressor) of ≤17 is considered suitable for transplant. A high PDRI score, based on donor sex, age, and race, is associated with a higher risk of graft loss.
- Recipient evaluation is similar to that in renal transplantation.
- The donor pancreas is implanted with vascular anastomosis to the common iliac artery and vein, with drainage into the urinary bladder, duodenum, or jejunum.
- Polyclonal anti-T-cell antibodies (ATG) or monoclonal anti-interleukin-2 receptor antibodies like Basiliximab are used for the induction of immunosuppression. Maintenance therapy typically involves Tacrolimus along with mycophenolate mofetil and prednisone.
- The success rate of pancreas transplant in the first year is close to 97%.
- Islet cell transplantation is a promising therapeutic approach for patients with type 1 DM. The procedure involves the transplantation of harvested islets from a donor pancreas into a recipient to restore endogenous insulin production and improve glycemic control.
- Islet autotransplant (IAT) is recommended after total pancreatectomy for benign diseases and trauma.
- One-third of adults become insulin-free after IAT, and in a significant number, the quality of life and glycemic control improve.
- Results of IAT in the pediatric subgroup are better than in adults.

Selected Reading

1. White SA, Shaw JA, Sutherland DE. Pancreas transplantation. Lancet. 2009;373:1808–17. https://doi.org/10.1016/S0140-6736(09)60609-7.
2. Weems P, Cooper M. Pancreas transplantation in type II diabetes mellitus. World J Transplant. 2014;4(4):216–21. https://doi.org/10.5500/wjt.v4.i4.216.
3. Esmeijer K, Hoogeveen EK, van den Boog PJ, et al. Superior long-term survival for simultaneous pancreas-kidney transplantation as renal replacement therapy: 30-year follow-up of a nationwide cohort. Diabetes Care. 2020;43:321–8. https://doi.org/10.2337/dc19-1580.
4. Witkowski P, Savari O, Matthews JB. Islet autotransplantation and total pancreatectomy. Adv Surg. 2014;48:223–33. https://doi.org/10.1016/j.yasu.2014.05.006.
5. Rickels MR. • Robertson, RP. Pancreatic islet transplantation in humans: recent progress and future directions Endocr Rev. 2019;40:631–68.

Part VII

Spleen

Splenomegaly and Splenectomy for Hematological Disorders

41

Anchin Kalia and Krunal Patel

Abstract

Spleen enlargement results from increased hematological or immunological activity or vascular causes. Laparoscopic splenectomy is recommended for small or moderately enlarged spleens but is contraindicated in cases of massive splenomegaly or portal hypertension. OPSS is rare, with a lifetime risk of 5%, but it carries a high fatality rate of 50–60%. Preoperative vaccination and prophylactic antibiotics are recommended to minimize the risk of OPSS.

Keywords

Splenomegaly · Hypersplenism

The spleen is a reticuloendothelial organ that develops from the dorsal mesogastrium by the fifth week of gestation. It moves to its permanent position in the upper left quadrant of the abdomen and connects to the stomach via the gastrosplenic ligament. In about 20% of individuals, splenic tissue does not fully consolidate into a single mass, leading to the formation of accessory spleens. The spleen plays a key role in quality control over red blood cells in the red pulp by removing old and damaged erythrocytes. The white pulp of the spleen produces antibodies. Additionally, the spleen helps clear antibody-coated bacteria and blood cells from the bloodstream. Splenomegaly refers to an enlarged spleen caused by increased activity, whether due to hematological or immunological reasons, or from vascular congestion when outflow is obstructed by thrombosis, stenosis, or portal hypertension (Table 41.1).

Table 41.1 Hematological causes of splenomegaly

Reticuloendothelial system hyperplasia	*Immune hyperplasia*
Spherocytosis	Infectious mononucleosis
Early sickle cell anemia	Viral infections (AIDS, cytomegalovirus, etc.)
Ovalocytosis	Hemophagocytic lymphohistiocytosis (HLH)
Thalassemia major	Disordered immunoregulation
Hemoglobinopathies	Autoimmune diseases (systemic lupus erythematosus, rheumatoid arthritis)
Paroxysmal nocturnal hemoglobinuria	*Infiltrative hematological disorders*
Pernicious anemia	Gaucher's disease
Bone marrow and hematological malignancies	Niemann-Pick disease
Myeloproliferative disorders (polycythemia vera, essential thrombocythemia)	Hodgkin's disease
Leukemias (acute, chronic, myeloid, lymphoid)	Myeloproliferative disorders
Lymphomas	

41.1 Pathogenesis

- *Extramedullary hematopoiesis*: In disorders like myeloproliferative diseases (e.g., chronic myeloid leukemia and polycythemia vera), the spleen acts as a site of extramedullary hematopoiesis. This compensatory process leads to splenomegaly.
- *Increased sequestration of abnormal blood cells*: Conditions like hemolytic anemias (e.g., hereditary spherocytosis, sickle cell disease, and thalassemia) cause the spleen to rapidly destroy abnormal red blood cells. The spleen filters these defective cells at a higher rate, which increases its workload and leads to hypertrophy. Additionally, the heightened activity of macrophages in

A. Kalia (✉)
Mahatma Gandhi University of Medical Sciences and Technology (MGUMST), Jaipur, Rajasthan, India

Mahatma Gandhi Medical college and hospital, MGUMST, Jaipur, Rajasthan, India

K. Patel
Mahatma Gandhi University of Medical Sciences and Technology (MGUMST), Jaipur, Rajasthan, India

M. Ibrarullah (ed.), *Recent Concepts in Gastrointestinal (GI) Surgery*, https://doi.org/10.1007/978-981-92-1118-0_41

removing damaged cells also contributes to splenic enlargement.

- *Immune hyperactivity*: In hematological disorders involving immune system dysregulation, such as autoimmune hemolytic anemia or immune thrombocytopenia, the spleen becomes overactive by removing antibody-coated blood cells. This heightened immune response leads to the proliferation of lymphoid and reticuloendothelial tissues within the spleen, resulting in its enlargement.
- *Malignant cell infiltration*: Disorders such as leukemias and lymphomas can cause malignant cells to infiltrate the spleen. In conditions like chronic lymphocytic leukemia (CLL) or non-Hodgkin lymphoma, the buildup of malignant lymphocytes within the spleen leads to its enlargement. As these abnormal cells proliferate, the splenic tissue expands, often resulting in significant swelling splenomegaly.
- *Portal hypertension and vascular congestion*: The spleen enlarges due to vascular congestion when outflow is obstructed by thrombosis, stenosis, or portal hypertension.
- *Storage of metabolic by-products*: In metabolic storage disorders such as Gaucher disease and Niemann-Pick disease, splenic enlargement occurs due to the accumulation of undigested substances, such as glucocerebroside and sphingomyelin, respectively, within splenic cells, leading to progressive splenic enlargement.
- *Infectious and inflammatory processes*: Infections associated with hematological conditions, such as the Epstein-Barr Virus (EBV) in infectious mononucleosis, can lead to splenomegaly. The immune response to these infections leads to the proliferation of immune cells within the spleen, resulting in its enlargement. Additionally, bacterial, parasitic, or fungal infections may cause splenic enlargement through a similar immune activation process.

41.2 Clinical Presentation

Patients may remain asymptomatic with mild splenomegaly. The most common symptoms include heaviness and pain in the left upper quadrant, which may radiate to the left shoulder. Pain can also arise from splenic infarction and perisplenitis. An enlarged spleen may compress surrounding structures like the stomach, resulting in early satiety.

41.3 Disease-Specific Symptoms (Table 41.2)

Table 41.2 Disease-specific clinical presentation

Hemolytic anemias Hereditary spherocytosis Sickle cell anemia	Jaundice and dark colored urine Fatigue and pallor Fever, bone, and joint pain in case of hemolytic crisis
Myeloproliferative disorders Polycythemia vera	Fatigue, headaches, and blurred vision Thrombosis or bleeding issues Gout and pruritus
Lymphoproliferative disorders Chronic lymphocytic leukemia Lymphomas	Lymphadenopathy Night sweats, unexplained weight loss, and fevers (B symptoms) Pallor, petechiae, or abnormal bleeding manifestations, and secondary infections
Autoimmune hemolytic anemias	Fever Fatigue, pallor, and tachycardia Jaundice and dark colored urine
Portal hypertension-related splenomegaly	Ascites, jaundice, and variceal bleeding, abnormal bleeding manifestations, and secondary infections

41.4 Diagnosis

The spleen must enlarge to twice its size to be clinically palpable. Imaging modalities, such as ultrasonography, CT, MRI, and liver-spleen radionuclide scans, are used to accurately measure splenic enlargement. Ultrasonography is the most frequently used technique for routine evaluation of spleen size (normal cephalocaudal diameter up to 13 cm) due to its high sensitivity and specificity. It is also safe, noninvasive, quick, and cost-effective. However, it is more important to determine the cause of splenomegaly than simply knowing its size.

41.5 Laboratory Assessment

The patient is advised to undergo basic laboratory tests, including a complete blood count, peripheral blood smear, reticulocyte count, liver function tests, renal function tests, lactate dehydrogenase, and haptoglobin levels. Based on the medical history, physical examination, and basic laboratory results, narrow the potential causes down to hematological

Table 41.3 Investigations for etiology of splenomegaly

Hemolytic anemia	
Autoimmune hemolytic anemia	Positive coombs test, spherocytes on smear
Sickle cell anemia	Sickled red cells on smear
Hereditary spherocytosis	Spherocytes on smear, positive osmotic fragility test
Thalassemia major	Microcytic anemia, target cells on smear, Hb electrophoresis
Myeloproliferative neoplasms	
Polycythemia vera	Raised red cell mass and hematocrit, JAK2 mutation
Primary myelofibrosis	Teardrop-shaped red cells on smear, bone marrow fibrosis
White blood cell disorder	
Chronic myeloid leukemia	Leukocytosis, Philadelphia chromosome present
Chronic lymphocytic leukemia	Lymphocytosis, smudge cells in smear
Acute leukemias	Immature blast cells on smear, anemia, thrombocytopenia
Lymphomas	
Hodgkin lymphoma	CD15+, CD30+, presence of Reed-Sternberg cells
Nodular lymphocyte-predominant Hodgkin lymphoma	CD45+, CD20+ presence of popcorn cells
Platelet disorders	
Essential thrombocythemia	Increased platelet count, JAK2 mutation
Immune thrombocytopenic purpura	Thrombocytopenia, giant platelets on smear

Advanced tests like bone marrow biopsy, flow cytometry, and genetic and molecular tests are used for further confirmation of diagnosis

issues (e.g., hemolytic anemias, leukemias, lymphomas, or myeloproliferative neoplasms) and other causes (e.g., infections such as malaria, viral infections, liver disease, or autoimmune conditions like systemic lupus erythematosus) (Table 41.3).

Splenectomy for hematological disorders fundamentally addresses three key issues: the excessive destruction of blood cells by the spleen, hypersplenism, and complications associated with splenomegaly, including infarction, abscess, and pain.

Table 41.4 Indications for splenectomy in hematological disorders

Indications	Incidence
Platelet disorders	*65%*
Immune thrombocytopenic purpura (ITP)	
Thrombotic thrombocytopenic purpura (TTP)	
Lymphoproliferative disorder *For diagnosis, staging, or complications of splenomegaly*	*25%*
Red cell membrane and hemolytic disorder	*10%*
Red cell membrane anomaly	
Hereditary spherocytosis	
Familial elliptocytosis	
Hereditary pyropoikilocytosis	
Hemoglobinopathies	
Thalassemia	
Drepanocytosis	
Pyruvate kinase deficiency	
Warm autoimmune hemolytic anemia (warm antibodies)	
Chronic myeloproliferative syndromes *For complications of splenomegaly*	
Hypersplenism[a]	
Portal hypertension	
Tropical splenomegaly	

[a]Hypersplenism is defined as (i) splenomegaly; (ii) anemia, leucopenia, thrombocytopenia, a decrease in at least two of the three components; (iii) Normal or hypercellular bone marrow, and (iv) reversal of blood picture after splenectomy

41.6 Preoperative Preparation

- Complete blood count, including platelet count and differential, along with PT and APTT to address any coagulation abnormality.
- Administer vaccinations at least 2 weeks before surgery, targeting *Streptococcus pneumoniae*, *Haemophilus influenzae*, *Neisseria meningitidis*, influenza, and COVID-19.
- Ensure optimum hemoglobin level, considering estimated blood loss during surgery (150 ml for laparoscopic; 250 ml for open procedures).
- Target platelet count should be ≥50,000/μl, although ITP cases may proceed safely with lower counts.
- Attempt to reduce glucocorticoid dosage before surgery to minimize infection risk.
- Consider stopping rituximab.

41.7 Open or Laparoscopic Splenectomy?

The spleen can be removed either via an open laparotomy or a minimally invasive technique, such as laparoscopic or robotic surgery. In centers with the necessary expertise, laparoscopic splenectomy is now often the preferred method. Relative contraindications to laparoscopic surgery are as follows:

- Massive splenomegaly
- Presence of portal hypertension
- Nonavailability of expertise and equipment
- Presence of accessory spleen since its identification is easier with open surgery

41.8 Important Considerations When Performing Splenectomy

- Massive splenomegaly, with or without portal hypertension, is better accessed through a long midline incision with thoracic extension.
- Division of the gastrocolic ligament and ligation of the splenic artery in continuity reduces the splenic volume and makes handling better.
- Mass ligation of splenic hilar structures should be avoided because it may not be secure and could also damage the pancreatic tail.
- In cases where splenectomy is performed for hematologic conditions, it is also important to thoroughly search for and remove any accessory spleens.
- Concomitant cholecystectomy may be required for documented gallstones that accompany certain hemolytic anemias.

Overwhelming Postsplenectomy Sepsis (OPSS) OPSS is a rare but often fatal complication, with a mortality rate of 50–60%, even with treatment. The annual risk of OPSS is estimated to be between 0.23% and 0.42%, and the lifetime risk is around 5%. Young children, elderly people, immunocompromised patients, and those with hematological disorders are especially vulnerable to developing OPSS, with 80% of cases occurring within the first 2 years after splenectomy. Although the risk is highest during the initial years after surgery, it remains throughout a person's life. Encapsulated bacteria, including *Streptococcus pneumoniae*, *Neisseria meningitidis*, and *Haemophilus influenzae*, are the primary cause of OPSS. Other bacteria, such as *Escherichia coli*, beta-hemolytic *Streptococcus*, *Staphylococcus aureus*, and *Pseudomonas* species, also carry significant risks.

Preventive measures for reducing OPSS risk are as follows:

- Vaccination with a polyvalent pneumococcal vaccine should be carried out 10–14 days before an elective splenectomy. Additional vaccines against *Haemophilus* and

Table 41.5 Complications of splenectomy

Intra-/postoperative	Short term	Long term
Hemorrhage	Deep vein thrombosis	Venous thrombosis
Gastric ileus	Spleno-portal thrombosis	Arterial thrombosis
Acute pancreatitis/ pancreatic fistula	Pulmonary atelectasis	Recurrent infection
Colonic injury	OPSS	OPSS
Subphrenic abscess		

OPSS overwhelming postsplenectomy sepsis

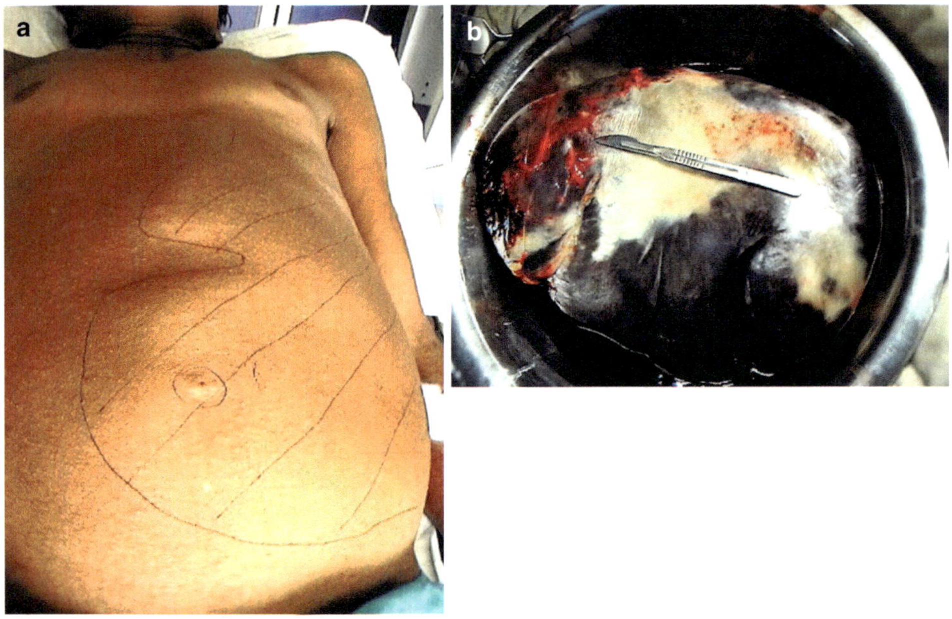

Fig. 41.1 (**a**) Massive splenomegaly (outlined in abdomen) in a patient with sickle cell thalassemia trait. (**b**) Splenectomy specimen

Neisseria are recommended. However, less effective vaccines can also be administered after surgery. Prophylactic antibiotics are crucial for patients in high-risk groups.
- Prompt antibiotic treatment at the first signs of infection.

Venous thromboembolism: Splenectomy is associated with an increased risk of venous thromboembolism (VTE), which encompasses portal vein thrombosis, splenic vein thrombosis, deep vein thrombosis, and pulmonary embolism. This heightened risk appears to be due to multiple factors, likely involving thrombocytosis, changes in vascular anatomy, increased blood viscosity, and coagulation alterations that may be linked to the underlying condition necessitating the splenectomy. An early postoperative CT scan (within the first week of surgery) is advised to monitor any progression of splenic vein thrombosis to the portal or superior mesenteric veins, facilitating timely adjustments in anticoagulation therapy. Severe thrombocytosis may necessitate prophylactic anticoagulation therapy.

Key Points
- Spleen enlargement results from increased hematological or immunological activity, or vascular congestion due to outflow obstruction caused by thrombosis, stenosis, or portal hypertension.
- Platelet disorders, lymphoproliferative disorders, and hemolytic disorders account for the majority of hematological causes for splenectomy.
- It is desirable to correct anemia and thrombocytopenia to an optimal level before surgery.
- Vaccines should be administered at least 2 weeks ahead of surgery.
- Laparoscopic splenectomy is recommended for small or moderately enlarged spleens, but is contraindicated in cases of massive splenomegaly or portal hypertension.
- OPSS is rare, with a lifetime risk of 5%, but it carries a high fatality rate of 50–60%. Young individuals, the elderly, immunocompromised patients, and those with hematological disorders are more prone to OPSS.
- Preoperative vaccination and prophylactic antibiotics are recommended to minimize the risk of OPSS.
- Splenectomy is associated with an increased risk of venous thromboembolism and may require prophylactic anticoagulation in selected cases.

Selected Reading

1. Weledji EP, et al. Benefits and risks of splenectomy. Int J Surg. 2014;12(2):113–9.
2. Jankulovski N, Antovic S, Kuzmanovska B, Mitevski A, et al. Splenectomy for haematological disorders. Pril (Makedon Akad Nauk Umet Odd Med Nauki). 2014;35(1):181–7.
3. Bonnet S, Guédon A, Ribeil JA, Suarez F, Tamburini J, Gaujoux S, et al. Indications and outcome of splenectomy in hematologic disease. J Visc Surg. 2017;154:421–9.

Splenectomy and Splenic Preservation

42

Shridhar G. Iyer

Abstract

Trauma and hematological disorders are the leading reasons for splenectomy worldwide. Preserving the spleen is increasingly recommended for its immunological functions. Partial splenectomy and splenorrhaphy, supported by topical hemostatic agents, can be attempted in cases of limited injury. In elective cases and when the spleen is mildly to moderately enlarged, laparoscopic splenectomy is the preferred procedure. Spleen-preserving distal pancreatectomy (SPDP) is recommended for benign or low-grade pancreatic tumors. The two recommended techniques for SPDP are the Kimura technique (splenic vessel-preserving) and the Warshaw technique (splenic vessel-sacrificing).

Keywords

Splenectomy · Splenic preservation

Splenectomy is performed for a diverse range of indications, broadly categorized into trauma, hematologic disorders, hypersplenism, infections, and as part of diagnostic or incidental procedures. Although splenectomy becomes unavoidable in specific clinical situations, preserving the spleen when possible is increasingly favored because of its immunological functions. Trauma remains the leading indication worldwide, especially in high-volume trauma centers, where splenic rupture from blunt or penetrating injuries requires urgent intervention. In nontrauma settings, the most frequent indications include *autoimmune and erythrocyte disorders* such as *immune thrombocytopenic purpura (ITP)* and *hereditary spherocytosis*, where splenectomy offers either curative or significant symptomatic relief. Patterns of indications vary by institution: *oncology-focused* centers report higher rates of incidental or diagnostic splenectomies, while *trauma hospitals* see splenectomy predominantly for injury. Across all settings, careful patient selection, vaccination, and consideration of spleen-preserving alternatives remain integral to modern splenic surgery (Table 42.1).

S. G. Iyer (✉)
National University of Singapore, Mount Elizabeth Medical Centre, ALPS Clinic, Mount Elizabeth, Singapore
e-mail: surisg@nus.edu.sg

M. Ibrarullah (ed.), *Recent Concepts in Gastrointestinal (GI) Surgery*, https://doi.org/10.1007/978-981-92-1118-0_42

Table 42.1 Indications for splenectomy

Category	Diagnosis	Indications for splenectomy	Presplenectomy requirements/ considerations	Response to splenectomy
Autoimmune/ erythrocyte disorders	Idiopathic thrombocytopenic purpura (ITP)	Refractory thrombocytopenia unresponsive to steroids or intravenous immunoglobulins	Confirm diagnosis; exclude secondary causes; trial medical therapy	Excellent response in >80% of cases; durable remission common
	Hereditary spherocytosis	Anemia, splenomegaly, gallstones, growth delay	Confirm diagnosis; delay until age ≥5 years	Curative in most cases
	Autoimmune hemolytic anemia (AIHA)	Failure of corticosteroids or immunosuppressive therapy	Confirm warm AIHA; exclude secondary causes	Good response if warm AIHA; less predictable in cold agglutinin disease
	Thalassemia (major/ intermedia)	Hypersplenism, transfusion overload, infarction	Evaluate disease burden; transfusion history	Variable; may reduce transfusion burden, but not curative
	Sickle cell disease	Recurrent sequestration crisis, infarction, symptomatic hypersplenism	Elective splenectomy after 2 years of age	Reduces crisis frequency; does not prevent long-term complications
Hematologic (malignant)	Hairy cell leukemia	Cytopenias or symptomatic splenomegaly in resistant cases	Confirm via bone marrow biopsy; splenectomy when chemotherapy fails	Effective in cytopenia control in chemo-refractory cases
	Chronic myeloid leukemia, chronic lymphoid leukemia, myelofibrosis	Massive splenomegaly, symptomatic hypersplenism	Confirm diagnosis; splenectomy is palliative; optimize counts	Palliative benefit: may improve symptoms but not the disease course
Trauma/iatrogenic	Splenic rupture (blunt/ penetrating)	Hemodynamic instability, high-grade injury	Follow ATLS protocol; angioembolization if stable; intraop assessment	Life-saving; no disease-specific outcome needed
	Iatrogenic splenic injury	Incidental during upper abdominal surgery	Decision based on the extent of injury and hemodynamics	Complication management; not disease-targeted
Hypersplenism	Gaucher disease, sarcoidosis, infiltrative/ neoplastic	Cytopenias, symptomatic splenomegaly	Confirm diagnosis; consider alternate therapy; vaccinate	Improves cytopenia and symptoms; disease persists
	Portal hypertension, splenic vein thrombosis	Hypersplenism, isolated gastric varices	Confirm via CT/MRI; evaluate liver function and operative risk	Improves varices and cytopenia; addresses secondary effects
Infective/ inflammatory	Splenic abscess	Failure of drainage, multiloculated/ruptured abscess	Confirm with imaging; attempt drainage; antibiotics	Resolves infection; definitive if drainage fails
	Hydatid cyst	Symptomatic, calcified, or ruptured cyst	Exclude liver involvement; perioperative albendazole	Definitive if cyst inaccessible or calcified; risk of rupture avoided
Congenital/ anatomic	Wandering spleen	Torsion, infarction, symptomatic mobility	Confirm with imaging; splenopexy if viable; total splenectomy if infarcted	Prevents torsion/ infarction; resolves pain/ mobility issues
	Nonparasitic splenic cysts	Large, symptomatic, or ruptured cyst	Confirm benign nature; partial splenectomy preferred if feasible	Relieves mass effect; definitive for large or symptomatic cysts
Incidental	During surgery for adjacent tumors/organs	Spleen removed due to anatomical proximity or oncologic need	Preserve spleen if oncologically safe; assess vascular involvement	Incidental; not therapeutic for splenic disease
Diagnostic/ staging	Lymphoma or unexplained splenomegaly	When less invasive diagnostics are inconclusive	Exclude biopsy alternatives; ensure splenectomy alters management	Enables diagnosis/ staging; no direct therapeutic role
Vascular	Splenic artery aneurysm	Large (>2 cm), symptomatic, ruptured, or pregnancy associated	Confirm via CTA/DSA; consider endovascular alternatives	Prevents rupture; definitive for large or symptomatic aneurysms

42.1 Evolution of Surgery for Spleen

- Traditional approach: Until the 1970s, splenectomy was the main procedure for splenic disease.
- Splenic preservation: Recognizing the high infection risk in asplenic and hyposplenic patients has led to spleen-preserving techniques like splenorrhaphy for trauma. Partial splenectomy may be considered in elective cases, such as hypersplenism, when total removal is unnecessary.
- Rise of minimally invasive surgery: In the past 15 years, laparoscopic splenectomy has become widely used for elective procedures. It is even employed in cases of massive splenomegaly. It is now considered the preferred procedure in most centers.

42.2 Splenic Trauma

The spleen is the most common intra-abdominal organ injured by blunt trauma. Historically, splenic trauma was uniformly managed by complete splenectomy.

42.2.1 Presentation

Signs and symptoms of an isolated splenic injury often include tenderness in the left upper quadrant of the abdomen. Focal tenderness over ribs 9 through 11 should raise suspicion of a possible splenic injury. Patients may experience referred pain to the left shoulder, known as Kehr's sign, especially when placed in the Trendelenburg position. A palpable mass in the left upper quadrant, indicating a contained or subcapsular hematoma, is known as Ballance's sign.

42.2.2 Diagnosis

Diagnostic findings may include a fall in hematocrit and hemoglobin, although initial levels might seem normal before volume resuscitation. Often, there is an initial leukocytosis ranging from 15,000 to 20,000/mm^3. Plain abdominal radiographs might reveal left rib fractures or displacement and a corrugated appearance of the stomach's greater curvature due to hematoma.

Focused assessment with sonography for trauma (FAST) may detect fluid or blood in the abdomen. Computed tomography (CT) with contrast is the most important diagnostic tool for hemodynamically stable patients, demonstrating splenic contour and extrasplenic blood. A staging system for splenic trauma is used, based on the degree of damage to the parenchyma and proximity to major vessels.

42.2.3 Management

The current trend in management is a nonoperative approach for lower-grade injuries, with operative management centered around splenic preservation when possible.

Factors influencing operative versus nonoperative management include the presence of peritonitis, associated injuries requiring surgery, overall injury severity, evidence of hypovolemic shock and ongoing bleeding, and the patient's age. Urgent laparotomy is required for patients with diffuse peritonitis or hypotension due to hypovolemic shock. Nonoperative management involves close observation in an intensive care unit, serial abdominal examinations, and repeated hemoglobin and hematocrit assessments. Follow-up CT scans may be performed, although routine scans might not change management if the patient remains stable. "Delayed splenic rupture" is considered a relatively rare event when patients are monitored prospectively. When operative management is chosen, the goals are to control ongoing bleeding, preserve as much viable splenic tissue as possible, and debride nonviable tissue. Minor peripheral splenic injuries can be managed with techniques such as primary repair, mesh repair, topical hemostatic agents (microfibrillar collagen, thrombins of Gelfoam, fibrin glue sealants), or the argon beam coagulator. Partial splenectomy may be considered based on the idea of segmental blood supply (Table 42.2).

Table 42.2 American Association for the Surgery of Trauma (AAST)—organ injury scaling (OIS) for spleen

Grade	Injury description	CT findings	Management
I	Subcapsular hematoma (<10% surface area)	Thin rim of hypodense fluid around the spleen	Nonoperative (98% success)
	Laceration (<1 cm depth)	Linear hypodensity	
II	Subcapsular hematoma (10–50% surface area)	Partial capsular disruption	Nonoperative (90% success)
	Laceration (1–3 cm depth) *without* vascular injury		
III	Subcapsular hematoma (>50% surface area)	Shattered appearance, active contrast extravasation	Nonop vs. embolization (60–80% success)
	Laceration (>3 cm depth) *or* trabecular vessel injury		
IV	Laceration involving segmental/hilar vessels *with* devascularization (>25% spleen)	Active bleeding, pseudoaneurysm	Embolization or splenectomy
V	Shattered spleen *or* hilar avulsion (complete devascularization)	No perfusion to the spleen	Splenectomy (100%)

42.3 Nonoperative Management of Splenic Trauma (Tables 42.3 and 42.4)

Table 42.3 Stepwise protocol for nonoperative management of splenic trauma

Step	Action	Details
1	Initial stabilization	Follow advanced trauma life support (ATLS) protocol; resuscitate, monitor vitals (MAP $\geq$ 65 mmHg, HR < 100)
2	Imaging	Perform contrast-enhanced CT to grade injury (AAST I–V), assess for contrast blush, pseudoaneurysm, or large hemoperitoneum
3	Monitoring location	Grades I–II: ward-level care; Grades III–V: ICU or high-dependency unit recommended
4	Hemodynamic and lab monitoring	Continuous vitals, serial abdominal exams, Hb/hematocrit every 4–6 h for the first 24–48 h
5	Angiography ± embolization	Indicated in cases with contrast blush, pseudoaneurysm, high-grade injury, or moderate hemoperitoneum
6	Failure criteria (triggers for surgery)	Persistent hypotension, transfusion >2–3 units, new peritonitis, dropping Hb, or rebleeding on imaging
7	Activity restriction	Grades I–II: no contact sports for 4–6 weeks; Grades III–V: restriction for 8–12 weeks
8	Follow-up	No routine imaging for Grade I–II if asymptomatic; repeat imaging in Grade III–V or if symptoms persist

Table 42.4 Indications for Surgery

Hemodynamic instability	Persistent hypotension despite adequate fluid/blood resuscitation Recurrent or worsening shock
Transfusion requirements	Need for >2–3 units of packed RBCs to maintain hemodynamic stability Ongoing transfusion requirement beyond 24 h
Worsening hemoglobin/hematocrit	Continuous drop in serial hemoglobin or hematocrit despite stabilization measures
New or worsening peritonitis	Emergence of guarding, rebound tenderness, or a rigid abdomen Suggests peritoneal irritation due to blood or visceral injury
Radiologic evidence of ongoing or delayed bleeding	Repeat imaging shows: Expanding hematoma New or enlarging contrast blush Development of pseudoaneurysm Increasing or persistent hemoperitoneum Splenic infarction with secondary rupture
Failure after angioembolization	Hemodynamic deterioration despite embolization Rebleeding requiring surgical control
Associated injuries	Polytrauma necessitating laparotomy for other indications
Delayed splenic rupture	Patient initially stable, but presents days later with new onset pain or hemodynamic compromise or sudden hemoperitoneum

42.4 Splenectomy for Trauma

42.4.1 Initial Steps (ATLS Aligned)

- Airway, breathing, circulation (ABCs) according to ATLS protocol.
- Insert large-bore IV access and initiate fluid/blood resuscitation
- Cross-match 4–6 units of blood.
- Monitor vitals continuously and assess for hemodynamic instability
- Insert urinary catheter and nasogastric tube if indicated
- If the patient is stable, perform a contrast-enhanced CT
- Prepare for emergency laparotomy if
  Hemodynamic instability persists
  Peritonitis is present
    Positive FAST + clinical deterioration

42.4.2 Antibiotics and Vaccination

- Broad-spectrum antibiotics preoperatively (e.g., cefazolin ± metronidazole)
- Ensure a plan for postoperative vaccination (pneumococcus, H. influenzae, and meningococcus) within 14 days if splenectomy is done

42.4.3 Splenectomy

In cases of trauma, because of the exigencies, an open approach is preferred over laparoscopic splenectomy. An upper midline incision allows quick access to the spleen and other parts of the abdomen for exploration and managing associated injuries. The spleen is brought out into the wound by dividing its posterior attachments. If identifying the splenic vessels at the hilum is difficult, they are double-clamped. After preserving the pancreatic tail, the splenic pedicle is carefully divided. The remaining perisplenic attachments and short gastric vessels are divided, and then the spleen is removed.

42.4.4 Spleen-Preserving Surgery

42.4.4.1 Indications

- Hemodynamically stable patient
- Isolated splenic injury (AAST grade I–III)
- Accessible splenic injury amenable to repair or partial resection
- Pediatric or young adult patients preferred

42.4.4.2 Operative Steps

Once the patient is positioned and a midline laparotomy is performed, a thorough exploration of the abdominal cavity is essential to exclude other intra-abdominal injuries. Mobilization of the spleen begins by dividing the splenocolic ligament, followed by the splenophrenic and splenorenal ligaments, to allow the spleen to be gently rotated medially into the laparotomy wound. The ligaments are divided using sharp dissection or diathermy, along with blunt dissection for the splenorenal ligament area. Care is taken not to further injure the spleen or the tail of the pancreas, which lies close to the splenic hilum. If necessary, a vascular clamp is applied to the splenic hilum or the hilum is pinched to temporarily control bleeding during the repair. With the spleen exposed, careful attention is given to identifying the location and severity of the splenic injury. If the injury seems suitable for preservation—usually AAST Grade I–III—and the patient remains hemodynamically stable, a spleen-preserving repair may be attempted.

Splenorrhaphy In cases of capsular or superficial parenchymal laceration, the preferred method is splenorrhaphy, where absorbable sutures (such as 3-0 chromic or 2-0/3-0 Vicryl coated) are placed across the defect using pledgets or Teflon felt to prevent suture cutting through. It is better to place all the sutures first and then tighten and tie them sequentially with a two-hand knot to avoid suture lacerations.

Topical hemostatic agents such as oxidized regenerated cellulose (e.g., Surgicel), gelatine sponge, or fibrin sealants can be layered over the repair to enhance hemostasis. Alternatively, a polyglactin (Vicryl) mesh wrap may be used to encase the spleen, holding it together and tamponading small bleeding sites.

Partial Splenectomy Partial splenectomy is considered for deeper lacerations or segmental devascularization. The procedure starts by identifying the segmental arterial branches to the injured part of the spleen, usually at the inferior pole. These branches are isolated, ligated, and divided, creating a clear line of demarcation between perfused and ischemic tissue. The nonviable tissue is sharply resected or removed with energy devices, and the cut surface is carefully oversewn with absorbable sutures, possibly with pledgets, and covered with hemostatic agents.

Once bleeding is controlled, the vascular clamp is released (if applied), and the spleen is carefully observed for 5–10 min to ensure that there is no ongoing oozing or arterial bleeding. A drain is placed only if there is concern about ongoing seepage or associated injuries; otherwise, routine drainage is avoided.

Intraoperatively, surgeons must remain vigilant for pitfalls such as missed hilar injuries, which can cause delayed hemorrhage or infarction. Excessive traction during mobilization risks damaging the pancreatic tail, and overly deep sutures can lead to secondary parenchymal tears. If bleeding cannot be controlled reliably or if the injury appears more extensive than initially thought, the surgeon should not hesitate to proceed with splenectomy.

42.5 Minimally Invasive Splenectomy: Laparoscopy/Robotic

Laparoscopic splenectomy has become the standard treatment for most elective cases because of its benefits, including less postoperative pain, shorter hospital stays, improved cosmesis, and fewer complications compared to open splenectomy. It is especially appropriate for conditions where the spleen is normal or moderately enlarged. Robotic splenectomy or computer-assisted surgery (CAS) was introduced into clinical practice in 2000, with its application to splenectomy reported from 2002.

Proposed Advantages of Robotic Splenectomy

- Increased instrument dexterity with wristed instruments and greater degrees of freedom than conventional laparoscopic tools.
- Enhanced optics: 3D high-definition vision improves depth perception, especially in anatomically complex areas.
- Stability: Tremor filtration and precision handling may reduce inadvertent injury, particularly around the splenic hilum or pancreas.
- Improved ergonomics: Especially for long or complex procedures.
- Perfusion assessment with Indocyanine green—Robotic platforms have the ICG camera integrated in the system. Although feasible with laparoscopic, with the current platforms offering an inbuilt system.

Limitations

- Increased operative time: Studies show a mean increase of approximately 30–45 min compared to conventional laparoscopy.
- High cost.
- Limited evidence of clinical benefit over laparoscopy.
- Questionable benefit for routine cases**:** No proven superiority in outcomes for standard splenectomy, leading many experienced laparoscopic surgeons to consider it unnecessary.

42.6 Complications (Table 42.5)

Table 42.5 Postsplenectomy complications

Complication	Presentation	Mechanism/risk factor	Management
Hemorrhage	Early	Injury to the splenic hilum or short gastric vessels	Intra-op hemostasis; post-op bleeding may need reoperation or angioembolization
Gastric stasis or early satiety	Early/late	Post-surgical adhesion or a large residual space	Conservative management with prokinetics and dietary adjustment
Injury to adjacent organs	Early	Pancreatic tail, stomach, or colon trauma	Drain fistulas; surgical repair if necessary
Pancreatic fistula	Early	Tail of the pancreas injured near the splenic hilum	Conservative; ERCP or surgery if persistent
Wound or intra-abdominal infection	Early	Hematoma, contamination	Empiric followed by culture-based antibiotics; drainage of abscess if needed
Subphrenic abscess	Early	Residual blood or necrotic tissue	CT-guided drainage; antibiotics
Pulmonary complications (atelectasis, pneumonia)	Early	Post-op splinting, poor respiratory effort	Incentive spirometry; chest physiotherapy; early ambulation
Venous thromboembolism (VTE)	Early/late	Reactive thrombocytosis, reduced mobility	Heparin prophylaxis; therapeutic anticoagulation if diagnosed
Overwhelming Post-Splenectomy Infection (OPSI)	Late	Loss of splenic immune surveillance (esp. encapsulated bacteria)	Emergency antibiotics; *vaccination*, education, ± lifelong penicillin
Thrombocytosis	Late	Loss of splenic sequestration	Usually benign; aspirin if platelets >1 million or thrombotic risk
Splenosis	Late	Seeding of splenic tissue in the peritoneum post-trauma/surgery	Often incidental; treat only if symptomatic

42.7 Spleen-Preserving Distal Pancreatectomy (SPDP)

42.7.1 Indications

Kimura and Warshaw techniques are the commonly described methods of spleen-preserving distal pancreatectomy. Situations where resection of the distal pancreas is necessary but spleen preservation is preferable include the following:

- Benign or low-grade malignant tumors (e.g., intraductal papillary mucinous neoplasms, mucinous cystic neoplasms, and neuroendocrine tumors)
- Preservation of immune function, particularly in young or immunocompromised patients
- Avoidance of OPSI risk
- Patients at a higher risk of postsplenectomy complications (e.g., hematological malignancies in remission)
- Desire to prevent gastric varices or portal hypertension, especially when the splenic vein is normal

Kimura technique The procedure preserves both the splenic artery and vein, preserving the spleen's direct blood supply. Key surgical steps include identifying the pancreas and the splenic artery/vein at the superior and posterior aspects of the pancreas in the mid-body or at a suitable location, carefully dissecting the pancreas away from the splenic vessels, transecting the pancreas with a linear stapler (or ultrasonic shear in open surgery), and completing the dissection of the pancreas from the splenic vessels up to the tail.

Pitfalls of this procedure include the risk of vessel injury, which may result in bleeding requiring conversion to the Warshaw technique (see below) or splenectomy, longer operative time, and increased technical demands. The procedure is not feasible if the tumor involves or encases the splenic vessels.

Warshaw technique It involves ligating the splenic artery and vein, relying on the short gastric and left gastroepiploic vessels for splenic perfusion. The operative steps include ligating the splenic artery ± vein near the pancreatic neck or body using clips or a stapler. The short gastric vessels are carefully preserved to maintain splenic blood flow. Distal pancreas transection is carried out using a stapler or a scalpel. The reported pitfalls of this procedure are the risk of splenic infarction or abscess (~2–10%), potential for gastric varices due to splenic vein ligation, and the possibility that it may require delayed splenectomy if infarction occurs.

Key Points

- Trauma and hematological disorders are the leading reasons for splenectomy worldwide.
- Preserving the spleen is increasingly recommended for its immunological functions.
- CECT abdomen is the primary diagnostic tool for splenic trauma in hemodynamically stable patients.
- Overall injury severity, peritonitis, related injuries requiring surgery, signs of hypovolemic shock, and ongoing bleeding are indications for emergency laparotomy and splenectomy.
- Conservative management is appropriate for low-grade injuries in hemodynamically stable patients.
- In trauma cases, due to urgency, an open approach is preferred over laparoscopic splenectomy. An upper midline incision allows quick access to the spleen and other abdominal quadrants for exploration and treatment of associated injuries.
- Partial splenectomy and splenorrhaphy, supported by topical hemostatic agents, can be attempted in cases of limited injury.
- In elective cases and when the spleen is mildly to moderately enlarged, laparoscopic splenectomy is the preferred procedure.
- Spleen-preserving distal pancreatectomy (SPDP) is recommended for benign or low-grade pancreatic tumors.
- The two recommended techniques for SPDP are the Kimura technique (splenic vessel-preserving) and the Warshaw technique (splenic vessel-sacrificing).

Selected Reading

1. Atkins K, Schneider AB. Splenic salvage: is there a role for splenorrhaphy in the management of adult splenic trauma? Am Surg. 2023;89:5599–56.
2. Granieri S, Bonomi A, Frassini S, et al. Kimura's vs Warshaw's technique for spleen preserving distal pancreatectomy: a systematic review and meta-analysis of high-quality studies. HPB. 2023;25:614–24.

Part VIII

Surgery for Tropical and Infectious Diseases

Surgical Complications of Enteric Fever

43

Kaushik Bhattacharya

Abstract

Perforation and lower GI bleeding are the most common complications of enteric fever that require surgery. These complications usually arise in the third week of fever. Simple closure of the perforation and peritoneal lavage suffices in a stable patient. In lower GI bleeding, surgery is required for an ongoing exsanguinating bleed.

Keywords

Enteric fever · Typhoid complications

Surgical complications usually occur 2–3 weeks after the onset of enteric fever. About a quarter of laboratory-confirmed, hospitalized patients with typhoid face surgical issues like perforation or bleeding. The overall rate of enteric perforation in children is approximately 10%, which increases to as much as 30% by age 12 (Table 43.1).

Table 43.1 Surgical complications of enteric fever

Typhoid intestinal perforation(TIP)
Lower gastrointestinal (GI) bleed
Acute acalculous cholecystitis and its complications (gangrene and perforation)
Intraabdominal abscesses
Rare complications: pancreatitis, hepatic and splenic abscesses, pleural effusion, and orchitis

43.1 Etiopathogenesis of Complications

The terminal ileum is predominantly affected in typhoid fever due to several anatomical and immunological reasons:

- A high concentration of Peyer's patches in the terminal ileum is responsible for immune surveillance and initiating immune responses to gut pathogens. *Salmonella typhi* enters the M cells of Peyer's patches, leading to infection, inflammation, and eventual necrosis.
- Low flow rate and stagnation in the terminal ileum enable *Salmonella typhi* to remain longer in the area, increasing its chances of colonization and penetration into the mucosa.
- The unique vascular supply of the terminal ileum, distinct from other parts of the gut, combined with inflammatory edema, makes the terminal ileum vulnerable to ischemia, ulceration, and perforation.

K. Bhattacharya (✉)
Mata Gujri Memorial Medical College and LSK Hospital,
Kishanganj, Bihar, India

M. Ibrarullah (ed.), *Recent Concepts in Gastrointestinal (GI) Surgery*, https://doi.org/10.1007/978-981-92-1118-0_43

43.2 Diagnosis of Enteric Fever (Table 43.2)

Table 43.2 Diagnostic tests for enteric fever

Investigation	Result	Comment
Hematological and biochemical tests	Leukopenia, anemia, thrombocytopenia, raised C-reactive protein, raised ESR, and liver function test abnormalities	Leukocytosis is noted in cases of perforation and peritonitis
Blood culture	Growth of *Salmonella typhi* or *Salmonella paratyphi*	The gold standard of diagnosis in the first week of illness Sensitivity is highest in the first 7–10 days before antibiotic use
Widal test	H agglutinin titer ≥ 1:160 and O agglutinin titer ≥ 1:80, toward the end of the first week, is considered positive	Serological test that detects antibodies against *Salmonella typhi* Sensitivity is 50–70% and specificity is 80–90% False-positive results may be due to prior infections or vaccinations
Typhidot and Tubex M	Positive	Rapid serological tests Detects IgM and IgG antibodies specific to *Salmonella typhi* Useful for early diagnosis
Enzyme-linked immunosorbent assay (ELISA)	Positive	It is a quantitative (titer) test that detects IgM and IgG antibodies against *Salmonella typhi* Specificity and sensitivity are more than 95%
Polymerase chain reaction (PCR)	Positive	Detects *Salmonella typhi* DNA Specificity and sensitivity are more than 90%

43.3 Diagnosis of Complications

X-ray of the abdomen in the erect position can detect free air under the diaphragm, a hallmark of intestinal perforation. It may also show signs of intestinal obstruction or air-fluid levels in cases of severe ileus.

Ultrasound is particularly helpful to detect complications like acute cholecystitis, liver abscess, or splenic abscess.

Computed tomography (CT) scan of the abdomen is indicated to confirm or exclude enteric perforation and generalized or localized peritonitis, particularly in a patient presenting with ambiguous abdominal signs and symptoms. CT angiography may be helpful in a patient presenting with massive lower GI bleeding.

Upper GI endoscopy and/or *colonoscopy* are part of the diagnostic work-up in patients presenting with GI bleeding.

43.4 Enteric Perforation

The incidence of intestinal perforation in typhoid fever ranges from 0.8% to 18%. Perforation usually occurs during the third week of fever, although it can occur as early as the second week in cases of fulminant disease. The onset of severe abdominal pain, guarding, and rigidity is followed by distension with absent bowel sounds. If not treated promptly, it can lead to sepsis, shock, and multi-organ failure. Significant guarding and rigidity may be absent in cases of severe sepsis. A subclinical perforation may present with focal tenderness, abdominal distension, persistent ileus, and signs of sepsis (Fig. 43.1).

43.4.1 Management

Diagnosis is confirmed with a plain X-ray of the abdomen in an upright position. If gas under the diaphragm is not visible on the plain X-ray, a CT scan may be necessary to verify a subclinical perforation. Initial resuscitation involves intravenous fluids, nasogastric suction, and broad-spectrum antibiotics to treat enteric fever and peritonitis. The preferred parenteral antibiotics for enteric fever are fluoroquinolones, ceftriaxone, and amoxicillin, while those for peritonitis include carbapenems or cephalosporins combined with ami-

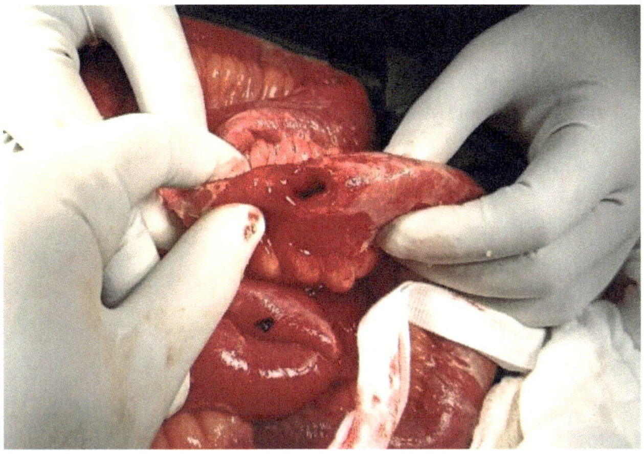

Fig. 43.1 Enteric perforation at laparotomy

noglycosides and metronidazole or tinidazole. During laparotomy, the affected segment of the terminal ileum is identified. Although multiple ulcers may be present, perforation is usually single. Rarely, more than one perforation or a thinned-out ulcer base with impending perforation can be identified in the intestine. Closure of the perforation with interrupted sutures in two layers, along with peritoneal lavage and drainage, suffices in most cases. However, non-healing ulcers and dehiscence can lead to intra-abdominal abscesses or fecal fistulas, especially in septic and hypotensive patients. In such cases, exteriorizing the affected segment as an ileostomy is a safer option. The ileostomy is closed later when the patient has fully recovered. Alternative treatments, such as segmental resection with anastomosis, perforation closure, and ileo-transverse bypass, have been described but with limited success.

43.5 Lower GI Bleeding

Lower GI bleeding occurs in 10–12.5% of patients with typhoid fever. The bleeding is usually mild but can be severe in 2–5% of cases. The typical presentation includes a sudden onset of melena or hematochezia. The standard protocol for investigating lower GI bleeding involves upper GI endoscopy, colonoscopy, CT angiography, and RBC scintigraphy, depending on the severity of bleeding. Colonoscopy is considered reliable for diagnosis in more than 90% of patients. In enteric fever, involvement of the cecum and ascending colon is observed in over 20% of cases. Part of the ulcer-bearing terminal ileum can also be examined during colonoscopy.

43.5.1 Management

The patient is initially managed conservatively to restore hemodynamic stability. Blood transfusion should be performed to maintain hemoglobin around 8 g/dL. Antimicrobial treatment for enteric fever should start with intravenous ceftriaxone or fluoroquinolones. Surgery is indicated for an ongoing exsanguinating bleed, persistent hemodynamic instability, or associated perforation. Right hemicolectomy involving the ulcer-bearing segment of the terminal ileum, cecum, and ascending colon is the preferred procedure. After resection, an end ileostomy with delayed reconstruction is the safer option in a hypotensive and unstable patient.

43.6 Cholecystitis and Gallbladder Perforation

Acute acalculous cholecystitis is a rare complication of enteric fever, with an incidence of 1.7–2.8%. Typical signs of acute cholecystitis, such as right upper quadrant pain and positive Murphy's sign, may be absent in a very sick patient. Diagnosis is confirmed with ultrasound and/or cholescintigraphy. A contrast-enhanced CT scan is recommended to rule out complications like gangrene and perforation. Uncomplicated cholecystitis generally responds to conservative treatment, while cholecystectomy is reserved for complications. CT-guided percutaneous cholecystostomy and drainage of collections may be considered in extremely ill patients.

43.7 Rare Complications

Liver abscess and splenic abscess are rare complications of enteric fever. Localized pain and high-grade, persistent fever are the usual manifestations. Failure of conservative treatment with antibiotics calls for CT-guided percutaneous drainage. Splenectomy is recommended for a deep-seated abscess that is considered unsafe for percutaneous drainage.

Key Points

- Perforation and lower GI bleeding are the most common complications of enteric fever that require surgery.
- These complications usually arise in the third week of fever.
- Simple closure of the perforation and peritoneal lavage suffices in a stable patient. Closure of perforation and exteriorization of the loop as an ileostomy is recommended for a very sick patient.
- In lower GI bleed, surgery is required for an ongoing exsanguinating bleed. Right hemicolectomy is the procedure of choice.

Selected Reading

1. Marchello CS, Birkhold M, Crump JA. Complications and mortality of typhoid fever: a global systematic review and meta-analysis. J Infect. 2020;81(6):902–10.

Abdominal Hydatid Cyst

44

Sadaf Ali and Younis Ahmad

Abstract

Hydatid cyst of the liver accounts for 60%–75% of cases, with 80% of the cysts located in the right lobe. Clinically, the cyst remains asymptomatic until it enlarges significantly or complications develop. Diagnosis is primarily based on imaging. Pharmacological treatment is recommended for disseminated hydatid disease, unfit patients, or as an adjunct to surgery. Preoperative administration for at least 2–6 weeks aims to sterilize the cyst and reduce the risk of contamination from intraoperative spillage. Puncture, aspiration, injection, and re-aspiration (PAIR) technique is recommended for unilocular cysts (CE1) or cysts with ruptured membranes (CE3a). Surgery is the most commonly practiced form of treatment. Conservative surgery, such as evacuation of contents and partial excision of the cyst, is a more widely performed procedure.

Keywords

Hydatid cyst · Echinococcus

Echinococcosis, or hydatid disease, is a zoonotic parasitic disease caused by the larvae of tapeworms (cestodes) of the genus *Echinococcus*. The cystic form, known as a hydatid cyst, caused by *Echinococcus granulosus*, is endemic in western China, Central Asia, South America, Mediterranean countries, and eastern Africa. More than 5000 new cases are diagnosed each year in Argentina, Brazil, Chile, Peru, and Uruguay. It has been declared eradicated in New Zealand and Tasmania, Australia. *Echinococcus multilocularis* is an uncommon variant of the disease, primarily found in the North Central United States, northwestern Alaska, northwestern Canada, and northern Japan over the past 40 years. Mass screening using ultrasound (US) and serology in China has confirmed a high prevalence of this variant in the Tibetan Plateau (Qinghai, Sichuan, and Tibet). The other rare variants, *Echinococcus vogeli* and *Echinococcus oligarthrus*, which cause polycystic disease, are limited to South America. *Echinococcus canadensis*, which causes cystic disease, is found in North America.

44.1 Pathogenesis

Hydatid cyst, caused by *Echinococcus granulosus*, is the most common form of the disease worldwide. Carnivores act as definitive hosts for the adult tapeworms, while their herbivorous prey serve as intermediate hosts. Humans become accidental intermediate hosts by contracting the disease. The life cycle of echinococcus granulosus is described below as how definate host pass on infections to humans (Fig. 44.1).

S. Ali (✉) · Y. Ahmad
Sher-i-Kashmir Institute of Medical Sciences,
Srinagar, Jammu and Kashmir, India

M. Ibrarullah (ed.), *Recent Concepts in Gastrointestinal (GI) Surgery*, https://doi.org/10.1007/978-981-92-1118-0_44

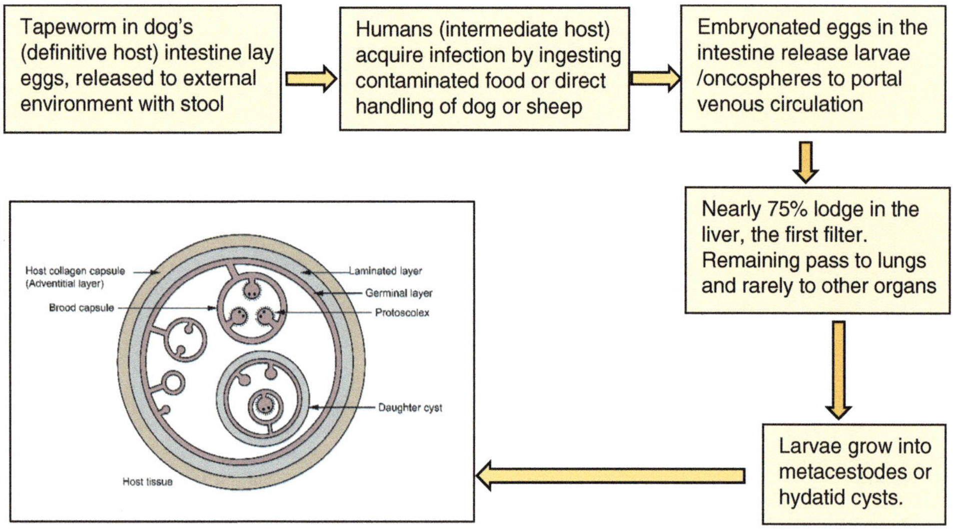

Fig. 44.1 A prototype hydatid cyst with all its components and pathogenesis

44.2 Hydatid Cyst of Liver

Hydatid cyst of the liver (HCL) accounts for 60%–75% of cases, with 80% of the cysts located in the right lobe.

44.3 Clinical Presentation

Clinically, the disease remains mostly asymptomatic until the cyst enlarges significantly or complications develop. When symptoms do occur, they are nonspecific and may include upper abdominal pain or a sensation of heaviness in the right upper quadrant, dyspepsia, or vomiting. The most common sign is hepatomegaly or a palpable, nontender, rounded cystic mass originating from the liver.

44.4 Complications

- Infection
- Pressure effect on adjacent structures
- Rupture
  Acute rupture
  Intrabiliary rupture
  Intrathoracic rupture

44.4.1 Infection

Approximately 25% of the HCL may become secondarily infected after rupturing into any luminal structure. Pain and fever are common symptoms, along with signs related to the communicating structure.

44.4.2 Pressure Effect

HCL typically grows at a rate of 2–3 cm per year. A large cyst may compress the extrahepatic bile duct, leading to obstructive jaundice. Depending on its location, the cysts may compress the hepatic veins or IVC, causing secondary Budd-Chiari syndrome. Portal vein obstruction is a rare complication when cysts are near the hepatic hilum.

44.4.3 Acute Rupture

Acute rupture can occur spontaneously or after trauma. The patient typically presents with acute abdomen and shock, requiring prompt resuscitation and surgical intervention. An acute rupture into the pleural cavity or bronchial tree may manifest as a sudden cough, dyspnea, and the extrusion of hydatid membrane in sputum (in cases of cysto-bronchial communication) (Fig. 44.2).

44.4.4 Intrabiliary Rupture

Intrabiliary rupture occurs in longstanding HCL due to stretching and erosion of the biliary radicles by the expanding cyst. The incidence of biliary communication is up to 80% in cysts larger than 7.5 cm in diameter. Small communication may remain quiescent, manifesting as a bile leak only after cyst decompression. Large communication leads to the extrusion of hydatid material into the biliary system, causing obstructive jaundice and cholangitis.

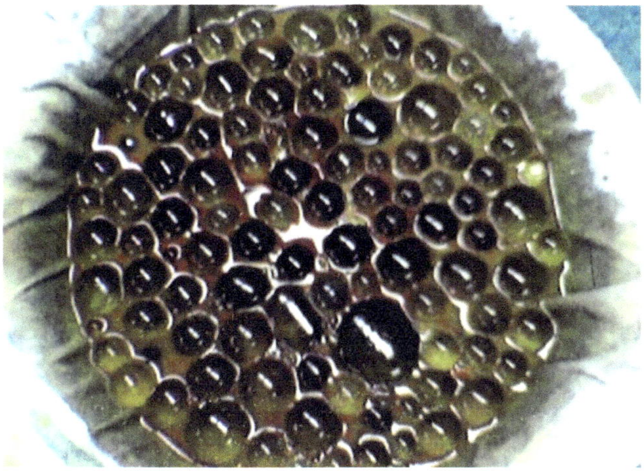

Fig. 44.2 A case of a ruptured hydatid where a bucket full of daughter cysts was evacuated from the peritoneal cavity

44.4.5 Intrathoracic Rupture

Large HCL abutting against the diaphragm may erode into the pleural cavity and/or bronchus, establishing cysto-bronchial communication. It may present with chronic cough and extrusion of hydatid membranes or daughter cysts in the sputum. Raely, a centrally located cyst can erode into the posterior mediastinal structures, such as the esophagus.

44.5 Diagnosis

Diagnosis of hydatid cyst is based on imaging, serology, cyst fluid microscopy, and biopsy of the surgical specimen (Figs. 44.3, 44.4, 44.5, and 44.6; Widely used classifications to describe the disease and plan appropriate treatment with USG Based Gharbis classification which is subsequently further confirmed with CT or MRI classification Tables 44.1 and 44.2).

Serology
The indirect hemagglutination test and the enzyme-linked immunosorbent assay (ELISA) are the preferred screening tests, with an overall sensitivity of 80%. ELISA and radioallergosorbent test (RAST) can also detect specific IgE antibodies. ELISA is especially useful for detecting recurrence. Antigen 5 (Arc-5) and antigen B8 are the major parasitic antigens of diagnostic importance. Immunodiffusion and immunoelectrophoresis demonstrate antibodies to antigen 5 and provide specific confirmation of reactivity. The limitations of serological tests are that negative serology does not rule out hydatid disease; these tests are not site-specific and do not indicate whether the cyst is dead or active. Therefore, despite extensive description, serological tests are rarely used in clinical practice.

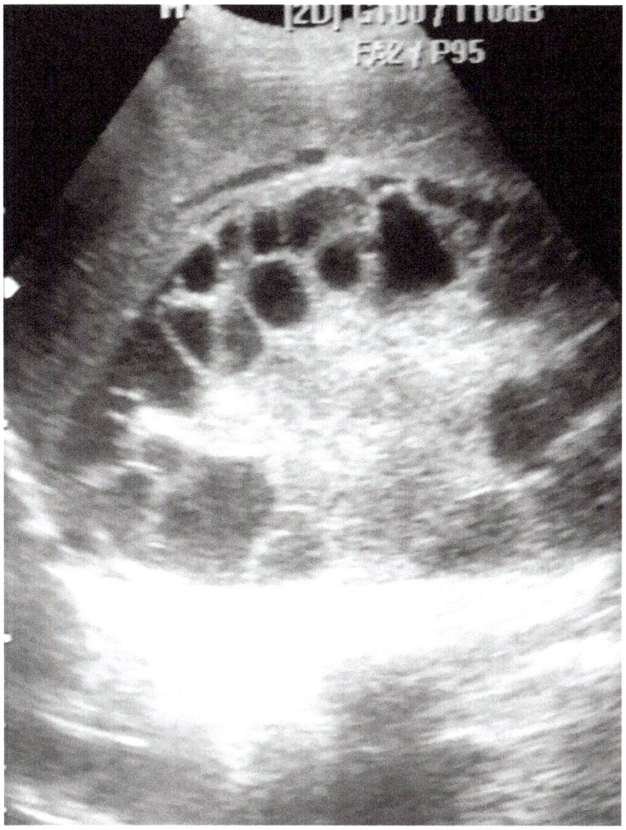

Fig. 44.3 USG appearance of hydatid cyst type CE2

Casoni Test
The Casoni test, an intradermal skin test formerly used, has a sensitivity of 70%. It has been discontinued in favor of more effective methods due to its low accuracy and the risk of severe local allergic reactions.

Cyst Fluid Microscopy
Microscopy of cyst fluid can reveal the following diagnostic features in suspected hydatid cysts:

- *Hooklets*: Appear birefringent under polarized light and can be stained with Ziehl-Neelsen or Fite-Faraco stains.
- *Protoscolices*: Identifiable by their mushroom shape and hooklets.
- *Laminated membrane*: Fragments of the laminated membrane stain pinkish-red with hematoxylin-eosin stain.

Hematological and Biochemical Tests Eosinophilia occurs in about a quarter of patients with hydatid cysts. Elevated liver enzymes, especially serum alkaline phosphatase and gamma-glutamyl transpeptidase, may be seen in cases of intrabiliary rupture or compression of the bile duct(s).

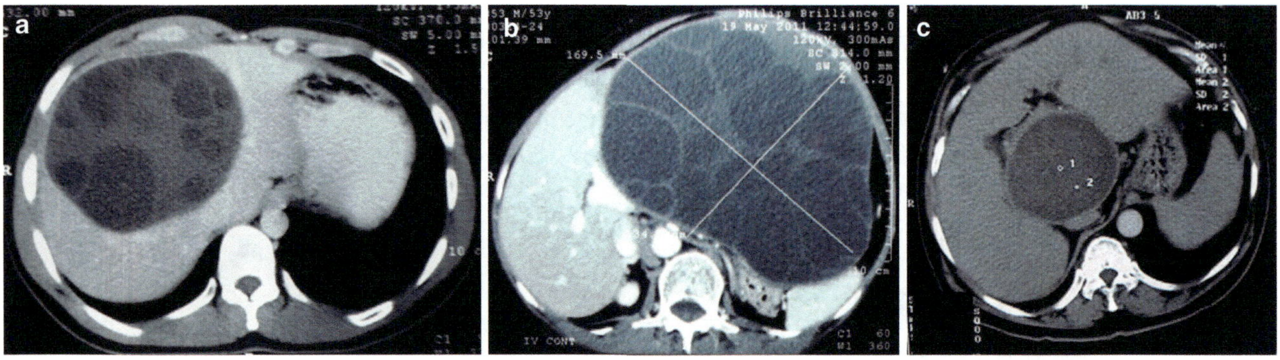

Fig. 44.4 CECT appearance of the hydatid cyst of the liver, in various locations: (**a**) right lobe, (**b**) left lobe, (**c**) caudate lobe

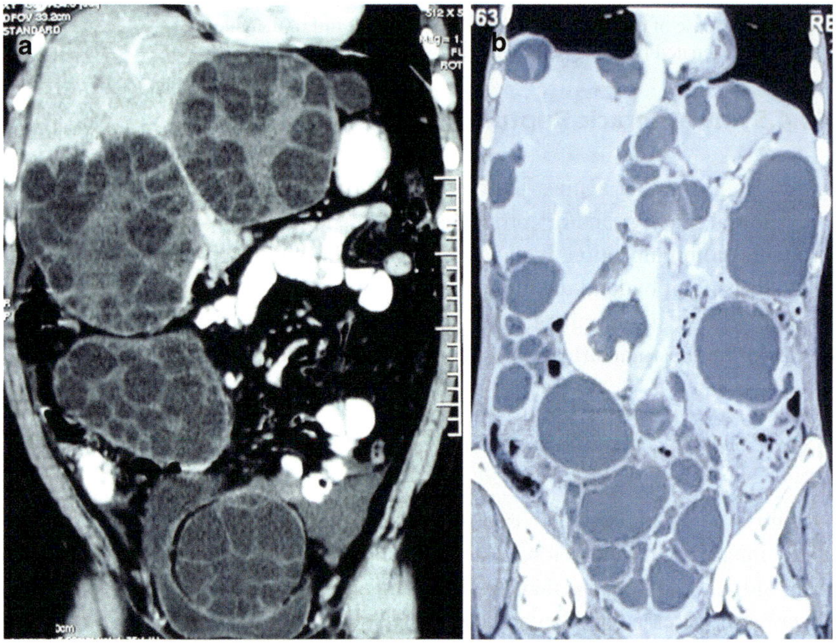

Fig. 44.5 Disseminated hydatid cyst in the liver and the peritoneal cavity: (**a**) CECT view, (**b**) magnetic resonance image

Treatment Options for the Hydatid Cyst of the Liver
Treatment modalities available for hydatid cysts are as follows:

- Pharmacological treatment
- Nonsurgical intervention: Puncture, aspiration, injection, and re-aspiration (PAIR)
- Surgical

44.5.1 Pharmacological Treatment

Pharmacological treatment is recommended for disseminated hydatid disease, unfit patients, or as an adjunct to surgery. Preoperative administration for at least 2–6 weeks aims to sterilize the cyst and reduce the risk of contamination from intraoperative spillage. Benzimidazoles, such as Albendazole and Mebendazole, are the preferred medications. Both are equally effective, but the dose and duration of Mebendazole are higher compared to Albendazole. Albendazole is administered at a dose of 10–15 mg/kg/day. The total treatment duration ranges from 3 to 6 months. An interruption of 2 weeks is advised after completing 1 month of treatment to lower the risk of adverse effects. Monitoring complete blood cell (CBC) counts and liver function tests every 2 weeks for the first 3 months, then monthly afterward, is recommended to detect any adverse drug effects. The medication is less effective in large cysts (>10 cm), calcified cysts, and deep-seated HCL. Treatment success is achieved in less than 60% of cases. However, when combined with surgery, the success rate exceeds 90% with 3 months of therapy. Another drug, Praziquantel, an isoquinoline derivative given at 40 mg/kg/week, has been used occasionally, especially in cases where intraoperative spillage has occurred.

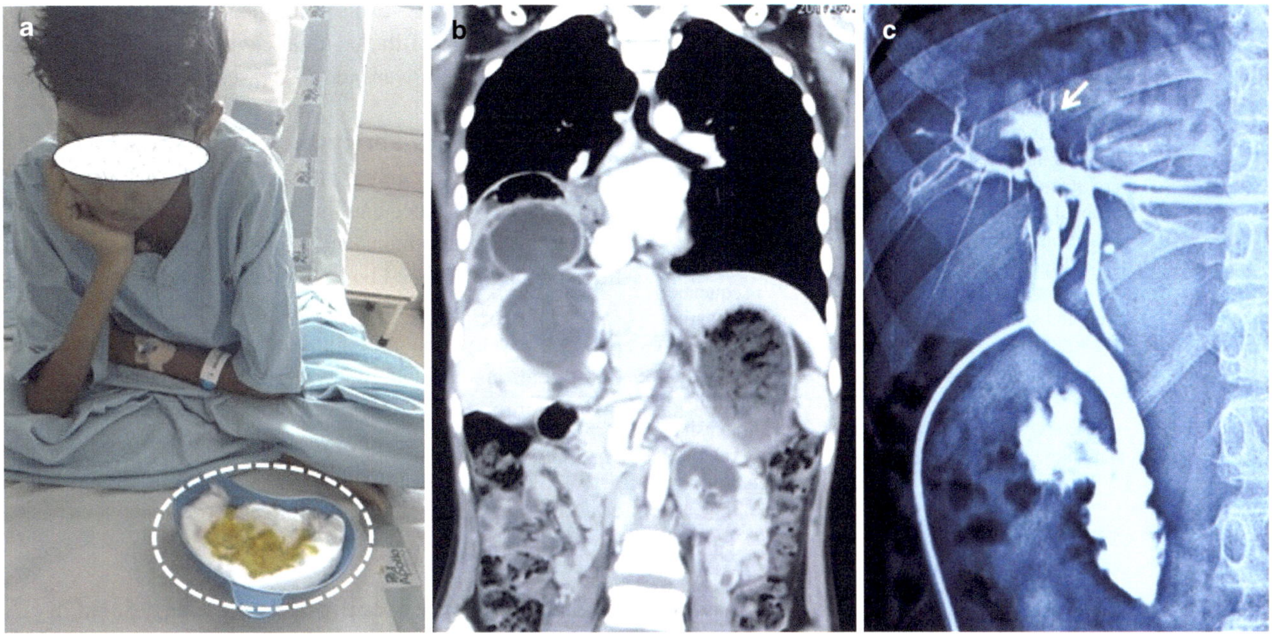

Fig. 44.6 Intrathoracic and biliary rupture of the hydatid cyst. (**a**) The patient, a young boy, presented with cough and bilious sputum (dotted circle). (**b**) Coronal section of CT showing intrathoracic rupture of the cyst. (**c**) Postoperative T-tube cholangiogram confirming the site of biliary communication (arrow)

Table 44.1 WHO-IWGE (informal working group on Echinococcosis)-2003 classification: ultrasonogram (USG) appearance of HD based on its natural history

Types	USG appearance	Disease activity
CE1	Uniformly anechoic cyst with double line sign. Fine internal echoes representing hydatid sand (fluid and protoscolices originating from a ruptured vesicle)	Active
CE2	Internal septation, multivesicular, rosette, or honeycomb appearance due to the presence of daughter cysts	Active
CE3a	Detached laminated membranes (water lily sign)	Transitional
CE3b	Daughter cysts within a solid matrix	Transitional
CE4	Absence of daughter cysts Mixed hypoechoic and hyperechoic matrix, resembling a ball of cotton	Inactive
CE5	Solid cyst with calcified wall	Inactive

44.5.2 Nonsurgical Intervention

Puncture, aspiration, injection, and re-aspiration (PAIR) technique is recommended for unilocular cysts (CE1) or cysts with ruptured membranes (CE3a). Contraindications for this treatment include peripherally located cysts (due to risk of rupture and spillage), cysts with biliary communications, predominantly solid contents, or calcified cysts. The procedure involves ultrasound- or CT-guided aspiration of the cyst contents, injection of a scolicidal agent for at least 15 min, and reaspiration of the cyst contents until the return is clear. The cyst is then filled with normal saline. The modified catheter technique (MoCaT) is recommended for CE2 and CE3b cysts to facilitate the removal of solid contents. Albendazole is mandatory for at least 4 days before and 1–3 months after the procedure. Potential complications include anaphylaxis and biliary sclerosis. Experience with this treatment approach is limited.

44.5.3 Surgical Treatment

Hydatid cysts tend to grow and eventually cause symptoms. Therefore, the presence of a cyst at any stage of detection is an indication for treatment. However, a deep-seated asymptomatic cyst or a dead cyst is a contraindication to surgical intervention. Conservative surgery, such as evacuation of contents and partial excision of the HCL, is more commonly performed than radical cysto-pericystectomy. A preoperative course of Albendazole is likely to sterilize the cyst and reduce the risk of recurrence from accidental spillage during surgery.

44.5.3.1 Cyst Evacuation and Partial Excision

The basic steps of this form of treatment are as follows:

The cyst is isolated with surgical mops soaked in scolicidal solutions to sterilize any spilled fluid. The various scolicidal solutions that can be used include hypertonic saline (14.2% NaCl), ethanol (95%), povidone-iodine (1%–2%),

Table 44.2 Classification of hydatid cyst based on contrast-enhanced CT (CECT) and MRI

Types	CECT	MRI
1: Initial phase	Well-circumscribed, unilocular cystic lesion with no internal architecture, with or without internal septations or hydatid sand. Frequent contrast enhancement of the cyst wall and septa	Low signal intensity on T1-weighted images (T1WIs) and a high signal intensity on T2-weighted images (T2WIs) with a low signal intensity rim "rim sign." the DWI sequence can differentiate hydatid cysts from simple liver cysts
2: Active phase	Cysts with multiple septa representing the daughter cysts	Daughter cysts appear on a low signal intensity or are isointense relative to the matrix on both T1WIs and T2WIs
A	Spoke-wheel appearance: Multiple daughter cysts arranged peripherally inside the mother cyst. High-density central matrix	
B	Rosette appearance: Multiple irregularly arranged daughter cysts inside the mother cyst	
C	Hyperdense matrix and occasionally calcification or daughter cysts	
3: Dead phase	Calcified cyst: Round hyperdense lesion on CT	Low signal intensity rim
4: Complication phase	Mass effect, biliary rupture, air bubble indicates infection, peritoneal rupture	Same as CT scan

hydrogen peroxide (3%), and silver nitrate (0.5%–1%). Hypertonic saline and povidone-iodine are most commonly used due to their availability and lower risk of tissue damage compared to other solutions. The cyst is aspirated with a thick-bore needle, and the aspirate is checked for any bile staining. Aspiration reduces intracystic pressure, causing the cyst to collapse. The cyst fluid is then replaced with a slightly smaller amount of scolicidal solution. After waiting a few minutes, the pericyst is incised, and the contents are evacuated, taking care to prevent spillage. Any protruding pericyst is excised. A surgical mop soaked in hypertonic saline (povidone-iodine masks any bilious staining) is left in the cyst cavity to monitor for bile leakage. Any biliary communication identified in the cyst wall must be meticulously sutured. The residual cavity can be managed with various techniques, such as omentopexy, capitonage, introflexion, marsupialization, capsulorrhaphy, and external drainage. However, deroofing—excision of the superficial pericyst and external drainage of the residual cavity—is technically feasible and straightforward in most cases.

44.5.3.2 Cysto-Pericystectomy

Excision of the cyst along with the pericyst is recommended to decrease recurrence and the morbidity linked to cyst evacuation. Both anatomical and nonanatomical hepatic resections can be performed based on the cyst's location and size. A review of existing studies indicates that cysto-pericystectomy results in significantly lower recurrence and complications because the cyst is completely removed with no remaining cavity. However, the technical simplicity of cyst evacuation, which an average general surgeon can perform, outweighs the benefits of cysto-pericystectomy, a more complex procedure that requires experience and skill (Fig. 44.7).

44.5.3.3 Laparoscopic Surgery for Hydatid Cyst

Despite initial concerns about technical feasibility and cyst spillage, laparoscopic surgery is now widely accepted in managing hydatid cysts. Special cannulas are used to facilitate cyst evacuation and laparoscopic inspection. Biliary communications are more clearly visualized under a magnified laparoscopic view. Cysto-pericystectomy has also been attempted for superficial and small cysts. Deep-seated cysts without surface protrusions and very large cysts pose limitations for the laparoscopic approach.

44.5.4 Postoperative Complications

- Residual abscess
- Biliary fistula
- Disease recurrence

An infected collection in the undrained residual cavity may manifest with fever and leucocytosis. Confirmation on CT scan and guided percutaneous catheter drainage usually suffices in the majority (Fig. 44.8).

A bile leak from an unsuspected cysto-biliary communication may present as a postoperative bilioma or biliary fistula via drain. A controlled fistula should be managed conservatively. If the fistula persists, it should be evaluated for CBD obstruction caused by any hydatid material. Endoscopic retrograde cholangiogram is the preferred method because any obstruction can be cleared and the CBD is stented during the same procedure. The fistula usually closes with endoscopic treatment, although the process can sometimes take longer than expected.

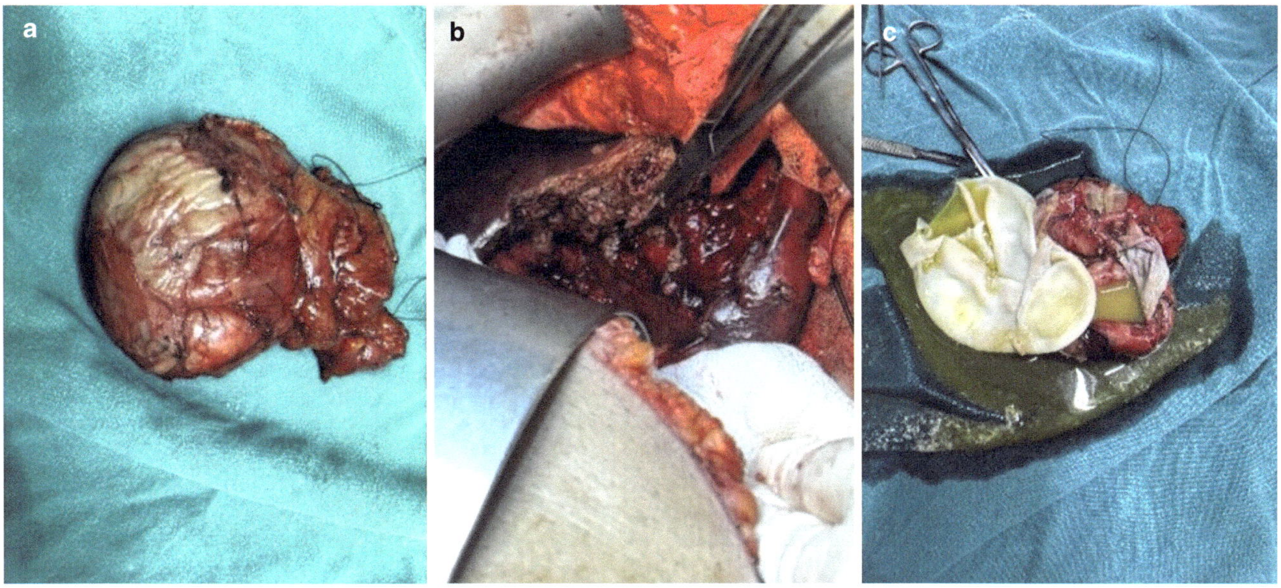

Fig. 44.7 (**a**) Cysto-pericystectomy of HCL. (**b**) Liver surface after resection. (**c**) Laminated membrane after excision

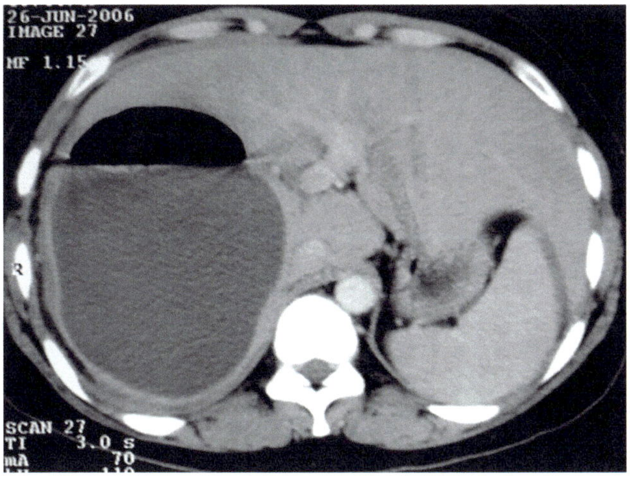

Fig. 44.8 An infected residual cavity; note the air-fluid level

44.6 Hydatid Cyst of the Spleen

Hydatid cyst of the spleen (HCS) is uncommon, accounting for about 0.5%–8% of all hydatid disease cases and 1.5%–3.5% of abdominal hydatids. Up to 30% of HCS cases may be asymptomatic. When symptoms are present, they are non-specific, such as vague, dull aching pain, heaviness, or a mass in the left upper abdomen. Diagnosis relies on serological tests and imaging studies. Serological tests, including ELISA and indirect hemagglutination, can achieve diagnostic accuracy exceeding 90% when used with imaging techniques. Ultrasound typically shows well-defined cystic hypoechoic lesions, while CT scans can provide detailed information about the size, number, and potential complications of the cysts.

The management of splenic hydatid cysts is primarily surgical, with the choice of procedure depending on the cyst's size, location, and whether there are complications like rupture or infection. Surgical options include total splenectomy, partial splenectomy, cyst enucleation, and unroofing with omentopexy.

In cases of small, superficially located cysts, spleen-preserving techniques may be used, especially in children, to reduce the risk of post-splenectomy consequences (Fig. 44.9).

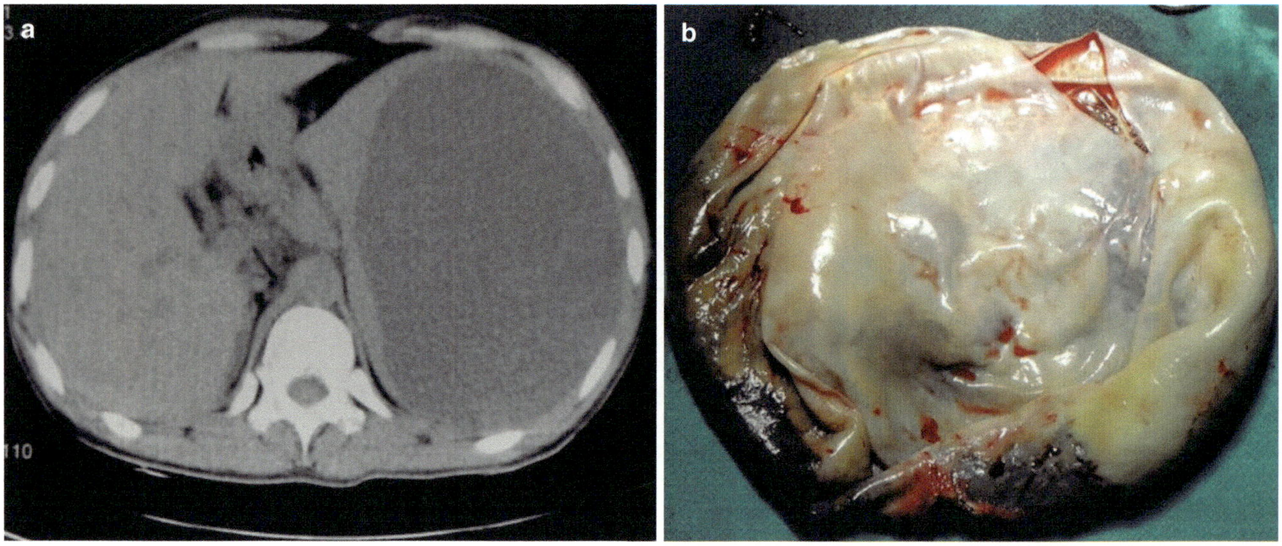

Fig. 44.9 (**a**) CT scan of a hydatid cyst of the spleen. (**b**) Excised cyst (splenectomy)

44.7 Hydatid Cyst of the Pancreas

Hydatid cyst of the pancreas (HCP) accounts for roughly 0.14%–2% of all hydatid cyst cases. Most of these cysts are found in the head of the pancreas (50%–58%), followed by the body (24%–34%) and tail (16%–19%). The symptoms of pancreatic hydatid cysts can vary greatly, with many patients remaining symptom-free until the cysts grow large enough to press on nearby structures or cause complications like pancreatitis or obstructive jaundice. Symptoms may include abdominal pain, nausea, vomiting, and signs of pancreatitis, which can be mistaken for other pancreatic conditions such as pseudocysts. In some cases, patients may develop jaundice due to bile duct obstruction caused by cysts in the head of the pancreas. The slow progression of the disease often leads to delayed diagnosis, as symptoms can be nonspecific.

The diagnosis of HCP is based on imaging studies combined with serology and diagnostic aspiration. However, the latter procedure carries the risk of cyst rupture and spillage.

The management options include cyst enucleation, partial cyst excision, and cyst evacuation. Radical surgeries such as Whipple's pancreaticoduodenectomy or distal pancreatectomy are reserved for undiagnosed cases (Fig. 44.10).

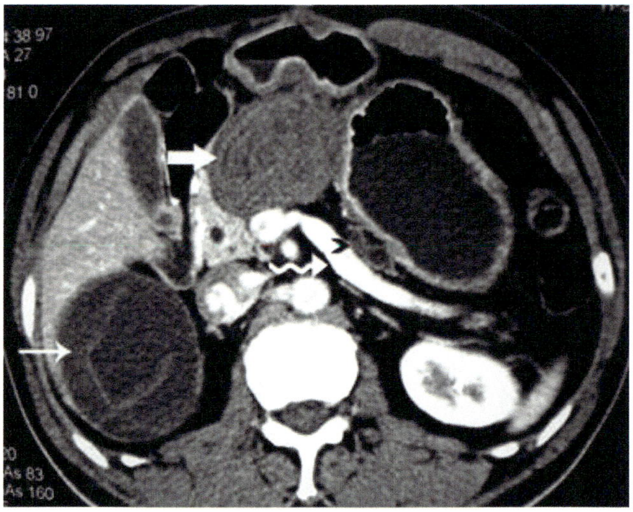

Fig. 44.10 Hydatid cyst of the pancreas (thick arrow) and liver (thin arrow)

Key Points

- Hydatid cyst of the liver accounts for 60%–75% of cases, with 80% of the cysts located in the right lobe.
- Clinically, the cyst remains asymptomatic until it enlarges significantly or complications develop.
- The usual complications are infection, pressure on adjacent structures, and rupture.
- Diagnosis is primarily based on imaging.
- Pharmacological treatment is recommended for disseminated hydatid disease, unfit patients, or as an adjunct to surgery.
- Albendazole is the preferred drug for treatment.
- Preoperative administration for at least 2–6 weeks aims to sterilize the cyst and reduce the risk of contamination from intraoperative spillage.
- Puncture, aspiration, injection, and re-aspiration (PAIR) is recommended for unilocular cysts (CE1) or cysts with ruptured membranes (CE3a).
- Contraindications for this treatment include peripherally located cysts, cysts with biliary communications, predominantly solid contents, or calcified cysts.
- Surgery is the most commonly practiced form of treatment. Conservative surgery, such as evacuation of contents and partial excision of the cyst, is a more widely performed procedure.
- Cysto-pericystectomy results in significantly lower recurrence and complications because the cyst is completely removed with no remaining cavity. However, the technical simplicity of cyst evacuation outweighs the benefits of cysto-pericystectomy, a more complex procedure that requires experience and skill.

Selected Reading

1. Gómez I, Gavara C, López-Andújar R, Belda Ibáñez T, et al. Review of the treatment of liver hydatid cysts. World J Gastroenterol. 2015;21(1):124–31.
2. Kahriman G, Ozcan N, Dogan S, Karaborklu O. Percutaneous treatment of liver hydatid cysts in 190 patients: a retrospective study. Acta Radiol. 2017;58(6):676–84.
3. Greco S, Cannella R, Giambelluca D, et al. Complications of hepatic echinococcosis: multimodality imaging approach. Insights Imaging. 2019;10:113. https://doi.org/10.1186/s13244-019-0805-8.
4. Govindasamy A, Bhattarai PR, John J. Liver cystic echinococcosis: a parasitic review. Ther Adv Infect Dis. 2023;10:20499361231171478. https://doi.org/10.1177/20499361231171478.

45 Abdominal Ascariasis

Nissar Hussain Hamdani, Sumyra Qadri, and Sanjay Debakshi

Abstract

Adult *Ascaris* worms live in the lumen of the small intestine, specifically in the jejunum and middle ileum. Symptomatic cases present with abdominal pain, acute or recurrent intestinal obstruction, appendicitis, intestinal perforation, or peritonitis. Biliary ascariasis is more common in females. It may present as biliary colic, acute cholecystitis, obstructive jaundice, cholangitis, or acute pancreatitis. Recurrent pyogenic cholangitis (RPC) involves biliary endothelial damage caused by *Ascaris* and secondary bacterial infection. It presents with intrahepatic brown pigment stones, multiple biliary strictures, cholangitis, and hepatic fibrosis.

Keywords

Ascariasis · Round worm

Ascariasis is a parasitic infestation caused by the nematode *Ascaris* (commonly known as roundworm). It is the most common helminthic infection in humans. Humans are primarily affected by the species *Ascaris lumbricoides*, which causes a range of clinical symptoms. Another species, *Ascaris suum*, mainly infects pigs but can occasionally infect humans.

N. H. Hamdani (✉)
Government Medical College, Srinagar, Jammu and Kashmir, India

S. Qadri
Sher-i-Kashmir Institute of Medical Sciences, Srinagar, Jammu and Kashmir, India

S. Debakshi
Calcutta Medical Research Institute, Kolkata, West Bengal, India

45.1 Disease Burden

Ascariasis is particularly prevalent in underdeveloped countries with poor sanitation and the practice of open-air defecation. In developed nations, however, most cases occur among refugees, immigrants, or travelers returning from endemic areas. It is estimated that around 500 million people are affected globally, particularly affecting children (aged 2–10 years) and people living in rural communities or in regions with lower income and human development indices. Regions with increased mean annual relative humidity, precipitation, and environmental temperature tend to have a higher prevalence of ascariasis.

45.2 Life Cycle and Pathogenesis

Adult *Ascaris* worms live in the lumen of the small intestine, specifically in the jejunum and middle ileum, for about 10–24 months. A female worm produces approximately 240,000 eggs per day, fertilized by nearby male worms, before being excreted in the feces. Fertilized eggs become infective (embryonated) in suitable soil—moist, warm, shaded—within 2–3 weeks and can remain viable for up to 10 years. (Studies suggest that 45% of infected individuals shed only fertilized eggs, 40% shed both fertilized and unfertilized eggs, and 20% shed only unfertilized eggs, with unfertilized eggs making up only 6–9% of total egg shedding. Unfertilized eggs may be ingested but are not infective.) Infection occurs through the oral ingestion of food or water contaminated with soil containing embryonated eggs from human or pig feces or by directly consuming infected, uncooked chicken or pig liver containing larvae. After ingestion, the eggs or larvae hatch in the duodenum. The larvae then penetrate the intestinal mucosa and are carried initially via the portal circulation and then systemically to the liver, heart, and lungs. Within the alveolar capillaries of the lungs, the larvae further mature over 10–14 days, penetrate the alveolar walls, ascend the bronchial tree to the throat or oro-

M. Ibrarullah (ed.), *Recent Concepts in Gastrointestinal (GI) Surgery*, https://doi.org/10.1007/978-981-92-1118-0_45

pharynx, and are then swallowed back into the small intestine, where they mature into adult worms (with separate sexes) that mate and release eggs into the stool. The life cycle of *Ascaris lumbricoides* lasts about 2–3 months, and adult worms can live for 1–2 years.

45.3 Clinical Features and Complications

- Most cases are asymptomatic, and patients may pass worms with stools or live worms per rectum, mouth, or even nostrils.
- Patients often present with recurrent non-specific abdominal pain, malnutrition (especially in children), or iron deficiency anemia.
- In surgical practice, ascariasis may present with typical features of an acute abdomen.
- Acute or recurrent intestinal obstruction: An entangled worm bolus typically blocks the distal ileum or ileocecal valve, presenting as colicky abdominal pain, vomiting, and distension.
- Acute appendicitis: Worms may enter the lumen of the appendix, causing obstruction, inflammation, or even perforation.
- Perforation and peritonitis: Due to perforation of the bowel or appendicular wall by obstructed worms and/or wandering worms.
- Occult or frank lower GI bleeding.
- Biliary ascariasis: Biliary ascariasis is more common in females, possibly due to progesterone-induced relaxation of the sphincter of Oddi. For the same reason, prior sphincterotomy is another risk factor for worm migration into the biliary tree. Worms migrate into the duodenum and through the ampulla of Vater into the biliary system, causing severe biliary pain, obstructive jaundice, recurrent cholangitis, acute cholecystitis, acute pancreatitis, or a liver abscess.
- Recurrent pyogenic cholangitis (RPC): RPC, similar to oriental cholangiohepatitis, results from damage to the biliary epithelium caused by *Ascaris* and secondary gram-negative bacterial infection. It is characterized by intrahepatic brown pigment stones, strictures, and eventual hepatic fibrosis.

45.4 Diagnosis

- Appearance of adult *Ascaris* in excreted feces by patient or within the bowel lumen during routine ultrasonography or gastrointestinal endoscopies.
- *Stool examination*: Confirming ascariasis involves microscopically detecting *Ascaris* eggs in stool samples. However, eggs may not be present in the stool for up to 6 weeks after infection, and some infestations may involve only male worms that do not produce eggs.
- *Complete blood count*: Peripheral eosinophilia may occur during the tissue migration phase of the infection.
- *Ultrasonography (USG) abdomen*: USG abdomen is a very effective modality that may demonstrate worms within the intestine or in the hepatobiliary or pancreatic ducts (Fig. 45.1). The various USG findings in the case of biliary ascariasis are

  Presence of linear or curvilinear, single or multiple echogenic structures in the biliary tract—the "stripe" sign and the "spaghetti" sign, respectively.

  "Tram track" appearance inside the common bile duct (CBD): This is due to the echogenic wall of the worm with a central anechoic tube—the "inner tube" sign.

  Movement of the live worm can often be observed in real-time ultrasonography, which is the definitive confirmation of the diagnosis.
- *Magnetic Resonance or Endoscopic Retrograde Cholangiogram*: Linear or curvilinear filling defect in the biliary tree is suggestive of ascariasis. The presence of live worms across or in the vicinity of the ampulla of Vater is diagnostic (Figs. 45.2 and 45.3).

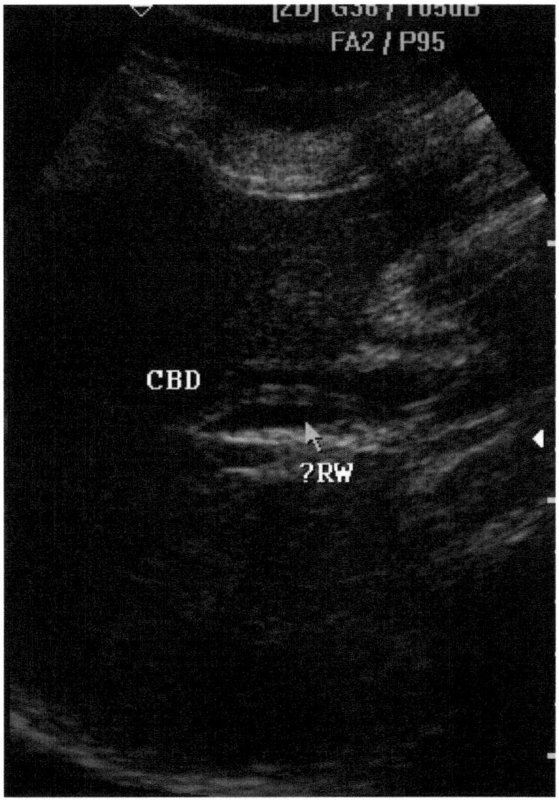

Fig. 45.1 USG abdomen showing *Ascaris* inside a dilated CBD. Note the "tram-track" appearance with the hypoechoic "inner tube" sign

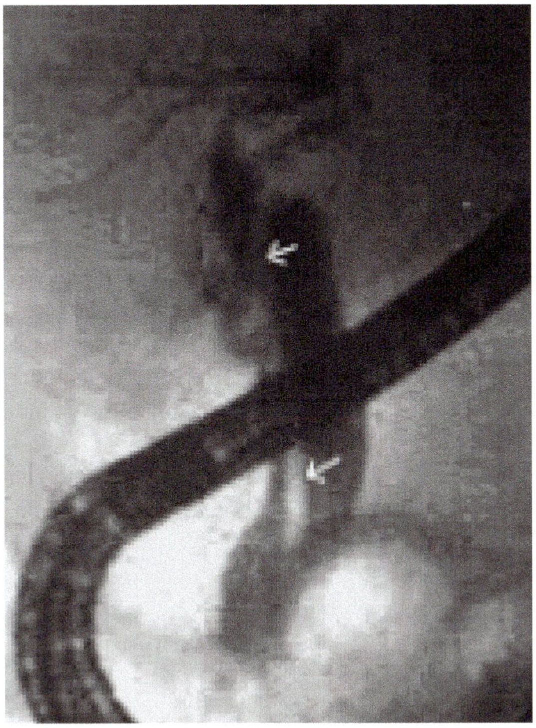

Fig. 45.2 Endoscopic retrograde cholangiogram showing a linear filling defect (arrows) inside a dilated CBD, suggesting the presence of *Ascaris*

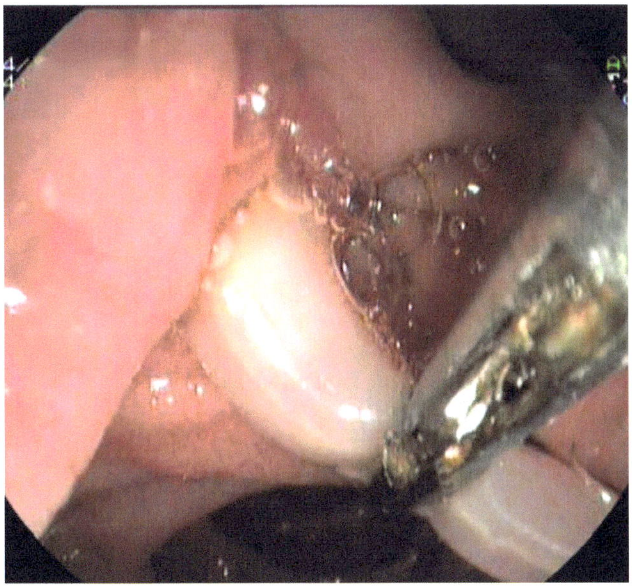

Fig. 45.3 A live worm being extracted across the papilla with the help of endoscopic forceps

45.5 Management

Every patient with intestinal ascariasis (even asymptomatic) needs to be treated to prevent the development of complications.

45.5.1 Pharmacological Management

- Albendazole (adult/age > 2 years: 400 mg orally single dose; age < 2 years 200 mg single dose)
- Mebendazole (100 mg orally twice a day for 3 days or 500 mg orally once)
- Ivermectin (200 mcg/kg orally single dose)

Since all the above are Category-C (potentially teratogenic) medications, they should be avoided during pregnancy. A safe alternative during pregnancy is Pyrantel pamoate 11 mg/kg Pyrantel base or 30 mg/kg Pyrantel pamoate (maximum daily dose, 1 gm pyrantel base) (1 mg base = 2.9 mg pamoate form).

45.5.2 Acute Abdomen

For an acute abdomen without signs of peritonitis, a conservative trial with oral restriction, intravenous fluids, and antispasmodics is recommended. Hypertonic saline enemas have been shown to increase the success rate of conservative treatment for intestinal obstruction and to reduce hospital stay. Anthelmintics should be avoided in the acute setting to prevent failure to dislodge the worm bolus in the small intestine if the worms have been rendered dead. Emergency laparotomy may be needed for unremitting intestinal obstruction or perforation and peritonitis. During laparotomy, the worm bolus should be removed through enterotomy. Removal of the worm bolus may also be required in the case of suture closure of perforation for the hypothetical possibility of suture disruption by the leftover worms.

45.5.3 Biliary Ascariasis

Conservative treatment and oral antihelminthic drugs are effective in over 80% of patients with biliary ascariasis. However, some authors recommend early intervention to prevent complications. Surgical options include cholecystectomy and/or CBD exploration with complete removal of the worms. Synchronous enterotomy and worm removal are advised to avoid re-infection. When facilities are available, endoscopic extraction of the worms appears to be a better alternative, providing quick relief from cholangitis and the severe pain some patients experience. To reduce the risk of recurrence, it is recommended to perform endoscopic balloon dilation of the papilla instead of sphincterotomy before extracting worms from the CBD.

45.5.4 Acute Pancreatitis

Conservative treatment is recommended in line with the management of acute pancreatitis from any other cause.

Key Points

- Ascariasis is particularly prevalent in underdeveloped countries with poor sanitation and the practice of open-air defecation.
- The adult Ascaris worms live in the lumen of the small intestine, specifically in the jejunum and middle ileum.
- Symptomatic cases present with abdominal pain, acute or recurrent intestinal obstruction, appendicitis, intestinal perforation, or peritonitis.
- Biliary ascariasis is more common in females. It may present as biliary colic, acute cholecystitis, obstructive jaundice, cholangitis, or acute pancreatitis.
- Recurrent pyogenic cholangitis (RPC) involves biliary endothelial damage caused by Ascaris and secondary bacterial infection. It presents with intrahepatic brown pigment stones, multiple biliary strictures, cholangitis, and hepatic fibrosis.
- Mild abdominal symptoms due to Ascaris are managed conservatively. Emergency laparotomy may be needed for unremitting intestinal obstruction or perforation and peritonitis.
- Acute biliary symptoms require therapeutic endoscopic intervention in the form of ERCP and clearance of the biliary tract.

Selected Reading

1. Shah OJ, Zargar SA, Robbani. Biliary ascariasis: a review. World J Surg. 2006;30:1500–6.
2. Ibrarulllah M, Mishra T, Dash AP, Upadhaya UN. Biliary ascariasis—role of endoscopic intervention. Trop Gastroenterol. 2011;32(3):210–3.

Part IX

Miscellaneous

Ischemic Disorders of the Gastrointestinal Tract

46

Shikhar Tripathi, Amitabh Yadav, and Samiran Nundy

Abstract

Acute mesenteric ischemia (AMI) is often caused by embolism, thrombosis, or vasospasm and presents with sudden and severe abdominal pain disproportionate to physical findings. Chronic mesenteric ischemia is characterized by postprandial pain, food aversion, and progressive weight loss, often due to long-standing atherosclerosis of the mesenteric arteries. Mesenteric vein thrombosis (MVT) can have an acute or insidious onset. AMI requires immediate revascularization through endovascular procedures like angioplasty and stenting or surgical methods such as embolectomy. Chronic mesenteric ischemia may benefit from angioplasty with stenting or bypass surgery to restore adequate blood flow and alleviate symptoms.

Keyword

Mesenteric ischemia

Ischemic disorders of the gastrointestinal (GI) tract include a broad spectrum of diseases affecting the arterial and venous systems within the abdominal cavity. Their presentation ranges from life-threatening emergencies to chronic, subtle abdominal symptoms. These disorders often mimic other intra-abdominal conditions, such as inflammatory bowel disease, appendicitis, or pancreatitis, which demands a high level of suspicion and careful evaluation. Furthermore, because the arterial and venous systems in the abdomen are interconnected, isolated problems in one vessel can cause widespread effects, frequently involving multiple organ systems. The variety of these conditions makes their detection and treatment essential parts of abdominal surgery, with outcomes largely depending on early diagnosis and prompt intervention. In recent decades, advances in imaging technology and endovascular procedures have greatly changed how these disorders are diagnosed and treated. These developments underscore the importance of an integrated, multidisciplinary approach in diagnosing and managing abdominal vascular disorders.

46.1 Acute Mesenteric Ischemia

46.1.1 Pathogenesis

Acute mesenteric ischemia (AMI) is characterized by a sudden decrease in blood flow to the intestines, leading to ischemia and, if not treated, gangrene and necrosis. Arterial embolism accounts for about 50% of AMI cases, often originating from cardiac sources such as atrial fibrillation, myocardial infarction, or valvular heart disease. Emboli usually lodge in the superior mesenteric artery (SMA), causing abrupt ischemia. Arterial thrombosis makes up 15–25% of cases, resulting from in situ thrombosis superimposed on atherosclerotic plaques within the mesenteric vessels. Risk factors include chronic hypertension, hyperlipidemia, and smoking. Nonocclusive mesenteric ischemia (NOMI) accounts for a small percentage of cases and results from splanchnic vasoconstriction due to low cardiac output states, hypotension, or vasopressor use, without an arterial blockage. Mesenteric venous thrombosis (MVT) accounts for 5–15% of AMI cases in Western countries but up to 45% in India. It may be associated with hypercoagulable states, abdominal infections, or malignancies.

46.1.2 Clinical Presentation

Patients with AMI usually present with sudden, severe abdominal pain that is disproportionate to physical examination findings. As the condition advances, signs of peritonitis, like rebound tenderness and guarding, may develop, indicating bowel infarction. Systemic signs, including fever, tachycardia, and hypotension, can occur in later stages.

S. Tripathi (✉) · A. Yadav · S. Nundy
Sir Ganga Ram Hospital, New Delhi, India

M. Ibrarullah (ed.), *Recent Concepts in Gastrointestinal (GI) Surgery*, https://doi.org/10.1007/978-981-92-1118-0_46

46.1.3 Diagnosis

Early and accurate diagnosis of AMI is essential to prevent irreversible bowel damage and enhance survival outcomes. AMI is often challenging to diagnose in its initial stages due to the nonspecific symptoms and overlapping with other abdominal conditions. Maintaining a high level of suspicion is vital, especially in patients presenting with severe abdominal pain that seems out of proportion to physical exam findings and who have risk factors like atrial fibrillation, cardiovascular disease, or recent episodes of hypotension.

eLaboratory tests offer initial clues but are not conclusive. Elevated serum lactate levels, indicating anaerobic metabolism and ischemia, are common in AMI. However, this finding is nonspecific and can be seen in other conditions causing hypoperfusion or sepsis. Leukocytosis is another common marker, reflecting systemic inflammation, but its diagnostic usefulness is limited. D-dimer levels may be elevated in cases involving thromboembolic events, but they are not specific for AMI.

Imaging studies play a pivotal role in confirming the diagnosis of AMI. Computed tomography angiography (CTA) is the gold standard and should be performed without delay in suspected cases. CTA provides a detailed visualization of mesenteric vessels, identifies embolic or thrombotic occlusions, and allows assessment of bowel viability through secondary signs such as bowel wall thickening, pneumatosis intestinalis, or portal venous gas. It also enables differentiation from other causes of acute abdominal pain, such as bowel obstruction or perforation. In hemodynamically stable patients, CTA is indispensable for guiding therapeutic decisions, including the feasibility of endovascular interventions.

In cases where CTA is contraindicated or unavailable, Doppler ultrasonography may serve as an adjunctive modality, particularly in evaluating mesenteric blood flow in chronic ischemia or nonocclusive mesenteric ischemia (NOMI). However, its sensitivity is limited in acute settings, especially in obese patients or those with extensive bowel gas. Magnetic resonance angiography (MRA) may offer an alternative in selected cases, but is not routinely used due to time constraints and limited availability in emergency settings.

Early identification of vascular occlusions allows for prompt therapeutic intervention, significantly improving patient outcomes and reducing the risk of complications such as bowel infarction or sepsis.

46.1.4 Management

Managing AMI requires quick and decisive action to restore intestinal blood flow and prevent irreversible bowel necrosis. The therapeutic approach is tailored based on the underlying etiology—arterial embolism or thrombosis, NOMI, or MVT—and the patient's condition.

46.1.4.1 Initial Resuscitation

Immediate resuscitative measures are critical to stabilize the patient and optimize mesenteric perfusion:

- Fluid Resuscitation: Administration of isotonic crystalloids to correct hypovolemia and maintain adequate blood pressure, thereby enhancing splanchnic circulation.
- Electrolyte Correction: Monitoring and normalization of electrolyte imbalances to prevent cardiac and neuromuscular complications.
- Broad-Spectrum Antibiotics: Prophylactic antibiotics to mitigate the risk of bacterial translocation and sepsis secondary to mucosal barrier compromise.

46.1.4.2 Endovascular Interventions

Endovascular techniques have transformed the management of AMI, offering less invasive options that improve outcomes.

- Percutaneous Transluminal Angioplasty (PTA) with or Without Stenting: This procedure involves inserting a balloon catheter to dilate the narrowed segment of the mesenteric artery, often followed by placing a stent to maintain vessel patency. PTA is especially useful in cases of arterial thrombosis or embolism, restoring blood flow with less perioperative morbidity compared to open surgery.
- Catheter-Directed Thrombolysis: This technique entails the infusion of thrombolytic agents directly to the thrombus site via a catheter, facilitating clot dissolution. It is primarily indicated for MVT and selected cases of arterial thrombosis, provided there are no contraindications such as active bleeding or recent surgery.

46.1.4.3 Surgical Treatment

Surgery is indicated for patients with peritonitis, bowel infarction, or when endovascular approaches are unfeasible:

- Embolectomy: Surgical removal of an embolus from the mesenteric artery is performed via an arteriotomy, followed by extraction using a Fogarty catheter. This procedure is indicated in cases of embolic AMI, aiming to promptly re-establish blood flow.
- Thrombectomy: Similar to embolectomy, this procedure involves the removal of thrombotic material from the mesenteric vessels. It is applicable in arterial thrombosis and extensive MVT, especially when thrombolysis is contraindicated or ineffective.

- Mesenteric Artery Bypass: When arterial blockage is extensive or not suitable for endovascular treatment, bypass surgery is performed to establish an alternative route for blood flow. Common grafts include autologous veins or synthetic grafts, anastomosed from the aorta or iliac arteries to the distal mesenteric artery.
- Bowel Resection: Necrotic segments of the intestine are surgically excised. The extent of resection is assessed during surgery. Conservative removal of the gangrenous segment, while sparing potentially viable part for a reassessment at second-look laparotomy within 24–48 h, is recommended. This approach is especially important when removing a large segment may lead to short bowel syndrome or be incompatible with normal life.

46.1.4.4 Postoperative Management

Postoperative care focuses on monitoring for complications, ensuring adequate nutrition, and addressing the underlying cause of AMI:

- Nutritional Support: Initiation of enteral nutrition as tolerated to promote gut integrity and function. Parenteral nutrition may be necessary if extensive bowel resection precludes adequate enteral intake.
- Anticoagulation Therapy: In cases of MVT or hypercoagulable states, anticoagulation is continued postoperatively to prevent recurrent thrombosis. The duration and choice of anticoagulant are tailored based on individual risk factors and etiology.
- Surveillance Imaging: Follow-up imaging studies, such as duplex ultrasonography or CTA, are employed to assess vessel patency and detect any recurrence of ischemia.

Despite advances in diagnostic imaging and interventional techniques, the mortality rate of AMI remains alarmingly high, ranging from 50% to 70%, depending on the stage at diagnosis. Even with prompt intervention, patients may face postoperative complications such as short bowel syndrome following extensive resection. This condition, marked by malabsorption and nutritional deficiencies, presents long-term challenges that require specialized nutritional support, including parenteral nutrition in severe cases.

Additional postoperative issues include anastomotic leaks and infections. These complications often necessitate reoperation and prolong recovery. For patients managed with endovascular techniques, risks such as restenosis or reocclusion of the treated vessels must also be considered, highlighting the need for close postoperative surveillance with imaging.

46.2 Chronic Mesenteric Ischemia

46.2.1 Pathogenesis

Chronic mesenteric ischemia (CMI) results from a progressive decrease in blood flow through the major splanchnic arteries, mainly caused by atherosclerotic occlusive disease. This condition primarily impacts the coeliac artery (CA), superior mesenteric artery (SMA), and inferior mesenteric artery (IMA), leading to the inadequate perfusion of the intestines, especially during times of increased metabolic demand such as the postprandial state.

The mesenteric arterial system has a rich collateral network that can compensate for significant stenosis in one or even two of the main arteries. However, symptomatic CMI usually appears when there is significant narrowing or blockage in two or more of these vessels, exceeding the ability of collateral pathways to compensate. This critical drop in blood flow causes the key symptoms of CMI, including postprandial abdominal pain, fear of eating (sitophobia), and weight loss.

Risk factors for atherosclerosis in mesenteric vessels are similar to those in other arteries and include advanced age, smoking, hypertension, hyperlipidemia, and diabetes mellitus. The gradual narrowing of arteries often leads to late diagnosis because patients may change their eating habits to lessen symptoms, which makes clinical recognition more difficult.

46.2.2 Clinical Presentation

The classic triad of CMI includes the following:

- Postprandial Abdominal Pain: Usually occurring 15–60 min after eating and lasting for 1–2 h, this pain results from increased metabolic demands of digestion in the context of reduced blood flow.
- Weight Loss: Patients often experience significant weight loss due to "food fear," where the anticipation of postprandial pain leads to decreased food intake.
- Abdominal Bruit: An abdominal bruit may be detected on physical examination, indicating turbulent blood flow through narrowed mesenteric vessels; however, its absence does not rule out the diagnosis.

It is important to note that although this triad is typical, not all patients will exhibit all three features. A high level of suspicion is needed, especially in individuals with risk factors for atherosclerosis who show unexplained abdominal symptoms.

46.2.3 Diagnosis

The initial step in diagnosing CMI involves a thorough clinical evaluation. Patients often present with postprandial abdominal pain, unintentional weight loss, and food aversion. A detailed history and physical examination are essential to identify these hallmark symptoms and to exclude other potential causes of abdominal pain and weight loss.

46.2.3.1 Imaging

Imaging plays an important role in confirming the diagnosis of CMI and planning suitable treatments. The following imaging methods are commonly used:

- Duplex Ultrasonography: This noninvasive method evaluates blood flow velocities in the mesenteric vessels. Elevated peak systolic velocities in the celiac artery and superior mesenteric artery can signal significant stenosis. However, its accuracy may be affected by the patient's body habitus and the operator's skill.
- Computed Tomography Angiography: It provides high-resolution images of the mesenteric blood vessels, enabling detailed visualization of arterial structures and detection of stenotic or occlusive lesions. It is especially valuable for assessing the extent of atherosclerotic disease and aiding in preoperative planning.
- Magnetic resonance angiography: It offers detailed images without ionizing radiation and is beneficial for patients with contraindications to iodinated contrast agents used in CTA. It effectively delineates vascular anatomy and can identify flow-limiting lesions.
- Diagnosis of CMI should be considered in patients presenting with appropriate clinical symptoms and evidence of significant stenosis (>70%) in the CA and/or SMA. The guidelines recommend using imaging studies to confirm the presence of such stenoses within the context of the clinical presentation.

46.2.3.2 Additional Diagnostic Considerations

In some instances, adjunctive diagnostic procedures may be warranted:

- Invasive Angiography: Though less frequently used, catheter-based angiography remains the definitive method for assessing mesenteric arterial anatomy. It offers both diagnostic evaluation and therapeutic procedures, such as angioplasty and stenting, in a single session.
- Functional Testing: Emerging techniques, such as visible-light spectroscopy during endoscopy, can assess mucosal oxygenation and aid in diagnosing CMI, especially in ambiguous cases.

46.2.4 Management

Management of CMI focuses on restoring adequate blood flow to the affected intestinal regions to relieve symptoms and prevent progression to acute mesenteric ischemia. The main treatment options include endovascular therapy and open surgical intervention, with the choice of treatment tailored to the patient's clinical condition, anatomical factors, and comorbidities.

46.2.4.1 Endovascular Therapy

Endovascular interventions have become the preferred initial treatment for CMI because of their minimally invasive nature and favorable outcomes. The main method used is percutaneous transluminal angioplasty (PTA) with stenting. This procedure involves inserting a balloon catheter into the narrowed section of the mesenteric artery through a percutaneous approach. The balloon is inflated to expand the stenosis, and a stent is placed to support the vessel and maintain patency. PTA with stenting has shown high technical success rates and provides symptom relief in patients with CMI. According to the Clinical Practice Guidelines of the European Society of Vascular Surgery, endovascular revascularization is recommended as the first-line treatment for most CMI patients because it has lower perioperative risks compared to open surgery.

46.2.4.2 Surgery

Open surgical revascularization is reserved for patients who are unsuitable for endovascular procedures, have complex arterial anatomy, or experience recurrent symptoms after endovascular treatment. The primary surgical options include mesenteric artery bypass and endarterectomy.

- Mesenteric Artery Bypass: This procedure involves creating an alternative pathway for blood flow to bypass the blocked or narrowed segment of the mesenteric artery. A conduit, either autologous (usually the saphenous vein) or synthetic, is anastomosed proximally to a source of adequate blood flow, such as the aorta, and distally to the mesenteric artery beyond the obstruction. The choice of conduit and anastomotic sites depends on factors like the location and extent of arterial disease, the patient's anatomy, and the surgeon's expertise. Mesenteric artery bypass has been linked to long-lasting patency and symptom relief.
- Endarterectomy: This procedure involves the direct removal of atherosclerotic plaque from the affected mesenteric artery to restore the lumen diameter and improve blood flow. Endarterectomy is usually considered when the disease is localized and accessible and when bypass

options are limited or contraindicated. However, it is less commonly performed than bypass surgery due to technical challenges and the risk of arterial wall injury.

46.2.4.3 Postoperative Management and Follow-Up

Regardless of the revascularization method used, careful postoperative care is essential to optimize outcomes. This involves antiplatelet therapy to prevent graft or stent thrombosis, control of cardiovascular risk factors (such as hypertension, hyperlipidemia, and diabetes mellitus), and lifestyle changes like quitting smoking. Regular follow-up with clinical exams and imaging tests, such as duplex ultrasonography or computed tomography angiography, is vital to detect restenosis or complications related to grafts or stents.

46.2.4.4 Complications

Chronic mesenteric ischemia (CMI) is a progressive condition characterized by insufficient blood flow to the intestines, primarily due to atherosclerotic narrowing of the mesenteric arteries. If left untreated, CMI can lead to significant complications, notably the progression to acute mesenteric ischemia (AMI) and severe nutritional deficiencies.

46.2.4.5 Progression to Acute on Chronic Mesenteric Ischemia

Untreated CMI can progress to ACMI, a life-threatening emergency. This sudden event may occur due to thrombosis superimposed on existing atherosclerotic lesions or embolic phenomena. The abrupt onset of AMI requires immediate diagnosis and treatment to prevent extensive bowel infarction and high mortality rates. The progression from CMI to ACMI highlights the importance of the early detection and management of chronic mesenteric ischemia. Prompt intervention can prevent acute complications and reduce the risk of severe nutritional deficiencies, leading to better patient outcomes.

46.2.4.6 Nutritional Deficiencies and Cachexia

Patients with CMI often experience postprandial abdominal pain, leading to food aversion and subsequent chronic malnutrition. Over time, this can result in significant weight loss and cachexia, further compromising the patient's overall health and quality of life.

46.3 Ischemic Colitis

46.3.1 Pathogenesis

Ischemic colitis (IC) results from a temporary reduction in colonic blood flow, causing inflammation and damage to the colon. This condition mostly affects the "watershed" areas of the colon, such as the splenic flexure and the rectosigmoid junction, which are especially vulnerable to hypoperfusion because of their limited collateral blood supply. Several factors can trigger the reduced blood flow typical of ischemic colitis.

- Systemic Hypotension: Episodes of low blood pressure, whether from dehydration, heart failure, or shock, can reduce perfusion to the colon. The colon receives between 10% and 35% of the total cardiac output; a reduction exceeding 50% can precipitate ischemia.
- Atherosclerosis: The buildup of atherosclerotic plaques in the mesenteric arteries can narrow these vessels, limiting blood flow to the colon. This occlusive type of ischemia is often caused by arterial embolism or thrombosis.
- Localized Vascular Compromise: Conditions such as vasculitis, hypercoagulable states, or the use of vasoconstrictive drugs can cause localized reductions in blood flow. Vasospasm of colonic vessels, either from systemic hypoperfusion or the vasoconstrictive effects of certain substances, can also be a contributing factor.
- Mechanical Factors: Colonic obstructions caused by tumors, volvulus, or strictures can increase intraluminal pressure, impair mucosal blood flow, and lead to ischemic injury.
- The development of ischemic colitis involves multiple factors, often including both systemic and local influences that reduce blood flow and lead to subsequent colon damage. Understanding these processes is essential for prompt diagnosis and proper treatment of the condition.

46.3.2 Clinical Presentation

The clinical presentation is often divided into three progressive stages: hyperactive, paralytic, and shock. Moving through these stages highlights the importance of early detection and prompt treatment of ischemic colitis to prevent permanent damage and related complications. Healthcare providers should remain highly alert, especially in patients with risk factors like advanced age, cardiovascular disease, or conditions that increase the risk of hypoperfusion. Early diagnosis and proper treatment are vital to changing the disease trajectory and enhancing patient outcomes.

46.3.2.1 Hyperactive Phase

The initial phase features sudden abdominal pain, typically in the left lower quadrant. Patients might also feel an urgent need to defecate, along with passing bloody stools or hematochezia, which signals mucosal or submucosal damage. This phase shows the body's immediate reaction to reduced blood supply and may resolve on its own if blood flow is quickly restored.

46.3.2.2 Paralytic Phase

If ischemia continues, the condition may advance to the paralytic phase, characterized by diffuse abdominal pain and tenderness. Bowel motility decreases, resulting in abdominal distension and absent bowel sounds on examination. Patients might experience nausea and vomiting due to the buildup of intestinal contents and gas. This phase indicates worsening ischemic damage and requires prompt medical intervention to prevent further decline.

46.3.2.3 Shock Phase

In severe cases, prolonged ischemia can lead to the shock phase, marked by systemic signs such as fever, tachycardia, hypotension, and leukocytosis. These symptoms indicate systemic inflammatory response syndrome (SIRS) and potential complications like necrosis and sepsis. Patients may show signs of peritonitis, including rebound tenderness and guarding, which suggest transmural infarction and perforation. This stage requires urgent surgical assessment and intervention to prevent life-threatening outcomes.

46.3.3 Diagnosis

Accurate diagnosis of IC requires a high level of clinical suspicion, supported by targeted laboratory tests, advanced imaging techniques, and, when appropriate, endoscopic examination. This comprehensive approach is essential for differentiating IC from other causes of abdominal pain and rectal bleeding, such as infectious colitis, inflammatory bowel disease, and diverticulitis.

46.3.3.1 Laboratory Assessments

While no laboratory test is definitive for IC, specific findings can help support the diagnosis.

- Leukocytosis: An increased white blood cell count is often seen, indicating an inflammatory or ischemic process.
- Elevated C-Reactive Protein (CRP): Higher CRP levels indicate systemic inflammation and may be linked to the severity of ischemia.
- Metabolic Acidosis and Elevated Serum Lactate: In severe cases, these signs indicate serious tissue hypoperfusion and anaerobic metabolism, highlighting the need for urgent intervention.

46.3.3.2 Imaging

Contrast-Enhanced CT This modality is preferred for its ability to delineate bowel wall abnormalities and assess mesenteric vasculature. Characteristic findings in IC include the following:

- Bowel wall thickening often shows the "thumbprinting" sign, indicating submucosal hemorrhage or edema.
- Pneumatosis Intestinalis: Gas within the bowel wall, indicating advanced ischemia.
- Mesenteric fat stranding indicates inflammation or swelling in the nearby mesenteric fat.

CT angiography can be used to exclude major arterial blockages, especially when there is clinical suspicion of concurrent mesenteric ischemia.

46.3.3.3 Endoscopic Evaluation

Endoscopy serves as a valuable tool for direct visualization of the colonic mucosa and for obtaining biopsy samples:

Colonoscopy: allows for a comprehensive assessment of the colon. Endoscopic findings in IC may include the following:

Pale, friable mucosa, indicating compromised blood flow and mucosal integrity

Ulcerations: vary from superficial to deep depending on the severity of ischemia

Submucosal hemorrhage: appears as petechiae or larger bleeding areas beneath the mucosa

It is imperative to exercise caution during colonoscopy in patients suspected of having IC, especially if the risk of perforation is present. In such cases, less invasive imaging methods should be preferred to reduce the chance of worsening the condition.

46.3.4 Management

Management of IC depends on the severity of the condition, ranging from conservative medical therapy to surgical intervention. Early and accurate assessment is crucial for identifying the appropriate treatment and minimizing potential complications.

46.3.4.1 Conservative Management

For patients with mild to moderate IC, conservative treatment is often effective. The main goals are to stabilize the patient, restore proper colonic perfusion, and prevent the worsening of ischemic damage. Key elements include the following:

- Bowel Rest: Implementing nil per os (NPO) status minimizes metabolic demands on the colon, thereby reducing ischemic stress and facilitating mucosal healing.
- Intravenous Fluid Therapy: Administration of isotonic crystalloids is essential to restore blood volume and

improve mesenteric blood flow, tackling the root cause of hypoperfusion that leads to ischemia.
- Antibiotic Prophylaxis: Empirical broad-spectrum antibiotics are advised to prevent bacterial translocation and subsequent sepsis, especially when mucosal integrity is compromised. This strategy is supported by clinical guidelines that focus on preventing infectious complications in IC.

Close monitoring of clinical parameters and laboratory markers is imperative during conservative management to promptly identify any signs of deterioration that may necessitate surgical intervention.

46.3.4.2 Surgical Management

Surgical intervention is necessary for patients with severe IC, especially those showing signs of peritonitis, bowel perforation, or gangrenous changes, as well as in cases that do not respond to conservative treatments. The main goals of surgery are to resect necrotic tissue, restore gastrointestinal continuity, and prevent systemic complications. Surgical options include the following:

- Segmental Colectomy: This procedure involves resection of the affected segment of the colon and then connecting the healthy bowel ends. Primary anastomosis is possible when the patient is stable and the bowel ends are well vascularized. However, in cases of hemodynamic instability or significant contamination, creating a diverting stoma may be necessary to prevent anastomotic complications.
- Subtotal or Total Colectomy: In cases of extensive colonic involvement or when ischemia affects multiple segments, a more extensive resection might be needed. This procedure is linked to higher morbidity and demands careful patient selection and postoperative care.
- Stoma Creation: When primary anastomosis is not advisable due to patient instability or poor bowel condition, creating a stoma (such as a colostomy or ileostomy) allows for fecal diversion, promotes healing, and lowers the risk of intra-abdominal sepsis. This approach is especially useful in emergency situations where delayed anastomosis can be considered after the patient's condition improves.

46.4 Mesenteric Venous Thrombosis

46.4.1 Pathogenesis

Mesenteric venous thrombosis (MVT) is rare in the West but a significant cause of mesenteric ischemia in India, resulting from thrombotic occlusion of the mesenteric venous system. The development of MVT is multifactorial, with several predisposing conditions:

- Hypercoagulable States: Both inherited and acquired thrombophilias significantly increase the risk of MVT. Inherited conditions include Factor V Leiden mutation and deficiencies in natural anticoagulants such as protein C, protein S, and antithrombin. Acquired hypercoagulable states include malignancies, especially hematological cancers, and antiphospholipid syndrome. These conditions promote thrombin generation or impair fibrinolysis, leading to thrombus formation within the mesenteric veins.
- Local Factors: Inflammatory processes within the abdomen can trigger MVT. For example, acute pancreatitis can spread inflammation to nearby mesenteric vessels, causing thrombosis. Intra-abdominal infections and direct trauma to the mesenteric vessels are additional local factors that can lead to thrombotic events.
- Portal Hypertension: Chronic liver diseases, such as cirrhosis, lead to increased portal venous pressures, which predispose to thrombosis in the portal and mesenteric venous systems. The slowed blood flow in these conditions promotes thrombus formation.

The interaction of these factors results in the blockage of the mesenteric veins, leading to decreased venous return, bowel wall congestion, and subsequent ischemic damage. Recognizing these risk factors early is crucial for quick diagnosis and treatment in cases of MVT.

46.4.2 Clinical Presentation

MVT presents with a clinical spectrum that often differs from the sudden, severe signs of arterial mesenteric ischemia. The gradual onset of MVT can make diagnosis difficult, requiring a high level of suspicion, especially in patients with risk factors.

- Diffuse Abdominal Pain: Patients with MVT usually experience abdominal pain that is diffuse, mild to moderate in intensity, and progressively worsening over days to weeks. This pain is often accompanied by abdominal distension due to bowel wall edema and venous congestion. Unlike arterial ischemia, where pain is sudden and intense, MVT-related pain develops slowly, indicating the gradual buildup of venous blockage and subsequent ischemia.
- Diarrhea: Mucosal congestion from impaired venous drainage can cause diarrhea, which may be tinged with blood.

- Lower GI Bleeding: Compromised mucosal integrity may cause bleeding, presenting as hematochezia or melena. Severe bleeding is rare but can occur if mucosal ulceration develops.

The gradual onset and nonspecific nature of these symptoms often result in delayed diagnosis. Clinicians should maintain a high degree of suspicion for MVT in patients presenting with these symptoms, especially those with risk factors such as hypercoagulable states, intra-abdominal infections, or recent abdominal surgery. Early recognition and appropriate imaging are crucial to confirm the diagnosis and initiate timely management, thereby reducing the risk of complications such as bowel infarction and sepsis.

46.4.3 Diagnosis

46.4.3.1 Laboratory Tests

Initial laboratory investigations, while not definitive for MVT, provide supportive evidence and help identify underlying etiologies.

- D-dimer Levels: Elevated D-dimer concentrations may indicate active thrombotic processes; however, this marker lacks specificity and can be elevated in various conditions, limiting its diagnostic utility for MVT.
- Complete Blood Count (CBC): Leukocytosis is a common finding in MVT, reflecting an inflammatory or stress response.
- Metabolic Panel: In advanced cases, metabolic acidosis may be present, signifying systemic effects of ischemia.
- Coagulation Profile: Assessment of prothrombin time (PT), activated partial thromboplastin time (aPTT), and fibrinogen levels is essential for evaluating coagulation status and identifying potential coagulopathies.
- Thrombophilia Screening: Given the association of MVT with hypercoagulable states, testing for inherited or acquired thrombophilias, such as Factor V Leiden mutation, protein C or S deficiency, and antiphospholipid syndrome, is recommended.

46.4.3.2 Imaging

- Computed Tomography (CT) Venography: Considered the gold standard for MVT diagnosis, CT venography provides high-resolution images that can detect thrombus formation within the mesenteric veins, bowel wall thickening, and signs of ischemia. The use of intravenous contrast enhances the visualization of vascular structures, enabling accurate assessment.
- Doppler Ultrasonography: As a noninvasive and easily accessible modality, Doppler ultrasound can identify changes in blood flow within the mesenteric vessels. It acts as a primary screening method, especially in stable patients; however, its sensitivity depends on the operator and can be affected by patient body habitus or overlying bowel gas.
- Magnetic Resonance Imaging (MRI): MRI, especially with MR angiography, provides detailed images without using ionizing radiation. It is helpful for patients who cannot have CT contrast agents, although its availability and longer scan times can be limiting.

46.4.3.3 Endoscopic Evaluation

While not routinely used in diagnosing MVT, endoscopy can be instrumental in assessing mucosal integrity and identifying ischemic changes. Direct visualization of the gastrointestinal mucosa may reveal edema, erythema, ulcerations, or necrosis, indicative of venous congestion and ischemia. Endoscopic findings can help determine the extent of bowel involvement and guide therapeutic decisions.

46.4.4 Management

Management of MVT focuses on restoring venous patency and addressing the underlying cause to prevent bowel ischemia and infarction. The treatment approach includes both conservative and interventional strategies, tailored to the severity of the condition and the patient's overall health status.

46.4.4.1 Conservative Management

- Anticoagulation Therapy: Initiation of anticoagulation is the cornerstone of MVT treatment. Unfractionated heparin or low-molecular-weight heparin is typically administered initially to inhibit further thrombus formation and facilitate endogenous fibrinolysis. Following stabilization, patients are transitioned to oral anticoagulants such as warfarin or direct oral anticoagulants (DOACs) for long-term therapy. The underlying cause determines the duration of anticoagulation; transient risk factors may warrant a finite course, whereas chronic conditions like thrombophilia or malignancy often require indefinite anticoagulation.
- Supportive Care: Maintaining adequate mesenteric perfusion is crucial. Intravenous fluids help stabilize hemodynamics and improve splanchnic circulation. Nutritional support is also important, especially if oral intake is limited due to abdominal pain or ileus. Enteral nutrition is preferred to maintain gut integrity, but parenteral nutrition might be necessary in cases of severe bowel dysfunction.

46.4.4.2 Interventional or Surgical Management

- Catheter-Directed Thrombolysis: In severe MVT cases or when anticoagulation alone is not enough, catheter-directed thrombolysis can be used. This method involves inserting a catheter into the mesenteric vein under imaging guidance, through which thrombolytic agents are directly infused to dissolve the thrombus. This approach can quickly restore venous flow and is especially helpful for patients with extensive thrombosis or worsening clinical conditions.
- Surgical Thrombectomy: Surgical intervention is generally reserved for patients who do not respond to medical therapy or who have complications such as bowel infarction. Thrombectomy involves surgically removing the thrombus from the mesenteric veins to restore blood flow and prevent further ischemic damage. This procedure is considered when less invasive measures fail or are contraindicated.
- Bowel Resection: If ischemia has progressed to bowel necrosis, resection of the affected intestinal segments is necessary. The principles of conservative and relook surgery are the same as those for acute mesenteric ischemia.

Key Points

- Acute mesenteric ischemia (AMI) is often caused by embolism, thrombosis, or vasospasm and presents with sudden and severe abdominal pain disproportionate to physical findings.
- Chronic mesenteric ischemia is characterized by postprandial pain, food aversion, and progressive weight loss, often due to long-standing atherosclerosis of the mesenteric arteries.
- Mesenteric vein thrombosis (MVT) can have an acute or insidious onset.
- Diagnostic advancements have revolutionized the management of these conditions.
- Computed tomography angiography (CTA) and magnetic resonance angiography (MRA) provide high-resolution visualization of vascular anatomy and abnormalities.
- Doppler ultrasound provides a non-invasive assessment of blood flow dynamics, particularly in chronic conditions.
- Biomarkers like D-dimer, lactate, and procalcitonin are valuable adjuncts, aiding in the evaluation of thrombotic activity, tissue hypoperfusion, and ischemic complications.
- AMI requires immediate revascularization through endovascular procedures like angioplasty and stenting or surgical methods such as embolectomy.
- Chronic mesenteric ischemia may benefit from angioplasty with stenting or bypass surgery to restore adequate blood flow and alleviate symptoms.
- MVT is mainly treated with anticoagulation to prevent thrombus progression and facilitate recanalization.
- Surgical intervention is reserved for cases complicated by bowel infarction.
- Long-term anticoagulation is indicated to prevent recurrence of thrombosis.

Selected Reading

1. Gnanapandithan K, Feuerstadt P. Mesenteric ischemia. Curr Gastroenterol Rep. 2020;22(4):17. https://doi.org/10.1007/s11894-020-0754-x.
2. Bala M, Catena F, Jeffry Kashuk J, et al. Acute mesenteric ischemia: updated guidelines of the World Society of Emergency Surgery. World J Emerg Surg. 2022;17:54. https://doi.org/10.1186/s13017-022-00443-x.

Indocyanine Green Dye and Its Applications in Gastrointestinal Surgery

47

Erin Yan Qing Wee, Matthias Yi Quan Liau, and Vishal G. Shelat

Abstract

ICG enhances visualization of blood flow and anastomotic perfusion, possibly decreasing complications. ICG allows accurate anatomy mapping, tumor pinpointing, lymphatic pathway identification, and resection margin marking, which may enhance oncologic results.

Keywords

ICG dye · Fluorescent cholangiogram

Indocyanine green (ICG) dye is an anionic, small (776 Da), non-toxic, water-soluble tricarbocyanine dye developed by Kodak Research Laboratories for infrared photography. It was later approved for assessing hepatic function and cardiac output. Due to its rapid hepatic clearance, low toxicity, and ability to provide real-time imaging during surgery, ICG has applications across various surgical fields. Additionally, ICG has a high affinity for human albumin and largely remains within the intravascular compartment. Increased access, availability, advances in imaging, and affordability have expanded its use.

47.1 Properties of Indocyanine Green Dye

ICG becomes fluorescent when excited by light between 800 and 820 nm. The wavelength emitted by indocyanine green dye is near-infrared, allowing the overlying tissue to remain transparent while deeper vessels can be visualized with an infrared camera. It does not cross the placenta and is not detected in fetal cord blood, making it potentially safe for use during pregnancy.

E. Y. Q. Wee · M. Y. Q. Liau
Lee Kong Chian School of Medicine, Nanyang Technological University, Singapore, Singapore

V. G. Shelat (✉)
Department of General Surgery, Surgical Science Training Centre, Tan Tock Seng Hospital, Singapore, Singapore

47.2 Applications in Gastrointestinal Surgery

Although ICG is widely used in many specialties, such as evaluating cardiac output and ophthalmic angiography, it has significant roles in gastrointestinal surgery. These include assessing hepatic function and perfusion for hepatic resection, imaging the biliary tract, assessing colorectal anastomotic perfusion, locating gastrointestinal tumors, mapping lymphatic tissue, and identifying the ureter during colon surgery.

47.2.1 Adequacy of Future Liver Remnant

ICG clearance can be evaluated by giving a single intravenous dose of about 0.5 mg/kg and measuring the blood level after 15 min. An ICG retention of more than 15% at 15 min is generally considered a contraindication for major liver resection, which is defined as resection of two or more liver segments. This assessment is clinically useful because posthepatectomy liver dysfunction and failure can be associated with substantial morbidity and mortality risk.

47.2.2 Biliary Tract Surgery

Fluorescent cholangiography can be performed by intravenous administration of ICG 30 min before surgery. This allows time for its biliary excretion and facilitates intraoperative visualization of biliary structures. Alternatively, ICG can also be delivered via the intrabiliary route by inserting a catheter into the gallbladder, enabling subsequent visualization of the biliary tree during laparoscopic cholecystectomy. This technique potentially enhances intraprocedural safety by clearly defining the biliary anatomy. This technological advancement has allowed high-quality fluorescence imaging for safer cholecystectomy procedures (Fig. 47.1).

M. Ibrarullah (ed.), *Recent Concepts in Gastrointestinal (GI) Surgery*, https://doi.org/10.1007/978-981-92-1118-0_47

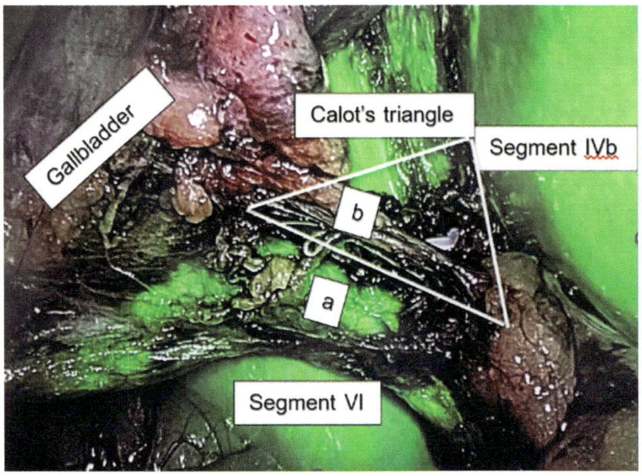

Fig. 47.1 Dissection of "critical view of safety" after intravenous injection of ICG dye. Cystic duct (a) and cystic artery (b)

47.2.3 Positive and Negative Staining During Liver Resection

ICG can help visualize tumors and differentiate cancerous tissues from healthy surrounding tissue, guiding precision surgery. The dye is usually given several hours to days intravenously before surgery, allowing absorption by hepatocytes. The ICG is then excreted into the bile and cleared from healthy hepatocytes within a few hours. In contrast, cancerous hepatocytes metabolize ICG slowly and remain illuminated during the procedure (positive staining), aiding in achieving appropriate resection margins. Similarly, injecting ICG after isolating and clamping a segmental Glissonean pedicle results in no illumination of the clamped segment, thus facilitating segmental liver resection (negative staining).

47.2.4 Application in Colorectal Surgery

ICG fluorescence angiography (ICG-FA) is an essential method for the real-time assessment of anastomotic perfusion in colorectal surgeries, effectively reducing the risk of leaks associated with poor blood flow, which can lead to serious complications. Studies have shown that ICG-FA enhances the safety of vascular ligations during ileal pouch-anal anastomosis procedures. Additionally, ICG-FA is valuable in managing pedicled omentoplasty and evaluating surgical flap perfusion, enabling necessary modifications and adjustments during complex surgeries.

Although rare, ureteral injuries during colorectal surgeries can result in increased mortality, morbidity, longer hospital stays, and higher healthcare costs. Intraureteral administration of ICG can assist in identifying the ureters during surgery, reducing the risk of iatrogenic injuries and allowing the early detection of ureteral damage for prompt repair. This is achieved by injecting 5 mL of 2.5 mg/mL ICG through a ureteral catheter, which offers 4–12 h of ureteral visibility.

ICG shows a natural affinity for lymphatic tissues, making it crucial for lymphatic mapping during D3 right hemicolectomy, as it helps increase the lymph node harvest. There is emerging evidence of using ICG lymph node mapping to identify sentinel nodes before routine lateral pelvic lymph node dissection (LPLND) in rectal cancer surgery. Avoiding routine LPLND may lead to lower morbidity and better patient quality of life. ICG-coated endoclips are reported to reduce the drawbacks of ICG injections for both tumor and polyp tattoos used for localization.

A diluted solution of 25 mg of ICG in 250 mL of water injected transanally through a rectal catheter can help identify anastomotic leaks during surgery. Additionally, peritumoral injections of ICG may help locate the total mesorectal excision resection plane and the presacral fascia during rectal cancer surgery.

47.3 Limitations of Indocyanine Green Dye Use

The usefulness of ICG fluorescence depends on patient factors such as obesity and inflammation. Dye aspects, including dose, concentration, timing, and route of administration, affect dye uptake and fluorescence intensity for lymph node detection. Additionally, issues like accessibility, cost, equipment limitations, and variations in fluorescence assessment methods make reliable use of ICG more challenging.

ICG dye has become a valuable tool in gastrointestinal surgery, providing surgeons with improved visualization and real-time feedback. Its uses demonstrate its versatility and potential to enhance surgical outcomes. As technology advances and more surgeons become familiar with its use, ICG is likely to play an increasingly prominent role in the future of gastrointestinal surgery, ultimately benefiting patient care and increasing surgical precision.

Key Points

- ICG enhances visualization of blood flow and anastomotic perfusion, possibly decreasing complications.
- ICG allows accurate anatomy mapping, tumor pinpointing, lymphatic pathway identification, and resection margin marking, which may enhance oncologic results.

Selected Reading

1. Preziosi A, Cirelli C, Waterhouse D, et al. State of the art medical devices for fluorescence-guided surgery (FGS): technical review and future developments. Surg Endosc. 2024;38(11):6227–36. https://doi.org/10.1007/s00464-024-11236-5. Epub 2024 Sep 18.
2. Lim ZY, Mohan S, Balasubramaniam S, et al. Indocyanine green dye and its application in gastrointestinal surgery: the future is bright green. World J Gastrointest Surg. 2023;15(9):1841–57. https://doi.org/10.4240/wjgs.v15.i9.1841.
3. Borg L, Portelli M, Testa L, et al. The use of indocyanine green for colorectal anastomoses: a systematic review and meta-analysis. Ann R Coll Surg Engl. 2025;107(6):390–6. https://doi.org/10.1308/rcsann.2024.0002.

Tumor Markers in Abdominal Malignancy

48

Ankur Punia

Abstract

Tumor markers are critical in diagnosing, managing, and surveilling abdominal malignancies. These markedly improve the ability to detect and monitor cancer.

Keywords

Tumor markers · GI malignancies

Abdominal malignancies remain a major global health concern, with cancers of the stomach, liver, pancreas, and colorectal region among the leading causes of cancer-related morbidity and mortality. The detection, monitoring, and treatment of these cancers have improved considerably over the years. Tumor markers play a crucial role in identifying these cancers and aiding in disease management.

48.1 Definition

Tumor markers are biological substances, such as proteins, hormones, mRNAs, and other molecules, produced by tumors or by the body's response to tumors during cancer development. They are primarily found in blood, urine, or tissues.

48.2 Key Tumor Markers in Abdominal Malignancies

48.2.1 Alpha-Fetoprotein (AFP)

Associated Cancer: Primarily hepatocellular carcinoma (HCC) and germ cell tumors.

A. Punia (✉)
Mahatma Gandhi University of Medical Sciences and Technology (MGUMST), Jaipur, India

Clinical Significance: AFP levels are elevated in the presence of HCC, providing a tool for early diagnosis, especially in high-risk populations such as individuals with chronic liver disease or hepatitis. These are elevated in germ cell tumors, especially yolk sac tumors.

48.2.2 Carcinoembryonic Antigen (CEA)

Associated Cancer: Colorectal cancer is the most common, but CEA can also be elevated in gastric, pancreatic, and lung cancers.

Clinical Significance: CEA is often used as a marker for diagnosis and monitoring therapeutic responses. Elevated CEA levels can indicate the presence of colorectal cancer or its metastasis, while normal levels may suggest a good prognosis.

48.2.3 CA 19–9

Associated Cancer: Primarily pancreatic adenocarcinoma, cholangiocarcinoma, and colorectal cancers.

Clinical Significance: This can be used to monitor the treatment response and recurrence after surgery for pancreatic cancer. Elevated levels often correlate with advanced disease and a poor prognosis.

48.2.4 CA-125

Associated Cancer: While primarily known as a marker for ovarian cancer, CA-125 can also be elevated in some abdominal malignancies, including those affecting the peritoneum.

Clinical Significance: It helps monitor treatment response and detect recurrence in ovarian cancer. It can occasionally assist in evaluating other malignancies like endometrial and cervical cancer, but is less frequently elevated in these tumors.

M. Ibrarullah (ed.), *Recent Concepts in Gastrointestinal (GI) Surgery*, https://doi.org/10.1007/978-981-92-1118-0_48

48.2.5 Human Chorionic Gonadotropin (hCG)

Associated Cancer: Germ cell tumors and certain trophoblastic diseases.

Clinical Significance: Elevated levels of hCG can help diagnose specific types of testicular or ovarian cancer. It is also valuable in identifying gestational trophoblastic neoplasms.

48.2.6 Lactate Dehydrogenase (LDH)

Associated Cancer: Lymphomas and germ cell tumors.

Clinical Significance: This is not a specific marker, as it can be raised in many benign conditions. However, it is helpful in certain germ cell tumors, like seminoma and embryonal tumors. It also helps to prognosticate patients with non-Hodgkin lymphomas.

48.2.7 Others

CA15–3, CA72–4 & CA27–29: breast cancer and stomach cancer
5-Hydroxyindoleacetic acid (5-HIAA): carcinoid tumors
PIVKA II: HCC
miR-371a-3p: germ cell tumors

48.3 Importance of Tumor Markers

Diagnosis: Tumor markers can help diagnose specific types of cancer, identifying the presence of disease in a patient.

Monitoring Treatment: These markers can help monitor the effectiveness of cancer treatments by indicating whether the cancer responds to therapy.

Surveillance: After treatment, tumor markers can be used to check for signs of cancer returning, allowing prompt intervention if necessary.

Prognosis: These provide information about the disease's likely outcome, helping inform patients about recurrence risk.

48.4 Limitations and Challenges

Despite their usefulness, tumor markers have limitations:

Low Specificity: These can be elevated in certain benign conditions, leading to false-positive results. For example, elevated CEA levels can occur in smokers and those with inflammatory diseases.
Variability: Individuals' levels of markers vary depending on their unique biology, and values might differ based on the reagent used in laboratories, making standardization challenging.
Low Sensitivity: Not all tumors produce detectable levels of tumor markers, which can sometimes lead to false-negative results.
Cost and Accessibility: These tests are becoming more available, but because of their specialized methodology, they are not available to everyone. Therefore, the cost and access to these markers may pose significant barriers to proper diagnosis.

48.5 The Future of Tumor Markers

Ongoing research continues to explore the potential for new tumor markers and the enhancement of existing ones. Advances in genomic and proteomic technologies hold promise for discovering novel markers that may provide increased specificity and sensitivity. Liquid biopsy technologies, which analyze circulating tumor cells and nucleic acids in the blood, signify an exciting frontier in refining tumor marker utility.

Here are some of the promising new markers that are under investigation:

*Protein biomarkers: circulating tumor cells (CTCs) and exosomes
*RNA biomarkers: microRNAs (miRNAs), long noncoding RNAs (lncRNAs)
*Genomic and epigenomic markers: circulating tumor DNA (ctDNA) and methylation patterns

*Metabolomic markers: Metabolites in urine, saliva, and blood
*Immunological markers: tumor-infiltrating lymphocytes (TILs) and checkpoint proteins

*Research is ongoing for novel markers, and some markers have shown promise, but clinical validation and standardization are crucial before they can be widely used in practice.

Key Points

- Tumor markers are critical in diagnosing, managing, and surveilling abdominal malignancies.
- These markedly improve the ability to detect and monitor cancer.
- Understanding these markers empowers healthcare professionals and patients to make informed decisions about cancer care, paving the way for more personalized and effective treatment strategies.

Selected Reading

1. Jakob Z, Günther SC, Marie-Christine S, Sebesta C. Clinical relevance of tumor markers in gastrointestinal cancers: a critical analysis and literature review. JSM Clin Oncol Res. 2024;12(1):1073.

49 Statistics in the Practice of Abdominal Surgery

Akash Mishra

Abstract

Understanding statistical concepts is vital for critically analyzing the surgical literature and conducting newer research. Applying appropriate statistical methods ensures that research findings are reliable and meaningful in advancing the field of abdominal surgery.

Keywords

Biostatistics

Statistics play a crucial role in modern abdominal surgery, influencing surgical decision-making, optimizing procedures, and improving patient outcomes. For practicing surgeons, a strong understanding of statistics is essential for critically assessing clinical research, refining surgical techniques, and providing evidence-based care. Abdominal surgery encompasses a wide range of procedures, from appendectomies to complex cancer resections. Statistics help evaluate outcomes, complication rates, and survival, enabling surgeons to compare techniques, predict complications, and identify risk factors for better prognoses and safer surgeries through clinical trials and cohort studies. This section introduces key statistical concepts, with examples specifically related to abdominal surgery.

Types of Data: Data could be either categorical or continuous variables.

Categorical Data: It represents distinct groups or categories. Examples: "gender" (male/female), "surgical approach" (open/laparoscopic), and "postoperative complications" (yes/no).

Continuous Variables: It represents measurable quantities with an infinite number of possible values within a range. Examples: "age" (in years), "body mass index (BMI)" (kg/m^2), and "duration of surgery" (in minutes).

Note: Understanding the type of variable is essential for selecting appropriate statistical measures and tests.

49.1 Descriptive Statistics: Measures of Central Tendency and Dispersion

Measures of central tendency are mean and median, and measures of dispersion are standard deviation (SD) and interquartile range (IQR). These are key components of descriptive statistics that summarize data.

Mean It represents the average value, while SD quantifies the variation or spread of the data. For example, the mean hospital stay for laparoscopic surgery may be 3.1 days (SD ± 1.2), compared to 4.5 days (SD ± 2.3) for open surgery. The mean and SD are reported when the data follow a normal distribution.

Median It is the middle value, and the IQR, which shows the range of the central 50% of the data, is used. For instance, the median blood loss during surgery might be 150 ml, with an IQR of 100–250 ml, indicating that 50% of surgeries resulted in blood loss between 100 and 250 ml. When data are skewed, the median is calculated.

49.2 Sample Size

Accurate sample size calculation is crucial to ensure that a study is adequately powered to detect a meaningful difference between groups. The sample size depends on factors such as the expected effect size, variability, desired significance level, and power. It also depends on the study's objective and design. Depending on the objectives, the study design may be a comparative cross-sectional, cohort, case-control, or RCT (including noninferiority, superiority, and

A. Mishra (✉)
Mahatma Gandhi University of Medical Sciences and Technology (MGUMST), Jaipur, Rajasthan, India

M. Ibrarullah (ed.), *Recent Concepts in Gastrointestinal (GI) Surgery*, https://doi.org/10.1007/978-981-92-1118-0_49

equivalence trials). A smaller measure value requires a larger sample size, while a larger anticipated difference means that a smaller sample size is needed for the same significance level and power. For example, in RCTs comparing recurrence rates after laparoscopic versus open hernia repair, a larger sample size is needed to detect a significant difference in recurrence rates.

Hypothesis Testing and *p*-Values Hypothesis testing is used to assess the statistical significance of findings, helping to determine whether to support or reject a hypothesis. The *p*-value indicates the probability of observing the data, or more extreme results, under the assumption that the null hypothesis (no effect or difference) is true. For example, a *p*-value of 0.03 in comparing postsurgical complications between two procedures means there is a 3% chance that the difference observed is due to random variation. Typically, a *p*-value less than 0.05 is considered statistically significant.

Common Statistical Tests Choosing the appropriate statistical test depends on the type of variables and the distribution of the data. If the variable under comparison follows a normal distribution, parametric tests are applied; otherwise, nonparametric tests are more suitable.

S.no.	Problem	Case scenario	Parametric vs. nonparametric tests
1	Comparison of quantitative outcomes between two independent groups	Is there a significant difference in the postoperative recovery time between patients undergoing laparoscopic cholecystectomy and open cholecystectomy for gallstone disease?	If the recovery time is normally distributed in both groups *Independent Student t test* Otherwise *Mann-Whitney U test*
2	Comparison of quantitative outcomes between two dependent groups/related groups	Is there a significant difference in patients' hemoglobin levels before and after abdominal surgery?	If differences between hemoglobin levels before and after surgery follow a normal distribution *Paired t test* Otherwise *Wilcoxon Signed Rank test*
3	Comparison of quantitative outcomes between more than two independent groups	Is there a significant difference in recovery times among patients undergoing three different types of abdominal surgery: open, laparoscopic, and robotic?	If the recovery time for each group follows a normal distribution *ANOVA test* Otherwise *Kruskal-Wallis test*
4	Comparison of quantitative outcomes between more than two dependent/related groups	How do pain levels change at different time points (preoperative, 24 h postoperative, and 1 week postoperative) in patients undergoing abdominal surgery?	If the differences between the repeated measures approximately follows normally distribution *Repeated measures of ANOVA* Otherwise *Friedman test*
5	Relationship between two quantitative variables	Is there a correlation between preoperative BMI and postoperative recovery time in patients undergoing abdominal surgery?	If both variables are approximately normally distributed *Karl Pearson correlation* Otherwise *Spearman rank correlation*
6	Measure of association between two or more categorical variables	Is there an association between the type of abdominal surgery (open vs laparoscopic) and the incidence of postoperative complications?	*Chi-square/ Fisher's exact test*
7	Comparison of two dependent/related categorical groups	Is there a significant change in the proportion of patients who experience complications before and after implementing a new surgical technique in abdominal surgery?	*McNemar's test*

Cohort Studies It can help to determine how certain factors (e.g., patient characteristics, surgical techniques, and preoperative conditions) influence postoperative outcomes. For instance, it can be used to assess whether preoperative nutritional optimization reduces the risk of postoperative complications in patients undergoing major abdominal surgery.

Randomized Controlled Trials (RCTs) RCTs are the gold standard for comparing surgical techniques and interventions, as they minimize bias and provide robust evidence. For example, RCTs comparing laparoscopic to open surgeries have transformed abdominal surgery, proving the benefits of minimally invasive methods in terms of faster recovery and lower complication rates.

49.3 Diagnostic Measures (Sensitivity, Specificity, and Predictive Values)

These measures help clinicians assess how well a diagnostic tool can detect true cases of a condition (such as complications or infections) and differentiate them from noncases. A 2 × 2 contingency table is made to compute the sensitivity, specificity, positive predictive value (PPV), and negative predictive value (NPV) of a diagnostic test as presented below:

	Gold standard test		
Diagnostic test	Diseased	Disease-free	Total
Test positive	TP	FP	TP + FP
Test negative	FN	TN	FN + TN
Total	TP + FN	FP + TN	TP + FP + FN + TN

where

- TP: true positives (correctly identified number of disease individuals)
- FP: false positives (missed diseased number of individuals)
- FN: false negatives (missed disease-free individuals)
- TN: true negatives (correctly identified disease-free individuals)

Sensitivity It is the proportion of correctly identified diseased subjects by the diagnostic test:

$$\text{Sensitivity} = \frac{\text{TP}}{\text{TP}+\text{FN}} * 100$$

Example A model designed to predict surgical site infections after abdominal surgery that has a sensitivity of 90% correctly identifies 90% of the patients who will develop infections but misses 10%.

Specificity It is the proportion of correctly identified disease-free subjects by the diagnostic test:

$$\text{Specificity} = \frac{\text{TN}}{\text{TN}+\text{FP}} * 100$$

Example A test with 95% specificity for detecting postoperative leaks correctly identifies 95% of patients who do not have a leak, with 5% being incorrectly flagged for further testing.

Positive Predictive Value (PPV) It is the proportion of correctly identified diseased subjects from among all identified as positives by the diagnostic test:

$$\text{PPV} = \frac{\text{TP}}{\text{TP}+\text{FP}} * 100$$

Example A model with a PPV of 85% for predicting intra-abdominal infections postsurgery indicates that 85% of patients predicted to have an infection actually develop it.

Negative Predictive Value (PPV) It is the proportion of correctly identified disease-free subjects from among all identified negatives by the diagnostic test:

$$\text{NPV} = \frac{\text{TN}}{\text{FN}+\text{TN}} * 100$$

Example An NPV of 95% for predicting no postoperative bleeding after surgery suggests that 95% of patients predicted to have no bleeding actually avoid this complication.

Classification Accuracy It refers to how well a diagnostic test or model predicts outcomes:

$$\text{Classification Accuracy} = \frac{\text{TP}+\text{TN}}{\text{TP}+\text{FP}+\text{FN}+\text{TN}} * 100$$

49.4 Statistical Analysis Approaches

Univariate analysis Only one variable was considered at a time to assess its association with the outcome. Example: examining the effect of age alone on postoperative complication rates.

Multivariable analysis More than one variable was considered to assess the effect of each variable. This approach adjusts for the effect of confounding variables and assesses the independent effect of each one separately on the outcome. Example: a logistic regression model to determine independently associated variables with postoperative infections, adjusting for the effect of variables like age, BMI, and surgical duration.

Survival Analysis Kaplan-Meier and actuarial methods in survival analysis are used to analyze time-to-event data, such as time to recurrence of disease or time to death after surgery. The Kaplan-Meier curve is a graphical presentation of survival data, showing the proportion of patients surviving over time. Example: comparing 5-year survival rates after liver resection for patients with and without preoperative chemotherapy.

49.5 Measures of Causal Association

Relative Risk (RR) It quantifies the association of an outcome with an exposure. It represents the ratio of occurrence rate in the exposed group relative to the unexposed group. This is computed in cohort studies. For example, an RR of 2.5 for complications in laparoscopic surgery compared to open surgery indicates a 2.5-fold higher risk of complications in laparoscopic surgery.

Odds Ratio (OR) The OR also quantifies the association between an exposure and an outcome. It represents the ratio of odds of exposure among those with the presence of outcomes relative to those with the absence of outcomes. This is computed generally in case-control studies. For example, an odds ratio (OR) of 0.30 indicates that the odds of developing a surgical site infection are three times lower in robotic-assisted surgery compared to open surgery.

Hazard Ratio (HR) The HR represents the relative risk of an event (e.g., death and recurrence) occurring at any point in time between the two groups. In a study comparing postoperative survival following two methods of abdominal surgery—laparoscopic surgery and open surgery—an HR of 1.8 indicates that patients who underwent open surgery had an 80% higher risk of death compared to those who underwent laparoscopic surgery.

Confidence Intervals (CI) It is an essential inference for all statistical measures that provide a range of values within which the true population parameter is likely to fall, with a specified level of confidence, typically considered 95%. For example, if the OR for complications is 2.5 with a 95% CI of 1.8–3.5, this means that the researcher is 95% confident that the true OR lies between 1.8 and 3.5.

Key Points

- Understanding statistical concepts is vital for critically analyzing surgical literature and conducting newer research.
- Applying appropriate statistical methods ensures that research findings are reliable and meaningful in advancing the field of abdominal surgery.

Selected Reading

1. Ram Jyothis AB (ed) Essentials of biostatistics for medical students: including manual on statistical analysis using SPSS, Kindle edition. https://www.amazon.in/Essentials-Biostatistics-Medical-Students-statistical-ebook/dp/B0D3B8M35W

GPSR Compliance

The European Union's (EU) General Product Safety Regulation (GPSR) is a set of rules that requires consumer products to be safe and our obligations to ensure this.

If you have any concerns about our products, you can contact us on ProductSafety@springernature.com

In case Publisher is established outside the EU, the EU authorized representative is:

Springer Nature Customer Service Center GmbH
Europaplatz 3
69115 Heidelberg, Germany

Batch number: 10683589

Printed by Printforce, the Netherlands